Principles of Paediatric Nursing

This book is dedicated to Carole and Marion and
to the many other children from whom I have
learned so much.

Principles of Paediatric Nursing

Rosa M. Sacharin

BA, RSCN, RGN, SCM, Dip N (Lond), RNT, CBiol MIBiol
Senior Tutor, (Paediatrics) Ayrshire and Arran College of
Nursing and Midwifery, Crosshouse, Kilmarnock, Ayrshire

Foreword by Olive Hulme

MBE, RSCN, RGN, SCM
Divisional Nursing Officer,
Royal Hospital for Sick Children, Yorkhill, Glasgow

With Contribution from
Eleanor J. Martin

RSCN, SRN
Nursing Officer, Neonatal Surgery and Cardiac
Medicine/Surgery Wards,
Royal Hospital for Sick Children, Yorkhill, Glasgow

SECOND EDITION

CHURCHILL LIVINGSTONE
EDINBURGH LONDON MELBOURNE AND NEW YORK 1986

CHURCHILL LIVINGSTONE
Medical Division of Longman Group UK Limited

Distributed in the United States of America by Churchill
Livingstone Inc., 1560 Broadway, New York, N.Y. 10036,
and by associated companies, branches and respresentatives
throughout the world.

First edition 1980
Second edition 1986

ISBN 0 443 03301 3

British Library Cataloguing in Publication Data
Sacharin, Rosa M.
 Principles of paediatric nursing. — 2nd ed.
 1. Pediatrics 2. Pediatric nursing
 I. Title II. Martin, Eleanor J.
 618.92′00024613   RJ245

Library of Congress, Cataloging in Publication Data
Sacharin, Rosa M. (Rosa Mary)
 Principles of paediatric nursing.
 Bibliography: p.
 Includes index.
 1. Pediatric nursing. I. Martin, Eleanor J., RSCN,
SRN. II. Title. [DNLM; 1. Pediatric Nursing.
WY 159 S121pa]
RJ245.S22 1986   610.73′62   85–11685

Produced by Longman Group (FE) Ltd
Printed in Hong Kong

Foreword

During this century the rapid changes in society have led to an increased awareness of the quality of life, and to advances in technology, science, and medicine.

In recent years, child health has been in the forefront of debate, discussion and legislation. A comprehensive service of health care for children is still awaited, although improved facilities for their care at home and in hospital are slowly evolving. In order to provide the nursing component of such a service, ever-increasing numbers of nurses effectively educated and experienced in the special needs of children are urgently required. Nurse training is at a 'cross-roads' and it is important to think not only of the present, but also of the future.

The publication of this textbook for paediatric nurses, written by Mrs R. M. Sacharin, a practising paediatric nurse teacher, fulfils a great need. I commend it to all nurses interested in children, and feel sure it will quickly become a 'must' for all sick children's nurses.

Glasgow, 1980   Olive Hulme MBE

Preface to the Second Edition

Since the publication of the first edition there have been changes in the philosophy of child care. There is now greater awareness of the needs of the child in health and disease with much emphasis on prevention of ill health.

Chapters 1, 3 and 4 have been rewritten to emphasise the importance of the child's growth and development and the environment in which he can achieve these. Chapter 6 has been extended to include the nursing management of the acutely ill child.

The understanding of the nutritional needs of children is necessary for the maintenance of health and the treatment of disease and so a chapter on nutrition in infancy and childhood has been included. Further new material includes a brief introduction to pathology and the healing process, medical genetics and some inherited disorders. Where necessary, the text has been updated and enlarged and many new drawings have been added.

New and updated material on the surgical neonate has been written by Miss E. J. Martin, a Nursing Officer at the Royal Hospital for Sick Children, Glasgow, who has extensive experience in that field of nursing.

It is therefore hoped that the book will be a valuable reference for the qualified nurse, working with children, and a comprehensive textbook for the nurse in training.

Glasgow 1986   R.M.S

Preface to the First Edition

It is often stated that the child is a miniature adult, that the difference between adult and child is one of scale and that the nursing of sick children does not differ from the nursing of the adult. While this is true to some extent, it overlooks the anatomical, physiological and psychological variations.

The term 'child' includes the neonate (1st month of life), infant (from the 1st month to 1 year), toddler (1 to $2\frac{1}{2}$ years), pre-school child and school attender, each group requiring its own approach, treatment, nursing management and technique. Even a relatively simple procedure such as 'taking a pulse' is different. In the neonate and very young infant the apical heart beat is taken for greater accuracy, since with the conventional method the beat may be missed or obliterated, due to the high pulse rate and easy compressibilty. The digestive system of the infant is not fully developed and this influences the type of food to be given and the technique of feeding. The sick children's nurse must also concern herself with many special procedures such as incubator care, administration of oxygen and injection technique, to name but a few. Likewise, there are disease and abnormalities encountered in the child which are not found in the adult, such as some congenital abnormalities, agenesis of organs, severe forms of spina bifida and hydrocephalus. Even when the conditions are the same in adults and children, the inability of children — particularly the very young — to communicate necessitates special skills of observation and interpretation.

Many aspects of child care are discussed, but the emphasis is primarily on the care of the sick child, whether at home or in hospital. Home care of the sick child has always been the responsibility of parents, and this is how it should be. The sick children's nurse, however, can extend her expertise to provide a support service for home nursing, thereby limiting the number of children requiring admission to hospital. Many of the tasks performed in hospital can be performed successfully in the home, provided this medical and nursing support service is efficient.

This book is divided into four parts. Part 1 discusses the growth and development of the child and the care of the healthy child, since it is necessary to know the normal in order to recognise the abnormal. Part 2 considers the child in hospital and the associated nursing care. Part 3 describes the child's biochemical and physiological environment. Part 4 deals with disorders of the systems of the body, including discussions of the normal and abnormal body structure and function and of the principles of treatment and nursing management in relation to the presenting features. Each chapter concludes with specific procedures relevant to the system. Hospital methods vary widely, however, so procedures may have to be adapted and modified. The emphasis in this book is, therefore, on the principles of paediatric nursing. Provided that these principles are understood and observed, the methods may vary considerably.

Although this book is intended primarily for those who specialise in the nursing of sick children, it is also meant for all nurses — both student and qualified — who work in the field of paediatrics, whether in hospital or in the community.

Glasgow 1980 R. M. S.

Acknowledgements

I wish to express my thanks to all my colleagues who have so generously given me information. I am indebted to Mr J. Devlin of the Medical Illustrations Department, Royal Hospital for Sick Children, Glasgow, and his staff, and Mr. E McNulty, Area Medical Photographer, Crosshouse Hospital, Kilmarnock, for photographs. I would like to thank the Ayrshire and Arran Health Board for permission to use the photographic facilities, and Miss Diane Auld for typing some of the material.

I would also like to thank the staff of Churchill Livingstone, Edinburgh for help and constructive criticism.

Figures 12.7, 17.10, 23.1, 23.3, 23.4 and 23.7 have been reproduced, by kind permission, from *The Physiology of Disease* (1975) by I. C. Roddie, MD, FRCPI, and W. F. M. Wallace, MD, MRCP, London, Lloyd-Luke (Medical Books).

R.M.S.

Contents

Part 1 The Healthy Child
1. Growth and development of the child   3
2. Care of children   34

Part 2 Social Aspects of Child Care
3. Child-care systems   47
4. Child health services   58

Part 3 The Child in Hospital
5. Hospitalisation   73
6. Nursing the sick child   84
7. General surgical nursing principles   128
8. Neonatal surgical nursing principles   156
9. Administration of drugs   163
10. Care of pre-term and low-weight babies   178

Part 4 The Biochemical and Physiological Environment (normal and abnormal)
11. Nutrition in infancy and childhood   189
12. Fluid and electrolyte balance   223
13. Micro-biology and the process of disease   234
14. Medical genetics   253
15. Inborn errors of metabolism   262
16. Disorders of the endocrine system   270

Part 5 Childhood Disorders and Their Management
17. Disorders of the nervous system   289
18. Psychopathological conditions   316
19. Mental retardation   326
20. Disorders of the visual system   330
21. Disorders of the auditory system   341
22. Disorders of the throat   355
23. Disorders of the respiratory system   362
24. Disorders of the cardiovascular system   399
25. Haematological disorders   429
26. Disorders of the alimentary tract, liver and pancreas   466
27. Disorders of the genito-urinary system   523
28. Disorders of the skin   567
29. Disorders of the skeletal-muscular system   573

Glossary   600

Bibliography   604

Index   607

Part 1
The healthy child

Chapter 1
Growth and development of the child

This chapter deals with very early life, tracing the progress of normal growth and development from conception to maturity. A knowledge of the normal, and of variations from it, is necessary in order that those who care for children can recognise the abnormal. The nurse is often confronted with children of all ages who vary in their appearance, behaviour, aptitude motor and sensory ability and intelligence. It is, therefore, important that she should be able to recognise these variations and contribute to an accurate diagnosis so that the decision for treatment and subsequent care will be the correct one for the child.

A superficial study of child development shows that a child's actions and behaviour is linked with age, and the terms 'milestones' or 'stepping stones' are often used to describe these age-linked developments. This emphasis on 'milestones' or 'stepping stones' produces a rigid concept about development and does not take into account the variations which exist between normal children. Growth and development should be seen as a continuous dynamic process which begins at the moment of conception.

A precise definition of growth is difficult, but a reasonably satisfactory one is 'the increase in weight or size of all or part of an organism', while development is 'the increasing sophistication in the use of the body'.

Biological basis of growth

Life begins with the union of two cells, the female egg cell and the male sperm cell. When the cells unite the new structure will not only contain similarities of the parents, but also a chain of inheritance. Each of these cells contains substances which will determine the future individual. With the use of a beam of electrons, it is possible to examine a cell under magnification ranging from 10 000 up to one million or more and to study the structures of a cell in very fine detail. The organisation and constant activity of the cell depend on the many structures and substructures within it.

Living tissues, mature or embryonic, consist of cells and intercellular material and much of embryology is concerned with changes in the construction, relative position and activities of cells. Despite these changes during the developmental life of the organism, and the differentiation which results from them, most cells have certain features in common. Some of these are illustrated in Figure 1.1.

Growth of the embryo
Once the ovum has been fertilised the contents of the nuclei of these two cells combine. The pronuclei of each cell carries 23 unpaired chromosomes, so that the fertilised ovum will have 46 paired chromosomes in a single nucleus, just like all the other cells in the human body. A few hours later the chromosomes reproduce and split apart, beginning the division of the ovum. Growth of the early embryo is associated with accumulation of serous fluid and the formation of the blastula. Propulsion of the blastula along the fallopian tubes to the uterus is by contraction of smooth muscle, contraction in the uterine tubes and the action of the cilia. By the time the ovum reaches the uterus, the cell mass has increased to about 16 or 32 cells and these cells have also begun to differentiate. This process takes about 3 to 4 days. When the blastula reaches the uterus it is implanted into the uterine mucous membrane. Changes which take place in the uterine lining accompany the implantation of the embryo. The cells around the blastocea invade the uterine lining and become the

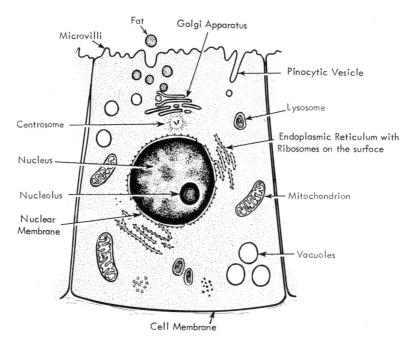

Fig. 1.1 Basic cell structure.

trophoblast. At about the 13th day the embryo is almost entirely buried in the uterine lining and the trophoblast begins to put out root-like structures which grow until they form an extensive system of branching rootlets implanted into the uterine lining. The embryonic blood vessels grow outwards and are brought into intimate contact with the maternal blood; this enables the fetus to receive nutritive substances and to transfer waste products into the maternal blood. The placenta is then formed and it unites the embryo to the uterus of the mother. It mediates the metabolic exchanges of the developing embryo through an intimate association of embryonic tissues and of certain uterine tissues. Nutrients, oxygen and antibodies, as well as other materials in the mother's blood, are carried to the uterus by the uterine arteries. These break up into smaller arteries in the uterine wall and empty into the spaces in which the embryonic villi lie. The materials diffuse into the embryonic and later fetal blood in the capillaries of the villi; nitrogenous wastes and carbon dioxide diffuse out of these capillaries into the maternal blood and are carried into the uterine veins and back to the mother's lungs where she eliminates the carbon dioxide, and to her kidneys where she eliminates the nitrogenous wastes.

As the embryo grows, differentiation of cells and tissues gives rise to specific tissues such as bones, muscles and other tissues. The shape of the embryo changes, gradually assuming a human appearance. It is possible to identify various structures and organs at different ages (ovulation age). For example, at 27 days it is possible to see a head with barely visible optic and auditory vesicles (future eyes and ears) (Fig. 1.2). The heart can also be seen through the transparent skin.

The growth of the embryo is at first rapid but the rate of increase slows down towards the end of the 3rd week as pregnancy advances.

Development of the fetus

By the end of the 7th or 8th week the developing organism is called a fetus. From the time of conception two things were occurring simultaneously to the zygote. Firstly, it was multiplying so that increasing numbers of cells were produced within the uterus. Secondly, the form of the cells was changing so that different parts of the fetus were becoming differentiated for different purposes.

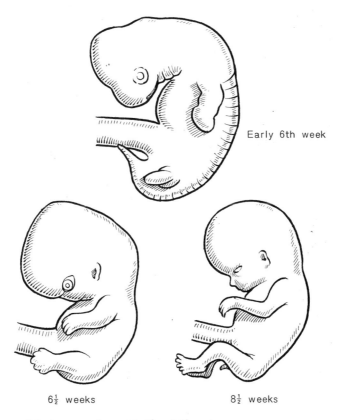

Early 6th week

6½ weeks   8½ weeks

Fig. 1.2 Size and development of the human embryo at 6, 6½ and 8½ weeks.

A number of general theories have been formulated on the way growth and development occur. One such theory is that the direction of development is governed by the cephalocaudal principle. This takes as evidence that the head of the fetus is longer and better developed than its legs and that in the development of the fetus, arm buds appear before leg buds. This cephalocaudal principle proposes that the development trend is from the head down to the feet.

It is also suggested that sequence of development in the arms proceeds from the shoulder to the arm to the hand and then to the fingers. This observation gives rise to the proximodistal principle, which states that growth and development proceed from the central vertical axis of the body outwards.

Different tissues and different regions of the body mature at different rates. Growth in length proceeds at a predetermined rate, the peak velocity of length being reached at about 4 months' gestation. Growth in weight follows the same general pattern as growth in length except that the peak velocity is reached much later, at approximately 34 weeks' gestation.

The rate of growth of the fetus compared with that of the child is largely due to the fact that cells are still multiplying. The proportion of cells undergoing mitosis in any tissue becomes progressively less as the fetus gets older. Intra-uterine growth as determined by body weight or length depends on factors inherent in the fetus, the placenta and the mother.

Fetal factors
These are inherent in the fetus and thus constitute the growth potential of the fetus. These factors may be genetic or imparted to the fetus earlier than the third trimester. Fetal disease may retard growth, e.g. fetal rubella.

Placental factors
The placenta is a fetal organ and, as already described, it is the vital link between fetus and mother. It is, therefore, essential that the placenta is healthy and functionally competent. Occasionally stunting of fetal growth may occur by primary placental hypoplasia, but extensive pathogenic changes such as infarcts interfere with the exchange between fetus and mother.

Maternal factors
Many maternal characteristics or abnormalities have been found to be associated with poor fetal growth and well-being, as demonstrated by low birth-weight in relation to gestational age.

Other factors include primiparity, heavy smoking, short stature, small heart volume, chronic or pre-eclamptic hypertensive disease.

By 12 weeks, muscles are already formed and he is able to move. The nervous system is developing and a number of reflex activities are possible. Facial features are forming; eyelids are present and fused; external sex identification is possible and tooth buds are forming. Fetal length is about 11.5 cm and weight is about 20 g.

13th to 16th week
Length is about 19 cm and weight about 100 g. Calcification of skeleton has taken place and increasing breathing movements can be detected by sonogram. Scalp hair is visible and the fetus is active.

17th to 20th week
Length is about 22 cm and weight has increased to 300 g. Eyebrows, lanugo and vernix appear.

24th week
Progress continues and this stage is currently accepted as the lower level of viability. All the features are clearly identified. The heart beat is louder; his muscles are stronger and he will accumulate a little fat under his skin.

24th to 42nd week
The fetus gains most of his birth-weight during this period. The hair on his head grows longer and most of the downy lanugo is shed from his body.

His length increases from 37 cm to 51 cm and his weight increases from 1000 g to 3200 g.

The fetal circulation
Oxygen supply is vital for the developing fetus, and diffusion of oxygen from the maternal to the fetal blood is facilitated by the difference in oxygen tension which is approximately 10 mmHg. Maternal oxygen tension is about 40 mmHg and fetal oxygen tension is 30 mmHg. Haemoglobin in fetal blood is different from adult haemoglobin and has about 30 per cent greater afinity for oxygen. There is also a greater concentration of haemoglobin, i.e. it is about 50 per cent higher than in maternal blood. Diffusion of oxygen is further facilitated by carbon dioxide tension. It will, therefore, be appreciated that any interference with maternal or fetal circulation or with placental function will have a harmful effect on the development of the fetus.

There are a number of features which are different in the fetus from those in the adult. For example, fetal lungs are not functional until after birth; fetal kidneys, alimentary canal and exocrine glands are also comparatively inactive during fetal development. The fetal circulation is not the same as in the adult and the following list will show the essential differences:

1. The lungs are by-passed since they are non-functional.
2. The right and left atria share blood via the foramen ovale.
3. A duct connects the pulmonary artery to the aorta (ductus arteriosus).
4. A duct (ductus venosus) connects from the umbilical vein to the fetal inferior vena cava.

The supply of blood to the fetus is obtained indirectly from maternal uterine blood vessels and fetal umbilical vessels. Blood containing nutritional substances passes from the fetal side of the placental membrane via the umbilical vein to the fetal liver, thence via the inferior vena cava to the right atrium and ventricle. This blood is oxygenated by diffusion of oxygen from the maternal red blood cells and loses carbon dioxide to the maternal placental membrane.

From the right atrium of the fetal heart, the blood passes via the foramen ovale into the left atrium where it is joined by blood from the pulmonary veins. The mixture passes into the left ventricle and is ejected into the aorta where most of this relatively well-oxygenated blood reaches the arteries of the heart, head, neck and arms. The residue traverses the isthmus aortal to join the stream from the ductus arteriosus.

The remainder of the inferior caval stream joins the blood from the superior vena cava and coronary sinus in the right atrium proper and enters the right ventricle. Some of the blood from the right ventricle goes to the lungs via the pulmonary artery. The remainder by-passes the lungs via the ductus arteriosus and joins the stream from the isthmus aortal in the descending aorta for distribution partly to the lower parts of the body but mainly via the umbilical arteries to the placenta. The umbilical vessels — one vein, two arteries — constitute the umbilical cord. A diagrammatic summary of the fetal circulation is shown in Figure 24.1 (p. 401).

Sexual development
Sexual development in the embryo involves two processes: sex determination and sex differentiation.

Sex determination
This is a genetic phenomenon and depends on the constitution of the sex chromosomes. The ovum and spermatozoa each contain 46 chromosomes. Of these the ovum contains 44 autosomes and two sex chromosomes, which are similar in form and are called the X chromosomes or *XX*.

In the male the sex chromosomes are dissimilar. One is an X chromosome and the other, although much smaller, is actively male-determining and is called the Y chromosome. The chromosomal complements of the female are 44XX and for the male 44XY.

When oocytes undergo reduction division the chromosomal number is halved so that each ovum finally contains 23 (i.e. 22+X). When spermatozytes undergo reduction division there are two resulting secondary spermatozytes which become spermatozoa, each containing 23 chromosomes. One type contains 22+X and the other contains 22+Y. The ovum may be fertilised by either kind of sperm with the following sex genotypes:

Sperm X and ovum X offspring XX = female
Sperm Y and ovum X offspring XY = male

Thus genetic sex is determined exclusively by the sperm and is quite independent of the ovum.

The sex genotype can be identified by a cytological test. The most suitable cells which can be tested are the epithelial cells of the epidermal spinous layer, buccal mucosa, vagina and the blood leucocytes. The nuclei of somatic cells in the female contain a *chromatin* mass about 1 μm in diameter which lies against the inner surface of the nuclear membrane. This sex chromatin is thought to result from apposition of certain regions of the XX chromosome pair. The chromosome pair of the male forms no detectable mass.

Sex differentiation
Sex differentiation in the embryo usually harmonises with the genetic sex, but environmental influences can lead to discordant development so that the apparent sex may not accord with the genetic sex.

Abnormalities of sex development
Aberrations of sexual development can arise from changes in sex chromosomes or from abnormalities in sex differentiation due to hormonal or environmental causes.

For example, in Klinefelter's syndrome the apparent male with small testes is characterised by the presence of feminine stigmata. The sex chromosome pattern is usually XXY making a total of 47 instead of the normal 46 chromosomes. The sex chromatin test is positive, that is genetically female.

In Turner's syndrome there is retardation of growth and of sexual development. There is usually only one X chromosome and a total chromosome number of 45. The sex chromatin test is negative. There may also be an extra X chromosome making an XXX pattern with 47 chromosomes.

True hermaphroditism
In this condition, both ovarian and testicular tissue is present, sometimes an ovary on one side and a testis on the other. Numerous variations in male and female differentiation can occur affecting

various structures. The sex chromatin test may be positive or negative.

Pseudohermaphroditism

Male and female pseudohermaphrodites are individuals in whom normal gonadal development has occurred in accordance with their chromosomal sex, but with later development of heterosexual characteristics. A common type of female hermaphrodite has ovaries, female ducts and varying degrees of masculine differentiation of the external genitalia. The chromosomal sex is female.

Growth after birth

The birth of the normal full-term infant completes a phase of growth which starts with fertilisation of the ovum during the embryonic phase. Cellular division is the main cause of growth which gradually develops into differentiation of function until the fetus is capable of maintaining a relatively independent existence, i.e. organ function is achieved. After birth the emphasis shifts to enlargement of existing cells and the laying down of intercellular matrix. For example, although nerve cells are present at birth, it is only after birth that communication with other nerve cells is vastly increased in number and complexity.

Growth is a continuous dynamic process depending on time and varying in rate. The duration of postnatal growth seems to be correlated with the age at which sexual maturity is reached and the greater that age, the longer the period of growth. In man, this may be up to 20 or more years.

The degree and rate of growth are influenced by many factors including:

1. The *inherent properties of the fertilised ovum itself,* which depend on the characteristics present in the chromosomes of both the sperm and ovum. It is now recognised that there is a genetic function during cell growth. Some genes occur continuously during the period of growth while others occur in a specific sequence. An increase in the rate of growth depends on the production of enzymes involved in protein synthesis.

   There are variations in growth in different races and in different members of a race. The internal and external environment of the body can at best bring out the growth potential to the full, but can normally do no more; however, poor environment may lead to a failure to realise the maximum inherent growth possibilities.

2. *Social factors.* There is strong evidence that the physical as well as mental development of disadvantaged children is adversely affected by the social conditions they live in. Socially disadvantaged children tend to be of shorter stature than those living in a better environment. They tend to suffer more ill health and emotional disorders and they also tend to suffer more accidents such as burns and scalds. These are primarily due to cramped accommodation and poor amenities. From studies made by the National Children's Bureau there seem to be three distinct factors which constitute social disadvantage: (a) family composition, e.g. the larger the family, the less chance the child has to develop satisfactorily. If this is allied to (b) low income and (c) poor housing then the problems are compounded.

3. *Ill health,* from any cause, may temporarily depress general growth. This lost ground is made good again during recovery, to a greater or lesser extent.

4. *Nutrition.* A great deal is known about dietetic factors influencing growth. If the diet is deficient in any way, growth will be impaired. It is possible that the present so-called 'normal' standards for height and weight do not represent the maximum potentialities but are average findings in people whose nutritional intake was not perfect. In many instances supplementary intakes of high-quality foodstuffs, such as milk, have produced higher growth standards in seemingly normal children.

5. *Role of the endocrines.* Disturbances of growth frequently accompany clinical disorders of the endocrine glands, e.g. growth depends on the building up (anabolism) of proteins which involves retention of nitrogen in the body. Protein build-up is encouraged by the combined actions of the anterior pituitary growth hormone, thyroid hormones (thyroxin, thyrocalcitonin and triiodothyrosine), insulin and androgens from the adrenal cortex and the testis. Protein breakdown (catabolism) is

favoured by the adrenal glucocorticoids (cortisol) (p. 278).

The baby at birth

At birth the baby is about 50 to 55 cm long and weighs about 2.8 to 4.5 kg with an average of 3.5 kg (Figs. 1.3 and 1.4).

The nervous system

It has been calculated that the newborn has all the nerve cells and that they number about 10^{10} to 15^{10}. This number does not increase, but the cells will increase in size and become myelinated. While he is not capable of co-ordinated movement he exhibits a number of reflexes.

The tone of the flexor muscles exceeds that of the anti-gravity muscles and the resting posture of the newborn is therefore a modification of the fetal attitude of generalised flexion. From this posture, the newborn makes spontaneous movements which, for the first week or two, are mainly random and generalised. His movements are reflex in action and there are about 70 primitive reflexes which have been described. Some of these will be described in more detail. These primitive reflexes are possible because myelination of nerves has not yet occurred and as myelination proceeds so greater control of movement and posture is possible.

Oral reflexes

Reflexes from the maxillomandibular area are well developed in the newborn. The 'search' or 'rooting' reflex is a response to peri-oral touch. When the baby's cheek contacts the mother's breast or other parts, he 'roots' for milk. It enables him to find the nipple without being guided to it. When the baby's mouth is lightly touched, the bottom lip is lowered on the same side and the tongue moves forward towards the point of stimulation (Fig. 1.5).

Eye reflexes

A number of eye reflexes are present. For example, the *blink* reflex can be elicited by various stimuli such as a bright light, a painful touch or stroking the eyelashes. *The pupil reflexes* are

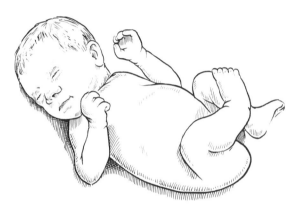

Fig. 1.3 Newborn baby.

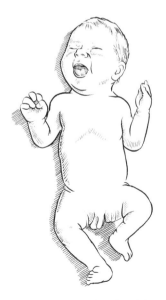

Fig. 1.4 Full-term baby, supine, flexed position.

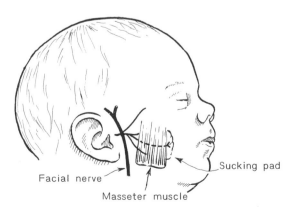

Facial nerve

Masseter muscle

Sucking pad

Fig. 1.5 Sucking pad in the newborn.

produced in response to light, the *doll's eye* response — so named because there is a delay in the movement of the eyes after the head has been turned. If the head is turned slowly to either side the eyes do not normally move with the head.

Moro reflex

The reflex consists of abduction and extension of the arms. The hands open, but the fingers often remain curved. This is followed by adduction of the arms as if in an embrace. At the same time it is accompanied by crying, extension of the trunk and head with movements of the legs. The Moro reflex is present in premature babies, except the very small ones. The Moro response is a vestibular reflex. It disappears by about 3 or 4 months of age. The Moro reflex can be elicited by holding the baby's hands and raising him gently a little way off the table. Rapid release of the hands causes the sudden movement of the cervical region which initiates the reflex.

The startle reflex

This reflex is obtained by causing a sudden loud noise or by tapping the sternum. The elbow is flexed and the hand remains closed. This reflex disappears by 4 months of age (Fig. 1.6).

The grasp reflex

When the palm is stimulated the fingers flex and grip the object (Fig. 1.7). Once the grasp reflex has been obtained the finger can be drawn gently upwards. As this is done, the grip is reinforced

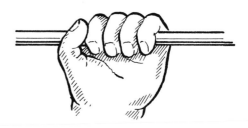

Fig. 1.7 Grasp reflex.

and there is a progressive tensing of the muscles from the wrist to the shoulder, until the baby hangs from the finger momentarily. A similar response can be elicited by gently stroking the sole of the foot behind the toes. The grasp reflex is assessed partly with regard to intensity, partly with regard to symmetry and partly with regard to persistence after it should have disappeared by 4 months of age

The tonic neck reflexes

These reflexes can be observed when the infant is in the supine position and not crying. He may be seen to lie with the head turned to one side with the arm extended to the same side. The contralateral knee is often flexed. The tonic neck reflexes are asymmetrical and symmetrical and are important in determining the posture of the neonate. They are more marked in spastic babies and persist longer than in normal babies. Another function of these reflexes is that they prevent the baby rolling from prone to supine or vice versa in the early weeks.

Placing and walking reflexes

The placing reaction is elicited by bringing the anterior aspect of the tibia or ulna against the edge of a table. The baby lifts the leg up to step on the table, or raises the arm to place the hand on the table. The reflex is present in full-term babies weighing over 1800 g. It can also be elicited in preterm babies weighing over 1700 g, after the first 24 hours.

The walking reflex is obtained by holding the baby upright over a table, so that the sole of the foot presses against the table (Fig. 1.8). This initiates flexion and extension of the legs, simulating walking. The walking reflex can also be elicited from premature babies but they tend to

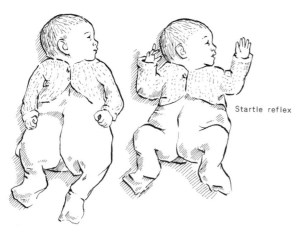

Startle reflex

Fig. 1.6 Startle reflex.

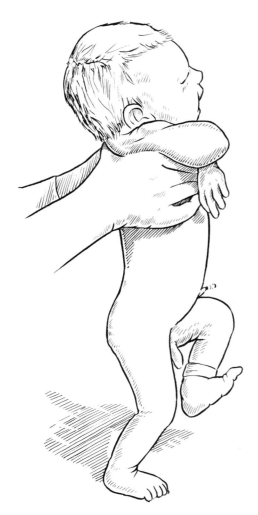

Fig. 1.8 Walking reflex.

walk on their toes. The walking reflex disappears in normal babies by the age of 5 or 6 weeks.

Righting reflexes

These enable the infant to roll from prone to supine and vice versa. They help him to get on to his hands and knees and to sit up. They are responsible for the ability to restore the normal position of the head in space and to maintain the normal postural relationship of the head, trunk and limbs during all activities. They include the following:

1. The neck righting reflex. This is present at birth and is strongest at 3 months of age.

Turning of the head to one side is followed by movement of the body as a whole.

2. Labyrinth righting reflex acting on the head. This is present at 2 months and strongest at 10 months of age. It enables the infant to lift the head up in the prone position, when he is about 1 to 2 months old and later when he lies in the supine position.

3. The body righting reflex acts on the body. It modifies the neck righting reflex and plays an important role in the young child's early attempts to sit and stand. It appears at 7 to 12 months of age.

Parachute reflex

This can be elicited at 6 to 9 months of age and persists throughout life. It can be elicited by holding the infant in ventral suspension and suddenly lowering him towards a surface (bed or couch). The arms extend as if to protect himself from falling. In infants with cerebral palsy, the reflex is absent or incomplete due to the strong flexor tone in this position.

Other reflexes which are present in the newborn and a young infant include tendon reflexes (Fig. 1.9), ankle clonus, abdominal reflexes and sucking and swallowing reflexes. The absence of the last two suggests a neurological defect.

Movements

Two types of movements can be detected, spontaneous and provoked. Spontaneous movements include tremors, twitching and sudden movements without apparent stimulus. The Moro and startle reflexes are examples of provoked movements.

Head and skull

The infant's skull bones are not united and this allows for moulding and overlap. This facilitates

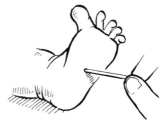

Fig. 1.9 Plantar response.

the passage of the head through the birth canal. The seven bones of the skull are divided by narrow spaces, called sutures. At the point where these bones meet are irregularly-shaped spaces called fontanelles. There are six fontanelles (Fig. 1.10), the larger anterior fontanelle, the small posterior occipital fontanelle and the small paired fontanelles called the sphenoidal and mastoid fontanelles. The fontanelles are sheets of membrane. The anterior fontanelle is of most interest clinically, since its size, tension and time of closure can be affected by disease. For example, increased intracranial pressure in infancy can be recognised by bulging of the fontanelles, and delayed closure may indicate rickets or cretinism. Closure of the posterior fontanelle occurs at about 6 weeks of age, while the anterior fontanelle closes between 17 and 19 months of age.

Head circumference

The head circumference is related to the size of the baby. A large baby is likely to have a larger head than a small baby while a small baby will probably have a smaller head than a large baby. For example, the range of normal head circumference for a normal child is between 33.8 and 37 cm with a mean of 35 cm. There are also slight variations between boys and girls. The head circumference is measured round the occcipito-frontal circumference (the largest circumference). A disposable paper tape or a fibreglass tape measure should be used, since a linen tape measure stretches and therefore produces inaccurate results.

Behaviour of the newborn baby

The newborn full-term infant shows alertness, eye following and responds to sound. He lies on his side with arms and legs flexed. When he is placed on his back he rolls to one side or the other. His limbs are flexed and the pelvis is raised from the surface he is lying on with his knees drawn up high under the abdomen (Figs. 1.3 and 1.4).

The cry of the infant

Crying is a means of communication. Each baby has his own characteristic cry and only experience will help to identify what he is trying to communicate. Normally the infant cries if he is uncomfortable, hungry or unhappy. The first cry enables the lungs to expand and generally accompanies the first breathing movement following birth. From the moment of birth, babies cry if they are in pain, either caused by wind or some external source. Overstimulation such as loud noises or sudden bright lights, varying tastes or being too hot or too cold will result in crying. Crying can be halted by picking the baby up and cuddling and in the very early weeks of life a variety of continuous, rhythmical movements predispose infants to sleep.

The respiratory system

The first and most important task of the newborn is to breathe so that he can oxygenate his own red blood cells. Breathing movements probably begin late in fetal life although there is no ventilation before birth.

Breathing of the newborn is mainly abdominal

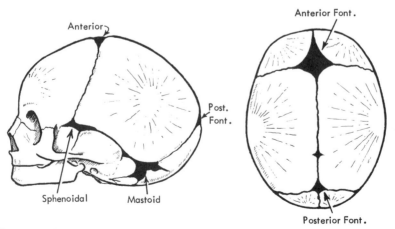

Fig. 1.10 Fontanelles and cranial sutures in the newborn.

and diaphragmatic and becomes thoracic when the infant begins to sit up by about 6 months of age. Breathing is quiet and shallow at a rate of between 30–60 per minute.

The cardiovascular system

With the birth of the baby, changes occur within the heart which alters the circulation of the blood (see p. 400). In the newborn, blood does not circulate readily to the extremities; therefore the hands and feet may have a bluish hue and feel cool, while the rest of the body is pink and warm. Blood pressure is characteristically low and can be difficult to measure. Normal pressure is about 80/46 mmHg at birth rising to 100/50 mmHg by the 10th day.

Body temperature

The infant's heat-regulating mechanism has not fully developed and his temperature tends to be unstable. He also has a relatively greater skin surface and this leads to a relatively greater loss of heat. Immediately after birth the infant's temperature decreases to about 35.5 °C. This is a normal reaction to the change from the warm uterus to the outside environment of the room and, since the infant's body is also moist, heat loss will be due to evaporation.

The digestive system

In utero the fetus obtained nourishment passively. When born he must perform sucking and swallowing actions. Both these actions are closely co-ordinated. Although the gastro-intestinal tract has not been active, it is functional at birth.

Sucking, biting and swallowing are activities of the mouth. The infant is capable of forming a seal around the nipple or teat. The seal must be airtight if the baby is to suck. When he sucks, his tongue is firmly opposed to the palate, so he can only breathe through his nose.

Sense of *taste* and possibly *smell* is present in the newborn baby. He can distinguish acceptable and unacceptable flavours.

The saliva does not contain the starch-digesting enzyme for the first 3 months.

At birth, the volume of the stomach is 25 to 50 ml but by the 10th day it can hold 100 ml plus the same volume of air. Air is always present in the stomach, but if the milk flows freely less air is swallowed.

Digestion

The stomach is never completely empty and in early infancy it does not have an important digestive function. As stated above, the saliva contains few enzymes. At birth the pH value is 6 but falls to 2.5 within a few hours after birth. Most digestion takes place in the small intestine. In the newborn, food reaches the caecum in 3 to 4 hours. Some is evacuated in 8 hours, the rest within 24 hours.

Elimination

Meconium, the first stool, is passed between 8 to 24 hours after birth. Meconium is a sticky, greenish-black substance composed of bile, mucus, cellular waste, intestinal secretions, fat, hair and vernix caseosa swallowed during fetal life with the amniotic fluid.

Renal systems

Most of the nephrons are present but not all function adequately. The amount of urine produced and passed will depend on (a) the level of renal development and (b) the amount of fluid taken. Urination usually occurs soon after birth but may be delayed until the 2nd day in about 8 per cent of newborn babies. Initially the amount of urine passed is about 20 ml but this will increase as the fluid intake increases.

Genitalia

In the male, the prepuce tends to adhere to the glans of the penis. In the female the labia minora appear relatively large and the infant may also have a slight mucoid blood discharge exuding from the vaginal orifice. The large appearance of the labia minora and the exudate are due to maternal oestrogens.

The skin

The premature newborn has fine downy hair, called *lanugo*, which covers the skin, but this should have disappeared in the full-term infant. A cheese-like, greasy substance, vernix caseosa, may cover the skin. This is believed to protect the skin during uterine life.

Growth after birth

Growth in height

At birth the baby is about 50 to 55 cm long and, to reach adult height of about 175 cm he has to grow three and a half times his initial length.

Growth in height is not uniform throughout life. For example, the maximum rate of growth occurs before birth in the 4th month of fetal life, with a progressive slowing down thereafter. However, at birth the infant is still growing very fast indeed compared with the infant and child.

Measurement of height in children and adults presents some difficulties. Some of these are related to the variation in width of the intervertebral discs of the vertebral column, as these become compressed by the gravitational strain imposed by the upper part of the body as the day goes on. This results in a decrease in height in the evening as compared with the morning. It is, therefore, important that measurements of height should be made at the same time of the day. For research purposes it is also desirable that the same person should make every measurement. This at least minimises errors.

Charts of height for age are available and invaluable, but it is important to recognise some of the limitations when comparing a child's height with a standard chart (Fig. 1.11).

In the first year after birth, body length increases by about 50 per cent and in the second year another 12 or 13 cm or so are added. Thereafter growth in height settles down to a rate of about 5 to 6 cm every year.

At about the time of adolescence the fairly steady rate of increase in height rises suddenly. This begins about the age of 10 to 11 years in girls and 12 to 13 years in boys. This spurt is followed by a rapid slowing of growth; girls reach 98 per cent of their final height by the average age of 16 to 17, whereas boys do not reach the same stage until the age of about 17 to 18. There are, of course, wide variations around the mean, depending on such factors as genes, race, nutrition, ill health and endocrine function.

Growth in weight

At birth, a full-term baby weighs on the average 3.5 kg within a range of about 2.7 to 4.5 kg. Weight is more variable than length and depends

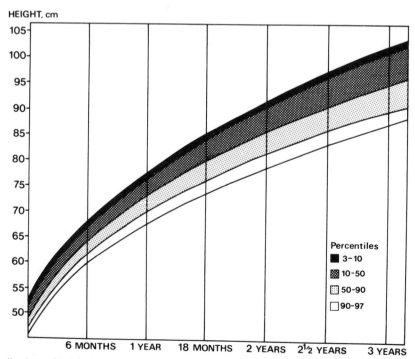

Fig. 1.11 Percentile chart of height increase.

more on the maternal environment than on the genetic factors of the child. Full-term females are on the average about 140 g lighter than full-term males and a twin weighs about 680 g less than a single baby. Rank of the child in the family is a factor in its birth-weight; later children tend to be somewhat heavier than first-born.

Unless there has been severe malnutrition, birth-weight is independent of the mother's diet, since the fetus will draw on the mother's tissues for its needs. However, there is evidence that women who smoke during pregnancy are more liable to have smaller or low-weight babies than those who do not smoke. The mean birth-weight of infants is regarded as one of the indices of the health of a people. In highly-developed countries a high mean birth-weight will be found, whereas where malnutrition is common a low mean birth-weight will be found.

The weight gain of a baby on average is for the first 3 months about 200 g per week, for the second 3 months 150 g per week and in the second year 42 g per week.

By the end of the first year, the birth-weight has approximately trebled and by the end of the second year it has quadrupled. After this, annual weight increase is relatively steady, about 2.25 to 2.75 kg a year until the onset of adolescence when boys may add about 20 kg to their weight and girls about 16 kg (Fig. 1.12).

The development of the child

Many studies of child development have been done by Gesell and his colleagues in America and by Illingworth & Sheridan in Britain. Certain landmarks of development have been described and charts and tables have been produced to help in the assessment of children at different ages. However, any table or chart should be considered as approximate and may not be applicable to every child.

Development is intimately related to the maturation of the nervous system. For example, the infant will not be able to pick up an object until the nervous system has developed to the point where muscular co-ordination is possible. In spite of the large size of the central nervous system at birth, it is functionally incomplete and requires a considerable time to develop to the stage at which it can be used efficiently.

Each aspect of development will be discussed separately. However, to provide a complete logical sequence of events and to emphasise the interrelationship between the different aspects of devel-

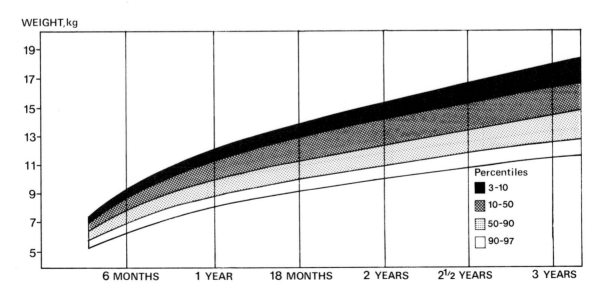

Fig. 1.12 Percentile chart of weight increase.

Table 1.1 Summary of developmental progress (birth to 5 years)

Age	Motor/Sensory	Social/Understanding	Speech	Manipulative
Birth to 1 month	Primitive reflexes. Can suck, grasp, responds to sudden sounds			
1–3 months	Holds head up momentarily; makes crawling movements when prone	Smiles responsively		
3–4 months	Lifts head from prone position for short periods. Turns head towards sound	Smiles	Makes sounds when spoken to	Begins to watch own hands; can hold rattle
6–9 months	Rolls from side to side when lying on back. Turns head to person talking	Shows pleasure with crowing and cooing	Vocalises — grunting sounds, sounds like 'da' 'ma'	Begins to pass objects from hand to hand. Able to manipulate objects
9–10 months	Sits up from lying position; moves about; crawls	Recognises and rejects strangers; imitates. Shouts for attention	Babbles and vocalises; says words like mum-mum, da-da	Picks up objects between finger and thumb
1 year	Crawls well; pulls himself upright; may walk with support	Obeys simple commands. Imitates adults. Shows varied emotions	Says single words	Holds cup to drink
1½ years	Walks unsupported; climbs stairs or furniture (chairs)	Wants to play near other children. Asks for potty. Recognises pictures of animals. Knows several parts of his body	Has use of about 20 intelligible words	Scribbles, turns pages, play with building bricks constructively
2 years	Able to run, climb, walk upstairs, open doors	May begin to play with other children	Begins to put two or three words together	Dresses himself; not able to tie or fasten buttons
3 years	Runs confidently; jumps; rides tricycle	Knows his name and sex; can be reasoned with; plays constructively and imitatively	Talks in short sentences	Draws circle; draws recognisable figures
4–5 years		Knows many letters of the alphabet; knows nursery rhymes; can count up to 10	Recites and sings	

opment these will be shown in table form (Table 1.1, p. 16).

Motor development (Fig. 1.13)

One of the principles of development is that generalised mass activity is replaced by specific individual responses. Another principle is that development is in the cephalocaudal direction, i.e. head control must be achieved before walking is possible.

When the newborn infant is held in *ventral suspension* with the hand under the abdomen, there is almost complete lack of head control. By about

6 weeks he is able to hold up his head momentarily in the same plane as the rest of the body. By 8 weeks he can maintain that position and by 12 weeks he can maintain the head well beyond the plane of the rest of the body. The elbows are largely flexed and there is some extension of the hips with flexion of the knees.

By about 2 to 3 months his limbs are more pliable and the movements become smoother and more continuous. His hands are more loosely open. When lying in the prone position he can lift his chin off the couch. By 8 to 12 weeks he holds his chin and shoulders off the couch with his legs

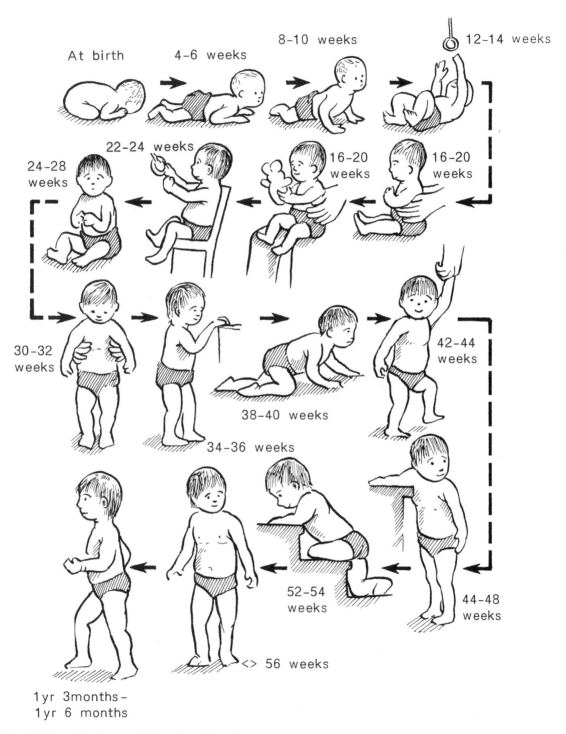

At birth

4–6 weeks

8–10 weeks

12–14 weeks

22–24 weeks

24–28 weeks

16–20 weeks

16–20 weeks

30–32 weeks

34–36 weeks

38–40 weeks

42–44 weeks

44–48 weeks

52–54 weeks

<> 56 weeks

1yr 3months – 1yr 6 months

Fig. 1.13 Motor development, birth to 1 year 6 months.

fully extended. When held in the sitting position he holds his back straight, except in the lumbar region. When held standing with his feet on a hard surface he sags at his knees.

Between 12 weeks and 24 weeks he should be able to lift his head from a pillow, gradually supporting his head. He should be able to sit supported by pillows in a cot or pram and move his head from side to side. Arm movements are more purposeful and towards 6 months he can hold his arms up to be lifted. He may also be able to pull himself up when his hands are held. He should be able to roll over and kick his legs strongly using alternate legs.

Between 24 weeks and 36 weeks he should be able to sit alone for increasing time up to 10 to 15 minutes. He can look sideways by turning his body and will attempt to grasp dangling toys or to pick up an object. For example, when holding a cube it is held against the thenar eminence at the base of the thumb (Fig. 1.14). He can almost bear his own weight by 24 weeks, and by 36 weeks he can stand holding on to furniture. He can also pull himself up to the standing position but cannot let himself down.

From 36 to 48 weeks progress continues and he is able to sit up for increasingly longer periods of time until by 40 weeks he not only pulls himself up to the sitting position but can sit well for a long time. Crawling will be attempted by some at 34 weeks but by 40 weeks he should be able to crawl on all fours. He can pull himself to the standing position and is able to lower himself while holding on. He should also be able to walk while holding on to furniture or to people and some are able to stand alone for a few minutes. During this period of development the infant is able to manipulate objects by using the index finger with the help of the ring and little finger. By about 48 weeks he can walk holding on to furniture. He can place objects into and out of baskets, boxes and should cease to place objects into his mouth. He is also ready to give objects such as toys to others. Some children will be able to pick up a cup, know its use and drink from it. They are also able to put it down without spilling its contents.

From 12 to 15 months

He should be able to twist round and pick up objects. He begins to creep upstairs. He can walk steadily with his feet wide apart. He can start walking alone but is frequently stopped by falling or bumping into furniture. He can let himself down from standing to sitting by collapsing backwards with a bump, or occasionally falling forward on his hands and then back to sitting. He can build

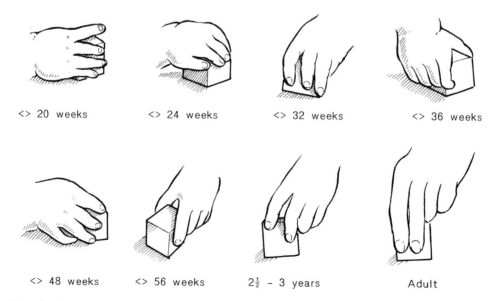

<> 20 weeks   <> 24 weeks   <> 32 weeks   <> 36 weeks

<> 48 weeks   <> 56 weeks   2½ – 3 years   Adult

Fig. 1.14 Motor development (hand control).

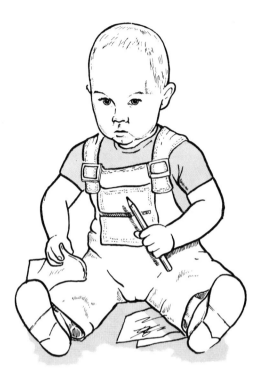

Fig. 1.15 Jon Paul, drawing at the age of 1 year.

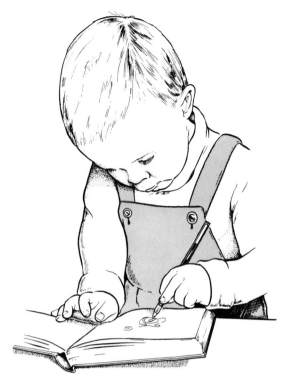

Fig. 1.16 Jon Paul, drawing at the age of 1 year 10 months. (Note control achieved.)

a tower of two to three cubes and is able to manipulate a pencil with his whole hand (Fig. 1.15).

From 15 to 18 months
He usually walks well with his feet only slightly apart, and starts and stops without falling. He runs stiffly upright with eyes fixed on the ground 1 to 2 metres ahead. He is able to push and pull large objects, i.e. toys, pans, boxes, etc. round the floor and can carry objects while walking. Many are able to climb on to a chair and sit on it. They are able to walk upstairs with a helping hand and creep downstairs backwards. Occasionally they bump down a few steps on buttocks while facing forward. They are beginning to achieve greater control of fine movements, for example holding and handling a spoon and pencil and beginning to scribble.

From 18 months to 2 years
He runs safely on his whole foot, stopping and starting with ease and avoiding obstacles. He can climb stairs holding on to the rail or wall using two feet to a step. He is able to throw a ball without falling. He can pick up fine objects, e.g. thread. He makes greater use of a pencil by attempting line drawing (Fig. 1.16). He can feed himself with a spoon without making too much of a mess. He is able to turn a door knob and unscrew lids. He should also be able to put on shoes, socks and pants.

From 2 to 2½ years
He should be able to walk upstairs alone without holding on to a wall or rail but when going down-stairs he will still hold the rail and use two feet to a step. He can push and pull large toys skilfully but may have difficulty in steering them round obstacles. He is able to jump with two feet together and attempts to stand on tiptoes. He can hold a pencil with thumb, forefinger and middle finger and begins to draw (Fig. 1.17). He can manipulate cubes and build a tower of seven cubes.

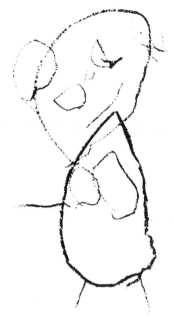

Fig. 1.17 Drawing by a child aged 2 years 6 months.

From 2½ to 3 years
By this stage he can walk upstairs with alternating feet but downstairs with two feet to a step, often jumping down the last step. He is able to ride a tricycle and can walk on tiptoes. He can build a tower of nine to 10 cubes. He can dress and undress fully and begins to manage buttons. Manipulation of a pencil progresses further and he is able to copy circles.

From 3 to 4 years
He walks alone up- and downstairs using one foot per step. He is able to hop on one leg and can stand on one leg for a short time. He shows great dexterity of hands and fingers.

From 4 to 5 years
He is active and skilful at climbing, sliding and swinging. He is able to skip on alternate feet. He can stand on one leg for a longer period and can hop forward on each foot separately. He can write letters and draw an incomplete man and houses.

Visual development
At birth the baby shows visual perception and will follow a moving person with his eyes. The eyes of the newborn tend to move independently.

Binocular vision begins at 6 weeks and is fairly well established by 4 months. He is unable to focus and can follow a dangling ring with difficulty. There is little convergence before 6 weeks of age. By 4 weeks he begins to watch his mother's nearby face when she feeds or talks to him. By 3 months he can fixate well on near objects. He is visually alert and moves his head deliberately to look around him. He watches the movement of his own hands held before his face.

By 6 months he moves his head and eyes eagerly in every direction and his eyes move in unison. He fixes immediately on objects within 15 to 30 cm. When toys fall from his hand he either forgets them or searches vaguely around him. By 9 months he is able to search in the correct place for toys dropped within reach of his hand. He watches other people's activities. By 12 months he looks in the correct place for toys which have rolled out of sight. He recognises familiar people and objects quite a distance away. His visual acuity improves with age; by 4 months it is 3/60; by 6 months 4/60; by 1 year 6/60; by 18 months 6/24; by 2 years 6/12; and by 5 years 6/6, i.e. he can read size 6 letters at 6 metres.

Development of hearing
The newborn full-term baby can hear; he may respond to sound by a startle reflex, by crying, by blinking, by a momentary catch in his breathing and by calming or quieting if he is crying.

By 1 month he may move his eyes towards sound. If a sound is made from a distance of 7 to 10 cm for a short time, movements may cease. By 3 to 4 months the infant turns his head towards the sound and his eyes look in the same direction. By 5 to 6 months he turns immediately to his mother's voice even when quite a distance away. About 6 to 8 months he is able to turn his head in a curving arc towards the sound source. From about 9 months the baby learns to control and adjust his responses to sounds. He may delay or inhibit altogether his response.

Development of speech and language
Babies vocalise from the time of birth. Initially the sounds they produce are simple vowels like 'a', 'e' sounds. The number of vowel sounds increases in

the first weeks of life until sounds like 'g', 'k', 'l' and 'r' can be clearly heard.

The infant's means of communication is mainly by crying, which is stimulated by discomfort, hunger or the crying of other infants even when very young. With increasing vocalisation the infant's lips, tongue and palate assume different positions, depending on the type of communication, e.g. hunger. Although the infant is able to recognise and respond to sounds from birth, a positive specific response like smiling or vocalising occurs at about 2 months of age. He will gradually respond to different tones of speech, i.e. whether friendly or unfriendly.

Between 3 and 6 months, his attempts to vocalise when spoken to will be more constant and he will also initiate vocal exchanges. By 6 months he vocalises tunefully using single syllables, e.g. ka, muh, goo, der.

By 9 months he can vocalise deliberately as a means of interpersonal communication. He will shout to attract attention and makes babbling sounds like mam-mam, bab, dad and repeats these.

Between 9 and 12 months some may be able to say one or two recognisable words. With increasing age the number of words spoken increase and they become clearer. As the child matures, the vowels become progressively differentiated and more like the speech he is hearing. By 18 months he may use six to 20 recognisable words, and may echo prominent words or the last word addressed to him.

The rate of vocabulary gain varies from child to child and is related to innate factors and the amount and type of speech which the child hears.

By 2 years he may use more than 50 recognisable words and can join two or three words together to form simple sentences. He tends to talk to himself continually as he plays and obviously practises words. Echolalia is almost constant with one or more stressed words being repeated. He makes use of 'I', 'you' and 'me'.

By $2\frac{1}{2}$ years he has greatly increased vocabulary and knows and uses 200 or more recognisable words. He continually asks questions beginning with 'what', 'why' and 'where', and is able to recite a few nursery rhymes.

By 3 years the child is able to provide normal speech but occasionally there are infantile phonetic substitutions. He can use plurals and pronouns and language has moved from the holophrastic phase to the complex sentence formation. He can carry on conversations of varying complexities and asks many questions. He likes to listen to stories and is often able to improvise.

By 4 years language acquisition has reached a high level. He can give connected accounts of recent events and experiences. He is able to play with words, knows their meaning and is constantly asking questions.

By 5 years speech is fluent and vocabulary is very extensive. He loves stories and acts them out.

Language and environment

The influence of environment to the development of language is extremely important. It begins remarkably early and its effects last a long time. The stimulating effect of a normal family environment cannot be overemphasised. Investigations have shown that children who have been socially, emotionally and intellectually deprived have a distinct disadvantage in language acquisition. The effects of a linguistically poor environment appear by the age of 18 months, while children living in a stimulating environment tend to have a richer vocabulary and two- and three-word sentences appear earlier. There is also good evidence that the attitude of parents and family habits are extremely important for a child's linguistic development. Although the stress has been on environmental factors this does not mean that hereditary factors are of less significance. Much of the acquisition of language occurs before the child goes to school, while the school enlarges the child's knowledge of language mainly by listening and by learning other ways of using it, for example through reading and writing.

Children are exposed to language in a variety of ways. For example: (a) live language directed to the child; (b) live language overheard by the child; (c) TV language; and (d) radio and records. In all these examples, children appear to be attending primarily to language experience per se. In other situations, language may be involved but the child appears to have other purposes in mind.

Many investigations have shown that during the first few months of life infants can discriminate differences in the voicing of languages foreign to their home environments. These cross-language findings suggest that perhaps these voicing categories are not acquired within the developmental stages of the individual infant but within the development of the human species. It is suggested that since the production of the full range of speech sounds is unique to the human species, it may be that human beings have evolved special auditory perceptual capabilities that are optimally correlated with their categories of speech sound production.

Much of the literature on infant speech perception suggests that normal infants are able to group many of the important basics of the human speech code at a very early age. There are also some indications that premature infants or those who have experienced a variety of stresses during pregnancy or during delivery have a greater chance of later developing problems in language acquisition.

General understanding

Some sign of understanding can be recognised in the first few days when he begins to watch his mother when she speaks to him. He responds in a variety of ways, for example, he quietens down, opens and closes his mouth.

By 4 to 6 weeks he begins to respond with a smile and vocalises.

By 12 weeks he recognises his feeding bottle and gets excited as it approaches his face. He is also able to imitate his mother's mouth movement or tongue protrusion. He also shows considerable interest in his environment. He is excited when a toy is presented to him.

By 16 weeks he anticipates when his bottle or the breast is offered by opening his mouth when he sees it approach. By 20 weeks he smiles at his mirror image and looks where a dropped object has gone. At about 24 weeks he shows evidence of response to different emotional tones of his mother's/father's voice. He lifts up his arms in expectation of being lifted up. He imitates acts such as a cough and uses it to attract attention.

By 32 weeks he responds to 'no' and knows when to imitate 'bye-bye' by 40 weeks. He repeats a performance that is laughed at.

By 48 weeks he shows an interest in books and words. At 11 to 12 months he laughs at funny situations and understands phrases such as 'where is your hat?' By 15 months he understands and obeys simple commands, e.g. give me the ball. By 18 months he shows his own hair, shoe, nose and enjoys nursery rhymes. By 2 years he shows and repeats parts of his body, e.g. hand, feet, nose, eyes, etc. As his speech develops his understanding also increases. By $2\frac{1}{2}$ years he continually asks questions and can give quite sensible answers to simple questions. He understands the concept of numbers. By 3 years he listens eagerly to stories and asks for favourite ones. He understands showing of things. By 4 years he begins to understand the need to co-operate, particularly at play but also in relation to adults. By 5 years he is able to define concrete nouns by use and asks the meaning of abstract words.

Intellectual development

What we call intelligence is manifested in behaviour in many different ways. Indeed there are many different kinds of intelligence, for example, the ability to make social contacts, linguistic ability or technical ability. These characteristics may be present in one and the same individual. They are known as intra-individual differences. These intra-individual differences increase with age and their development is complex.

Piaget & Werner both postulated ideal states of intellectual development toward which a child is supposed to be progressing. Piaget's theory rests on the fundamental notion that the child develops through stages until he arrives at the stage that resembles an adult. The stages according to Piaget are as follows.

1. *Sensorimotor stage* which lasts from birth to 18 months. By the end of the sensorimotor period, children show considerable insight into their environment. They can use simple tools to obtain objects. They can anticipate the relatively immediate consequences of actions and can recognise the causes of events that occur. They are able to make use of such external forces as gravity or they can employ the agency of other people to accomplish the results they want. All of these abilities are limited but that they exist at all is quite an achievement. To obtain these accomplishments

they must have achieved a degree of internal control which finds expression in sequences of behaviour involving motor acts.

In addition children must recognise some major characteristics of their environment. During infancy they come to assume that external objects are relatively permanent and continue to exist even when not directly perceived. The sensory information changes radically whenever children close their eyes or turn their heads and also when the objects in the environment themselves move or change shape. Piaget calls the assumption of a permanent identity of objects, the 'object concept'. When children look away, or when an object goes out of sight, the children must be able to return to it, to look for it, and to anticipate its reappearance. To be able to determine that the vanished object still exists, they must be able to organise their information about it, so that they can look for it in an appropriate way. They must understand the characteristics of the world about them. They must be able to use all their senses and be able to interpret these. For example, if a marble disappears behind a screen and rolls to a stop, the child will go after it rather than waiting for it to reappear. They will have to learn that different paths can be taken to a point and be able to retrace their steps. Children learn to handle problems involving cause and effect. For example, the child may kick his feet in the air and by doing so set a rattle into motion. It may not always produce the same effect however, if the same effect is achieved repeatedly then he will realise that kicking produced that effect.

2. *Pre-operational period* which extends from 2 years to 7 years of age. According to Piaget this is a period during which the child's internal cognitive picture of the external world, with its many complexities, is gradually growing. This period is considered to be a transitional one, not marked by a stable equilibrium. It is a period where thought is rather limited but is, nevertheless, a distinct advance on the previous stage.

The child is able to represent the environment in symbolic form and to distinguish between himself and objects in the world around him. Both his language and his thought are characterised by egocentrism. He tends to be 'self-centred' in the liberal sense that he is unable to understand the view that other people may possess. He behaves and speaks in a manner that assumes that what is known to him must be common knowledge to all. For example, when he explains an episode which he has experienced, he usually does not set the scene or describe the participants, but assumes that the listener already knows these. At this stage he is also limited to handling only one attribute of a stimulus at a time and this tends to be of a very physical nature. He is also unable to master the idea of sameness, particularly related to numbers. He is not able to think logically about problems, but in the free-play situation he tends to show sensible and logical behaviour.

3. *Stage 3* is considered to be the stage of concrete operations and is seen in the 7- to 12-year-old children.

Thought processes become much more stable and reasonable. The children can, for example, arrange objects in order of size and fit new ones into the series. They can understand that the equality of number of two sets of objects depends upon a one-to-one correspondence between the objects in the two groups. They show understanding of many of the simpler relationships between classes of objects and they can understand what will happen to the sequence of objects if they are rotated. They can distinguish between the distance of two objects and the length of path between them. By this time, therefore, they have acquired a rudimentary conception of time, space, number and logic, those fundamental conceptions in terms of which our understanding of events and objects is ordered. The concrete operational child shows what is called the ability to conserve. For example, he can state that liquids and solids do not change their amount or quantity merely because their external shape changes.

4. *Stage 4* is considered to be the stage of formal operations beginning at about the age of 12. It reveals the adolescent's ability to think about hypothetical problems that are not necessarily in accord with his experience. He shows willingness to think about possibilities. The adolescent is said to generate a number of possible solution hypotheses to a particular problem. Basically it is an orientation toward problem solving. Formal

thinking is rational and systematic. Another aspect of adolescent thinking is that it is often brooding in type and he tends to be self-conscious about his introspections.

Some psychologists believe that Piaget's concept of cognitive development in infancy is relatively simple. More recent literature about cognitive development indicates that babies given experience in visual search tasks show accelerated success in coping with manual search tasks. It is proposed that the infant can cope with abstract solution and that there is a 'conceptual store', a memory for abstract solutions. There appears to be good experimental evidence that the baby has the ability to think, deduce and reason. Certain important ideas have been formulated which have general applicability to cognitive development. For example:

1. Cognitive development does not follow a necessary sequence.
2. Conflict is important in generating development, i.e. the baby is presented with a conservation task and knows two things: the same objects always weighs the same and longer objects weigh more than shorter objects. Before his very eyes he sees an object become longer, and yet there is no replacement of one object by another. This is an obvious conflict for the baby, a conflict that can only be resolved by deducing a concept of conservation.
3. There are several behavioural patterns to the same developmental end, and each of these behavioural patterns reflects the same conceptual path.
4. Processes of schematisation make behaviour highly efficient but inhibit transfer to new situations.
5. Early experience can facilitate later development.

The greatest change is perceived from the age of 3 to about 12 years of age. The richness of the child's supply of symbols, concepts and rules increases and his tendency to rely on images in problem solving decreases. The child shows growing concern with whether his concepts and rules agree with those of other children. He tends to appear more apprehensive about making mistakes and his memory function may show dramatic improvement.

Cognitive-developmental psychologists believe that the transition from one cognitive level to another is a cognitive reorganisation, that it occurs fairly rapidly over a period of a year or so, and that it is qualitatively discontinuous with the thinking that went on before the new stage. They view development as a result of interaction between the individual and the environment. Some psychologists recognise that there is a transactional process which supports the view that children influence their caretakers and the caretakers influence the children.

It is a long and tenuous path that leads from infancy to symbolic knowledge. It is wonderful that the path is pursued successfully to its conclusion by the majority of children and how seldom any one of the many components fails to make its contribution at the right time. The growth of human understanding is indeed one of the most intricate and amazing phenomena in life.

Emotional development

The word 'emotion' is used to describe a state of excitement in the organism characterised by alteration of feeling tone and by physiological changes. Anger, fear, sorrow and joy are typical emotions. However, emotional life does not only consist of powerful and violent feelings but also of a calm and temperate emotional state.

Emotional development depends on a number of factors: Gesell believes that it depends chiefly on maturation and is genetically predetermined. Others, such as Jones & Hebb, support the environmental theory. It is suggested that there is a sequence of emotion. For example, the emotional content of the first month of life is designated 'excitement'. By this is meant that specific reactions cannot be detected during the first weeks. Only very general and uncontrolled muscular activity can be observed.

During the first months, distress and delight are differentiated, though distress can be identified earlier than delight. Between 3 and 6 months the infant is capable of expressing anger, disgust and fear. By about 7 months to 10 months the infant can exhibit anxiety, surprise, obstinacy, dissatisfaction and anticipation. By about the end of the first year there is evidence of satisfaction and affection for grown-ups and children. By 18 months he can show jealousy and by 24 months there is evidence of joy.

Most emotional expressions appear to be learned and can be elicited during various maturational phases. Emotional expressions such as crying, laughing, excitement and startle pattern could be considered innate elements of emotion. The stimuli which elicit these behaviours vary with each individual and so does the degree of expression of emotion. As the child develops, and as a result of training, he will learn to modify the expressions of emotions and here social and cultural factors play an important part.

Emotional development, like all other aspects of development, is related to age. He has to learn to deal with frustration which is described as a state characterised by baffled impulses giving rise to irritating dissatisfaction. The individual is subjected to such frustration at all stages of development, e.g. the baby is frustrated when his needs remain unsatisfied. There are three main types of frustration behaviour: fixation, aggression and regression.

In *fixation* the behaviour pattern cannot be modified and may seem unintelligent. It does not allow adjustment to a specific situation. Such behaviour can sometimes be observed in children with strictly formed habits. Difficulties with a school subject can lead to the form of resigned disinclination.

Aggression means that the individual makes blind attacks as a reaction to frustration. It is not always directed against the immediate cause of the frustration. A young child who has been frustrated often finds relief in temper tantrums, or the schoolchild will work off his frustration by kicking a wall or banging a door.

Regression is a form of behaviour where the individual returns to an earlier and more primitive form of behaviour. Behaviour such as thumb-sucking or marked dependence on the mother at a stage when dependency has usually been overcome.

There are other defence mechanisms which the child can adopt against internal tensions: rationalisation, compensation, projection, repression and withdrawal.

Rationalisation is the justification of an act after it has been performed, to avoid feelings of guilt.

Compensation means that failure in one field of endeavour leads to greater efforts to succeed in another and thereby gain approval. For example, the child who fails or finds it difficult to succeed in one area at school will work hard to be successful in another area.

Projection is a method of avoiding guilt feelings by transferring one's own mistakes and bad features to others.

Repression is a process by which a person attempts to protect himself against painful impulses by transferring them to the unconscious.

Another defence mechanism often used by children is to withdraw within oneself. This form of behaviour can be seen in very young children, e.g. during hospitalisation when the conflict situation becomes too painful.

Defence mechanisms begin to function early and their use depends on many factors. Some of these are due to external stimulus situations, others are internally induced.

Emotional maturity

As the child grows older, the emotional behaviour seems to be better integrated. He is able to govern and control emotional impulses to a greater extent so that he can use them spontaneously and for life-enhancing purposes. In an effort to achieve improvement of control of emotionality he needs to learn how to direct the stimuli received, i.e. the one function which directs the response reaction and determines the path the arousal should take. This means that it is important to provide an environment which will ensure emotional stability. The care of the child should be such that his physical and mental well-being is assured since this should reduce emotional stress. The attitude of the parents is of primary importance. For example, allowing the child ample opportunities for his own activities, accepting his playmates and allowing him a share in decision making.

Personality development

Personality is a term which denotes a whole range of attributes that an individual may be said to possess, and which finds expression in his modes of behaviour and thought. The nature of a personality, which is the product of heredity and environment, is always unique and decisive for behaviour in any given situation.

Personality development is a dynamic process with the goal of the individual to be able to work, to play, to master personal problems, to love and be loved; to be creative, socially acceptable and to feel personally gratified. Personality development is a complicated process involving all aspects of the individual and his environment.

Each individual is born with specific potentialities and these are developed by the individual's experiences as he matures. Although all experiences are individual it is possible to identify two broad classes: (a) the common experiences shared by most individuals growing up in a given culture, and (b) unique or individual experiences.

The process of growing up includes learning to behave in ways expected by our society. The child has to learn to accept group values and he will recognise the roles assigned to him. Some roles are of own choosing but even they are patterned by the culture.

Each person reacts in his own way to social pressures upon him and this is in part due to biological make-up of the individual. The biological potentialities of the child are influenced by his parents, his siblings, his peers and others. It is those persons who transmit the culture in the precise form in which it makes an impact upon the individual. They impose social roles and provide the models which show how the roles are played. They give and withhold satisfaction of primitive impulses. They give food to satisfy hunger and use force to prevent undesirable behaviour. They show approval and disapproval of the child's behaviour. As the child comes to seek approval and disapproval, he becomes capable of hindsight and foresight and begins to see himself as a responsible agent. He gradually develops a conscience whereby he judges his own behaviour according to ideals he has acquired.

Identity formation

The many diverse influences and experiences which impinge on the child must become unified or integrated before the child emerges as a recognisable personality structure. The child goes through various steps or stages before he finally achieves an adult identity. This the child achieves by identifying himself with significant people in his environment. As long as these different identifications remain, the personality is made up of parts, often not self-consistent. He is therefore torn into a variety of roles, and this Erikson calls *role diffusion*. Role diffusion is normally characteristic of early adolescence when the young have not yet achieved an identity. The processes by which identity is finally achieved are various but they all involve some experimentation with various experiences and roles.

Infancy

As the infant grows and develops there is a growing awareness of himself as an entity separate from his environment. During the first year psychological development is interrelated with physical development. As his senses mature he will be able to discriminate between self and non-self.

The newborn infant is at first aware only of his bodily needs. The pleasure of relief from discomfort gradually becomes associated with mothering and later with the mother. He derives a feeling of security when his needs are satisfied and from contact with his mother. If he is deprived of the security and affection necessary to produce a sense of trust he may respond with immobility, listlessness, indifferent appetite, appearance of unhappiness and difficulty in sleeping.

Early childhood (18 months to 5 year)

The child's horizon widens. Increased body control makes possible the development of many physical skills. He now begins to have feeling of autonomy, self-direction and initiative. It is a time when the child will want to assert himself while at the same time he has to learn how to become a self-respecting, likeable and socially responsible adult.

Later childhood (5 to 12 years)

In this period the child achieves a rapid intellectual growth. Primitive drives have become fairly successfully controlled and are expressed in a socially acceptable way, or they are repressed. Preoccupation with fantasy gradually subsides and the child wants to be engaged in real tasks he can carry through to completion. He desires to become a member of a larger group consisting of his equals and this tends to make for qualities of co-operation and obedience to the will of the group. Towards the end of this period he tends to question parental values where these differ from those of the group.

Early adolescence (12 to 16 years)

With great physical changes in body size and configuration comes a new confusion about the physical self. Sexual maturation brings with it resurgence of the strong instinctual drives which have been successfully repressed for several years. The calm emotional adjustment is disrupted and the child has to learn again to control strong feelings such as love, hate, and aggression. Relationships are changing, for example, the demand for independence from his parents and yet the need for some measure of dependence. The changes in behaviour and personality traits are not necessarily those of the future adult. They tend to be erratic and extreme in their behaviour.

Late adolescence (16 to maturity)

By the 16th year most children have again achieved relative equilibrium. Body growth is slowing down and they have had time to adjust to the new body image. They will have achieved comparative mastery over biological drives to the extent that they can now be channelled into more constructive patterns. There is a tendency towards heterosexual social activity and the relationship to the parents is now more mature. They are now learning rapidly and there is active preparation for adulthood.

Personality theories

There are a number of theories relating to personality and some of these are dealt with in Chapter 18. Each theorist discusses different aspects of personality, its dynamics and components. According to Freud, personality develops and grows as a result of a variety of processes, stresses and experiences, such as maturation, deprivation, conflict and anxiety. Freud believed that every human personality passed through a series of fixed stages called psychosexual stages of development. For example, the oral stage occurs in infancy, where the primary focus of the infant's existence is on the mouth. So the infant derives pleasure and satisfaction from sucking, biting, chewing and vocalising.

At the beginning of the second year the child enters the dual stage where the primary focus is on elimination. This is the period of toilet training and it is usually during this stage that the child is confronted by conflict. As the anal stage fades the child gradually enters the phallic stage of development. This stage lasts from 3 to 5 years. During this period the child may experience intense guilt and conflict.

The latency stage or period corresponds to the middle years of childhood ending with puberty. During this stage the child tends to be relatively unaware of sexuality until he reaches adolescence when sexual feelings become more urgent and bring the latency period to an end. The final stage he considers to be the genital stage when sexual needs are reawakened and lead to mature love for those of the opposite sex.

Carl Rogers' self theory deals with the individual as a whole. According to Rogers the individual constantly strives to develop and expand the self. The aim is for self-actualisation and, in order to achieve that goal of self-growth, four conditions are necessary. First, the choices available to the individual must be clearly perceived. Second, the choices must be clearly symbolised. That is, the individual must not only be aware of the alternatives but he must also have a clear idea and full understanding of choices. Third, he must be loved and respected by others and this leads to self-regard, that is the person must have faith in and respect for himself.

According to Cattell there are trait clusters, that is groups of trait that tend to go together. If an individual has one of the traits from a cluster, he will probably have the others. For example, if a person is characteristically honest, he is also likely to be trustworthy. The traits tends to be highly correlated. He also categorised the traits of personality along more substantive psychological dimensions into *ability*, temperament and dynamic types.

Hans J. Eysenck claims that there are just two fundamental trait dimensions of personality, normal-neurotic and introversion-extraversion. The normal-neurotic dimension refers to the general adjustment of a person to his circumstances and the stability of his behaviour over time. The introversion-extraversion dimension reflects the degree to which an individual is generally outgoing and participative in his inter-actions with other people.

He believes that personalities, traits and actions in general, are a product of learning, especially early conditioning. He also assumes that learning ability is determined by the structure and func-tion of the nervous system. During infancy and early adolescence some people are 'overcon-ditioned' by their environments and others are 'underconditioned'.

Personality can then be seen as the way in which a person relates to his environment and circum-stances. It is a combination of the knowledge, skills and intentions reflected in a person's actions as evaluated by others. A process which begins in infancy and continues into adulthood.

Moral development

Standards of conduct are set by societies to control the behaviour of their members. These are in the form of moral codes which exist in every society however primitive it may be and involves the manner in which an individual should behave with respect to his fellow men. It includes rules of conduct concerning property, sexual behaviour and the resolution of interpersonal conflict. Moral codes are deeply embedded in the beliefs of a culture, so that members state that they know they should behave in a certain way without being able to explain that belief.

According to Piaget, who investigated children's use of rules and views of justice, it is stated that children below the age of 6 showed little conscious awareness of any rules. Even those which they accepted did not seem to constrain their behaviour in any way.

From 6 to 12 years the child is subject to increasing laws imposed from outside. Rules are fixed by others and they tend to be sacred and unchanging. Whilst they constrain behaviour within a given situation they will not change a child's conduct in other situations because he is not aware of the meaning of the role, only its application. Subsequently, rules are seen as compacts between individuals, for the purpose of fostering co-operation and reciprocity. Rules are not negotiable but are essential for a purpose.

Piaget also looked at the way children viewed justice. By about 6 to 10 years of age the child's view of justice changed from one of realism to one of relativism, i.e. he initially equated the serious-ness of a misdemeanour with the extent of the outcome or the severity of the punishment. Gradu-ally this gives way to relativism in which the child is able to consider mitigating circumstances.

Kohlberg suggests that there are six develop-mental changes in morality — two at each level.

1. Premoral level I contained two stages charac-terised by the view that cultural rules and evalu-ative labels denote pleasant and unpleasant consequences or reflect the influence of those who exercise power.
2. Level II is described as 'Conventional Role Conformity' in which the child actively main-tains the expectations of family and friends as values in their own right.
3. Level III or 'Self-accepted Moral Principles', is concerned with defining moral values and principles without reference to the authority of those imposing them, but seeing them in terms of contractural obligations which all human beings must observe. Development is seen as a gradual decrease in the number of lower level responses and an interrelated increase in those at a higher level, although stage 6 (latter half of level III) is often not reached.

Other studies suggest that moral behaviour may be situation-specific in that a child may be honest in one situation and dishonest in another. It is considered that this does not negate a develop-mental trend. It is still possible to observe an organised progression.

Social development

Social development begins early in an infant's life. Smiling can be considered a 'social' response. At first the smile is elicited in response to strangers as well as to known faces. After the age of 6 months his smile is more selective, i.e. mainly towards his mother, father and siblings. He will also be shy with strangers. Increase in social exchange is rapid when he begins to speak. During this time, the development of motor skills such as walking and fine manipulation enables the child to explore and master his immediate surroundings.

By the age of 18 months, he may be able to let his mother know when he needs the toilet, though control of bladder and bowel may not be complete until the age of 2 or 3 years. He will learn to give as well as take and to mix with and be near to other children, at first for short periods and gradually for longer periods.

Relationships with his parents become more complex and by about 3 years of age his behaviour is characterised by what is termed 'negativism', that is active resistance to requests or instructions. Social play is already found in 2- and 3-year-old children. Play is associated with being with or near other children and during this period the child tends to converse with himself revealing the individual, and the self-centred world in which he lives.

The main social change occurs when the child begins school, when the relationship shifts from that with adults to that with other children of his age. For some this change is more difficult than for others. He has to learn to compete and co-operate. He will learn to accept or reject standards of behaviour and will switch relationships and join groups or gangs.

Belonging to a small group helps to develop the child's sense of belonging to a community outside his home, but there are also children who remain outside such intimate groups and find it easier to form a one-to-one relationship. The transtition from this stage of childhood to full social maturity lasts a considerable time. It varies with each child and is generally achieved with varying degrees of emotional stress and social upheaval.

The importance and functions of play

Play is defined as activity in which the individual can:

1. Practise and perfect skills. This includes manipulation involving motor and sensory function as well as social skills.
2. Give expression to thought. In this sense it is used in problem solving and as a means of mental development.
3. Be creative, i.e. be able to use his mental processes to develop his imagination and give expression to creative thinking.
4. Perfect language. The child uses the language learned extensively during the play situation. He plays with language as a skill and as a means of communication.
5. Be indoctrinated into the culture in which he lives and learn to accept its values and morals.
6. Be prepared for adult behaviour and roles. In play the child acts out the roles of adults and begins to model himself on adult behaviour.

According to this definition it is possible to further categorise play into distinct developmental areas, i.e. the impact that play can have on his physical, emotional, intellectual, educational and social development. For example, while practising and perfecting skills he uses his body extensively and this is essential for physical development. The more a muscle is used the better and precise will be its function. In that sense it can also be considered *functional* play. This tends to dominate the first year of life when there is adaptation of reflex action and assimilation. An example of functional play is playing with hands, mouthing, knocking down and building up. In *imaginative* play, the child tends to give meaning to actions and events. The toddler and pre-school child uses 'pretend' situations with the creation of imaginary people and things. This involves a number of developmental areas such as emotional, intellectual, educational, social and physical development. Another form of play recognised is constructional or constructive play where the child uses existing objects and constructs others. It implies the use of thought, imagination, language. Indeed it is difficult to isolate any specific aspect of play since it is developmentally interrelated and any defined part is included.

Progression of play

Play can also be seen to progress along a well-defined path and is closely related to the different stages of development. This is particularly relevant if one looks at the *social* content of play.

Initially the child tends to play on his own, i.e. *solitary play*. Indeed, this form is the only possible form for the youngest children. The child is primarily concerned with physical development in relation to neuromuscular maturation. He has not yet perfected language and tends to listen and practise speech rather than using it as a means of communication. Solitary play in an older child implies the will to be independent and alone with the material available to others too. It may also imply possessiveness.

By about 2 to 2½ years of age the child tends to watch others at play which may mean that verbal contact is made. This is often associated with 'parallel play' when children play side by side rather than joining with other children. By about 3 to 3½ years he still tends to play outside the group interest but ideas, toys, books and tools are borrowed from or lent to each other. They still tend to follow their own inclination. Around the age of 4 and 5 years of age play becomes much more organised. There appears to be conscious co-operation between members of a group.

Play has also a social function. Throughout life people live by rules and laws, and modification of these takes place from time to time. Even without official legislation there exist codes of behaviour which are obeyed to the letter and indeed it may be dangerous to violate such codes. The same seems to apply to many aspects of play. The child learns to recognise and accept these rules, particularly in relation to games and this is an important stage in social development.

Up to the age of 3 there are rarely any hard and fast rules in his play but, after that age, rule making begins. This is related to the progression of play because by that age the child begins to join other children in play. However, rules are changed constantly to suit any given situation and individual. When a rule changes it is usually the more dominant members of the group who make and alter the rules of the game.

At a later stage rules are fixed once and for all and may not be changed. The final stage may be considered as *realistic* when rules are subjected to discussion. This begins in the early adolescent period when other actions and elements of behaviour are also debated and questioned.

The developmental phases of play

Infant play
This is primarily physical, e.g. play with hands, handling objects, manipulation of objects, feeling objects, sucking and chewing.

From 4 to 7 months he can hold and handle, at first one toy or object then two at a time. All these are motor/sensory activities which enable the child to develop his motor/sensory system.

Toddler play (18 to 24 months)
This can be called 'practice' play. When a new skill is acquired he tends to repeat the actions repeatedly. This is partly due to the fact that the child has a surplus energy of play and it serves also an important function in the development of the child's perception of the relation between his own actions and their results. For example, hide and seek. Hand-eye co-ordination is quite well developed; eye movements are more rapid and he can recognise objects. He can also judge distance and depth.

2-to 3-year-old child
At this stage language develops rapidly; the neural system is well developed and manual dexterity has reached a high level. Play becomes more organised and tends to be imitative, and social play is dominant. Examples of play: play with dolls, washing, building bricks, play with words, repetition of words.

3-to 5-year-old child
Joins other children to a greater or lesser extent. The older child of 4 to 5 years ventures and seeks the compnay of other children, particularly if he has already met them. Play tends to have a learning function.

When school begins play extends into school where it becomes part of the learning process. Play also assumes a seasonal aspect, i.e. certain games are played at certain seasons, e.g. skipping during springtime; marbles and rolling games during summertime.

Play activities and the young child
As can be seen play activity and the mechanics of play follow a complex pattern of behaviour which is closely related to physical, mental and emotional development. For example, judging distances and depth or anticipating the position of a wrong object are not simple matters. Hand and eye co-

ordination is necessary to be able to touch and handle objects competently. The combination of perceiving, moving, progressive adaptations, modification and refinement are the main developments in the first 18 months of life.

There also appear to be phases of play activity which follow a relatively constant pattern. For example, water and sand play are favourites with toddlers (2 to 4 years). Building with bricks from simple to more complicated construction may start early, about 2 years and may continue until about 10 years of age. A child's first drawings are as unrecognisable shapes, that is, they are not recognisable to the adults but appear to be so to the child.

Drawings start as scribbling, but when the skill of holding and manipulating the pencil begins, recognisable forms and clear composition of subject matter emerge. This takes a long time to develop, from $1\frac{1}{2}$ to 16 years of age (Fig. 1.17).

The question of boredom in children and what it constitutes is relevant in deciding when and how to introduce change. Should change be initiated by the child or imposed on him? How can we recognise boredom and is it the same as adult boredom? This involves selection of information or stimuli which the child should receive in order to change his environment and/or activity. Normally, a child does not sit or stand still for any length of time, and the younger the child, the more active he will be.

The kind of stimulus to provide for the young child presents a problem. It is difficult to identify what stimulus is either required or suitable at any particular time. The response elicited by any particular stimulus varies with each child and should meet the needs of the moment. Young children are more easily distracted than older ones and too frequent change can be as disturbing as too little change. The attention of the young child is easily attracted by change of environment or activity, but whether it is sustained depends on factors such as freedom from anxiety, familiarity and personality.

Make-believe play and fantasy are suggested to represent expression of feeling. Feelings such as anger or frustration affect make-believe and fantasy play, that is they can make play less constructive and coherent. Make-believe play has other functions for the child, for example testing and exploring his feelings, decreasing his fears and experimenting with the adult world and the many rules adults appear to have. Imitation plays a big part and much of it belongs to role-playing and re-enacting behaviour and events. This type of play is most common betwen the ages of 2 and 8 years. As the child grows, play takes on different forms but basically it is used as a means of learning and preparing for adulthood.

Adolescent growth and change

The basic developmental problems of adolescence are the sudden physical changes, the intensity of the young person's emotion, and the impact of new social demands.

The age at which puberty occurs can differ widely within a given population. It is not uncommon in Great Britain to find girls of 10 approaching puberty and others of 13 or 14 who are not yet sexually mature. This variation is accepted as normal and an equivalent variation occurs in boys about 2 years after the girls.

Physical changes

The years 11 and 12 are regarded as the last years of childhood, and puberty marks the upper limit. There is an increase in the production of sex hormones leading to a spurt in height and changes in sex organs. While this growth spurt occurs, other physical attributes such as brain volume remain stable. In girls the breasts begin to bud, followed by the appearance of underarm, then pubic hair. Menstruation begins between 11 and 13 years on average.

The growth spurt in boys begins around 13 years of age. The first change is the growth of the genitalia and this is followed by the appearance of pubic, underarm and facial hair, deepening voice and the first ejaculation of semen by about 13 to 14 years.

Clumsiness is often observed in early adolescence. This is not due to lack of motor control over the body, which has new physical dimensions, but rather to increased awareness of bodily activities. This acute awareness of self characterises much of adolescent behaviour.

Psychological development

The teenager strongly needs to be liked by his peers. During this time the parents' influence diminishes and the influences of the peer group are greatly increased. There is also a greater interest in the opposite sex. Peer friendships are important to the adolescent because friends will allow experimentation with new identities. He is constantly anticipating reactions from others, reaching to imaginary audiences in his fantasy. The adolescent also tends to overemphasise his own feelings and assume they have a special intensity and quality; he assumes that his experiences and emotions are unique.

Behaviour and attitudes at different ages

The 12-year-old tends to have an enthusiastic approach to life. His self-knowledge increases and his social skills improve. He is capable of thinking hypothetically-deductively, that is, he can draw conclusions.

The 13-year-old has periods of uneasiness. This is due to hormonal activity and also is part of the maturational process. The behaviour is often characterised by attitudes of opposition and resistance to authority. The choice of friends or companions is often made more deliberately and is often confined to one or a few friends. Some may experience difficulties in social contacts. There may also be shyness and an inclination to withdraw into himself. The 14-year-old may show a different pattern of behaviour. He finds it easier to make social contact and he tends to have a greater circle of friends. Verbal comprehension and verbal fluency are an important feature of this age.

The 15-year-old may again show reserve which can be identified as an increase in inner strain. There is an urgent need for independence which makes the individual both vulnerable and often aggressive.

By the age of 16 many of the conflicts have been resolved. Though still striving for independence he has a more stable outlook towards the future and at this time plans for the future take on a more realistic form.

There is evidence that personality is relatively stable during adolescence and it is not accepted today that adolescence automatically involves emotional tension and strain. It is, however, believed that adolescence represents a time of role transition and at such times the individual tends to be prone to emotional disturbance. It can be prevented if the social circumstances are such that the requirements of the new role can be met and if the adolescent is shown tolerance and support during the transition period.

FAILURE TO THRIVE

In the previous section the growth and development of the child was discussed and the conditions necessary for this dynamic process were identified. However, there are children where growth and development fails to meet realistic expectations and this is broadly described as 'failure to thrive'.

Growth and development in infants, children and adolescents are sensitive indicators of their general state of health. In infants it presents as insufficient weight gain; in children, as insufficient gain of both weight and height; and in adolescents, as shortness of stature and lack of sexual and emotional development. Failure to thrive may be due to genetic, physical and psychosocial factors and each can influence specific spheres of growth and development.

Aetiology

Any pathological process, if it is severe enough to interfere with normal metabolism, will inhibit growth. If the interference is of short duration, it will not have any long-term effect on growth or development. However, if frequent or prolonged abnormalities are present, then growth and development can be impeded and in some cases this can have a permanent effect. The areas involved can be physical, psychological or psychosocial or a combination of these. Failure to thrive may be only one of many manifestations of complex disease processes. It is worthwhile to look at the various factors and the effects they produce.

Genetic factors

The child can inherit certain characteristics, e.g. tall parents tend to have tall children, short parents, short children. Children also inherit a pattern for growth and development, e.g. parents whose own growth pattern was slow or delayed but who continued to grow beyond the usual accepted age may have children who have the same pattern of growth.

Chromosomal abnormalities

Certain chromosomal abnormalities affect growth. For example, in Turner's syndrome children do not grow well and have birth-weights below those expected for the gestational age. These children also tend to have multiple congenital abnormalities.

Physical factors

Defects in function of major organ systems will have an effect on growth and development. For example:

Endocrine system. Deficiency of thyroid hormone or growth hormone leads to profound growth retardation and, in addition, deficiency of thyroid hormone leads to developmental delay. Excessive adrenocortical hormones interfere with growth.

Central nervous system. Damage to the brain can lead to feeding difficulties. It can also cause changes in endocrine functions which affect growth and development.

Cardiovascular and respiratory systems. Metabolic processes will be disturbed and tissues fail to grow and function effectively if there is breakdown in the delivery of nutrients and oxygen to the tissues and removal of waste products and CO_2.

Haematopoietic system. Oxygen is necessary for optimal cell metabolism and normal growth. Any defect in the oxygen carrying and delivery system, as found in moderate or severe anaemia, will lead to tissue hypoxia and affect growth.

Genito-urinary system. The kidney's function is to help to maintain normal cellular electrolyte concentration and pH, and to remove toxic waste products of metabolism. Any interference in these functions, e.g. chronic renal failure or renal tubular defects, congenital or acquired, will disturb the cellular environment to such an extent that normal growth and development cannot take place.

Gastro-intestinal system. Structural lesions such as pyloric stenosis, where vomiting is an important feature, or mucosal malfunction or absence of digestive enzymes (as in malabsorption syndromes), may reduce the amount of food which reaches the tissues and thereby interfere with the growth process. *Malnutrition* is closely associated with failure to thrive and can be caused by inadequate intake of food, malabsorption or faulty metabolism. Not only general malnutrition but also specific deficiency of essential nutrients may cause serious growth defects or retardation, e.g. marasmus, kwashiorkor or rickets.

Psychosocial and environmental factors

To enable the child to grow and develop satisfactorily, it is essential to provide a supportive, loving relationship. If the infant and young child is physically or emotionally deprived, growth will be interfered with. Parental withdrawal, rejection or hostility can cause emotional deprivation and this can lead to failure to thrive.

The socio-economic status of the family may affect the growth of the child since it can affect the quality of nutrition, living conditions and parental attitudes. Other environmental factors which may interfere with growth include infections, parasitic infestations and intoxication by a variety of foreign substances. This also includes drugs in lactating mothers. For example, corticosteroids, when given in large doses to the mother can attain high concentrations in milk and pose a danger of suppressing growth in the infant. Any stressful event, such as a family move, hospitalisation or some intercurrent illness can also delay growth and affect development.

It can be seen that there are many factors which can affect growth and development and no doubt other causes could be cited. It is important that early diagnosis is made and, where defects are found, relevant treatment is given or investigations instituted to identify the cause.

Chapter 2
Care of children

The care of children varies in different societies, but in all societies there are fundamental needs which must be met to enable the child to develop satisfactorily. The aim of achieving an acceptable standard of care involves an understanding of the basic needs of the child and an appreciation of the norms of that society. This chapter looks at methods of child care as generally accepted (with some variation) by most Western societies. The methods vary with the age of the child, and since the human baby is such a helpless being his care and management provide the greatest challenge, involving not only understanding of the physical needs of the infant but also a recognition that each infant must be handled as a unique being who has a different make-up and will respond in his own individual way.

Bathing

BATHING THE INFANT
While bathing an infant the aims are:

1. To bath the infant as quickly and safely as possible.
2. To ensure that there is as little body heat loss as possible.
3. To use a method which is suitable for the situation.

Preparation
The preparation for infant bathing should include the following:

1. Clothing should be warmed and arranged in sequence of being used. It should be suitable for the season, condition and age of the infant, e.g. nappies — for the newborn and neonate, muslin with turkish towelling are suitable. In hospitals and at home disposable nappies may be the choice. For older babies, either towelling nappies or disposable ones and nursery safety pins are appropriate.
2. The room should be warm.
3. All the equipment required should be available and easily accessible, i.e. soap (in a soap dish) or soap solution, powder, barrier cream, cotton wool balls, sterile water (for newborn babies' eyes), and a container, disposal bag, scissors (nail), covered pail for used linen, brush and comb, bath towel.
4. Baby bath on a stand or ideally a large sink designed for bathing at a suitable height should be available.
5. A low chair should be on hand if a baby bath is used.
6. A protective apron or gown should be worn.
7. Bath water should be ready at about 40.6 °C.

Method
Two methods will be described and the advantages and disadvantages considered. The initial stages are the same for both and are as follows.

The infant is undressed except for the nappy (this is to prevent wetting or soiling while the head is washed). He is then wrapped in the bath towel exposing the head only.

Eyes. These are washed first. For the new-born and neonate, warmed sterile water should be used, whereas clean bath water can be used for the older baby. A cotton wool ball should be used in either case. The moistened cotton wool is held lightly on the eyelids and the swab gently moved from the inner to the outer aspect of the eye, using one swab only for each manoeuvre and discarding it. If the eye is clear, one moist swab is sufficient. The last swab should be a dry one. If the eye is sticky or discharging, treatment will be as described on page 338.

Nose. If the nostrils are clear and clean, it is not necessary to clean them. Should they require cleaning, the following method is useful. A small piece of cotton wool is rolled until it is of sufficient thickness to be inserted into the nostril. It should be kept long enough to retain a grip on it. Some hospitals use a cotton wool carrier, but it must be stressed that the cotton wool must be firmly attached to the carrier and sufficient cotton wool left protruding. This will prevent damage by the carrier to the inner lining of the nostrils.

If one nostril is blocked, the cotton wool can be inserted into the clear nostril. This will cause the infant to sneeze, which will dislodge the plug of mucus. It is not considered safe practice to use the cotton wool in an attempt to dislodge the mucus plug, as this may be pushed further in and inhaled. However, it can be eased out by inserting the cotton wool along the inside wall of the nostril and gently scooping it out.

Ears. The inside of the ears should be left alone, but the outer ear can and should be washed with moist cotton wool. Drying the ear is important, particularly the fold behind the ear, since moisture can lead to excoriation of the skin.

Normal wax secretion is orange in colour and there is no need to remove it from the external auditory meatus. Once it has worked itself to the outer ear it can be removed easily.

Face. The face is washed using either moist cotton wool or a soft face cloth. Soap is generally not used, but if the bath water contains a substance like Infa-care it can be used. The face is dried gently, using either cotton wool or a soft towel.

Hair and scalp. While the baby is young it is usual to wash his hair daily but opinion varies. However, it does help to keep the hair and scalp clean, particularly if matting of hair is a problem or if he sweats excessively. Soap can be used, but there are several mild shampoos available which have the added advantage in that they do not sting the eyes.

The baby, still wrapped up, is held under the nurse's left arm (if right-handed) or right arm (if left-handed) and the head is supported with that hand. This provides good control of the baby, while the free hand washes and rinses the head. The hair and scalp is then dried gently.

Method 1 (washing the baby's body)

The baby is unwrapped and the nappy removed. If he is soiled the faeces are removed and the area cleaned, using cotton wool. The infant is then placed in the bath water, his head resting in the crook of the nurse's arm. While the body is immersed, it is washed all over. For the very young baby, the soapy hand is all that is required. It is easier to feel the amount of force and pressure applied to the infant's skin using the hands rather than a cloth, which tends to be more rough. Turning the baby on its abdomen involves a relatively simple manoeuvre of the hands. The following method is satisfactory.

With the infant lying on his back nestling in the crook of the nurse's arm, the nurse places her free hand under the child's left armpit. She then slips her left arm towards the infant's right armpit. While holding the baby under the armpit he is gently rolled over on his abdomen, the shoulders and head resting on the nurse's left arm. The back can now be washed, paying particular attention to the buttock fold. When he is clean and rinsed, the manoeuvre is reversed and the baby is lifted out of the bath, with head, back and pelvis being supported.

He can now be dried thoroughly but gently, paying attention to all areas where two skin surfaces meet. If powder is used it should be dusted off to prevent caking. The baby's nappy is put on and he is now dressed. A soft baby brush can be used to tidy the baby's hair.

The advantage of this method is that the infant is immersed in warm water during the washing process and cooling of the body is less likely. Although the manoeuvre described may appear complicated, with practice it is quick and safe and involves only two position changes.

Method 2

After unwrapping the baby and removing the nappy, etc. the baby's body is soaped all over, the abdominal part first, and then turned over to wash the back. He is then placed in the bath and the soap rinsed off. Turning the infant involves similar manoeuvres as in Method 1. After the baby's body has been rinsed, he is lifted out of the bath, dried and dressed as described in the previous method.

This method, although frequently used, has

some disadvantages. (1) It involves four position changes, i.e. two on the nurse's lap and two in the bath. (2) The baby is soaped on the nurse's lap which means that his body tends to lose heat fairly rapidly. (3) It is not so easy to hold the baby while his skin is soapy.

Care of the umbilical cord
The umbilical cord is the vital link between mother and baby via the placenta. After the baby is born, the cord is clamped or tied approximately 2.5 cm from the umbilicus. Another clamp is attached a short distance from the first and the cord between the clamps is cut. The clamp nearer the umbilicus is left in position. The cord dries and shrivels, separating spontaneously after a few days. To ensure that the cord separates without difficulty, it is necessary to keep it dry and clean. After bathing the baby, the cord is dabbed dry. Normally neither dressing nor powder is applied but if there is any moisture, methylated spirit or a sterilised antiseptic powder may be applied.

Cleanliness of the napkin area
Nappy changes take place usually before and sometimes after feeding. It may, however, be necessary to do so more often, particularly if frequent stools are passed. It should be realised that nappies are not only changed when the infant has defaecated, but also when he has urinated. The same method should therefore be used.

Method
Any nappy change requires equipment necessary to wash the infant's napkin area. Warm water and soap should be used to cleanse the area, removing all traces of urine and faeces. The soap should be rinsed off and the napkin area well dried. If the area is healthy looking, baby powder can be applied. Otherwise it may be necessary to apply a thin coating of barrier cream.

BATHING OLDER BABIES AND TODDLERS
This age group can be safely bathed in an ordinary bath. Bath time should be fun and should hold no terror for the child. It can, however, be an extremely dangerous one. No small child should ever be left alone in the bath. As in the case of the infant, everything should be prepared beforehand, and all the equipment required should be placed in a convenient place and readily available. A small waterproof toy is very useful and can help to make bath time a happy event. If the child is frightened to go into the bath, it is best not to force him into it. It requires a great deal of patience and gentle persuasion and rather than forcing the issue it is better to wash him, either standing in the bath or at the basin. Watching other children having a bath may help him to overcome his fear.

The bath water should be run in before the child goes into the bath, again taking care that the water is at a safe temperature (approximately 40.6 °C). When the child has been washed and dried he is dressed in suitable clothes. Hospital clothes tend to look rather institutional, particularly if they are too long, so it is important to find clothes which are appropriate for the child.

OLDER CHILDREN
Supervision should be provided up to 10 or 11 years of age. At home the child would probably still be bathed, or at least supervised by his mother. The sick child in hospital also requires supervision, not only from the safety aspect but also in relation to his condition, e.g. the epileptic child may have a convulsion.

The older child or adolescent may be allowed to bathe himself, provided it is safe for him to do so. However, each hospital will have its own rules and policies.

Sleep

The newborn infant tends to alternate rather frequently between sleeping and waking; gradually one period of sleep is lengthened, although there are still naps. Eventually the night-and-day rhythm tends to be established.

There is as yet no satisfactory definition of sleep, but it is accepted that sleep is affected by many factors including social conditions, the 24-hour day and the level of sensory input. Procedures which minimise sensory stimulation favour the onset of natural sleep, e.g. a darkened room, relaxed muscles, comfortable environmental temperature and quietness. But the problem is more complex, because sleep is more likely when the individual is tired even though the environment is not conducive to sleep. Sleep therefore is believed to have important functions. For example, during sleep dreams will take place. Dreaming is apparently a universal phenomenon and studies carried out indicate that interruption of dreaming can lead to psychological distress. It is also suggested that dreaming is a device whereby the brain runs over the events of the day to remove the trivia and repetitions that might otherwise clutter it and reduce its efficiency. Sleep is the natural time for dreaming since the brain is then relieved of many of its waking functions. The same pattern of sleep has been observed in infants, yet there seems to be little that an infant could dream about. It may therefore be an important function in helping to develop the nervous system.

The sleeping requirements of babies and young children vary from child to child, though a pattern can be recognised. Gradually the amount of sleep required decreases.

The following list shows a breakdown of the generally accepted hours of sleep required according to age:

Birth–2 months: about 21 hours
2–4 months: 19–20 hours
4–6 months: 19 hours
6–12 months: 16–17 hours

Although sleep is a natural phenomenon which often takes place despite non-conducive conditions, every endeavour should be made to promote it by creating a satisfactory environment. For example, the infant should not be disturbed unnecessarily, toddlers and older children should not be allowed to waken an infant (they may look upon him as a doll).

As the baby grows there will be a greater need for more exercise and a growing awareness of his surroundings. This means that the infant will stay awake for longer periods. It is important at this stage to set a pattern, that is to show that there are times in the 24 hours for sleeping and times for being active.

Disturbed sleep

This can be quite a problem. There are many causes for this. Some are readily dealt with, others are more difficult to understand.

Infant. The newborn baby has to adjust himself to a new environment. The adjustment is both psychological and physiological. For 40 weeks the unborn child has lived in a special environment where temperature is constant, nutrients are supplied as and when required and where the process of elimination also occurs.

This relatively stable state is changed at the moment of birth. The infant has to wait for food and comfort and is dependent on warmth from outside sources. Hunger is probably the most common cause of disturbed sleep in the newborn. As he becomes more satisfied with the feeding regime and the amount he gets, his sleep will also be more regimented. There is a mistaken view that a baby should be allowed to cry, particularly at night, so that he will 'learn' that there are times when his cry will not be recognised and that his needs may be only partially satisfied. For example, instead of being fed he is given water to drink. Water will not satisfy a hungry infant, and if the crying is due to hunger it will not stop his cry.

Pain. This is another reason for disturbed sleep. Any type of pain in any part of the body will interfere with sleep. It may only be transient but may be an indication of some abnormal conditions.

Psychological cause. Both infants and older children can be subject to anxiety and this is a recognised cause of disturbed sleep in either group. It is more difficult to identify in infants than in toddlers and older children. Observation of the sleeping problem of the child is an important function of the nurse, though not an easy one. The mother is by far the most important and reliable informant and it is important to listen and assess the presented evidence. While the child is in hospital, observation of his sleeping behaviour should be reported accurately, as this is an important aspect of the progress or otherwise of the child. (See observations and their interpretation p. 91.)

Feeding of infants and children of all ages

FEEDING INFANTS
The purpose of feeding is to provide nourishment for the infant so that he can grow and develop

satisfactorily. For the newborn infant, as for the newborn of any mammalian species, the milk of its mother is the natural food.

Production of milk

During pregnancy the breasts enlarge greatly and become changed in structure. During the first half of pregnancy there is a further duct development and many alveoli appear to form lobules. No milk is secreted by the gland cells at this stage. During the second half of pregnancy the epithelial cells swell and there is a gradual initiation of secretory activity with the accumulation of milk.

Lactation consists of two distinct processes:

1. Milk secretion, i.e. the production of milk by the alveolar epithelium and its passage into the lumen of the gland.
2. Milk ejection, i.e. the discharge of milk from the breast. This depends not only on the suction exerted by the infant but also on a contractile mechanism in the breast which ejects milk.

Milk

Milk is a naturally balanced food containing about 55 g of first-class protein per litre, mineral salts (especially calcium and phosphorus for bone and tooth formation), practically all the vitamins, fat and soluble carbohydrate.

The fluid secreted during the first three days after parturition is called *colostrum*. It is yellow in colour and rich in protein and salts. It contains large granular bodies called colostrum corpuscles which represent either discharged alveolar cells of the gland or leucocytes loaded with fat. These are abundant in the first few days and disappear at the end of the second week. It is important to look at the differences in composition of colostrum, mature human milk and cow's milk. Indeed the differences between human and cow's milk are quite striking, as Table 2.1 shows.

The protein content of milk — which is made up of lactalbumin and caseinogen — is highest in colostrum (8.5 per cent and falls during the first few weeks until it reaches a steady level of about 1.25 per cent.

The proportions of lactalbumin and caseinogen are different in human and cow's milk. In human

Table 2.1 Difference between colostrum, mature human and cow's milk

	Protein (g/100 ml)	Lactose (g/100 ml)	Fat (g/100 ml)
Colostrum (human)	8.5	3.5	2.5
Mature human milk 65 kcal (0.26 MJ)/100 ml	1.0–2.0	6.5–8.0	3.0–5.0
Cow's milk (average) 65 kcal (0.26 MJ)/100 ml	3.5	4.75	3.5

milk there are about two parts of lactalbumin to one of caseinogen whereas in cow's milk the caseinogen is six times in excess of lactalbumin. The caseinogen of cow's milk forms large masses in the stomach which are relatively insoluble.

The quantity and composition of milk is directly related to the mother's diet. For example, if the diet is inadequate the yield of milk is reduced in later lactation.

Drug intake by the mother will also affect the baby, though not all drugs are equally effective. For example, bromides may cause drowsiness, and addiction to morphine has been reported in children of mothers addicted to the drug. Purgatives like phenolphthalein may also affect the baby.

Method of breast feeding

Before feeding the baby, the mother should wash and dry her breasts. Hands too should be clean. Comfort is important for both mother and baby; therefore she should find a suitable low chair with a good supporting back. Privacy is equally important — privacy for both mother and baby, with little distraction for both. Feeding should take place in a relaxed atmosphere.

The infant is held closely in the crook of the mother's arm sitting comfortably on her lap. The lower part of the breast is supported leaving the nipple and areola (pigmented area) free to be inserted into the baby's mouth. It is important to prevent the weight of the breast from resting on the baby's face since this could obstruct his breathing (Fig. 2.1). The upper part of the breast is depressed with the thumb, again to prevent obstruction to breathing. The baby should not be

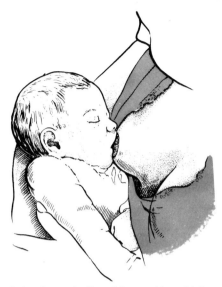

Fig. 2.1 Infant breast feeding. (Note position of infant; breathing should not be obstructed by the breast.)

allowed to play with the nipple. This could cause soreness and cracked nipples.

The length of feeding will vary with the age of the baby. The first feed may last 3 to 5 minutes at each breast and this is gradually increased until the sucking time is about 10 minutes at each breast. Some babies may require less time to get a sufficient amount of milk. The baby should be allowed to rest during the feeding period but should not be encouraged to go to sleep.

Amount of milk

It is not easy to decide the amount of breast milk the infant should get at each meal and in the course of the day. Investigations show that the amount of fluid taken by a healthy infant increases proportionately with his weight during the early months of life. It has been found that the 3.5 kg baby takes about 60 to 75 ml of breast milk for each 0.5 kg of body weight at the age of one week, but there are variations. In calculating the fluid requirement of a baby in the early months of life the upper limit is generally used, i.e. 75 ml per 0.5 kg of body weight. It is also important to consider the caloric requirement of a healthy baby.

Breast milk has a somewhat variable food value with a mean of about 19 kcal (0.07 MJ)/30 ml, but both cow's and human milk are calculated at 20 kcal (0.08 MJ)/30 ml. It is therefore suggested that a healthy infant takes between 80 and 100 kcal (0.32 and 0.4 MJ)/kg, or 40 and 50 kcal (0.16 and 0.2 MJ)/lb of body weight.

To determine whether a breast-fed infant receives adequate amounts, *test weighing* is carried out. The method is as follows. The baby, wearing his clothes, is weighed and the weight recorded. He is then fed for the prescribed period of time and then weighed again wearing exactly the same clothes. For example:

Weight after feed   7.255 kg
Weight before feed   7.200 kg
Amount of milk   0.055 kg or 55 g

Obviously there cannot be any rigid rules which apply to all infants. Low-weight infants tend to have a higher metabolic rate than normal-weight babies of the same age. They may require relatively more food per unit of body weight than the normal-weight infant.

Winding

This should be a gentle manoeuvre. There is no need to rub the baby's back vigorously. Each baby differs in the amount of air he swallows and in his response to the method of relieving his discomfort. Some bring up wind easily, others find it more difficult, and so it is important to study each baby's needs.

Feeding times

Opinion varies regarding when and how often a baby should be fed. One school of thought advocates 'demand feeding', that is the infant is fed when he wants. This is a useful method for the newborn and it is interesting to note that once feeding is established, the infant settles into a 4-hourly regime.

The other school advocates feeding by the clock, i.e. the infants is fed at intervals of 3 to 4 hours. This settles the infant into a routine early and is probably more realistic in hospital where an established routine is easier to fit into the routine of the ward.

The feeding times should be related to the infant's needs and weight. The lighter the infant the more frequent are the feeding times and the smaller is the amount to be given. Feeding times may therefore be 3 or 4 hourly, the latter being the interval for normal-weight, full-term infants.

It is also important to look at the times that feeding takes place. Normally the times are 6 a.m., 10 a.m., 2 p.m., 6 p.m., 10 p.m., though the young infant up to 1 to 2 months of age may still require a night feed.

Three-hourly feeding times are generally 6 a.m., 9 a.m., 12 noon, 3 p.m., 6 p.m., 9 p.m., 12 midnight. Feeding times at home are based on the routine of the home and the mother will no doubt organise her feeding session to suit her domestic arrangement. For example, the last feed at night may be about 11 p.m. As the baby grows, there will be less need for a night feed, the night sleeping pattern will develop and this will also give the mother a longer, undisturbed night.

Bottle feeding

When breast feeding has been attempted and there is an insufficient supply of breast milk, the feed may be *complemented* by a bottle feed. Generally this implies giving modified cow's milk, though breast milk is given under some circumstances, e.g. pre-term baby.

Before considering the different types of milk used, it is important to look at the problems involved when using cow's milk. The fetus receives its nourishment through the bloodstream via the mother's placenta. The change to intestinal digestion does not develop fully for several months. This presents certain hazards to the baby but more so if the baby is fed on cow's milk. The greatest problems are associated with the differences in composition between human and cow's milk, the difficulties in the preparation of feeds and the problems of infection and immunity.

The breast-fed baby absorbs some whole proteins which can be absorbed without digestion. In this way antibodies against some diseases may be absorbed intact from the mother's milk. The infant cannot readily digest starches until he is several months old.

Looking at Table 2.2 of comparative composition of human and cow's milk, it can be seen that there are some important differences.

For example, cow's milk contains relatively large amounts of inorganic calcium and phosphorous compared with human breast milk. Babies fed

Table 2.2 Comparative composition of human and cow's milk

Constituent	Human	Cow's
		(per 100 ml)
kcal (MJ)	67 (0.27 MJ)	66 (0.26 MJ)
Carbohydrate	7.0 g	4.8 g
Fat	3.8 g	3.7 g
Protein	1.2 g	3.3 g
Calcium	33 mg	125 mg
Iron	0.051 mg	0.045 mg
Magnesium	3.5 mg	13 mg
Phosphorus	14.1 mg	56 mg
Potassium	55 mg	138 mg
Sodium	15 mg	58 mg
Vitamin A	58 μg	40 μg
Vitamin C	4.3 mg	1.6 mg
Vitamin D	0.01 μg	0.06 μg

on cow's milk have been found to have, on average, a higher concentration of phosphate and a lower concentration of calcium in their blood than breast-fed babies (Oppé & Redstone, 1968). In the very young infant, this is believed to lead to a type of neonatal tetany, although it has also been found that babies adapt to the increased phosphorus load and the danger of tetany is diminished.

Other elements such as magnesium are also affected and are believed to be associated with convulsions in the newborn period. Sodium and potassium concentration are also higher in cow's milk than in human milk. Since newborn infants cannot excrete as adults do, re-absorption occurs. This leads to a decreased output of water and so to overhydration and hypertonicity. If there is an increased water loss or a decrease in the intake of water, hypertonic dehydration may result.

Other constituents also vary; for example, protein is higher in cow's milk than in human milk. However, there are differences in the two milks in not only the amount of protein, but also in the amino acid patterns of the protein mixtures.

Fats

Breast milk is richer in polyunsaturated fatty acids than cow's milk and this is considered important, for example, in the growth of the developing brain.

Despite these very important differences and the hazards which they may present, the great majority of babies adapt physiologically and develop satisfactorily.

Types of milk

There are a variety of artificial milks available on the open market, and in the UK the 1976 recommendation regarding compositional standards should make infant feeding safer. The essential factor is to make cow's milk resemble human milk.

There are pre-packed, sterilised, liquid feeds which are in use in hospitals but are not as yet economic or practical for domestic use. Most of the milks available require to be reconstituted, i.e. water is added to the dried milk powder. This presents many problems, such as risk of contamination during the preparation and incorrect dilution, which will affect the composition and concentration of the reconstituted milk. To help overcome these problems the manufacturer's instructions should be clearly printed and those feeding infants should be educated in the accurate method of preparing the feeds.

Calculation of feeds

Calculation of feeds is based on the food requirements of the infant. The growing child requires a continually increasing amount of nourishment. To maintain normal development food must be supplied to satisfy the following:

Basal requirements.
Growth.
Loss in elimination.
Muscular activity.

Table 2.3 shows the recommended daily energy intakes, based on growth potential, of infants of a certain weight. Using this table, in conjunction with how much energy a certain amount of milk provides, it is possible to calculate the total daily feed for a particular infant. This amount is then divided by the number of feeds an infant should receive daily to arrive at the amount of each feed.

Before showing two examples of calculations based on this information, we should note the following points. Because the newborn's digestion is incapable of dealing with various nutrients, he is given a half-cream milk. Between 2 to 3 months it is generally safe to change to a full-cream milk. A suggested regime using dried cow's milk is as follows:

For the *first month and up to 4 kg in weight* a half-strength milk is preferred. It is made up of full strength, i.e. 1:8 (12 g of powder to 100 ml water). This would supply 56 kcal (0.22 MJ). Some proprietary milk preparations have sugar already added, so that no further additions are necessary. If sugar is added, it should be in proportion of 1 part of sugar to 4 parts of dried milk powder.

Over 4 kg in body weight a full-cream milk is usually used. It is made up to full strength as with half cream, but the sugar is slightly reduced to 1 part to 6 parts of dried milk powder.

Now to return to how to calculate feeds. The following two examples demonstrate the calculation of feeds for a 4-week-old infant using half-strength milk and an 8-week-old infant using full-cream milk, assuming that a five-feeds-a-day regime has been prescribed. The information on the energy supply of milk is usually expressed on the basis of 100 ml of the feed, but since feeds are usually calculated on the basis of 30 ml (1 ounce), which is a simpler calculation, this figure has been used in the examples.

Table 2.3 Recommended daily energy intakes (1 kcal = 0.004 MJ)

Age (months)	kcal/kg of body weight	MJ/kg of body weight
Birth–3 months	120	0.48
3–6 months	115	0.46
6–9 months	110	0.44
9–12 months	105	0.42

Example 1

The data

Age and weight of infant	4 weeks old; 3.5 kg in weight
Energy needs (see Table 2.3)	120 kcal (0.48 MJ)/kg body weight
Number of daily feeds for that infant	5
Energy supplied by 30 ml (1 ounce)	17 kcal (0.004 MJ) therefore, 1 kcal (0.004 MJ) is supplied by $\dfrac{30}{17}$

The calculation
Multiply the infant's weight by the energy need per kg of body weight to find how much the infant requires in terms of energy

$3.5 \times 120 = 420$ kcal (1.68 MJ)

Multiply the energy requirements by the amount of feed needed to supply 1 kcal (0.004 MJ) of energy $\frac{30}{17}$ to find out how much the infant requires in 24 hours

$\frac{420 \times 30}{17} = 742$ ml per 24 hrs

Divide the amount required in 24 hours by the number of feeds prescribed to find out how much should be given per feed

$\frac{742}{5} = 148$ ml per feed

Example 2
The data

Age and weight of infant — 8 weeks old; 4 kg (0.48 MJ)

Energy needs (see Table 2.3) — 120 kcal (0.48 MJ)/kg body weight

Number of daily feeds for that infant — 5

Energy supplied by 30 ml (1 ounce) — 20 kcal (0.08 MJ) therefore, 1 kcal (0.004 MJ) is supplied by $\frac{30}{20}$

The calculation
Multiply the infant's weight by the enery need per kg of body weight to find out how much the infant requires in terms of energy

$4 \times 120 = 480$ kcal (1.92 MJ) (1.92 MJ)

Multiply the energy requirements by the amount of feed needed to supply 1 kcal (0.004 MJ) of energy $\frac{30}{20}$ to find out how much the infant requires in 24 hours

$\frac{480 \times 30}{20} = 720$ ml per 24 hrs

Divide the amount required in 24 hours by the number of feeds prescribed to find out how much should be given per feed

$\frac{720}{5} = 144$ ml per feed

An infant's food requirement is not only based on caloric needs but also on the infant's age and adequacy of intake. Another important factor to consider is *fluid requirement*. This is estimated to be *165 ml per kg*/day for a healthy normal infant. For a new-born infant, the fluid requirement is somewhat less, but fluid needs must be satisfied

and these take precedence over nutritional needs in the first few days.

To ensure that the infant receives an adequate amount of fluids, the above estimate of fluid requirements can be calculated, and the result compared with the amount of fluids the infants is receiving in the total daily feed. Then any deficiency can be made up by giving drinks of fluids such as orange juice between feeds.

To go back to Example 2, the fluid requirement of that infant is:

$$165 \times 4 = 660 \text{ ml}/ 24 \text{ hours}$$

We calculated that the infant will be receiving 720 ml per 24 hours, so in this case, the fluid requirement is satisfied.

Preparation of feed
Milk is a perfect medium for bacterial growth and it is therefore vital that the equipment before, during and after the preparation is kept in as clean an environment as possible. The dried milk powder, while in the closed tin, is sterile, but as soon as the tin has been opened it must be considered to contain micro-organisms, some of which may well be pathogenic. The ideal would be either to have the feed prepared in a sterile environment and have individual feeds pre-packed (as is now the practice in some hospitals) or to have individual dried milk packs to be used once only (economically not viable).

To prevent infection it is therefore incumbent on the operator, whether nurse, milk kitchen operator, or mother, to practise a technique which will minimise this danger.

Sterilisation of baby bottles
The type of baby bottle in use is cylindrical in shape with an opening at one end. The size of opening varies but can accommodate either a soft rubber teat or a screwed top with teat attached. The bottle can stand upright, which is useful if the milk is to be kept warm, cool, or to be heated. They are also easily cleaned with a special bottle brush. After cleaning and removing all traces of milk, the bottles are immersed in a solution of Milton 1:80. Teats should be cleaned with warm water, removing all traces of milk with salt. A

strong jet of water should be directed through the hole to ensure that it is patent.

The Milton solution should be changed once in 24 hours, or if milky looking.

Another method of sterilisation is by boiling. The bottles and teats should be immersed in a covered pan; the water is brought to boil and kept boiling for 20 minutes. The bottle and teat can be kept in the pan until required for the next feed.

Hole in the teat

The new teat is already holed, but it is often found that the hole is not adequate. The opening should be of sufficient size to allow milk to drip slowly (approximately one drop per second). If the hole is too small it can be increased in size by the following method.

A darning needle (medium size) or an intra-muscular needle may be used. To pierce the teat it should be made red hot over a flame. Unless the needle is red hot it will *not* pierce the rubber teat. Care should be taken not to make the hole too big as it can be difficult for the baby to control the rapid flow of milk and suck and swallow at the same time, leading to danger of inhalation of milk.

Preparation of feed

Aseptic technique is essential, therefore the following should be observed:

1. The area where the feed is prepared should be clean and should not be an area used for any other purpose, such as preparation or dismantling of dressing, injections, etc.
2. Windows should be closed to keep out insects.
3. If the nurse has a cold, she should wear a mask.
4. Hands must be washed and dried.
5. All equipment should be at hand.

Equipment required

1. Bottle with cooled boiled water.
2. Measuring jug.
3. Spoon for mixing.
4. Bottle and teats (teat may be left in small covered container until ready to feed).
5. Bottle cover.
6. Tin of milk powder with a scoop.
7. Sugar.

Method of preparing feed

The nurse washes and dries her hands and assembles the equipment. A bottle is filled with the required amount of boiled water. The prescribed amount of powder is mixed with a small quantity of this water and the mixture is then returned to the bottle. The required amount of sugar is added and care should be taken that is is properly dissolved. If the infant is to be fed immediately, the teat is attached. Otherwise the bottle is covered with a sterile cup or special sterile cover until required.

Feeding the infant

The temperature of the feed should be about 37 °C. If the bottle feels hot, the milk temperature can be tested on the back of the hand. The infant should have a bib/feeder round his neck and prior to feeding should have had a napkin change. The position of the infant is similar to that of the infant feeding from the breast. The important principles here are:

1. The infant should sit comfortably and be well supported, resting in the mother's or nurse's crook of the arm. (Fig. 2.2.). Physical contact is as important to the bottle-fed as to the breast-fed infant and this can be achieved by holding the infant's hand and gently talking to him.
2. The teat should always be filled with milk to prevent air being swallowed.
3. He should be allowed to rest between sucks and not allowed to fall asleep. Winding is an essen-

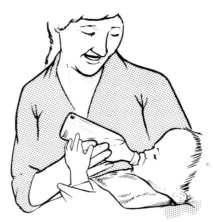

Fig. 2.2 Infant bottle feeding. (Note position of infant and bottle.)

tial part of feeding and each infant has his own method of breaking wind. Some find it easier than others. However, in all cases gentleness is the best way and there is no need to rub his back excessively. Indeed too rough handling might well produce regurgitation. After completion the bottle is cleaned as described above.

FEEDING CHILDREN OF DIFFERENT AGES

Infants are unique in that they rely on one food — milk. As already stated, where possible the mother should try to breast feed her baby for at least 2 weeks and ideally for 2 to 6 months. Milk feeds are not enough when the infant is older, but it is recommended that solid foods should not be introduced before 4 months of age.

From about 6 months the infant can be gradually introduced to infant cereal foods, pureed fruit and vegetables, egg yolk and finely minced meat. By about 12 to 18 months the infant can eat a mixed diet not very different from that of the rest of the family. Milk continues to be very important but as more solid food is eaten less milk will be drunk.

The amount to be given will vary with each child, but to begin with teaspoonfuls rather than a cupful of solids are better tolerated until the child has accustomed himself to the new tastes.

SCHOOLCHILDREN

Schoolchildren grow quickly and are also very active. For example, the food requirements of 9-to 12-year-old girls with regard to energy, protein, calcium and other nutrients are higher than those required by grown women in most occupations. The choice of foods should therefore be related to their nutritional value rather than bulk.

According to the recommended daily intake of nutrients (Department of Health and Social Security, 1969), young males of 9 to 11 years should have a protein intake of 63 g, while young females of 9 to 11 years should have a protein intake of 58 g.

Excellent sources of nutrients are: bread, milk, cheese, meat, fish, liver, eggs, fruit, green vegetables and potatoes. Milk is one of the best sources of calcium, riboflavin and protein.

Good eating habits should be taught from an early age and foods such as biscuits, sweets, soft drinks, chips and crisps should not be given instead of more useful foods, although they can be given in moderation. Indeed, eating between meals should be avoided and meals should be taken at regular intervals and in a pleasant, calm atmosphere.

Food fads and tantrums should, where possible, be avoided, but it is also important to recognise that food fads in children represent likes and dislikes which could be catered for. Tantrums during meals, particularly in the case of the very young school child, are often an expression of anxiety or rebellion. It is probably better to handle such situations calmly, as generally if a child is hungry he will eat.

ADOLESCENTS

The nutritional needs of this group are probably higher than most other groups. Healthy adolescents have big appetites and these must be satisfied with food of high nutritional value. During this stage, physical growth reaches it peak and at the same time physical and emotional changes are taking place and these will affect the overall behaviour of the individual. Some may be more lethargic, others very active and each state must therefore be assessed in relation to nutritional needs.

Recommended protein intake for males of 12 to 18 years is 70 to 75 g, and for females of 12 to 18 years, approximately 58 g. (See Table 7.1 for approximate daily nutritional needs.)

SCHOOL MEALS

In Britain and many other Western countries school meals have been provided for many years. For many children the school meal is the main meal for the day. In the UK, under the Provision of Milk and Meals Regulation 1969, school dinners should be suitable in all respects as the main daily meal. In many areas there is a selection of dishes available, while in others no choice is possible but a set dinner is provided. Allowing for losses of edible food during preparation, cooking and serving, it should be possible to supply at least one-third of the recommended daily intake of energy and between one-third and one-half of the recommended intake of protein.

Part 2
Social aspects of child care

Chapter 3
Child-care systems

The family unit

The basic social unit of human society is the family and within this unit the young are born. It is also within this unit that most of their developmental needs are met. Traditionally, at least in Western society, the needs of the child are met by the child's natural mother and father.

The immediate needs include nutrition, warmth, shelter and protection from danger, though the family must also provide an environment in which the child's physical, mental and social capacities are fully developed so that, when grown up, he is able to deal effectively with his environment.

The earliest interaction is between mother and infant and this satisfies the basic physical and psychological needs. The father too plays an important part in fostering the child's development. His role is twofold. Firstly, he provides the child with a second adult model. If the child is a boy, he can identify with a member of his own sex and, if a girl, she can learn about the behaviour and attitudes of the opposite sex. Secondly, the father's role is a supportive and protective one which reinforces the mother's role and thereby increases her confidence in mothering. This in turn will communicate itself to the child.

It is accepted that to develop normally, both physically and mentally, the infant and young child should experience a warm, intimate and continuous relationship with his mother. This close relationship has a beneficial effect on both mother and child.

If one of the basic needs is not met or is inadequately met, then development may be stunted or disturbed. Indeed it is likely that if one need fails to be met, others will be affected too. An essential ingredient for successful development is the provision of love and security. The lack of these may have serious consequences for the individual.

Functions of the family

While the formal structure of the family has remained more or less unaltered, its function has undergone considerable modifications.

At one time the family was a unit for both production and consumption; now it is primarily a unit of consumption only. As soon as children reach an age to work, they become external producers. They no longer need to co-operate with the family to maintain a common livelihood. If they remain a member of the household they do so only for convenience sake. They tend to have a looser tie which is based more on sentiment than interest. The young will form new links which often bind them closer to the stranger than to their own relatives. It is only in the rural setting that the family still possesses that kind of cohesion which is derived from shared interest, with the family acting as the unit of both production and consumption.

Personal or individual functions

An important function of the family — especially in Western society where there is much tension — is emotional security. Independent nuclear families are especially associated with intimacy and emotional interdependence. In Western culture, there is particular emphasis on the companionship between husband and wife, symbolising the modern equality of sex roles and based on a division of labour that gives the same value to male and female tasks.

Education

The primary and most important function of the family is the transmission of cultural norms from one generation to another. This is education in its widest form and will not change appreciably. As long as children are for some years in the care of their parents, the educational role of the parents remains supreme.

In the past, parents also had a secondary educational role. Children were taught skills of trade and hobbies by their parents. Even formal education could be obtained at home and, while this is still possible to a limited extent, the majority of children are sent to school to receive formal education. The home and the parental attitude to education have an important effect on children. The more learning is encouraged and respected, the greater will be the children's response to formal education. Where this encouragement is non-existent or at most limited, there will be a considerable strain on the children to adjust to the enforced formal education. This can have one of two effects: (a) the children will not respond, or (b) children will consider it a challenge and overcome the lack of parental interest. These children tend to succeed.

Religion
A man belongs to the religion into which he is born. However, some change from one religion or sect during some time in their adult life. Where religion is practised, it is primarily through the family that beliefs and dogmas are implanted. However, where the family is no longer the religion-centred institution it once was, religious instruction, like formal education, is largely left to the care of the school or church.

Recreation
At one time, recreation was largely family-based. This tended to make the family more cohesive, but now, increasingly, this takes place outside the family. The attraction of television does not make up for the disruption of family cohesion which recreational activities in the home helped to foster.

Health care
The family is still the prime unit where prevention and treatment takes place. The involvement and support is still to be found in the family without which rehabilitation would be more difficult to achieve. Much of the health care, though, has passed into more expert hands as far as diagnosis and specialist care is involved.

An individual feels a sense of physical security because of the family's willingness or duty to protect one another, to care for the sick or injured, to provide one another with shelter, warmth, food and clothing.

The family can, therefore, be seen as an essential social institution; irrespective of what type of family, it is the one permanent and unchanging feature of the social system. It is a universal institution and it is possible to see similarities between society and family, in that it is representative of society.

Attempts have been made to change the role of the family and this is usually associated with extreme ideologies. There are also varieties of child-care methods, some as part of the family system, others as an extension of that system.

Family disorganisation
In the above discussion it was shown that the family has a variety of different functions, each one having a profound effect on the developing child. It can also be seen as the source of the deepest sentiments a person can experience, as well as the source of the worst passions of which a human being is capable, such as hate, lust and violence.

No family can escape conflicts, but each family has its own way of handling them. Most of the conflicts emanate from within the marriage and have a direct effect on the children. When problems arise each partner generally attempts to solve them but if this is not possible then separation or divorce results. Separation means that husband and wife have agreed to live apart; one of them may have gone to court regarding the financial support of wife and children or the custody of the children. The laws of separation vary; for example, in Scandinavia, separation is the first step towards divorce and is meant to give the partners at least a year in which to try out the economic and emotional consequences of living apart.

Divorce is the legal dissolution of marriage and affects children in many ways and may threaten their socialisation if they are very young. This, however, may just as well be attributed to the strife leading to the divorce as to the divorce itself. Studies of maladjusted boys showed that a higher than normal percentage came from divorced families. There are probably also other reasons for the maladjustment with divorce being one element.

Courts tend to entrust the mother with the custody of the children unless there are serious reasons against this. Data suggests that boys who grow up with their mothers and without contact with their fathers or other male behaviour patterns to follow, may have difficulty in defining their own roles.

One-parent families

One-parent families are a very diverse group consisting of either mother or father with children. Today about 1.25 million children in Great Britain are being brought up in families in which there is only one parent. The reasons why parents become lone parents are varied. Primarily, it is due to the death of one partner or break-up of the family by divorce, but it can also be due to failure of partners to marry.

In most one-parent families, the mother is the parent responsible for the children and the largest number of one-parent families are those where the woman is separated from or deserted by her husband. Statistics show that there are about 600 000 families without a father and about 100 000 in which there is no mother and the father is responsible for trying to keep his home together.

The effect on children being deprived of a parent can vary. Some suffer lasting depression on the death of a parent and many suffer bitterness or divided loyalties when their parents have parted. Children are, however, resilient and many are able to overcome the changed circumstances. For others the trauma is extensive and this can express itself in a number of different ways and for example, disturbed or anti-social behaviour or failure to attend school or make satisfactory progress.

In 1976, the National Children's Bureau published the result of their survey of children in one-parent families. This research showed that it is not being brought up by one parent that puts children in one-parent families at a disadvantage, but their poverty and all the cumulative problems that go with it.

The Finer Report, which was published in 1974, made a number of comments and suggestions including the proposal that a special cash allowance should be given to all one-parent families as of right. The problems of the divorced woman were also highlighted in relation to maintenance by fathers. However, income is not the only problem, nor does the provision of income solve all these problems. While the child is in the pre-school period, he can be placed in a nursery while the mother or father is at work. The problem becomes greater when the child goes to school, as there is a period between return from school and parents' return from work. The Finer Committee recommended substantial extension of day-care services, not only nursery provision but also provision for the school child. While many of the recommendations have been rejected by the Government, a few have been accepted and acted on. For example, a child benefit scheme for all children is available with additional cash allowance for one-parent families and Local Authorities have been asked to provide housing for such families.

Maternal deprivation and its effect

Bowlby (1965) contends that the nature of the child's earliest emotional relationship to his mother is of vital importance and that he needs to establish a lasting 'bond'. If this bond is broken or has never been satisfactorily established, then physical, intellectual, emotional and social development may be affected.

The evidence for the relationship of maternal care to children's mental and physical health comes from clinical observations and from studies comparing the development of children from happy, loving and secure homes with that of children deprived of such a home. Bowlby states that if a bond is not formed in the first 3 years of life, it never can be formed, with the inevitable consequence of development of an affectionless character. He believed that the primary bond is the model that specifies all later bonds, and if it is very superficial, later relationships can only be superficial. Other studies were made, but in many cases it was not possible to determine the levels of adjustment and intellectual functioning in the parents, and therefore the possibility of inherited defects could not be ruled out.

Recent studies indicate that the attachment behaviour is made up of a number of interrelated features. Schaffer studied babies after their return home from two institutions to discover how long it took them to begin showing the attachment behaviours typical of their age. There were differences in the institutional environment but in neither institution was it possible for the infants to form specific attachments because there were no constant figures in these environments. He found that those babies who were cared for by a higher ratio of staff per baby were quicker to respond than those babies who were cared for in an understaffed institution. However, all of the babies did normalise their social interactions.

Rutter (1972), whilst acknowledging that genetic and organic factors are also involved, considers also the specific forms of deprivation and their consequences. He concludes that many children who are admitted to hospital or residential nursery immediately show acute distress. If these institutions are of 'poor quality' — for example, lack stimulation and give impersonal care — a long stay may result in intellectual impairment, and 'affectionless psychopathy', i.e. severe emotional impairment, may follow multiple separation experiences. Acute distress may be caused by severance of the bond with the care-taker, developmental retardation and intellectual impairment by inadequate perceptual and linguistic stimulation, short stature by inadequate nutrition, delinquency by family discord, and psychopathy by failure to form attachments in the early years of life. Not only are these physical and psychological mechanisms distinct in character, they are also related to the age at which deprivation occurs. In general, it appears that the longer the deprivation of an attachment figure continues, the harder it is to develop attachment to an individual. Ultimately, it may become impossible.

An interesting feature of 'maternal deprivation' is that some children seem to suffer severe damage, whilst others emerge from similar situations relatively unscathed. Evidence is now suggesting that children's temperaments equip them with different degrees of resilience to stressful situations.

Child-rearing

The child is reared within the family unit. However, the unit may take on different forms and be part of different cultures. Within these cultures the child will be brought up according to the specific pattern of that culture. Culture not only provides the values and attitudes but also affects the structure and dynamics of the personality.

Whatever the culture, the child has fundamental needs such as the need for warmth, security, love, nourishment and the chance to develop, and it is within each culture that those needs are satisfied. The pattern in which these needs are satisfied vary but one can identify certain similarities.

The more primitive the society the more elemental the pattern is, the more sophisticated, the more intellectual the approach. The aim however, is, the same and the end result will be an individual who will conform to that society and make his own contribution.

In the nuclear family the child is brought up by his parents according to their ideas, which in turn conform largely to the norms of that society or grouping. In a Western European setting the infant spends some time in his parents' bedroom but, if economic conditions allow, is soon placed in a room of his own. Feeding pattern varies from breast to bottle to solid food fairly early on and the process towards independence progresses steadily.

Educational needs are satisfied first within the home, later within the educational system. Much of the control of behaviour passes on to the school system, while primary control is maintained by the parents. The emphasis is towards independence and integration and this can often lead to conflict. However, the child has to conform to a pattern of behaviour suitable for the culture he is born into.

Britain contains a number of different ethnic groups and each tries to maintain its own traditions, which find expression in child-rearing. However, the child is also influenced by his external environment, e.g. school; these influences will have a marked effect and gradually each generation will absorb more of the alien culture and the individual become more like the society he lives in.

Child-training or rearing the world over is in certain important respects identical. In all societies the helpless infant must be changed into a responsible adult, obeying the rules of society. Child-training everywhere seems to be in considerable part concerned with problems which arise from universal characteristics of the human infant and from universal characteristics of infantile behaviour.

This seems to imply that there is a universal way of rearing children. While this may be true as far as the principles are concerned, it is also important to recognise that each culture has its own peculiarities and, since interaction with one's culture is all-embracing, it is also true to say that there will be variations in style and manner of child-rearing.

Child-rearing practices change over time. The attitudes of previous generations are no longer those of today. Some societies change more rapidly than others. In some, the change is due to inter-cultural influences. This is particularly true where West European influences have penetrated the social framework of those in, for example, Africa or , nearer home, have impinged on the culture of incomers such as Asians, Africans and West Indians. Each group has its own particularities, e.g. infant feeding, food variations, discipline and religious values. Indeed we borrow from other cultures and integrate that which is useful.

Whether children are breast-fed, bottle-fed, cup-fed or spoon-fed, they must eat with their mouths, learn to suck or drink, chew their food, swallow and learn to discriminate between that which is and which is not food. Learning to walk may be by different means, but they all walk within relatively close age ranges. It is possible to apply all these developments across cultural dimensions and it can be seen that these are recurrent biological similarities. Children will have to learn to live in houses, to use tools, to observe social rules, to respect the person and property of others.

There are some interesting differences in child-rearing. For example, weaning takes place at 3, 6 or 12 months or even at 2 years; in some societies the infant is kept wrapped and carried by the mother on her back, in others the infant is placed in a pram. There are also dietary variations — for example, special bread eaten by Indians, Pakistanis and Chinese and different approaches to

hygiene and clothes. As the child grows older and he makes contact with other cultures, his ideas, attitudes and behaviour will change to be as near the cultural variations and where possible allow children to live and grow up in their own cultural setting, it is not possible within an institutional setting to meet all their cultural needs. People recognise the need to conform within limits and tend to follow those tenets of behaviour which are least disturbing to their own philosophies and practices.

One function of the family is the socialisation of the child. In most cultures children are indoctrinated into the culture in a process whereby they pick up the necessary knowledge and lore. The period of socialisation ends in adolescence. In some cultures it is at that period that they assume adult responsibilities; in others obtaining the status and privileges of adults is only achieved after dramatic or painful passage rites, often interpreted as the killing of the boy and his rebirth as a young man. Girls tend to receive less attention and ill treatment, but their first menstruation is sometimes considered dangerous and may be associated with a period of isolation.

Each culture has its own beliefs and patterns of child-rearing. For example:

Bathing varies according to custom, e.g. while some use water, others use oil.

Feeding programmes also have a strong cultural bias. In some societies breast feeding is the norm, in others artificial feeding. In recent years changes have taken place in the philosophy of breast feeding and many more mothers have reverted to breast feeding. No doubt social norms or social pressures play an important part in influencing the attitudes of its members.

Discipline as far as discipline is concerned, it is the family's responsibility to ensure that the child's behaviour is acceptable. Discipline varies in each family and culture. While discipline is the domain of the family, society also takes a part in ensuring that the child behaves in an acceptable way.

It is generally accepted that the care and upbringing of a child belongs to its biological parents automatically, without regard to their qualification or suitability. There are, however, groups rearing their children in common (usually in tribal societies). Where there are areas of concern about the care of the child, then the state takes over that function, e.g. local authority. The parental system has been justified on religious grounds; an example is given of an Irish court action (decision) which stated that, 'The authority of a father to guide and govern the education of his child is a very sacred thing, bestowed by the almighty, and to be sustained to the uttermost by human law'. A criticism of this system is the inequality of opportunity and upbringing it can offer one child as compared with another. In our society public services and the educational system play an increasing part in the rearing of children, but the overall aim is to allow each child to achieve independence within the framework of the society.

Ill treatment of children (child abuse)

Child abuse or the 'Battered baby syndrome' was first described in 1946 by an American radiologist, but it was not until 1962 that C. H. Kempe first coined the term 'battered baby syndrome'. There are many families where children, wives and others are roughly treated or beaten. It is difficult to determine the number of children involved since only the more severely injured come to the notice of the authorities. There are certain identifiable characteristics of these families, e.g. ill treatment of children is most common at an age when a child is unable to communicate and is immobile. There is also a tendency for the first- or last-born child to be subjected to such treatment, as well as low-weight babies. There may also be associated organic disease or the child's personality and behaviour may contribute to such treatment. The mother is more commonly responsible than the father. The parents are often lacking in maturity and are unable to cope. When one parent is involved the other usually gives tacit consent. The adult tends to be an unhappy, aggressive, socially isolated young person who may have been subjected to similar treatment in childhood.

Those parents tend not to co-operate effectively with authorities and fail to attend for antenatal care and subsequently child health clinics. They tend to present themselves frequently at the general practitioner and this may indeed be a 'cry for help'. The home environment may be violent and contact with their own parents may be absent or limited. The biological father may be absent from home and another mate may share the home.

Clinical features or alerting signs

Many children will have bruises and injuries, not necessarily as a result of ill treatment. However, there are a number of features which should make the doctor or nurse alert to the possibility of ill treatment.

1. The child is generally brought in late for treatment and no explanation is offered, or the explanation may not support the injuries presented.
2. The injuries are multiple and of mixed types, e.g. bruises and scratches.
3. The lesions are of different ages, i.e. they are at various stages of healing.
4. The nature of the lesions include fractures (unusual in young infants), burns and scalds, dappling of the skin and coldness and blueness of the extremities in association with low weight. The latter occurs in emotionally depressed children.
5. The site of injuries such as petechiae of ear lobes (pulling and pinching ear lobes), ligature marks round the neck (attempt at suffocation), and cigarette burns. There may also be special injuries to the eyes — subconjunctival haemorrhage, globular vitreous haemorrhage and dental injuries.

Demeanour and behaviour of the children

The expression of the child should be studied since it can be of great value in assessing his emotional state. For example, his expression may be haunting, reproachful and accusatory, or may appear to show 'frozen watchfulness'. His eyes show the alertness of a wild animal, or there may be sustained gaze avoidance. It must be remembered that ill treatment can also be of an emotional nature where physical signs may be absent or minimal.

Sexual abuse in children

Sexual abuse in children is difficult to assess without the co-operation of the family members. However, there is an awareness that sexual abuse appears to be on the increase. It includes all inappropriate intrafamilial sexual relationships as well as incest as legally defined. In some families it is associated with husband- or wife-beating and violence towards children. If sexual abuse has been established, then it must be reported to the police.

Common signs of sexual abuse
1. There may be a history of sexual assault from the child or family member.
2. Where pregnancy or venereal disease occurs in a child aged 12 or younger.
3. There may be a conflicting history of genital trauma between child and adult.
4. If the child has painful micturition or defaecation, this may be the initial sign of sexual molestation.

Obtaining evidence by interviewing
There should always be a witness present and interviewing of parent and child should be done gently and carefully. It is also important to take the child's cognitive growth into consideration. For example, the young child up to the age of 7 or 8 years describes what he experiences and finds it difficult to describe something he hasn't experienced, and it is unusual for a girl older than 7 to 8 or even as adolescent to lie about sexual contact within the home. It is also important that the child is reassured that he is believed, and to allow him to talk without interruptions. Toys, preferably a doll, should be given to the child to handle. This is useful to refer to body parts. A warm and patient approach is essential and frank hostility to the parents should be avoided. It is desirable that the mother is interviewed alone and the perpetrator last. However, it must be realised that both parents can be perpetrators of the assault.

Exploitation of children
Apart from the intrafamilial abuse discussed above, there is also the problem of extrafamilial exploitation. While this is not so likely in this environment, there is increasing awareness of this problem in the Third World. A look outside the family reveals the existence of child labour under conditions deleterious to health and growth, boy and girl prostitution and child pornography. Another form of child abuse is the Munchausen syndrome. It derives its name from the Munchausen syndrome of adults, where patients are known intentionally to falsify symptoms and fabricate evidence leading to unnecessary medical investigation and treatment. The same deception is practised by parents on their children. Successful deception sometimes continues for years, and children suffer by being subjected to unnecessary tests and treatments. A difficult diagnosis to make is that of non-accidental poisoning. The administration of non-prescribed drugs to children for non-medical reasons may be likened to a form of non-accidental injury or chemical battering.

Neglect and abuse of children can be seen to take varied forms which may go unrecognised and therefore untreated. It is very important that all those who care for children must be constantly aware of the possibility that children can be mistreated by those who are responsible for their care.

Care of the abused child
There are two main routes in protecting the child. The first one tends to be via the general practitioner service, and the second one via the hospital service.

The primary care team will be initially involved if abuse has been recognised by the child health clinic, the health visitor or the general practitioner. However, many children are taken directly to hospital and, if ill treatment is suspected, then a recommended standing procedure is followed.

1. Further information should be sought from others, e.g. general practitioner, health visitor, social worker and from an officer of the National Society for the Prevention of Cruelty to Children who might be able to confirm or preclude the possibility.
2. If there is serious suspicion that non-accidental injury has occurred, then the child must be admitted to the hospital. Admission to hospital must also be arranged where the information provided indicates that there is a possibility or likelihood of injury to the child occurring.
3. In all cases, adequate records must be made of clinical findings, including sketch drawings and medical photographs (both colour and black and white).
4. If the parents refuse to have the child admitted,

contact should be made with the social worker on duty who will seek a Place of Safety order, under which the child can be detained in hospital against the wishes of the parents. This allows sufficient time for the case to be investigated. In an emergency, where speed is imperative, the police should be notified.

It is not always necessary to admit such a child to hospital, but there are a number of advantages for such an admission:

1. There is generally availability of a bed.
2. The child can be investigated and treated without delay.
3. Hospitals can resist parents more easily than can, for example, foster parents. There are also advantages, however, for admission to a children's home, or placing the child with foster parents, and these are:
   a. A foster home is more natural for the child and less frightening.
   b. A community problem is contained within the community.
   c. It is less expensive to place a child either in a children's home or with foster parents than to admit him to hospital.

The 'at risk' register
All local authorities are now maintaining 'at risk' registers. There are advantages and disadvantages of keeping registers of children who have been injured, or who are at risk of ill treatment, and these can be summarised as follows:

1. It provides ready access to professionals, i.e. social workers, doctors and health visitors, when confronted with a child exhibiting features of ill treatment.
2. Families tend to move from one area to another, and the register enables a follow-up of these families.
3. There are readily available data about incidence, prevalence and characteristics of families exhibiting characteristic features, and these statistics identify trends and highlight the need for changes in organisation.

The disadvantages involve the loss of confidentiality because information of an intimate nature is more widely available. There is always concern

at the presence of secret records or files and the possibility that non-authorised persons may gain access to the information.

Case conferences
In an effort to find a suitable method of dealing with the problem, case conferences are held at hospital and community level. A case conference consists of a local authority social worker, a representative of the National Society for the Prevention of Cruelty to Children (NSPCC), a consultant paediatrician, a paediatric registrar, the general practitioner, the health paediatrician, a police officer and perhaps a representative from the housing department. If the case conference is held at the hospital, the ward sister may also be included. It is important that all the members should have some knowledge of the family so that each can make informed contribution to the discussion.

The decision reached at these conferences should be based on a flexible, tolerant and compassionate approach which must be able to cope with the parents and suggest suitable care for the child. Such a team must have the power to apply for the removal of the child, by a court order, to a place of safety. Help should be available for the parents, and some regions have facilities where parents can meet and give expression to their feelings and where they are encouraged to speak about their behaviour.

In 1980, the Department of Health issued new guidelines on the use of risk registers. It was recommended that parents should be told when their child is put on the register and the scope extended to include mental and emotional abuse and failure to thrive. It also suggested that each area should appoint one officer as custodian of the register.

Consequences of child abuse
Studies are now available which indicate that child abuse can have serious consequences for children who have been ill treated. It is also recognised that a significant proportion of abused children start life as low-birth-weight babies. Pre-term babies handle differently; some have transient dystonia, feeling stiff and arching away when cuddled, with a grimace instead of a smile. Small-for-dates babies

look scraggy and anxious and are more likely to have unpredictable feeding and sleeping patterns. They may also be more difficult to live with throughout the first year of life.

The child's growth assessment is probably at the point of identification of abuse when many will be found to be below the mean for height and/or weight. There is, therefore, a relationship between failure to thrive and abuse.

It also appears that a number of children are physically and possibly mentally handicapped before they were abused. Stress is increased where parents suspect the presence of an abnormality which has not been diagnosed as such. There is, however, evidence that the number suffering permanent handicap is greater in those who have been abused. These handicaps have been divided into neurological classes.

Class 3: Serious and significant neurological abnormalities.

Class 2: Less severe neurological handicaps and abnormalities, e.g. clumsiness.

Class 1: Mild neurological findings, not severe enough for the child to show significant functional handicap, e.g. intention tremor.

Class 0: No neurological dysfunction, immaturity or damage.

Other physical handicaps which can result from abuse include deformities and scars, e.g. small flattened head, and defective vision and hearing. The study further showed that on intellectual and developmental assessments, 49 per cent of abused children showed definite evidence of developmental delay, e.g. delay in language development was pronounced, school performance was impaired and 19 per cent of those studied were mentally retarded. Behavioural studies in the follow-up period, using play periods, showed that these children exhibited aggressive behaviour, lack of imagination, tearfulness and lack of spontaneous and playful chatter.

Alternative care of the child

A number of social changes have affected the traditional family unit and this is reflected in the alternative caring systems which have evolved. Many of the systems are not new, but the philosophies governing their use have changed over the years. The first of these were the *nursery schools*.

The first one to be established in Britain was in 1816 when Robert Owen, the industrialist reformer of the New Lanark cotton mills, offered supervised care for children of women working at the mill. The emphasis was on education and children were admitted from the time they could walk and say a few words. They remained at the nursery school until they reached school age. The first nursery was a model of kindliness and good sense with a child-centred approach. The curriculum consisted of singing, dancing, marching, fife-playing and outdoor free play. No books or formal instruction were permitted. This school was the exception rather than the rule and it was unfortunate that Robert Owen's ideas were not accepted.

There were others such as Samuel Wilderspin whose pedagogical ideas were totally opposed to those of Robert Owen. He set up infant schools all over the country. They tended to be dreary environments where the children had to sit in tiered galleries and were taught the three Rs. This type of nursery education was typical until the beginning of the 1900s when the Board of Education condemned early schooling. Some toys were introduced and benches were replaced by movable desks. However, formal drilling of the three Rs continued until 1926 when the Code of Regulation for Public Elementary Schools in England stipulated that recreation periods for classes of children under 5 must be available but should not exceed 30 minutes.

In 1933, a report by the Consultative Committee on infant and nursery schools recommended that nursery schools emphasise children's physical well-being and intellectual development through a teacher-guided 'unfolding' of children's natural powers.

In the Education Act of 1944, the local education authorities were required to provide nursery school education for those who required it. During the 1960s much pressure had been applied for an increase in nursery school places and indeed many more nursery schools were opened, though in recent years economic constraints mean that fewer places are now available.

The function of the nursery school is to provide a safe and rich environment in which the young child can develop. The $2\frac{1}{2}$/3- to 5-year-old is given the right stimulus to enhance or to stimulate mental development. It is suggested that, in such an environment, the socially deprived child can obtain the same advantages as the child who is socially, economically and culturally better provided for. Also, the child is in company with other children and is introduced at an earlier stage to the discipline of community living.

These schools are staffed by teachers who may or may not be qualified in infant schooling and by specially trained nursery nurses. The time spent in the school may be a few hours in the morning, e.g. 9 a.m. to 12 noon, or in the afternoon, e.g. 1 p.m. to 4 p.m. In some areas the school day may be from 9 a.m. to 4 p.m., depending on the availability of places and the age of the child; the younger the child, the shorter the period. If the child attends for a full day, he will have a rest period after dinner. The emphasis is on play in a safe, supervised environment, creative activity and learning to live in an enlarged community.

Day nurseries

These cater for the very young children up to the age of 5. Day nurseries were already established in 1850 and then, as today, were primarily for those children whose mothers acted as breadwinners. This ensured that the children were well cared for and protected. These nurseries are open from early morning, e.g. 8 a.m., until early evening. The staff consists of nursery nurses with possibly a registered nurse in charge. The routine is based on that which the children may well experience in their own home.

Play groups

Play groups for pre-school children were started in New Zealand and the idea spread to Europe. Groups of mothers met regularly in one another's homes or a public hall to share activities with their children. By 1965 there were 500 such groups and by 1972 there were more than 15 000. Some are run by charitable organisations. Often some form of trained help or advice is available. One disadvantage of these voluntary play groups is the problem of discontinuing them when the more enterprising and active members send their children to school. Advice is available regarding formation of a play group and the type of equipment suitable. All play groups charging a fee must conform to regulations concerning premises and children's health and they must be approved by the local health authority. Play groups offer children enriching experiences through such activities as singing, games, stories and art.

Care in the child's home

Care may be provided by a number of different people while the mother is at work. These include: father (if unemployed), grandmother, older sibling, neighbour, friend, babysitter, nanny, housekeeper or an au pair. This form of care has not been studied. It is very private and varies from home to home. In many cases it is mainly an extension of the care received by the mother. There are a number of advantages to this type of care. The hours are flexible; there is no need for the child or parent to travel; the child remains in his own familiar place, and the mother is able, to some extent, to monitor the attitude and behaviour of the care given. It also keeps siblings together and the care-giver can give each child personal attention. It is a relatively economic way of arranging care and often includes additional services such as shopping and laundry. The disadvantages of this sytem are that the care-giver is unlicensed and unsupervised. In some instances it may not be a stable form of care-giving, particularly if there are frequent changes of personnel.

Home day-care (childminders)

All home day-care providers, called childminders, who are paid and who care for children for more than 2 hours a day at least one day a week, are required to register with the Social Services Department. This law is, however, not strictly enforced and it is not known how many unregistered childminders there are. There may be several children cared for in one home and this offers children less interaction with an adult than they would have with their own mothers.

There are many other care systems, like the 'crèches' which are similar to nurseries but which tend to be organised by industries for children of employees. A communal system of care, like that provided by the kibbutz in Israel, ensures that children are cared for by trained people and yet allows a close link between parents and their children.

Whatever system is used it must ensure that the child is cared for by caring, loving people and that the environment is safe and secure, rich and stimulating in experience so that the child can develop fully.

Chapter 4
Child health services

Children are a nation's greatest asset and the value it places on them is reflected in the way it provides for their well-being. The system of care has evolved over many years and one way of assessing the quality of care is by analysing statistical information. Infant mortality, the death rate per thousand live births in the first year of life, is an easily accessible index of child health in a country. Other indices can be used such as stillbirth rate and neonatal mortality rate. Figures available show that there has been a steady decline in the infant mortality rate, e.g. the infant mortality rate in Scotland has fallen from 25 per 1000 live births in 1961 to 13 per 1000 in 1981. This may indicate that there has been an improvement in the standard of health care, however, it is important to remember that this is only one measure and to obtain a more accurate picture it is necessary to analyse other factors. The findings of the Committee on Child Health Services, under the chairmanship of Professor Donald Court, indicated the shortcomings of the services and made many recommendations to improve them. Since the publication of the Court Report 1976, changes have taken place which no doubt have affected the care provided within the National Health Service.

While the family still retains some measure of control over the care and welfare of the children, the state has assumed a wide range of control. The family still has responsibility for the education and health of the children; the state, however, provides the means by which both are achieved.

This is embodied in the Education Act 1944, which not only ensured education for all children but also health surveillance of schoolchildren. In addition various Acts have been passed to give protection to children, e.g. the Children and Young Person Act 1969 which covers statutory care both of deprived and delinquent children, or the Children's Act 1975 giving power to any local authority to provide both short-term and long-term care for children in need.

OBJECTIVES OF CHILD HEALTH SERVICES

The health of children is of paramount importance and to monitor this it is necessary to have a well-organised service. The state provides such a service, which is continuous throughout childhood.

The Brotherston Report (1973) envisaged an integrated Child Health Service and made many recommendations. Three main objectives were stated:

1. To promote the health of infants and children so that they grow and develop as normally as possible, enjoy as happy a childhood as circumstances permit, and can profit by education to the limit of their abilities.
2. To ensure that children reach adult life in the best physical, mental and emotional health that can be achieved.
3. To give counsel and support to parents and relatives, always bearing in mind the well-being of the whole family and those with whom the child comes into daily contact at school and in play.

The importance of prevention of ill health and disabilities is also stressed as is the therapy, care and management of the ill child. To achieve these objectives requires a competent primary care and supporting domiciliary consultant service. All aspects of child-care services are highlighted and in particular the provision of paediatric hospital services for infants, children and adolescents in collaboration with the other specialties. It was also recommended that there should be continuity of care of the chronic sick and the handicapped into adult life.

No service can function effectively in isolation and it is important that there is consultation between other departments, e.g. education, social service, youth employment service and voluntary agencies. Many of the recommendations have been accepted and many improvements made in existing services for the benefit of the children.

Child health clinic

The function of the child health clinic is to apply paediatrics in its broad sense as a means of preventive medicine by maintaining vigilance over the health of the child from birth to school entry.

The clinic has important roles in observation and guidance on nutrition and growth; reassurance and explanation of minor problems; screening for physical neuro-psychiatric and metabolic disorders; immunisation against infectious disease; and health education. This is achieved by follow-up of the baby's progress at frequent and regular intervals; regular examination of the infant and toddler; provision of advice regarding feeding and general care of the baby; and referring to a specialist when necessary.

The birth of a baby is notified to the local child health services and the health visitor of that area visits the mother and the baby. The mother can attend the clinic or receive the same service from her general practitioner. Indeed it is important that there is close co-operation between the two services, since, should a problem arise, it is usually the general practitioner who will deal with it.

The child health clinic would also seem to be the obvious centre to promote health education. Accidents form the greatest single cause of death between the first birthday and the end of childhood and it is therefore pertinent that every effort should be made to prevent this. The parents must be made aware of the possibilities of domestic dangers and discussions as well as displays can be used to emphasise these and indicate how these can be prevented.

An additional important function of the child health clinic is the help which can be provided to immigrant parents. Child-care systems vary with different cultures and the system used may not be in the best interest of the child. Guidance may be required regarding nutrition and general care of the child. Language difficulties will further increase misunderstanding and the help of an interpreter will be very valuable.

The health of the schoolchild

The progress of any child at school depends on many factors; his home and his parents, his intelligence, his school environment and his health. Ill health or a serious physical or mental handicap or disability can affect his performance at school. The Child Health Services include both the National Health Service and local authority services and it is incumbent on the educational services in conjunction with the National Health Service to organise a special school health service. The aims and objectives of the School Health Service are:

1. To make sure that every child is as fit as possible so that he may obtain the maximum benefit from the educational programme. The school medical service includes an examination which aims at identifying any problems as early as possible and recommending suitable treatment. Any supportive treatment can involve the services of the speech therapist or remedial gymnastic therapist.

2. To promote health. In this sense it is involved in health education programmes. Lectures are given by various health personnel on topics such as cleanliness, nutrition and bodily functions (menstruation, sex education).

3. To help with the detection and treatment of various groups of handicapped children and those with disabilities or significant difficulties and children with learning difficulties, and to assist every child to gain the maximum benefit from his education. It includes those who are either partially blind or deaf, those who suffer from the effects of some serious congenital abnormalities such as spastic diplegia or spina bifida, or chronic ill health, and those who have serious behaviour problems and neurological conditions.

Pre-school examinations do not as a rule take place though some authorities have introduced that service. It is carried out a year before the child is due to attend school. The mother is invited to bring the child to a convenient centre where a full history is collected and a medical examination carried out. This also includes dental examination. A check on immunisations received is made and, if any are needed, these can be given before entry into school. The pre-school examination is a voluntary one and is not meant to replace the examination given on entry into the primary school.

School examinations and inspections

The present basis of the School Health Service is a combination of full routine examinations on all children either just before or immediately after entry into school combined with selective medical examinations during school life. There is a full examination at about 14/15 years of age, including a fitness test for employment. The school nurse has the responsibility to ensure that all the relevant information is available. It covers many areas such as developmental history, social development, home conditions, general muscular co-ordination and auditory memory.

At the age of 8 or 12 (the practice varies) questionnaires are completed by parents and teachers and as a result selective examinations are carried out on those children who are shown to have various problems.

A special room is set aside for the purpose and a rest room should also be available.

The School Health Service is basically a diagnostic service and treatment is not instituted; children are referred to their own general practitioner or other specialist services.

Sight testing is carried out on 5-year-olds, using the Keystone machine. This tests visual acuity, colour vision and muscle balance. If any defect is found a full ophthalmic examination is arranged. If any squint is discovered, investigation and treatment are started although many such cases will have been under treatment since infancy.

Hearing is also tested. This can be carried out by the school nurse using a sweep test with a pure tone audiometer, which is a light, portable machine producing sounds of varying volume at frequency ranging from 128 to 8000 cycles per second. Each ear is tested separately. The child is given a small wooden mallet and asked to strike the table each time a sound is heard. Tests are carried out at each frequency starting with a loud volume of sound and gradually reducing the volume.

The School Health Service should apply to children in List D schools, grant-aided schools and independent schools for handicapped children.

Access to health advice: parents and pupils should have ready access to the advice of both the school doctor and nurse. The means of contacting either should be made known to parents and pupils. In most circumstances the school nurse should be the first point of contact.

Every school should have a named school doctor, nurse and health visitor. The named doctor should visit the school sufficiently frequently to be known personally to the teaching staff. The named nurse should visit all schools for which she has responsibility not less frequently than once per week.

Examples of routine medical examinations

Normal child

He is examined when aged 5 years and 14 years. In addition, the school nurse visits the school each term to check on minor illnesses and cleanliness and questionnaires are completed by parent and teacher when the child is aged 8 and 12 years.

A child with constant disability

Examples of disabilities are scoliosis, vision defect or hearing defect. There should be follow-up examinations at least once a year, but more frequent check ups may be arranged.

Normal child on entry to school who later develops a severe illness

An example could be rheumatic fever. On return to school he would be seen by the school doctor at least once a year.

It can be seen that various groups of children will be seen during the routine inspection periods, for example:

1. Those in the various age groups selected for routine medical examination.
2. Any child seen previously and marked as needing to be seen that year.
3. Any child with recent serious illness or long absence.
4. Any child whom the parent, teacher or school

nurse desires the school doctor to see because of unsatisfactory progress or difficulty of any kind.

5. Any child aged 8 to 12 years whose parental or teacher questionnaire indicated medical, behavioural or educational problems.

CARE OF THE HANDICAPPED SCHOOLCHILD

With the publication of the Warnock Report in 1978 a number of changes have been suggested, some of which have been implemented.

Although the responsibility of medical services to school children is that of the Health Board, the responsibility for the ascertainment of pupils needing special education remains under section 34 of the Education Act 1944, i.e. with each local education authority. At present any LEA can legally insist on a medical examination of any child who they have reason to believe requires special education once the child has reached the age of 2 years, but this is likely to be altered to require any LEA to be given the power to require a multiprofessional assessment of children of any age (after due notice to the parents).

At the present, handicapped children are divided into 10 categories by disabilities: blind, partially blind (sighted), deaf, partially deaf, delicate, educationally subnormal (mild, severe), maladjusted, physically handicapped, epileptic, and those with speech defects. One criticism is that these categories do not indicate multiple handicaps such as blind and deaf (and therefore no special educational facilities may be available). There is a strong suggestion that the educational needs of the child should be determined, rather than categories of disabilities. When planning educational services it is important to recognise that a large percentage of children (16 to 20 per cent) may require some form of special education. This may involve special teaching techniques or equipment, or a specially modified curriculum.

To ensure that these children benefit from the educational system it is essential that diagnosis is made early and that the special education and care are started early. The aim should be to make the child as independent as possible, for eventual success in life is usually related to independence. Wherever possible, the child should be integrated into the ordinary school system. To ensure that the programme is suitable, a careful assessment of the child will be made at special assessment centres. Figures 4.1 to 4.5 illustrate one such centre and the facilities available.

Range of special education provided

The needs of children with disabilities or significant difficulties are extremely complex and varied. It may be possible to allow a disabled child to attend an ordinary school provided the physical

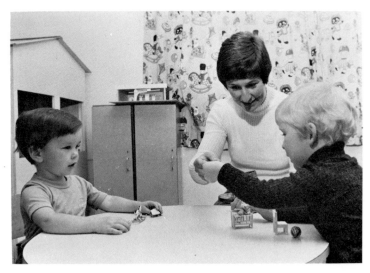

Fig. 4.1 Speech therapist giving language stimulation in a play situation (Balvicar Assessment Centre, Glasgow).

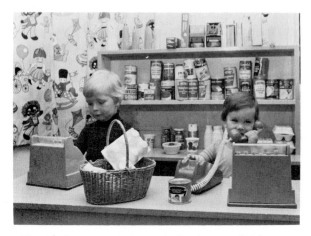

Fig. 4.2 Group speech therapy in the playroom (Balvicar Assessment Centre, Glasgow).

conditions are suitable, e.g. ramps, special equipment. In practice, special schools are needed for three groups:

1. Children with very severe or complex physical disabilities (blindness, deafness, spina bifida, spastic diplegia and progressive diseases such as muscular dystrophies).
2. Children with severe emotional or behavioural disorders who have difficulties in forming relationships with others.
3. Children who for various reasons do badly in ordinary schools and who need the more inti-

mate atmosphere of small teaching groups to make educational progress.

Integration

The idea is to integrate the disabled child with the ordinary school system. Three forms of integration can be identified:

Locational. A special school is sited within the same grounds as an ordinary school, but is still run, in the educational sense, as a separate school. This allows seriously disabled children to attend the same school as their brothers and sisters and,

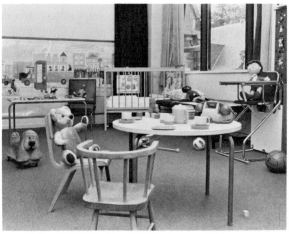

Fig. 4.4 Consulting room for developmental assessment at the Balvicar Assessment Centre, Glasgow.

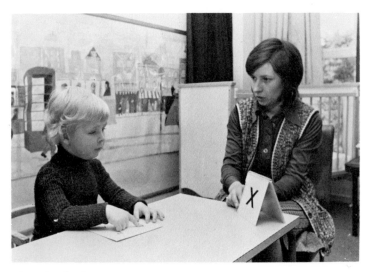

Fig. 4.3 Stycar vision testing using five letter test.

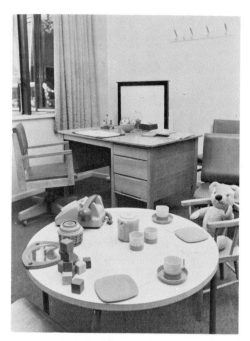

Fig. 4.5 A typical medical consulting room at the Balvicar Assessment Centre, Glasgow.

in addition, should help the children in the ordinary school to understand better the needs and problems of disabled persons.

Social integration. The children in the special unit play, mix and eat with children from the ordinary school; they may also share some of the out-of-class activities. However, there is still separate classroom teaching.

Functional integration. Achieves all the above but, in addition, the disabled children share some or most of their classes with ordinary children. Such an arrangement still allows some essential specialisation to be practised with the severely disabled children, but it also enables them to gain many of the advantages of not only mixing with normal children, but also having access to a wider range of teaching than is usually possible in a special school. The idea is to increase the expectations of the disabled child, particularly if he is intelligent, to a level which he would otherwise not have been able to achieve.

The child with reading difficulties

Reading is a complex cognitive process requiring visual, auditory and motor skills to enable the child to recognise words and symbols, to associate them with the appropriate sounds and to give them meaning derived from previous experience. When development in some area is slow or fails to reach a certain level, a child may be unusually slow in learning to read. The term 'dyslexia' is often applied by neurologists to describe severe difficulty in reading after a localised injury to the brain of an adult who had been a competent reader. The same term is applied to children, although only a minority of children are affected with severe reading retardation.

There is still controversy over the underlying cause of reading retardation, but in 1968 a research group meeting in Texas formulated the following definition of the disorder as 'dysfunction in the synthesis and interpretation of information coming into the brain through and by the eyes and ears, the cause of which is specific and essentially neurological'. This view is not necessarily accepted by paediatric neurologists since a number of associated difficulties are also found among children with the most severe reading difficulties.

The facilities and remedial help available vary from one local authority to another. Remedial treatment is approached on an individual basis related to the needs of the child.

Visual handicap

Defective vision is the most common defect among children, with the exception of dental disease, and it is frequently the cause of lack of progress in school. The type and prevalence of visual defect vary with age, and some, such as short-sightedness and squint, may be corrected by wearing glasses. These children attend ordinary schools but it is recommended that those who wear glasses should be put at the front of the class if possible.

Regulations under the Education Act of 1944 made the partially sighted a separate category of handicapped children. The blind were defined as 'pupils who have no sight or whose sight is or is likely to become so defective that they require education by methods not involving the use of sight'. The partially sighted were defined as 'pupils who by reason of defective vision cannot follow the normal regime of ordinary schools without detriment to their sight or to their educational development', but can be educated by special methods involving the use of sight'.

Provisions available

A visually handicapped child is usually referred to the local authority social services department by the hospital, general practitioner or health visitor. Certification and registration of the handicap are voluntary but are usually preliminaries to receiving services and benefits. Assessments are made by an ophthalmologist, an educational psychologist and a teacher of the visually handicapped. It is obvious that the blind person will be unable to do certain things and that he will need certain kinds of help at various stages in life. Whatever care is given, either physical or educational, his basic needs are for confidence, competence and independence.

It has now been recognised that the young blind child should be kept at home and that too early separation from the mother carries emotional hazards. As for sighted children, the social and emotional development of the blind child should be a gradual process of widening relationships.

Education

Various schemes are currently being explored — one is to provide for blind children in ordinary schools. There is evidence that in some cases this can be successful. However, at present, blind children are generally provided for in special schools.

In the UK, all special schools for the blind are boarding schools. The reasons are that (a) the total number of blind children is comparatively small and it is not possible to provide day schools within reasonable distance of all such children, and (b) the blind child needs education not only in academic and technical subjects, but also in the special techniques of everyday living, e.g. cooking, cleaning, etc.

It is nevertheless important that the blind child is gradually given a greater degree of independence and that he learns to live in the larger community. For this reason, it is worthwhile to consider letting the blind child join a neighbouring ordinary school for the last two years of school life.

The child with partial sight has to be dealt with according to the degree of useful sight. From the educational standpoint the partially sighted child is one who can be taught by visual methods but may need special aids or techniques unavailable to ordinary schools.

The partially sighted child has useful sight and it is important to prepare and train him for life as a sighted person, even though his sight may be limited. Depending on his intellectual capacity he can cover the same educational fields as the sighted child.

Deafness

There are wide variations of deafness depending upon the degree of deafness, the age and rate of onset and the presence of other handicaps.

The normally hearing child first develops auditory language before speech. The profoundly deaf child does not develop auditory language and will not develop spoken language unless given special education. He cannot converse in the ordinary sense of the term unless both parties have learned to use sign language. The moderately deaf child can converse and communicate imperfectly and with difficulty. This creates many problems and makes great demands on other people.

Assessment

Children learn through all the five senses and deficiency in any of these will affect their intellectual, emotional and social development. Hearing has a special importance. Man is not born with speech but with the potential ability to speak. We acquire speech by listening to and imitating others.

Any child with a hearing defect will be slow in learning to speak and if it is severe enough he will not learn to speak spontaneously.

It is, therefore, important to assess the degree and type of deafness, and to institute, as early as possible, a training programme so that the child can develop as fully as he can. Early screening should be carried out using simple methods like rattling a spoon or crumpling a piece of paper and noting whether he tries to look in the direction of the sound or shows any reaction to it.

Observations of any signs of deafness, for example slowness in speech development or in progress in learning, should be the responsibility of both home and school. Hearing tests are carried out in school and the type and extent of the hearing defect identified. Further tests will also be necessary, not only for hearing but also for attainment and intelligence.

Education

The positive approach to the deaf child is to make use of whatever hearing is present and to build on it using various techniques to develop the child's hearing skills, speech and use of language.

Hearing aids can be invaluable but they do have their limitations. The type used must suit the individual child and should be provided as soon as possible or practicable.

The aim of the education of deaf children should be to help them to achieve their full potential and to integrate them, as far as possible, into a 'hearing' society. Training should start as early as possible. The mother has an important part to play, although skilled, professional help and advice are essential. These children require special attention and it may not be possible for a mother with other young children to meet these extraordinary demands. Special nursery units give auditory training at the age of 2 or 3 years. Day units are preferred to boarding schools, but if a boarding school is chosen the child should be allowed home at weekends. The type of training and education varies, e.g. lip reading, sign language or aural training. Even where aural training has been given, it has been found that children tend to use sign language and lip reading when out of the classroom.

Provisions (in the community) for the maladjusted child

The term 'maladjustment' was first used in the 1920s and has only been widely adopted in this country since the Second World War. Maladjustment has existed throughout history but only in more recent years have the implications of the problem been recognised.

Although the worst effects of maladjustment are seen among adults, it has come to be regarded as a problem of childhood. This is because it is during childhood that the pattern of behaviour is set and events take place which may lead to maladjustment. At this time of life the individual has the greatest need of care and understanding, so that he can adjust to changing situations and conditions.

When dealing with maladjustment, the emphasis is on prevention, discovery and treatment. The first signs may be noted in school since this is the first community outside the family into which the child ventures. It is here that his reactions to his contemporaries and teachers can be evaluated. The degree of maladjustment varies widely and it is often difficult to determine the point at which it begins.

The method of dealing with this problem is through 'child guidance'. The term is believed to originate from the period of the First World War, although the idea of child guidance can be traced back to antiquity. It was not until the nineteenth century, however, that the need for a scientific approach was appreciated by men like Darwin, Bain & Spencer.

With the introduction of compulsory education in this country in 1880, it was realised that there were many children who could not benefit by the education offered, because of physical weakness or defect. This led to the setting up of a medical department by the Board of Education. Provision was made for children of subnormal intelligence, but it was also realised that there were many children who did not fit into this category but who were maladjusted. With the appointment of a psychologist in 1913 by the London County Council, child guidance became an area in which the behaviour problems in children were studied. An extension of this study was the recognition that there might be a relationship between early behaviour problems and delinquency. Gradually clinics were opened in various centres in Britain and the first Child Guidance Clinic was opened in 1932 in connection with the Birmingham Education Committee's special school service.

A further impetus to the treatment of maladjusted children was given by the Education Act 1944. This Act emphasised that every child should be educated in accordance with age, ability and aptitude, and that some children require special educational treatment either in ordinary or in special schools because they suffer from disabilities of body or mind, including emotional or psychological disorders.

Maladjusted pupils

Maladjusted pupils were defined in the Handicapped Pupils and School Health Service Regulations 1945/1953 as 'pupils who show evidence of emotional instability or psychological disturbance and require special educational treatment in order to effect their personal, social or educational readjustment'. The services which have been established to ensure that the maladjusted child is helped to overcome his difficulties are described in the next section.

Function of the child guidance clinic

Generally, the term 'child guidance' is used to describe the treatment of maladjusted children but, in the broadest sense, it is concerned with education itself. It involves not only the child but also his parents and the school.

The staff of a child guidance clinic includes psychiatrists, educational psychologists and psychiatric social workers.

The child is referred to a clinic and attends it with one or both his parents. The psychiatric social worker may have already visited the child's home and is in possession of information regarding the home background. The psychologist will obtain a report from the school and indeed may have seen the child there. He also assesses, through various tests, the child's capacity and attainment.

The psychiatrist will have access to the child's medical record from the School Health Service, but further medical examination will probably be carried out. It is the psychiatrist's responsibility to decide what form of treatment is to be given. He talks to the child and aims to uncover the emotional problems in his life.

Since this is team work, the clinic staff hold frequent discussions at which diagnosis may be made and programmes of treatment instituted.

Other forms of treatment involve the use of special day schools and classes. Most children can be treated without removing them from their normal school and home environment. However, if the relationship within the family becomes seriously disturbed, it may be necessary to remove the child to a hostel, foster home or special residential school.

A small proportion of maladjusted children are so acutely disturbed that they are unfit for any formal education and may need special medical investigation and treatment. Some children's hospitals have special units which are equipped to investigate and institute psychiatric treatment for these children. These units are under the control of a psychiatrist and the team includes clinical and educational psychologists, psychiatric social workers and nurses with special training in psychiatry or child psychiatry. These units also have teachers trained to work with maladjusted children.

Provisions for children with mental handicap

In an effort to ensure that the mentally handicapped child can develop to his full potential it is essential that provisions are made to foster his development.

Detection of mental handicap should be made as soon as possible. It may be obvious at an early age or it may require skilled examination and assessment over a period of time. The local area medical officer maintains a register of all children based on the notification of birth. These notifications are normally accompanied by details of any congenital abnormalities detected. Handicaps appearing in the weeks after birth are notified to him by the general practitioner and the clinic doctor. Some children develop severe mental handicap as a result of subsequent illness, and these are notified by the doctor treating or assessing the child.

Care and management

The mentally handicapped child, like all handicapped children, requires early assessment so that the necessary arrangements can be made for his care and education. The great majority of mentally retarded children look normal at birth, though some will show early signs of their defect in the first weeks of life.

Parents are often the first to recognise that there is something abnormal about their child and to seek help and advice. Some parents, however, find it difficult to accept that their child is mentally abnormal and this may prevent early modification of the child's educational programme. The basic care of the child will be the same. He has the same needs as any normal child and these must be satisfied. Feeding can sometimes present with problems. For example, he may be slow to feed, have difficulty with sucking and may be reluctant to change to solids. Patience will be needed and the mother advised to find a more suitable way, e.g. spoon feeding rather than bottle feeding. If there are associated physical abnormalities then the feeding regime will have to be modified (p. 311).

Love and security are as important to these children as to any other, and most will respond readily and lovingly. Auditory and visual stimulation play an important part in developing their senses and motor stimulation is important in developing motor skills (p. 30).

Education

Mentally handicapped children need particular and continuing attention from health, education and social services. Most of them live at home and attend nurseries and special schools. Some are resident in hospitals, but many of those whose families cannot look after them may only be in need of good residential care. Future plans envisage that more children will live in community homes and that hospitals will only look after those who need special assessment, medical and nursing care. Support, training and education may be needed from birth and may have to continue long after normal school-leaving age.

Provisions

Various provisions are available, for example *integration* in the ordinary school. This means the setting up of a group of classes for mentally handicapped children within the ordinary school. At present, however, most mentally handicapped children are educated in separate special schools.

The under-5s. Some children can be appropriately placed in ordinary play groups, nursery classes and schools. Some are so limited in ability that they present a special problem and separate play programmes have to be designed to meet their needs.

Schoolchildren. When the child attends a special school, the programme of education will be designed to meet his educational needs. Children in institutions will also receive schooling or training according to their stage of development and capability, while at the same time receiving medical and nursing care.

Older pupils. It has been demonstrated that many mentally handicapped adolescents can work effectively and consistently in closely supervised routine situations. The education and training are therefore geared to prepare the adolescent for adulthood, taking into consideration his limited opportunities and inadequacies. Behaviour variations have to be assessed and decisions made regarding social tolerance of variant behaviour.

In preparation for leaving school, simple skills, both manual and social, are included in the curriculum. Co-operation between school and industry is also important and here the careers officer can play a key role.

Although the minimum statutory school-leaving age for pupils in special school is 16 years, the education authorities may provide education up to 19 years of age.

Severely handicapped children

It is the duty of local education authorities to provide education for all children irrespective of the degree of their handicap. This may be either in a school or in a hospital. The children tend to form two sub-groups: those who have also psychotic features in their behaviour, are hyperactive, aggressive and self-destructive, and those with multiple physical handicaps in addition to mental defects. Different disciplines are usually involved in the caring and educational programme. In day schools, the medical officer, speech therapist, physiotherapist, teachers, school nurses and non-teaching assistants play a part. In hospitals, these workers join consultants in mental subnormality and nurses, to form the group from which team work will develop. It can be seen that a number of different departments are involved and if the children are to benefit, then co-ordination of the services offered by these departments will be essential. In addition to the official services available, there are also voluntary associations. These not only provide advice and encourage mutual self-help but also provide play facilities, transport for children and their parents and residential accommodation.

Social services

The importance of the home for handicapped children is well recognised. However, where social, economic and cultural factors are concomitants of mental handicap, the contact with the home may not be possible. The welfare services will then have an important role to play in maintaining contact between home and school.

The care and welfare of the mentally handicapped and their families is now the responsibility of the local authority social services departments. These are empowered to provide assistance in co-operation with area health authorities. There is a close link with hospital services and schools for the mentally handicapped. Where residential care is required, hostels and foster homes may be provided. The social services act as co-ordinator of all the services available including the voluntary services and this link ensures that the best possible use is made of the available services for the benefit of the mentally handicapped.

Provisions for physically handicapped children

Physical handicap covers a wide range of conditions which result in some disability. These include birth abnormalities, congenital heart defects, progressive muscular atrophy and handicaps resulting from accidental injury or the after-effects of diseases such as poliomyelitis.

The care and management largely depend upon the type of disability and when it occurred — whether congenital or acquired after birth. If it is present at birth, education and management starts early and is directed towards training the child to live within the limitations of his handicap. When the disability occurs later, the problems are different, in that the parents and the child have to learn to adjust to different patterns of life.

In the first instance, any physical defect, whether congenital or acquired, is dealt with within the medical/surgical services, depending on the type. Each case is assessed on the basis of long-term planning, particularly if the defect is a continuous one or if it requires prolonged treatment.

Care and management

Many physically handicapped children are cared for in their own homes. Depending on the actual handicap and the degree of disability the child may be able to join a nursery school or play group — though sometimes special provisions may be necessary. This applies particularly to children whose mobility is affected and structural adjustments may be required or the choice will depend on the availability of ramps or lifts.

As with all other handicaps, team work is required to treat all aspects of the disability, for example: physiotherapy, speech therapy and repeated hospitalisation to improve and correct the handicap; visits to orthopaedic departments of hospitals and adjustment and modification of splints and calipers. Financial help may be required with transportation and home modifications and here the social work services will be able to offer advice. If the home care of these children is to be effective then support should be available from the community paediatric service.

Education

The question of schooling for physically handicapped children must be seen in the context of the type of handicap and the availability of facilities.

In theory, a child can be educated in an ordinary school if his sight, hearing and intelligence are within normal limits and if he can use his hands or at least one hand for writing and drawing. It is also essential, however, to consider fundamental needs, such as acceptance by others and the need to find a role within the school community. In some cases it may be necessary to provide education in a special school or at home.

If the child is to attend an ordinary school then facilities such as ramps and special toilets should be available. If local arrangements are not satisfactory then the child can attend a special school which is usually purpose-built and where the education programme is planned to meet the needs of the child. Where possible, and when the disability becomes less, it may be possible to transfer the child to an ordinary school or to attend the special school as a day pupil if he had previously been residential.

Each handicap, whether skeletal-muscular, cardiovascular, respiratory or endocrinal, must be assessed carefully and the choice of care, management and education of the child related to its type and severity.

Transition from school to adult life

Throughout the child's life all the decisions made must take into consideration his potential for leading an independent adult life. It is therefore essential that all children with disabilities or significant difficulties have a careful assessment made of these difficulties so that the transition into adult life is less difficult. All who are involved in the care of the child, and this includes the parents, must play a part during this period. The transition period from childhood to adulthood is difficult for the normal, healthy child and must be even more so for the handicapped person who not only has to cope with his handicap but also with his growing awareness as a person. Every effort should therefore be made to make this transition period as easy as possible.

He will also require work preparation and he should be given the opportunity to discuss work opportunities and possibilities with the disablement resettlement officer and arrangements made to obtain work experience suitable to his handicap.

Part 3
The child in hospital

Chapter 5
Hospitalisation

An understanding of the hospital's function and the nurse's role in relation to the sick child would perhaps bring into perspective the relationship each has with the other.

The hospital

The function of the hospital is to provide an environment in which the sick child can be helped to overcome or to alleviate his illness. The aim is to cure (if possible) or to improve the child's physical and mental state so that he can develop within his limits. This involves team work, and essentially the hospital community is made up of a 'team' or a group of people each with a specific function and each contributing to the desired aim. Although the hospital community is a hierarchical system with clearly defined functions, unless the borders of each group merge, however imperceptibly, then the overall goal cannot be achieved.

Each group within the hospital provides a skill and expertise which should benefit the child and, generally, it is easy to define or recognise what the function of each is or should be. For example, the physician is concerned with diseases which can be treated by physiological re-adjustments; the surgeon performs the more mechanical aspects of healing involving change of structure or realignment (precision engineering); the physiotherapist deals with the rehabilitation of the body that can be achieved by massage, exercise, etc.

What of the nurse? Where does she fit in and what is her function? A nurse has been defined as 'one who tends a child; one who has the care of the sick, feeble or injured' (*Chambers Twentieth Century Dictionary*, 1975). This definition should now be revised and extended to include all the functions of the nurse.

The nurse

The nurse may be defined as a person who by virtue of training and experience is able to observe, interpret and assess suffering and discomfort and thereby alleviate a patient's state of ill health and help him to regain a level of physical and mental well-being commensurate with his capacity. This definition could be applied to others, such as the doctor, but whereas the doctor may see the patient only once or twice a day, the nurse is in almost continuous contact and it is the nurse who decides if and when medical assistance is necessary.

Observation
This function of the nurse is vital. It implies an ability to use all the senses — eyes, ears, nose, tactile and intuitive — to a very high degree. It also means that the person is able to identify the relevant and important in what has been observed within any given situation. Of equal importance is the continuity of the observation. The nurse is the only member of the hospital team who is in direct contact with the patient for a considerable period of time and she has the greatest opportunity to observe the patient under different circumstances and conditions. She is also the first person available to observe any deviation from the normal — that is, the perceived normal in the context of ill health or disease. In children's nursing, keen observation is an essential attribute. The infant and child cannot communicate by speech and is therefore dependent on the adult to observe any changes in behaviour and to respond in an appropriate manner.

Observation is normally the function of the mother, but in hospital the nurse must assume that function. In addition to observing normal behaviour, it is necessary to observe the sick child and recognise any deviation. There may be some subtle change in facial expression, cry or movement which can be observed, not only in the young infant or child but also in the sick child of any age.

Interpretation

Interpretation of signs and symptoms is generally the function of the medical officer. However, it is often not realised that nurses, too, have a role to play. The nurse must be able to act in situations which do not necessarily involve the doctor. For example, in the case of the reluctant feeder, she should be able to determine whether the infant is satisfied or whether his loss of appetite is symptomatic of some illness. Interpretation leads to assessment of the action to be taken. Can the nurse deal with the situation or is medical help needed?

Alleviation

The nurse's function is often said to be to comfort the patient and attend to his every need — for example, to provide an environment which is conducive to healing, to be a listener and to relieve some of the anxieties created by the patient's illness and the hospital environment. The ability to alleviate pain and to create a relatively happy yet disciplined environment is indeed an art and a skill, but it is also a question of personality and temperament.

It is important, however, not only to alleviate the state of ill health but also to ensure that improvement is maintained and to prevent, where possible, a recurrence of the condition or the development of another. Prevention is an important function of the nurse; fulfilling it involves all the aforementioned functions. In the hospital setting it involves prevention of accidents and cross-infection; in the community it includes provision of support and help which should to some extent prevent the onset of ill health or, where it has occurred, prevent deterioration.

The child in hospital

Since the publication of the Platt Report on the 'Welfare of Children in Hospital 1959', many changes have taken place in the care of children in hospital. Yet despite all the changes, many of which are a vast improvement on previous conditions, hospitalisation still presents many problems for the child as well as the nursing staff. However well intentioned and kind the staff may be, there is still fear and terror for many children. This is related to the child's age: the younger he is the more difficult it is for him to adjust to the experience of hospitalisation. This does not apply quite so much to the very young infant, whose problems are different, but who nevertheless still feels the separation.

Recognising these difficulties it is perhaps relevant to discuss them in relation to the age of the child and to look at ways in which one can improve the situation and create the best possible conditions. (It must also be noted that parents, too, have a problem and here it is vital to find some measure of understanding.) Children may be divided into five groups: the infant, the toddler (6 months to 2½ years); the pre-school child (2½ to 5 years); the school-child (5 to 12 years); the adolescent.

The infant

The infant is not capable of rational thought but he is capable of feelings. His life experiences are limited to the close family unit where he enjoys individual care, love and security. He is capable of responding to the care of his mother and is extending a close relationship which began in utero. It is difficult to appreciate and also to accept that the very young infant can be affected by separation, but it is easier to accept that the young infant thrives better in a one-to-one relationship.

The very young infant is susceptible to changes in environment which involve not only physical alterations but also differences in handling. In recognition of this, mothers are encouraged to stay in hospital and to participate in nursing the infant. Not all children's hospitals are equipped to accommodate mothers, but there may be free visiting, and during these periods the mothers can undertake some of the nursing functions. For the nurse, the infant presents few problems: normally, he feeds and sleeps and it is relatively easy for the nurse to mother him. But in order to prevent cross-infection, contact will be limited and the changing pattern of care will be felt by the infant. Some of the procedures are unpleasant and the infant, however young, is able to recognise and eventually anticipate these events.

Identification with mothering creates in the young nurse tensions and anxieties which are intensified by lack of experience and an overwhelming sense of helplessness. This feeling of helplessness can be disturbing for the nurse and she has to learn to deal with it in her own way. The danger always exists that the nurse will become so emotionally involved in the identification of the mothering role that she cannot sever it, and this may lead to conflict and unhappiness.

6 months to 2½ years old

The next two groups have certain characteristics in common, but the main one is that from 6 months to 5 years of age the child is still part of the closely knit family unit. His life experiences are still limited but his development is going through different stages and, within these stages, there are varying levels of understanding.

The 6- to 12-month-old has built up a close relationship with his mother and is not able to adjust quite so readily to others. Speech is just beginning and he has difficulty in communicating his needs. Frustration and deep-felt unhappiness occur and these are difficult to relieve. It is also difficult for the nurse to explain in simple terms what is to happen and why, and the child's feeling of mistrust and apprehension will increase, making the relationship between nurse and child even more difficult. It is impossible sometimes not to hurt the child and a struggling child increases the risk, but he should never be made to feel 'bad'. It is essential to recognise his fears and hold and comfort him, particularly after the event. Although he may seem to reject the nurse, he will still be glad to have her near him.

Parents can also be of help here, though not all parents feel able to watch some of the more difficult procedures, such as dressings or catheterisation. Many nurses feel that they can carry out procedures better without the presence of parents. Whichever way it is done, the child should be the first consideration.

Wherever possible, the mother should be encouraged to stay in or at least visit as often as possible.

Pre-school child

The pre-school child can already understand a great deal and is capable of quite complex language. It is therefore possible to explain in simple terms what is required of him. The difficulty arises with interpretation of the explanation: what seems clear and simple to an adult assumes a different complexion to the young child. He cannot build a mental picture on previous life experiences and thereby has to create one. This can be very distorted and frightening. We have to be very careful, therefore, in offering explanations which should be as near as possible to the experience of the child. Honesty is also important. For example, if something will be painful, the child should be told that he will feel some pain though care will be taken to be as gentle as possible. This will make it easier for him to believe when told that something will not hurt.

This age group has special needs, for example, perfecting many of the skills he has already acquired. This can be achieved within the hospital. The child's day can be so organised that he can play either by himself or in the company of other children, provided he is well enough to do so. The child in isolation, whether in the main ward or in a cubicle, needs toys for stimulation. He also requires human contact. Other children, particularly older ones, take an interest in younger children, but nurses as well as parents can read to them or play simple games.

Schoolchild

This group of children accepts admission to hospital with mild apprehension. Yet even some of them may resent going into hospital and openly fight against admission. The reaction depends on the level of intelligence and the condition from which the child suffers. Most are able to understand the reason for admission, and again honesty is essential. If the child is well enough, he can do some school work. This not only passes his day but keeps him up to date with his lessons. Play, too, is important and most children's hospitals make provision for play, either in each ward or a central play room, under the supervision of a nursery nurse or play leader.

Adolescents

Provision for this group of young people, which includes those from 13 to 16, has also to be considered. Many of these children have been in continuous care since early childhood and may, with the consent of their parents, wish to remain under the care of the paediatrician. This group's needs differ greatly from those of the younger child. Physically adolescents are developing rapidly, though emotionally the rate is not as fast. Privacy and quietness are necessary as the noise and crying of the younger children can be very disturbing for them.

Their day should include school work and any suitable occupational activity. Radio and television play an important part in passing the day and other older children will provide the company they need. However, they too can be apprehensive and anxious. Early recognition of this is essential to relieve their anxiety. It must be remembered that adolescents are still young and have difficulty in solving some of their problems. they should therefore be encouraged to talk about their fears and should not be made to feel inadequate or foolish when tears are the only way to obtain relief.

Admission of the child

Preparation for admission to hospital

It is believed that children accept admission to hospital better if they have been prepared beforehand. This again depends on the age of the child. The young child, as already indicated, has little life experience and cannot be expected to understand what hospitalisation means. Nevertheless, the prospect of leaving home and staying in such an institution must be explained in simple terms. It can be reinforced with little booklets in picture form which show the staff in their uniforms working in a hospital environment. This will prepare them mentally for the experience and take away some of the strangeness which many must feel. The child should be reassured that the hospital people are there to help him and that his parents will visit him every day, if this is possible,

or even stay with him. His favourite toys and other useful books or games can accompany him. In some hospitals children are allowed to visit the ward prior to admission and meet the ward staff. Obviously this can only be done with 'cold admission' or waiting list cases not with emergency admissions.

The child is not the only one who should be prepared for admission: the parents, too, should be able to express their anxiety. The hospital staff have a responsibility to explain matters of detail to the parents. Any problems should be freely discussed and every opportunity given to consult the medical officer about any worry regarding their child. The attitude of parents plays an important part in the care of the child. Mixed in with their natural distress at the separation from their child is a feeling of relief that he will receive treatment. Some parents, however, feel that hospital admission implies failure on their part in caring for the child properly and resent that others take over their role. Feelings of failure may be expressed in a somewhat hostile and critical attitude towards the staff. This can be very trying, but requires understanding and patience on the part of the staff.

Education of the public might also be useful, particularly in relation to introducing young children to the idea of hospitalisation. Children are often threatened with hospitalisation as a means of punishment. This is to be discouraged. Hospitals are frightening enough without introducing additional fears. The same applies to telling the truth regarding admission. Some children are told they are going on holiday. When they realise this is not so, it must shake their trust, not only in their parents, but in all adults. It also makes adjustment to hospital life and to members of staff very difficult.

First impressions are particularly important to the child as well as to the parents. The method will vary with the type of admission.

Planned admission

The child is admitted after waiting his turn on a list. He has usually been to the outpatient department and has met doctors and nurses. He therefore already has some experience on which to build his anticipated stay in hospital. The mother has also had an opportunity to prepare him mentally for separation from home and also to gather together his favourite toys.

The child arrives in hospital reasonably well, but anxious. The ward staff know of his admission and can organise a bed within a suitable area.

Reception of the child and his parents is extremely important. He should be welcomed and introduced to the other children in the ward. The task of admitting a child is often left to inexperienced nurses, but it may be worthwhile considering giving this task to a more experienced nurse. Admission to the hospital can be a traumatic experience and requires tact and understanding. If the child has had a bath at home, this is often dispensed with, but the decision must rest with the ward sister/charge nurse and will depend, among other things, on the reason of admission. The mother can be of help in undressing the child and seeing him safely settled down.

The sequence of events usually follows a routine pattern and no doubt each hospital, if not each ward, will have its own policy. The physical examination of the child is the responsibility of the medical staff but the nursing staff has its own part to play.

Observation and management during admission
This includes:

1. Taking the child's temperature, pulse and respiration (p. 98).
2. Checking the general condition of the child; whether well cared for or otherwise, presence of bruises, spots, any special features such as abnormalities.
3. Checking the state of hair — presence of lice and nits. This is an important observation which should be recorded. It not only serves as a record should the child subsequently become infested, but also, if the child is already infested, the parents should be notified and eventually guidance can be given on the prevention and treatment of verminous heads.
4. Looking for pressure areas — this is relevant where the child has been confined to bed at home or in the case of a chronically ill child where pressure sores may be expected. Infants may have a nappy rash or show frank excoriation and this must be recorded.

5 Weighing and measuring children on admission. This is useful in making the overall assessment of the child's development and growth and, as far as weight is concerned, is necessary for drug calculations.
6. Obtaining a specimen of urine. This too is part of the routine examination of the child. (See p. 547 obtaining specimen of urine.)

Once all the preliminaries have been completed and the necessary records made, the child may be allowed to play or may be put into his cot. This decision will be made by the ward sister/charge nurse and depends on his age, the reason for his admission and his condition.

Emergency admission
A child may be admitted without prior preparation either from home or as a result of an accident. Whatever the circumstances, the same principles apply as for planned admission. There are, however, additional problems to consider.

1. The reception of the child depends on his condition, e.g. he may be unconscious and the ward should be ready to deal with that situation.
2. The child will be much more anxious, again depending on the severity and type of illness; the approach will therefore be related to that state.
3. The choice of bed and area of the ward will also depend on the degree and type of illness, but he should be in a position where he can be observed closely.
4. The parents require a careful approach. They will be anxious and require sympathetic understanding and support. A room should be available for them and they should be allowed some privacy, but if they can be of help in any way, then this should be encouraged. Parents feel helpless and find it difficult to relinquish their caring role. It is also better for them to be occupied in some way rather than to sit and wait. Information should be readily available or given to them as soon as possible.
5. Since no preparation for admission was possible, the routine and policy of the ward should be explained to the parents.

Method of admission

This will vary according to the policy of the hospital. The basic sequence is the same as for a planned admission, except that the procedures are probably carried out in the bed which has been prepared when notice of the admission was received.

Observations, too, are the same, with some additions made necessary by the emergency nature of the admission, for example, breathing rate, rhythm and depth. There will also be greater activity in an attempt to diagnose and to make accurate assessments. Preparation for venepuncture and other investigations may be necessary.

During this time the child should not be left alone and constant encouragement and reassurance should be given. The degree of co-operation from the child will also vary and patience is important. It must be remembered that the child's behaviour is not necessarily that which he normally displays and allowances should therefore be made for uncooperative acts. Anger will rarely achieve the desired result, but firmness is necessary if anything is to be achieved. Parents can be helpful in this situation, though they often find it difficult to handle the child because of their own anxiety.

Interviewing the parents

This is an important aspect of the admission procedure and should be the responsibility of the nurse in charge of the ward. The purpose is to obtain as much information about the child as possible. The nurse must establish rapport with the parents so that they feel relaxed enough to discuss their child. Small children who have not as yet acquired 'adult' language are nevertheless able to communicate with their parents. Many children create their own words and attach meanings to them which the stranger finds difficult to interpret. Since communication in some form is essential, the nurse must know how the child speaks and what special words he uses and understands. It is quite distressing to watch the frustration of a young child attempting to indicate his needs and wants and failing to be understood. The following information from the parents will therefore be necessary:

1. By what name is the child known? It may well be a distortion of his real name.

2. What word does he understand and use when indicating toilet, needs, e.g. 'potty'?
3. Has he any special toys he would like to hold and play with?
4. Is he able to drink from a cup, use a spoon?
5. Has he any special likes and dislikes? Although it may be impossible to attend to these completely, simple likes and dislikes should be accommodated to keep conflict and tension to a minimum. It is all too easy for the nurse to impose her own opinions and to assume that they are superior. She must always remember her responsibility to respect and recognise the child's standards, while at the same time generally encouraging him to adapt to the norms of the hospital.
6. What is the relationship between mother and child? Can we learn something about it by listening to the mother?
7. What developmental progress has the child achieved and what are his special difficulties? This is particularly important in relation to young and handicapped children.
8. What is the personality of the child? Are there any special features which would help the nurse to understand him.

While talking to the parents, the nurse can assess them and obtain a glimpse of the complex relationships which make up a family. Nurses should be careful, however, not to make judgements based on a single interview. If doubt exists about a particular situation, it should be discussed with the medical officer. This applies particularly if doubt exists regarding child abuse.

The parents, too, will be assessing the nurses with whom they come in contact and forming opinions regarding their ability to care for their child. The parents' behaviour and attitude will be a reflection of the nurses'. Aggressive behaviour tends to elicit aggressiveness, while sympathy will elicit greater co-operation.

Information of diagnosis and prognosis should be the prerogative of the medical officer, but it is important that the nurse in charge should know of the content of the conversation so that she can clarify and often simplify the terms used. In emergencies, parents are often in a state of shock and fail to understand what is said to them. It is at this point that the nurse can take over and give accurate, yet simple, explanations.

Parent participation — rooming in

Preserving continuity between the child's home and hospital is the thinking behind the practice of admitting the mother with her child. This generally applies to children under 5 years of age. The idea is not new and has been used in various centres. Evidence for its value is the behaviour of children when returning home. Parents report that the children are less 'clinging' and aggressive and have fewer sleep disturbances than those who were separated from their parents for any length of time.

The success of this method is largely dependent on both the mother and the nursing staff, with the latter bearing the larger share of the responsibility. Some of the factors for success are:

1. The ability of the mother to adjust to the hospital environment and relinquishing part of her role. The parent's signature on the admission card giving permission for any treatment deemed necessary by the surgeon or physician as well as ward sister/charge nurse gives the staff a high measure of control, e.g. how and when to feed, bath or change the nappy of the child.
2. The ability of the nursing staff to accept the mother as part of the ward population, to recognise her needs and to be willing to accept that the role of the mother is specific and supportive, not dominant.
3. The extent to which the mother is given clearly defined instructions about the policy and routine of the ward and what is permissible. She should know the role of each member and whom to contact when help is required.
4. The degree to which the staff recognise that the mother has problems which may be personal or related to her child. She has a need to talk and to be kept informed of any treatment and the results of investigations. She should have access to the ward sister/charge nurse and should be given the opportunity to discuss any problems.

It is interesting to look at the areas where the mother can fulfil a useful function (Figs. 5.1 and 5.2). These include the following: bathing;

feeding; changing nappy; taking temperature; playing with her child and also being 'mum' to other children. There may also be a place for her to help in more specialist nursing activities, e.g. giving oral medicine to her child. This would be

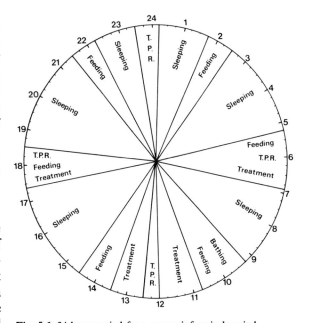

Fig. 5.1 24-hour period for a young infant in hospital.

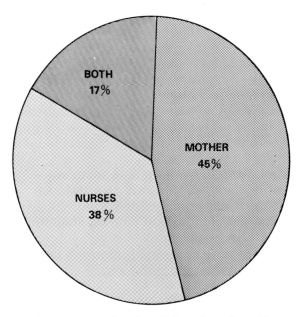

Fig. 5.2 Percentage of nursing which can be performed by the mother. (Parent participation.)

under the supervision of the nurse detailed to administer medicine.

Despite the many glowing reports, it is nevertheless also the case that parents 'rooming in' with their children and having unlimited visiting have created a great many problems. These are primarily caused by the mistrust between the nursing staff and the parents. The young inexperienced nurse feels insecure as a result of the presence of the parents, just as the parents feel subjected to supervision and find it difficult to relinquish their role. It must also be recognised that there is a greater amount of movement in the ward, which can be disturbing. Psychologically, this must create a great deal of tension for all concerned and it may be necessary to rethink the whole concept, so that all may benefit.

An important first step towards more harmonious relations may be to explain to the parents the nature of nurse training and to impress upon them that many nursing skills can only be acquired by practice. It is not easy for parents to accept that another person is better able than they to care for their own child.

There are many other difficulties which, if they can be overcome, could mean the creation of a situation which would be of benefit to all concerned in the care of the child.

Unrestricted visiting by parents

This means that parents are able to visit at any reasonable hour during the day. The times for visiting are usually arranged with the ward sister/charge nurse and are arranged to fit in with other family commitments. Fathers, too, are able to visit in the evening at times that coincide with specific events, such as feeding or tucking down for the night.

Some problems do occur, such as children being fed when they should not be, but these can be overcome with proper explanation and education. Despite the problems which are still present after many years of 'unrestricted visiting', it is recognised that children tend to be more satisfied and the ward is somewhat more relaxed.

The child's day

The routine of the ward generally depends on the type, but certain basic functions, such as infant feeding, other children's meal times, medicine times, treatment periods and doctors' visits, are performed at regular intervals. The child's day is therefore built around these events. For the infant the day is similar to one at home with some additional events.

The school age child, if he is reasonably fit, takes part in individual tuition. This not only passes the time but also, as already mentioned, helps to keep him up to date with his school work. This applies to both primary and secondary school age children. The time spent at school work is generally limited to 2 hours but is largely dependent on the child's condition.

Play in hospital

Among the many differences between a children's hospital and an ordinary one is the provision made for play. Play, as already stated, serves a most important function in a child's life. It is essential for his growth and development. In hospital play serves another important function — the relief of anxiety. For instance, by acting out his experiences in a game of make-believe, the child is able to come to terms with the situation and communicate his fears. Of course, the ability of a child to adjust to the hospital environment must depend to some extent on his personality, his life experience and his intelligence. And no doubt other factors could be added, such as his relationship to other people, both children and adults.

The hospital environment generates fears which cannot be totally avoided but which should be minimised wherever possible. Nurses, by the very nature of their work, are responsible for some of the pain inflicted on children, e.g. injections. It may be rightly claimed that the mother, too, inflicts pain at some time or other and yet she, unlike the nurse, is generally not resented nor is she considered the cause of anxiety in relation to the inflicted pain. The difference here lies in the relationship which exists between mother and child and what is equally important, the continuity of the relationship. The nurse, on the other hand, cannot establish such a relationship. She is distinctively dressed, assumes a specific role and is often associated with pain or discomfort.

In addition the child is looked after by many people, each with his own personality, standards and attitudes which must be very confusing. He must transfer loyalty and affection to constantly changing groups of people. The many nursing functions do not make it possible to give the child undivided attention.

The need for a stable person, whose function it is to ensure that the child is occupied and has the opportunity to play and be creative as well as find relief from his pent up feelings, has been recognised for some time. However, there is still no agreement on who such a person should be. Some hospitals employ people who have had some experience with children, perhaps their own, others utilise the services of nursery nurses who have been trained to look after young children and in the art of play. Another group who would qualify for this task are those who have been trained in nursery school work and are concerned with the early socialisation and education of the young child.

The advantage of having one individual looking after children's recreation in hospital is that it ensures relative permanency. Also, the person is not involved in any painful event and she therefore acts as a safety-valve. It does, however, mean that the nurse may be identified with painful and unpleasant events only. In such situations it is important that the nurse does not relinquish totally her comforting role.

Function of play leader

In some hospitals elaborate provisions are made to accommodate play. Usually it takes place either in each ward, where an area has been specially allocated for playing and for other activities, or in a play department, where children from all the wards are taken. The advantage of the former is that cross-infection can be limited to each ward, while the latter has the important advantage that the child is taken out of the ward environment and play can take place without the constant interruptions of ward activities. The same applies to school lessons which, in some hospitals, may be given in the ward and in others in a special unit outside the ward.

The play leader (for want of a better title) is responsible for ensuring that the equipment available is suitable for all ages and stages of development. Her role is not to show children how to play

but to create an environment suitable for play and other activities. Suitable equipment including books, dolls, toys which are well made, safe and suitable for most children, paper, pencils, crayons, paint, black-boards, nursery scissors (round-pointed), coloured paper, a sand pit and water. A play-house, with all the usual house equipment in miniature, is enjoyed by both boys and girls. The cost of the equipment is the responsibility of the hospital authority, but its maintenance and storage are the responsibility of the play leader.

The function of the play leader is not only to supervise play, but also to give comfort and support to the child, especially the anxious one. The young infant also requires stimulation. The ill infant is often left alone and it is forgotten that he too requires physical contact and reassurance. Whenever possible, he should be lifted out of his cot and comforted.

Children requiring bed-rest should be occupied in a way suitable for their position in bed and for their condition. For example, the child on traction should be given books to be read to: hand games are useful, particularly when played with other children.

Television and radio or cassette playing can also be used profitably to entertain the child in bed. Finger painting or moulding with plasticine is also useful but care should be taken to protect the bed. Games can be designed to give pleasure and also to be a part of the overall treatment, for example blowing bubbles or cotton wool balls (useful for breathing exercise).

The function of the play leader can thus be seen as an important one, but it should also be remembered that this is not a 24-hour service. The nurse should therefore be aware of the need for play and occupation for children of all ages, and she should accept some responsibility for this function, which is an integral part of the care of the sick child.

Discipline

Maintenance of discipline can be quite a problem when one is dealing with a group of children of varying ages, stages of development and intelligence, but is nevertheless essential if the ward is to be orderly. Children vary in their response to discipline even when it is fair, reasonable and firm. However, the real difficulty arises when too many people assume the responsibility of maintaining discipline. The ward staff consists of a number of adults, each with a specific role and each with her own standards. This can be confusing to the child. The tone of the ward should depend largely on the ward sister/charge nurse, who by her personality and ability to control her staff will also set the standards of behaviour acceptable to her ward. This implies that her requests or instructions should not be countermanded by someone else.

Tantrums, which can be very disturbing to other children, should be handled with patience but with firmness. The violent child should not be allowed to disturb the acutely ill children and it may be necessary to remove him from the ward. Isolation is not intended to be, nor should the child feel that it is a punishment. A nurse should stay with him until he has calmed down and only then will it be possible to ascertain the cause. Physical punishment must never be used. Parents can be of help in solving many discipline problems. Contradiction between staff and parents should be avoided, since this will create acute problems for the child.

Authority itself can create problems of discipline, and the nurse is inevitably an authority figure. The mature and experienced nurse will often find it easier than her less experienced colleague to show flexibility and understanding, assessing each situation as it arises and dealing with it in that context.

Preparation for returning home

The majority of children will be able to return home after treatment in hospital. This entails preparation for both parents and child. A certain amount of psychological disturbance should be expected. This may take various forms, for example:

1. *Regression* to earlier stages in the child's development. The commonest forms are loss of sphincter control, loss of speech and the need for excessive cuddling. Such behaviour may last from a few hours to several days, and varies in severity.
2. *Aggression.* Aggressive behaviour is a natural response to frustration and feeling hurt. While in hospital, the child finds it impossible to act out his aggression; he therefore stores it up and releases it at home.
3. *Night terrors* and sleep disturbance are also common reactions to stress of any sort. The child may fear a repetition of separation and the experience of hospital and may not be able to express these fears, leading to sleep disturbances. Inability to sleep alone causes restlessness and he will want to sleep with his parents to reassure him that they are still there. Parents should recognise that though disturbing for them, it is a real need and the child should be allowed to do so. Gradually he will feel more secure and these episodes will diminish until he is able to sleep on his own again.
4. *Difficulties at school* may also be expected and may be due to anxiety related to separation and the hosptial experience. Teachers should be aware of this possibility and should show understanding.

All these behaviour problems should be explained to parents so that they are prepared and are able to cope with the situation when it arises.

The time of discharge should be suitable to both the parents and the hospital. Transportation should be available, either private or public, depending on the condition of the child. Outpatient appointments should be made before discharge and any special care should be discussed in detail.

The general practitioner should be informed of the child's return home and information should be given regarding hospital treatment and suggested continued home treatment. If the health service functions adequately then the hospital liaison health visitor should also contact the district health visitor so that guidance can continue to be given. This applies particularly to the handicapped and the long-term-care children and also to those whose condition is related to social problems.

It may also be necessary to provide a supply of drugs until the parents can obtain the requisite prescription from the family doctor. Clear instructions should be given with any drug prescribed and a description of the expected side-effects should be given. It also helps if parents can feel free to contact the hospital if they are worried about any aspect of the child's condition.

If an operation has been performed, another factor to consider is the post-operative state of the wound. For example, if stitches are still present, the parents should be given guidance on how to handle the child, how much mobility is recommended and how to bath him. An appointment should also be given for the removal of the stitches. It is often not realised that stitches can be a cause of concern to parents, who may fear that the stitches may burst and that complications may follow. It is equally important that the parents understand not to tamper with the wound nor expose it to family and friends.

Discharge home requires the same careful preparation as admission, and the responsibility for it is with the hospital staff. To ensure that the care of the sick child is continuous and reaches a satisfactory conclusion, all the services involved must work in co-operation.

Chapter 6
Nursing the sick child

Role and responsibility of the nurse in the care of sick children

In the previous section, issues arising out of hospitalisation were raised and discussed. It dealt primarily with the event of admission and the preparation of both parents and child for it. This section considers the nurse-child relationship. This relationship is built on a more tenuous basis than that which the child has developed with his mother. The way the child reacts to any one individual depends on factors such as, the type and extent of the illness, the ability of the nurse to respond to the needs of the child and the degree of security he can obtain in this relationship.

It is also relevant to look at the way the nurse perceives her role. In the position of authority she has a certain amount of power which, to the child, may be a punitive one. However, she also has an important guiding role and takes over many of the functions of the mother. Illness and separation from parents cause stress, not only for the child but also for his parents. He has to adjust to a strange environment. This adjustment can be made easier when a good relationship with a nurse can be established and when the child knows that here is a person who feels for him and accepts him as he is. Firmness is an essential feature of caring but compromise should also be possible. Rules, though necessary, should be adjusted to the needs of the situation.

Demands made on the child should be such that he can cope with them — they should not increase his stress. Verbal communication is an important feature in human relationships. The way the nurse speaks to the child will, therefore, affect their relationship. The child should be spoken to without harshness, in a way that he can under-

stand and in words that he can understand. (Baby talk should be avoided however young the child). Physical contact is also important — how important depends on the age of the child and his emotional needs. This contact is easy to achieve with infants and young children who are dependent on the adult, but may be more difficult with the older child.

The role of the nurse is also that of a good listener. Children do not necessarily want explanations but they want to talk. Some find it difficult to express their feelings and by observation it is possible to detect repressed feelings. The child needs to know that the nurse is aware of his difficulties and is willing to listen. Some questions are difficult to answer, but the answer should nevertheless be as near the truth as possible. For example, the fear of pain is expressed in many different ways, according to the age of the child. The fact that pain is present should be recognised, just as that pain unavoidably caused, should be stated. There is no sense in stating that a procedure will not be painful when it is known to be so. It is also necessary to recognise that the threshold for pain varies with each individual and what is causing great pain to some, may not be so painful to others. Explanations given to the child should be appropriate to his level of understanding. For example, if a child of 5 years who is to have a tonsillectomy asks what the doctor will do, the answer does not have to be details of the technique, but that the doctor will remove the tonsils because they have caused a great deal of ill health and that he will not feel anything during the operation. However, he should be told that there will be some discomfort in his throat, but that this will not last long and that he will still be able to eat and drink. There may be some children who should be given more information. Again it must depend on each child, the type of question asked and how satisfied he appears to be with the explanation given.

PROTECTION OF THE CHILD

It was Florence Nightingale who stated 'that the hospital shall do no harm to the patient'. This statement is as important now as it was then. While the child is in hospital, the nurse's responsibility towards him involves prevention of accidents as well as professional integrity — the carrying out of nursing procedures with skill and understanding.

Prevention of accidents

Falling out of cots

This is a common accident in a children's hospital ward. The cot should be so designed that the cot sides are lockable and are sufficiently high that the toddler cannot climb over. The nurse should therefore ensure that the cot sides are locked after finishing a procedure.

A frequent cause of accident is the infant and young child left for an instant without the protection of the cot sides and the controlling hand of the nurse. This can happen when the nurse turns round without holding on to the child. It is important to remember that even the young infant who may look quiet and does not move about a great deal, can still roll over and fall out.

Bathing

Scalding and drowning are consequences of careless planning of procedures. The temperature of the water should therefore be safe for the child. To prevent drowning requires constant supervision during bathing, and the young child should not be left alone in the bathroom. It is not always possible to prevent children entering the bathrooms, as this depends largely on the lay-out of the ward. Children do not spend such a long time in bed now and have greater opportunity to move around freely and falling into the bath is therefore a real possibility. Each hospital will no doubt have its own rules regarding safety of children in the wards, but rules can only be obeyed if they are readily understood.

Medicines

Drugs and lotions. Any drug must be considered potentially dangerous and kept in a place of safety. The safe custody of drugs is a legal requirement which is binding on all nurses. During the medicine round, all medicines must be kept under the control of the nurse detailed for this task. (See administration of medicines, p. 165.) Lotions must not be left within easy reach of children. When not in use, they should be kept in a locked cupboard. While in use, care should be taken that the child does not handle or drink it.

Running around

The child who is not acutely ill and is allowed up will want to run about. This can easily lead to accidents. A ward is obviously not suitable for this type of activity and some restrictions will need to be placed on this form of play. The same applies to fighting, whether it is friendly or angry in intent.

Equipment (hospital)

Any equipment used must be in working order and mechanically and electrically safe.

Glass thermometers should be checked to ensure that the glass is not broken.

Toys. Many toys are supplied or bought by the hospital authorities. These should be of good quality, i.e. well made and suitable for children of all ages. Any broken toys should be either repaired (if that is possible) or discarded. However, many toys are bought by parents and here too it is important to ensure that they are safe to use. Some toys, particularly cuddly animals or dolls, are made with wires and it is important to examine these carefully and discard them (if necessary) or return them to the parents, if found in a dangerous state. Sparking toys should be used only in the play area, since they may be a source of danger in the vicinity of oxygen administration.

Syringes. Plastic syringes are often given to children to play with. This should be discouraged. There are dangers, for example, that of viral hepatitis being transmitted to children when a syringe has been used for removing blood containing the virus. It should also be recognised that there is a danger of the child building up

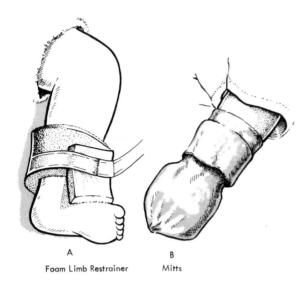

A
Foam Limb Restrainer

B
Mitts

Fig. 6.1 Limb restraints.

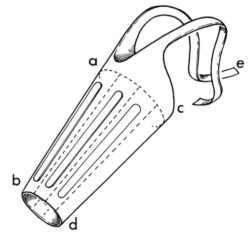

Fig. 6.2 Arm restraint. This can be made from strong cotton. Wooden spatulae are inserted into five slots in the sleeve. The following measurements are useful:

Measurements	Infant size	Toddler size
a–b	17.5 cm	20 cm
c–d	22.5 cm	25 cm
e–a	30 cm	37.5 cm
Circumference at b	14 cm	16.5 cm
Circumference at a	20 cm	23 cm

Note: Point 'a' is on the shoulder and tapes 'e' tie under the opposite arm.

resistance to antibiotics, if the syringe has been used for antibiotic treatment.

Restraints (Figs. 6.1 and 6.2). If these are used, they should be applied in such a way that there will be no constriction to any part of the body. Arm and leg restraints should be applied to allow some movement without affecting the purpose of their application, e.g. to prevent scratching, to prevent handling the infusion needle, etc.

Mistaken identity

Each child should be readily identified. It is easy to mistake a child's identity when one considers the number of people involved in performing some procedure with or on him. To know a child well is only possible when one is with him for some considerable time, and of all the people working in a hospital, the nurse is the only one who has continuous contact with him. Mistakes, however, do occur and most institutions have developed a system of identification of children. Rules have also been drawn up to ensure that the child receives the treatment or investigation which is intended for him.

Identi-bands are widely used. These can be applied to either wrist or ankle. They should contain the child's name, age, ward number and date of admission. The plastic band tends to cause sweating and it is advisable to change the identi-band once in 24 hours or more frequently. When changing the identi-band it is advisable to check that the correct one has been applied. All treatment should be checked against the name band and all documents relevant to the treatment should accompany each child to whatever department he has to attend.

Observation of the child

The nurse's function does not include that of diagnosis, but since she is with the child more than any other member of the caring team, she is expected to observe the child carefully and to report accurately her observations. However trivial the observations appear, it may be a link in the chain which will enable the doctor to arrive at some decision, either to investigate further or to prescribe treatment on the basis of the presenting symptoms. In some cases nurses have the responsibility to initiate treatment to relieve a distressing condition, but to do so she must have some understanding of the principles underlying the treatment, for example, giving oxygen when there is difficulty in breathing.

Observation of the child is also a routine everyday event which is generally done with little conscious effort. When nursing the sick child all the senses become more sensitive so that any change, however small, can be recognised and an assessment can be made of the observations and, where necessary, action taken. Whatever procedure is performed on the child and even where no active nursing is taking place, observations of some kind will be necessary. This section will therefore discuss the relevant observations and their interpretation.

OBSERVATION OF FACE AND SKIN

Face

Facial expression
The face is the most expressive part of the body and is extensively used as a means of communication. Points to note: is the expression alert, anxious, pained or quite placid? For example, constant grinning may be due to spasm of the masseter, found in tetanus.

Mouth
Presence of abnormality such as cleft lip, the condition of the lips, whether dry and cracked and the presence of sores such as herpes simplex.

Tongue
The tongue may be clear or coated and in conditions such as scarlet fever, the tongue has a strawberry appearance. There are other causes such as local infection, mechanical trauma or systemic disorder such as avitaminosis (particularly of the B group). Mucous membrane of the mouth: presence of white patches may be an indication of thrush. These white patches may look like milk flakes but, unlike milk, cannot be removed.

Gums
Gums should look healthy and firm, but if infected may be spongy and bleeding. Presence of pus should also be noted. Gingivitis can be due to several factors, e.g. long continued use of drugs like diphenylhydantoin.

Breath
The breath may be clean smelling or offensive (perhaps due to decomposition of food). In diabetic coma the breath will smell of acetone.

Teeth
This depends largely on the age of the child and the number of teeth (p. 95). The colour and state (healthy or decayed) of the teeth should be noted. Some children may have artificial teeth.

Skin

Colour of the skin
Pale as in shock or anaemia.

Flushed as in increased temperature though there may also be a pinkish flush in condition such as measles and scarlet fever.

Cyanosis. This is a bluish hue and indicates the state of oxygenation of the blood in the capillaries of the skin or mucous membrane. Cyanosis at birth may be due to cyanotic congenital heart condition.

Yellow. Discolouration of tissues occurs due to bile pigments and is found in jaundice.

Texture of the skin
The skin should be elastic and pliable but under certain conditions may be dry and lustreless, as in cretinism. There may also be excessive sweating, such as found in fibrocystic disease of the pancreas. There may be marks indicating previous operation scars or marks due to irritation caused by the itch mite (sarcoptes scabiei). Many infectious diseases can be recognised by the appearance of different types of spots and there may be subcutaneous bleeding in the form of petechiae or bruises.

POSTURE
Observation of posture can also indicate the state of health and level of ill health, for example:

1. Knees drawn up in an effort to relax the abdominal muscles indicate abdominal pain.
2. Lying sunken in bed may indicate extreme weakness.
3. Lying with head retracted and spine arched, may indicate cerebral irritation, as in meningitis.
4. Sitting up supported by pillows may ease

breathing, particularly in conditions affecting the heart and lungs.

OEDEMA

This is due to excessive fluid in tissue spaces. It is demonstrated by 'pitting', when applying pressure with the thumb or fingers. This may be found in the face, particularly the eyelids, in the sacral region and the extremities. It is also important to recognise different types of oedema, e.g. oedema surrounding an area of inflammation, or oedema caused by pressure from plaster of paris.

PAIN

This can be observed by the expression and behaviour pattern of the child. Only the patient can feel his pain and the nurse's function is to assess the level of pain and where it is felt most. Reporting pain should always be based on the information obtained by observation and the comments made by the child. It is not the nurse's function to minimise or maximise the discomfort nor to judge the behaviour of the child in response to pain.

Infant

The infant and very young child cannot yet express his feelings in language, but it is possible to learn a great deal from his behaviour. For example, the position adopted, the type of cry and the intensity of his cry; any specific movement indicating pain, e.g. head moved from side to side may indicate painful ears; drawing up legs and screaming may indicate abdominal pain.

Older child

The older child can usually describe the pain and indicate its location.

Duration of pain
Whether it is continuous or spasmodic.

The time when pain occurs
1. Its relation to food intake — whether intensified or relieved when taking food.
2. Before or after taking food.
3. Its relation to movement.

Character of pain
1. Smarting pain — burning sensation.
2. Shooting pains — involving nerve tissue.
3. Stabbing pain.
4. Colicky pain.

EYES

The nurse should note the following:

1. Colour of the sclera — whether bluish, yellow (as in jaundice) or bloodshot.
2. Discharge, may be watery or purulent. Presence of photophobia (dislike of light) found in conditions such as measles.
3. Pupils:
   a. Reaction to light.
   b. Whether equal or unequal. Not infrequently one pupil may be larger than the other. This may occur in bright light or in subdued light. In cerebral injury, this is an important point to note (see unconscious child).
   c. Dilated pupils may be associated with fear, excitement and atropine poisoning.
   d. Contracted pupils are found, for example, in narcotic poisoning.
4. Presence of squint (strabismus).
5. Ability to close lids.
6. Ptosis (drooping of the upper eyelid).

EARS

The nurse should note the following:

1. Ability to hear — does the child respond to sound?
2. Discharge — type of discharge, e.g. purulent (may be due to otitis media or a boil in the external auditory meatus).
3. Presence of pain and the area involved, e.g. behind the ear and accompanied by swelling may be due to inflammation of the mastoid bone.
4. Tinnitus — ringing or buzzing in the ears, may be associated with overdose of some drug, e.g. aspirin, but may also be due to wax in the ears.

CRY OF THE INFANT

The only way an infant can express himself is by crying. Each infant has his own characteristic cry and only experience will help to identify what he is trying to say. However, there are some common features in every baby's cry which can be recognised as having special meaning.

1. An angry cry with fists in his mouth denotes hunger.
2. An angry cry with excessive movements of hands and legs indicates frustration or anger.
3. A shrill, piercing cry — spasmodic as in pain.
4. A shrill, 'gander-like' cry is suggestive of meningitis.
5. A weak, whimpering cry denotes general weakness.

OBSERVATIONS RELATED TO FUNCTIONS OF THE DIGESTIVE TRACT

Appetite is the desire for food.

Anorexia is loss of appetite.

Excessive appetite is the need to eat constantly and greedily.

Pica is an abnormal, voracious appetite.

Meal times are suitable for making observations of:

1. The amount of food taken.
2. Variations in appetite and any obvious causes, e.g. anxiety, unhappiness and/or infection.
3. Dysphagia — difficulty in swallowing.
4. Vomiting — whether associated with food intake.
5. Manner of vomiting:
   a. Effortless.
   b. Projectile, i.e. forceful ejection as in pyloric stenosis.
   c. Accompanied by retching and pain.

Characteristics of vomitus

1. Small, mouthful, occurring frequently, e.g. in rumination.
2. Copious, sour smelling, e.g. in gastroenteritis.
3. Green fluid, e.g. postanaesthetic or intestinal obstruction.
4. Undigested food, e.g. in gastritis.
5. Yellowish-green (bile stained), e.g. in intestinal obstruction.
6. Brown fluid, e.g. in intestinal obstruction.
7. Brown faecal, e.g. in intestinal obstruction.
8. Coffee ground — blood altered by gastric juices, e.g. gastric ulcer.
9. Fresh blood — both (8) and (9) are described as haematemesis, e.g. in gastric ulcer.

Abdomen

Observations of the following features are important:

1. Distension of abdomen; this may be due to flatus or obstruction.
2. Retraction — as in dehydration.
3. Rigidity — tenseness — as in peritonitis.
4. Visible peristalsis — as in pyloric stenosis or intestinal obstruction.

Stools

Early detection of abnormal constituents is an important aid to diagnosis.

Points to note

Colour, quantity, odour and consistency.

Normal stool

The normal stool is brown in colour, well formed and has a characteristic odour.

An infant's stool should be light yellow and soft in consistency. As the child gets older and his diet changes from milk foods to solids, the stool will become brownish and more formed.

Odour. Abnormal constituents produce abnormal odours. In children suffering from coeliac disease and fibrocystic disease of the pancreas, it is very offensive.

Meconium. This is the term given to the first stool passed by the infant after birth. The stool is dark green, thick, tenacious and unformed. It consists of debris from the intestinal tract and contains mucus.

Abnormal constituents

1. *Blood* (fresh). A well-formed stool containing blood indicates a bleeding point in the rectum or at the anal sphincter, e.g. anal fissure.

   A loose stool containing blood may indicate disease affecting the colon, e.g. ulcerative colitis.

   A loose stool containing blood and mucus may indicate dysentery.
2. *Pus.* A yellowish mucoid material as found in infection, e.g. abscess.
3. *Mucus.* Slimy, found in colonic irritation or disease affecting the gastro-intestinal tract.
4. *Green stool.* Generally due to infection, particularly in infants.

5. *Fatty stool.* Found in coeliac disease and fibrocystic disease of the pancreas.
6. *Black tarry.* Can be due to iron intake.
7. *Melaena.* This stool also looks tarry but may show a tinge of red. It indicates presence of blood due to bleeding of the upper digestive tract, e.g. gastric ulcer.

Observation also involves the act of defaecation. Any difficulty experienced during defaecation, e.g. straining, should be noted and reported. If the child complains of pain or if pain is suggested by the behaviour of the child, e.g. screaming, this must be reported. Anal fissures are a common cause of pain during defaecation and are due to dilatation of the anus and further tearing.

OBSERVATION OF MICTURITION AND URINE
The following points should be observed indicating abnormal functions:

1. *Amount.* The amount of urine passed will vary with the age and condition of the child. (See normal kidney function, p. 527.) In some cases the urinary output is measured accurately as an indication of renal function. In the infant this can only be done accurately by applying a 'urobag' and draining it into a collecting bag. However, under normal circumstances it is possible to estimate urinary output by noting the degree of moisture of the nappy or sheet.
2. *Frequency.* This is closely related to amount but not necessarily so. If the child asks for a bedpan/urinal frequently or wets his bed excessively, it should be noted and reported.
3. *Odour.* Normal urine has a characteristic smell. In some diseases abnormal constituents will alter this, e.g. a fishy smell may indicate bacterial activity. New-mown hay smell indicates acetone, found in cases of diabetes mellitus or acidosis. Smell of honey may be indicative of phenylketonuria.
4. *Colour.* Normal urine is amber in colour, but the shade depends on the concentration. The deeper the amber, the greater the concentration, the lighter the lower the concentration. Some urine may look like water: this indicates low concentration and is usually also related to large amounts. This is found for example in diabetes insipidus.

Reddish colour usually indicates presence of blood.

Deep yellow colour may indicate presence of bile.

The act of micturition should also be observed. For example, pain when passing urine may be associated with inflammation of the bladder or urethra and may be due to presence of stones.

Terms used to describe amount and type of urine passed are:

1. *Anuria.* Absence of urine indicates:
   a. No urine excreted by the kidneys (renal failure), or
   b. Urine repressed, i.e. not passed.
2. *Oliguria.* Little urine passed (renal insufficiency, nephrosis).
3. *Polyuria.* Large amounts of urine passed (diabetes mellitus and insipidus).
4. *Incontinence.* Involuntary passing of urine.
5. *Retention.* Urine is retained in the bladder.
6. *Suppression.* No urine is excreted by the kidneys.
7. *Enuresis.* Bedwetting.
8. *Diuresis.* Increased output.
9. *Dysuria.* Pain in passing urine.
10. *Haematuria.* Blood present in urine.
11. *Glycosuria.* Sugar present in urine.
12. *Pyuria.* Pus present in urine.

OBSERVATION OF COUGHING AND ITS EFFECT
Coughing is a reflex action in an effort to discharge an irritant from the respiratory tract. There are a number of features about coughing which can indicate the type of condition responsible for the cough and the product of coughing.

The following characteristics can be observed:

1. Dry or moist cough. In early bronchitis the cough is dry but after one or two days it becomes moist.
2. Short and restrained, usually due to pain.
3. Short and frequent as in bronchiolitis.
4. Spasmodic as in whooping cough.
5. Barking as in laryngeal stridor.

The effect of coughing is to remove sputum from the inflamed respiratory tract. It may contain blood, mucus and pus.

The following observations are important:

1. Quantity: whether scanty or copious.
2. Time at which sputum appears to be more profuse, e.g. excessive amounts early in the morning as found in bronchiectasis.
3. Consistency:
   a. Fluid — clear.
   b. Tenacious — thick.
   c. Mucus.
   d Muco-purulent.
4. Colour:
   a. Blood as in haemoptysis.
   b. Greenish — indicating presence of pus.

OBSERVATIONS RELATING TO THE NERVOUS SYSTEM

Disorders of the nervous system require careful observation and accurate recording is essential. This involves recognition of the various levels of consciousness and the power or ability to move, and aspects of behaviour and mental state. Observation of sleep is also important as an indication of certain mental and physical states. The amount of sleep, whether sleep is restful or restless, whether sleep is disturbed by dreams and whether the child talks during sleep must be included in the observation.

Levels of consciousness. (See Chapter 17 for greater detail, in particular, the section on the care of the unconscious child, p. 302.) Observations should include the child's response to stimuli, whether he is disorientated, incoherent, or hallucinated.

Ability to move and the type and form of movement should be noted.

Inability to move (paralysis). The following points should be noted:

1. Mode of onset, i.e. whether sudden or gradual.
2. Areas involved: whether hemiplegic (one side only) and which side is involved or paraplegic (both lower limbs).

Inability to speak (aphasic) or loss of voice (aphoria).

Presence, type and location of convulsions

(p. 305). Observations include, the onset and duration of the convulsions; whether local, e.g. right arm, or generalised, i.e. affecting the whole body.

Routine nursing procedures

Routine nursing care includes procedures such as bathing and feeding infants and children of different ages as well as procedures which are necessary for the comfort of the child. Bathing and feeding of infants and children has been discussed in Chapter 2 and these procedures apply also to most sick children. There are, however, some children for whom different methods must be used, e.g. the child who is on bed-rest whose activity is limited, is a suitable case for a bedbath.

The following procedures will be discussed under routine nursing procedures:

1. Examination and care of a verminous head.
2. Tepid sponging.
3. Bedbathing.
4. Care of pressure areas.
5. Care of the mouth and teeth.
6. Toilet needs.

Care of the hair

Combing the child's hair is a routine activity which normally does not require detailed comment. However, the care of the child's hair involves not only routine combing, brushing and washing, but also examination for prevention of and treatment for vermin.

The presence of head lice is creating a problem which is proving difficult to solve. Theoretically it is simple enough through education to make the elimination of head lice a possibility, but it is not so simple because it needs only one infested child to transmit it to other children.

The number of people infested at any one time cannot be determined accurately because it is not a notifiable condition. It is easier to calculate the number of children infested since they are subject to regular inspection within the school system, but despite these examinations and the treatment available there appears to be an increase in the number infested.

Schools provide the ideal setting for the spread of infestation because children have close physical contact both in the classroom and during play.

The head louse inhabits that region of the hair nearest the scalp, approximately half an inch (1.25 cm) from the scalp surface. It can, however, be seen crawling further away and also to other hairy parts of the body, e.g. the eyebrows. The proximity of the scalp is necessary for feeding purposes.

The nits (eggs) are laid by female lice on the hair shafts near the scalp and each egg, measuring 0.8 × 0.3 mm is firmly attached to the hair. It is generally believed that the head louse is found only on people whose personal hygiene leaves much to be desired, but studies of lice behaviour suggest that the lice favour a clean environment.

Method of examination
Privacy is essential since this is embarrassing for the child. A plastic cape is placed round his shoulders, not so much to protect the child, but to gather any falling lice. Every child should have his hair examined for nits and lice. In the first instance visual examination would indicate the presence of nits. Newly laid nits are found near the hair insertion, older nits move up with the growing hair. Nits can be seen all over the hair but larger colonies can be found behind the ears, on the nape of the neck and on the crown of the head. It is also possible to see the lice crawling about.

Method of combing and treating the hair
The requirements are:

1. Ordinary comb.
2. Fine-toothed comb.
3. Gauze swabs or old, clean cotton material.
4. Disinfectant, e.g. chlorhexidine in alcohol.
5. Disposal bag.
6. Treatment lotion in current use, e.g. Prioderm.

Method. The child's shoulders are covered with a protective plastic sheet and the hair is combed normally, removing all tugs. Care should be taken to prevent lice falling all over the bed. Using a fine-toothed comb, each part of the head is combed, removing as many lice as possible. A moistened swab should be held in readiness as each comb sweeps down the hair. This is to collect the lice. The moistened material prevents further movement of lice and is discarded into the disposal bag. When the whole head has been combed, the lotion is applied according to instructions. Generally the lotion is sprinkled on to the head and is then massaged into the hair, where it remains for 12 to 24 hours, after which the hair is washed and re-examined. A further application may be necessary.

The female louse lays about seven to eight eggs a day. The nymph (newly hatched louse) sucks hard from the scalp immediately it is hatched. Each head louse lives on average, about 10 days.

To obtain food, the lice break the skin in order to feed by sucking blood. By doing so, they introduce saliva which produces irritation resulting in scratching. This almost invariably leads to secondary bacterial skin infection, e.g. impetigo.

Several substances have been found useful, though some, like DDT, have the disadvantage that the lice become resistant to it. Prioderm has the advantage that it stays on the hair sufficiently long to kill the lice and is also lethal to the eggs or nits. Death of the nits is said to occur within seconds of contact with this substance.

Tepid sponging
Pyrexia (increased body temperature) can occur due to increased metabolic activity in response to infection by micro-organisms. Chemotherapeutic agents, like aspirin or those more specific to the infection, e.g. antibiotics, are given. The action of aspirin is not clealy understood but it appears to have an anti-pyretic action, while antibiotics destroy micro-organisms which leads to a fall in temperature. Systemic treatment is sometimes suggested by local relief of pyrexia and the method of choice is tepid sponging. In some hospitals this is only done when required by the medical officer.

Principle
The principle of tepid sponging makes use of the fact that a moist body loses heat more rapidly than a dry one. Normally excess heat is lost by sweating and evaporation of water. In hyperpyrexia, sweating is not effective in decreasing body heat, particularly if the environment is hot and still and cannot take up moisture from the skin. Tepid sponging cools the air surrounding the skin

allowing evaporation of sweat and this decreases the body temperature.

Reducing the body temperature, when it is high, to a reasonable level, is important but is not without danger. A sudden rapid decrease leads to shivering (this increases temperature) and may also lead to shock which is indicated by pallor. The pulse rate increases and the volume of the pulse falls.

Requirements are the same as for bedbathing with the additional equipment:

1. Cool water at a temperature of 29 to 32 °C.
2. Several sponges or disposable cloths.
3. Clinical thermometer.

Method

If the child is old enough, the procedure should be explained to him. The temperature, pulse and respiration are taken first. This is important in assessing the effectiveness of the treatment.

The bedclothes and patient's clothes are removed and he is left covered with a cotton blanket or bathing sheet. The moist cool sponges are placed in the nape of the neck, the axillae and groin. As the sponges become warm they are changed and replaced with cool sponges. The body is sponged, leaving some moisture. The evaporation of this moisture should reduce the body temperature.

The temperature is taken again. A reduction of 0.5 to 1 °C is considered satisfactory. If there is no reduction, the procedure may be repeated. If the reduction in temperature is greater than 1 °C, the child should be observed carefully. The pulse and breathing rate are also checked. The child is dressed and the bed linen is changed, leaving the child comfortable.

Bedbathing

The child who is confined to bed will not be able to be taken to a bath, but nevertheless it is important that he is clean and fresh. Bedbathing is not as refreshing as a bath but it may be the only method applicable in certain circumstances.

The principles of bedbathing are:

1. To ensure that the child receives a bath in as short a time as possible.

2. To prevent excessive muscular activity and exertion, where applicable.
3. To prevent cooling of the body by avoiding excessive exposure.
4. To leave the child comfortable.

Requirements for bedbathing

1. Usual bathing equipment.
2. Sheets for changing bed linen.
3. Clean clothes.
4. Two bath sheets.
5. Basin and water jug.
6. Containers for used linen.

The temperature of the water should be hand hot, i.e. approximately 44 °C and if no sink is available, a pail should be available for the used water.

Method

An explanation should be given to the child and privacy should be provided. Draughts should be eliminated by closing adjacent windows and doors. He should be asked if he has any special likes or dislikes, e.g. he may not like soap on his face. It is also advisable to give him a bedpan or urinal before commencing.

The upper bedclothes are removed and the child is left covered with a cotton blanket or large bathing towel. Another bathing sheet/towel is placed under him. The child is then undressed and kept covered as far as is possible. One part of the body is washed and dried, before the next part is exposed and washed. Washing should be from above downwards, leaving the genitalis and anal region to the last. The front part of the body can be washed first, the child being gently turned to wash his sides and back. While in this position, pressure care can be carried out. If the child is old enough and fit enough, he may wish to wash his buttocks, etc. himself, however, it is still the nurse's responsibility to ensure that they are clean and to satisfy herself that there is no discharge or any other abnormality. Children of 10 and upwards are usually responsible enough to report anything unusual, but they may be shy or embarrassed to talk about it.

When the process has been completed, the child is dressed and the bed linen changed. Finger and toe nails should be cut and it is often appreciated by the child if he is allowed to place his hands in a basin of water, rather than having them washed with a cloth only.

Once the bed has been made, the hair is combed and tidied. Any observation made during the procedure should be noted. The equipment is removed and the area is left tidy.

Care of pressure areas

A pressure area is any part of the body which is subjected to pressure of the body on the bed (Fig. 6.3). The pressure is always present but becomes a problem when the child is unable or unwilling to move himself. The tissue concerned will gradually be deprived of blood, the skin becomes red and eventually breaks. Moisture and friction aggravate the condition, when the skin becomes soggy and soft and breaks easily.

There are several areas which are particularly prone to pressure sores and these are found where a bony part is prominent. The following areas are usually found to be subject to injury: shoulders; elbows; buttocks; vertebral column; sacral region; coccyx; knees; heels and ankles.

Prevention is by far the most important aspect of nursing, particularly since the healing of pressure sores requires considerable time and patience.

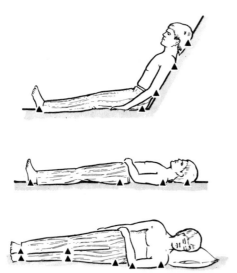

Fig. 6.3 Pressure areas. ▲ marks the areas which can be subjected to pressure.

General measures
These aim at improving the nutritional state and maintaining a good diet which includes high protein and high vitamin intake, particularly vitamin C. Physiotherapy is also useful and in appropriate cases passive or active exercises can be given.

Local measures
1. Turning or moving the child frequently, will relieve the pressure.
2. Cleanliness and dryness. Bedclothes are changed frequently. Sheets should be soft and free from wrinkles and crumbs. After a bath, the skin should be dried gently and to absorb moisture, fine talcum powder can be applied to the skin. Care should be taken to flake it off to prevent 'caking' since this could be a cause of pressure sores.
3. Use of special equipment to relieve pressure, e.g. ripple mattress, sheepskin pads.

Treatment for prevention of pressure sores
This involves more energetic prophylactic measures, e.g. stimulation of the circulation by gentle massage and protection of the skin by applying a suitable barrier cream, tincture benzoin compound or oil and spirit. The choice depending on the policy of each unit.

Treatment of pressure sore
A pressure sore may be treated conservatively or surgically. Again no specific agent can be said to be absolutely effective in every case. The sore should be treated as any wound using aseptic technique. (See Dressing technique, p. 137.) If slough is present, it should be removed. Enzymatic digestive agents such as trypsin or streptokinase solution may be useful. Anti-microbial lotions may help to combat infection locally and systemic application of antibiotics may also be given as a necessary adjuvant to local therapy.

Care of teeth

Dental disease is one of the commonest causes of ill health. It is responsible for a great deal of pain and discomfort as well as being debilitating and disfiguring. Since dental disease is preventable, it

Table 6.1 Dental development

Deciduous teeth (20 in number)	Number	Time of eruption (months)	Permanent teeth (32 in number)	Number	Time of eruption (years)
Lower central incisors	2	5–9	1st Molars	4	6–7
Upper central incisors	2	8–12	Incisors	8	7–8
Upper lateral incisors	2	10–12	Premolars	8	9–10
Lower lateral incisors	2	12–15	Canines	4	12–14
Anterior molars	4	12–15	2nd Molars	4	12–15
Canines	4	18–24	3rd Molars	4	17–25
Posterior molars	4	24–30			

is important to look at areas where the nurse can play a part in preserving children's teeth.

Teeth are of different sizes and shapes, but in any tooth, three parts may be distinguished, namely the *crown*, visible above the gum; the *neck* covered by the gum and the *root*, held in the socket of the maxilla or mandible. When the tooth is sectioned, it is found to be composed of an outer layer of very hard material, the *enamel*; this covers only the crown. Underneath the enamel crown, and covering the neck and root, is a less dense material similar to hard bone. This is called *dentine*. In the centre of the tooth is the pulp which is made up of nerve fibres and blood vessels. Between the dentine of the root and the bone of the jaw is a thin layer of modified bone called the *cementum*.

Man receives two sets of teeth. The temporary, milk or deciduous teeth appear normally after birth, though on rare occasions a baby may be born with one or more teeth already cut. The permanent teeth are present within the jaw though not fully formed until some years before the milk teeth fall out.

Dental caries

The teeth decay from without inward. Once the protective enamel is broken, the less resistant dentine is easily affected by bacteria which readily find their way to the pulp where the nerves are. This results in toothache (Fig. 6.4).

Causes of dental decay

No single microbial agent is believed to be responsible for dental caries but acidogenic bacteria and streptococci, for example, are capable of producing a pH of 5.5 or lower (normal pH is 7.2). Ferment-

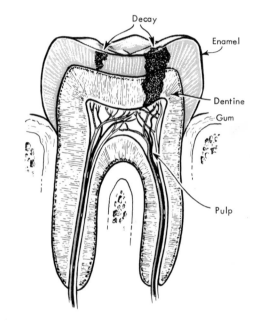

Fig. 6.4 Tooth decay.

able carbohydrates are used by bacteria, producing lactic acid. The bacterial plaque formed serves as an area which favours local acid production and this prevents the saliva acting as a buffer.

Carbohydrates are considered the single most important substance responsible for dental decay, but the frequency rather than the total quantity is important, for example, frequent between-meal snacks of sweets, biscuits and sticky sweet foods.

It should also be recognised that the condition of a child's teeth depends partly on heredity, partly on the diet of his mother during pregnancy, partly on the way he cleans his teeth and on his eating habits.

Prevention of dental decay

There are several ways in which prevention of tooth decay may be achieved.

1. Protection of teeth by *fluoridation* of water supply. It has been known that fluoridation of water supply considerably reduces the amount of dental decay among children. It has been suggested that when fluoride is added at a level of 1 part per million during the period when the teeth are being calcified, maximum benefit can be achieved. Fluoride becomes incorporated into the apatite crystal, forming the less soluble fluor-apatite. Excessive fluoride may cause mottling. Where fluoridation is not the policy, fluoride tablets have been recommended. They are taken last thing at night after brushing teeth.

2. Teeth may also be *scaled* using phosphoric acid and ultraviolet light technique. This is also considered a valuable method of protecting teeth.

3. *Brushing* is still the simplest way of protecting teeth, but unless it is done effectively, it will not fulfil its function. Children should be taught to brush their teeth at least after breakfast and last thing at night. The teeth should be brushed in a rolling motion, from the gums towards the biting surface and the bristles should penetrate the space between each tooth. This can be difficult if the teeth are too close to each other. In this case, older children in particular, can be taught to use dental floss to remove dental plaque or food particles. Rinsing the mouth is also of value and he can be taught to force the water between the teeth.

4. *Food eating habits.* From a dental point of view, children as well as adults eat too often and too many sweets and soft foods. It is suggested by dental experts that more hard fruits and vegetable should be eaten. For example, salted nuts, apples, carrots, celery, etc. However, it has also been recognised that foods which produce acidity in the mouth should not be eaten last thing at night, e.g. apples.

5. The child should *visit the dentist* at 6-monthly intervals. The habit of visiting the dentist should be started as early as possible so that expert advice can be given should any difficulties present themselves. For example, there may be overcrowding of teeth and this may require future orthodontal treatment. Early detection of tooth decay may prevent spread to other teeth and here too preventive care can be instituted.

Care of mouth and teeth of the sick child

The same care should be provided for the child in hospital as that provided at home. Each child should have his own tooth mug, toothbrush and toothpaste and tooth care should be part of the daily ward routine. There are, however, some differences in care where the child is unable to carry out this procedure himself.

The secretions of the mouth and tonicity of the tissue may be affected quite considerably when a child is ill. In health, these tissues are kept moist and clean by saliva secreted by the salivary glands and by the secretions of the small accessory glands of the mouth. In ill health, these functions may be disrupted and the aim of the nurse should be to keep the mouth and teeth clean and fresh and to prevent dental decay.

Infants

To maintain the healthy state of the mouth when the infant is febrile, toxic or dehydrated, small quantities of cooled boiled water should be given to drink between feeds. Sweetened water or drinks of concentrated rose-hip syrup given regularly between feeds is not advisable; the latter substance in particular alters the pH value which encourages bacterial plaque formation leading to dental caries. It is important to remember that developing teeth can also be affected before eruption.

Methods of oral hygiene for older children

The child who is confined to bed and is unable to sit up, can still manage to brush his teeth and wash out his mouth. A flexistraw can be used to suck up the fluid and a bowl provided to spit out the fluid. Protection for the child and the bed is necessary.

If he is unable to brush his own teeth the following methods can be used:

Swabbing the mouth

The following equipment will be required:

1. Dissecting forceps.
2. Small swab holding forceps or artery forceps.
3. Small swabs or dental rolls.

4. Lotions for use, e.g. glycothymoline.
5. Gallipots.
6. Glycerine.
7. Box of tissues.
8. Disposal bags.

Method. The nurse should wash and dry her hands. Privacy should be provided for the child. Protective sheeting or tissue is placed under the child's chin. Where possible an explanation should be given. The lips are smeared with glycerine to prevent the lotion entering cracks and causing unnecessary pain.

A dressed pair of forceps is used, care being taken to ensure that the forceps are covered and do not injure the child. Artery forceps are safer, because the swab or dental roll can be clamped, thus preventing the swab or dental roll from being pulled or sucked off and inadvertently swallowed. The mouth is gently opened and the inside of the cheeks, teeth, all crevices around the gums, the roof of the mouth and the tongue are swabbed. If the mouth is dirty, several swabs may be required. After swabbing, the lips are dried and again lubricated.

Irrigation of the mouth
This may be the method of choice when the child is unable to open his mouth adequately for cleansing. It may also be the method when trauma or infection is present. The following equipment will be required, and where the area to be treated is damaged, aseptic technique should be used:

1. Syringe with fine catheter No. 10 FG or 4 EG.
2. Jug containing lotion at a safe temperature, i.e. 37 °C.
3. Lotion thermometer.
4. Lubrication for lips.
5. Receptacle for used lotion.
6. Waterproof sheeting to protect the child and the bed.
7. Swabs or tissues.
8. Disposal bag.

Method. Where possible an explanation should be given to the child. The child is protected with the waterproof sheet and gently turned on his side. This is to allow the fluid to run out of his mouth into the receptacle. If he is able to sit up his head is bent forward over the receptacle. The lotion is tested for temperature and the syringe filled. The fluid is then gently introduced into the mouth. The flow of lotion should be directed from behind forwards, and the fluid is allowed to flow over the surface of the tissue but is not directed on to it.

Mouthwashes
Mouthwashes are used before, or in place of, other methods of cleansing to loosen debris from between the teeth. The child should be shown or instructed to swill the lotion around the mouth and to force it several times against the teeth before spitting out into a receptacle.

Gargles
These are excellent for cleansing and soothing purposes, but can only be given effectively to children of 7 years of age and upwards. The solution should be warm and the lotions given for mouth washes can be used for gargles.

Lotions for mouthwashes and irrigation
A variety of substances can be used and the action of each should be understood so that the right choice can be made.

Sodium perborate(Bocasan)
   Action: cleansing and active against anaerobic organisms.
   Strength: one sachet of powder is dissolved in the prescribed amount of water.
   Method: used as a mouthwash, but only for children old enough to understand how to use it. The child must hold the fluid in his mouth for one and a half minutes. If this creates difficulties, a dental roll soaked in the solution can be sucked, or the dental roll can be placed just inside the cheek alongside the gums. The substance should not be swallowed. Sodium perborate is effective while nascent oxygen is released. It is this effervescent action that is important and it is therefore of little value unless it can be retained in the mouth for the recommended length of time.
   Indication: infected mouth.
   Contra-indication: this substance should not be used where there is an open wound in the mouth, as it can drive micro-organisms into the raw surface.

Hydrogen peroxide
   Hydrogen peroxide 10 volumes
   Action: cleansing and active against anaerobic organisms.
   Strength: one teaspoonful of hydrogen peroxide to 5 ounces (150 ml) water.
   Method: indication and *contra-indication* are as for sodium perborate.

   Bicarbonate of soda
   Action: cleansing and fat solvent.
   Strength: 1 in 80.

Method: as a mouthwash, swabbing the mouth or as in irrigation.

Indication: (1) sores in the mouth; (2) following surgery 4 hours after all evidence of haemorrhage has ceased.

Hypertonic saline
Action: astringent.

Strength: one teaspoonful of sodium chloride to 300 ml of water.

Method: as a mouthwash, swabbing the mouth, or as in irrigation.

Indication: injury to the mouth and following surgery.

Glycothymoline
Action: mildly bacteriostatic, bacteridical and it is also refreshing.

Strength: 1 in 8.

Method: used as a mouthwash, swabbing of the mouth.

Indication: infections of mouth and throat. Tap water is adequate for making the solution unless surgery has been carried out when sterile water and sterile equipment should be used.

Toilet needs

When the older child enters hospital, he will surrender much of the independence he has achieved already. Some of the functions can be readily relinquished, others, and particularly the more personal ones, can produce difficulties. It is not so easy, for example, to micturate and defaecate on a bedpan, yet the child will have to learn to do so if he is not allowed out of bed. The child will also have to be able to make his requirement known. There is a great number of terms which he may use according to the environment of his upbringing. The older child will readily learn to accept, i.e. conform to the hospital pattern of speech but the toddler may well be confused and may continue to use the expressions he has learned from his parents. This means that the nurse has to learn the meaning of the terms which the child uses. Failure to do so can lead to intense frustration for the child and could also be attributed to regression of behaviour, e.g. wetting and soiling.

Methods of toileting depend on the age of the child. The toddler will find it easier to use a potty. It must be recognised, however, that the potty is not quite so stable on a mattress and this can add to the difficulties. The child should not be left alone while on the potty (this applies both to the bedfast child and to the ambulant one). Children cannot be expected to remain seated until they are removed. This often leads to spilling of contents either deliberately or accidentally. Generally as soon as he thinks he is finished, he gets up. It is therefore safer that the nurse should remain with him until he has completed this function.

The pre-school child presents little difficulty, but he may also require reassurance, particularly if not comfortable in the position he is placed. Privacy is also important and should be provided. If the child has difficulties, then the nurse should stay with him.

The older child may wish to cleanse himself, but here too there may be difficulties, he may be too shy to ask for help. Recognition of this difficulty is therefore necessary and steps should be taken to help him.

Hand washing after the use of bedpan or urinal is also necessary and should be part of the routine. Use of urinals for older boys may also require explanation if these have not been used previously. Little boys may find it difficult in bed and help should be given until they feel more confident in using them.

The helpless child

To place a child on a bedpan may require two nurses, one to raise the child's pelvis while the other slips the bedpan under him. Extra pillows may be used to raise him to the semi-sitting position.

Removal of the bedpan involves much the same technique in reverse. Cleansing and treatment of pressure areas are carried out to complete the procedure.

Measuring body temperature

Body temperature is relatively constant in man and the relatively accurate control is achieved by balancing heat loss against heat production. The controlling mechanism is found in the nervous system and the main structures involved are the anterior and posterior hypothalamus. The 'heat centre' in the anterior hypothalamus acts to cool the body, and the 'cold centre' in the posterior hypothalamus acts to warm the body. If the body temperature is increased, the hypothalamus induces sweating, increases breathing and cutaneous vasodilatation, while cooling induces vasoconstriction and shivering.

Heat is not produced uniformly throughout the body, but most of it is produced in the muscles, in the secreting glands and in the liver. It is lost mainly through the skin and lungs. The range of body temperature in a group of healthy persons is quite small and has been found to be from 35.8 to 37.3 °C with a mean of 36.1 °C. However, since the child's heat regulating mechanism is not fully developed until about the age of 3 to 4 years, there are greater fluctuations in his body temperature, particularly at the onset of an illness. There are also temperature variations in different parts of the body. The temperature of the *skin* is not uniform and that is due to the varying activity of different tissues. It will therefore be found that temperature variation will depend on the area measured, e.g. in the axilla or the groin.

Oral temperature can vary from 35.8 to 37.3 °C. It is highest in the evening (between 5 and 8 p.m.) and lowest in the morning (between 2 and 4 a.m.). These variations are related to alterations of environmental temperatures. Exercise may raise oral temperature by 1 to 2 °C. It can also be affected by hot or cold drinks and by the atmosphere, if the mouth is kept open when the nose is blocked. Oral temperature tends to be higher in children and lower in the elderly.

Rectal temperature has generally been assumed to be an accurate index of the temperature of the blood, but it has been found by experiment (Cranston, W. I. (1966) *British Medical Journal*, 2, 69) that the rectal temperature gives a poor indication of rapid changes in blood temperature. When the changes in temperature are slower (as found in infections), the rectal temperature is similar to mouth temperature. The new-born baby, particularly if pre-term, has a rectal temperature of about 1.1 °C below that of the adult. He reaches adult level when he is 10 to 14 days old.

Hyperthermia

A rise in body temperature is due to a disturbance in the heat regulating mechanism. It is most commonly caused by:

1. Infections due to bacteria, viruses or protozoa.
2. Tissue destruction, e.g. rheumatic fever. In pyrexia, there is an increase in heat production and a decrease in heat loss. At febrile tempera-tures, thermoregulation in response to heating or cooling the body is just as precise as in the normal state. This is attributed to resetting of the set point in the heat regulating centre (hypothalamus).
3. Pyrogens. These are substances which produce a rise of temperature. Endogenous pyrogens may be the main cause of many types of fever, e.g. certain steroids are pyrogenic (steroids formed during degradation of adrenocortical and sex hormones).
4. Excessive exercise. Physical exertion produces heat, but there is also a compensatory increase in heat loss. The blood flow through the skin is increased, leading to a rise in skin temperature. The main heat loss in exercise is due to increased secretion and vaporisation of sweat.

Hypothermia

When the temperature of the body is reduced to below 35 °C then a state of hypothermia exists. Hypothermia can occur if a new-born infant is exposed to a cold environment, particularly if he is also pre-term. Hypothermia may also develop rapidly in an infant suffering from acute infection, or from conditions such as respiratory distress syndrome, intracranial haemorrhage, congenital heart disease and hypoglycaemia.

Cold injury

Cold injury is the most serious form of hypothermia occurring in neonates, but is not confined to the first month of life. The causes are similar to those found in the new-born baby, with the additional cause of malnutrition, when the infant has little subcutaneous fat and loses heat rapidly.

Effects of hypothermia (Fig. 6.5)

When the body temperature falls, all the body systems will be affected and the lower the body temperature, the more severe will be the effects.

Nervous system. Cooling of the body depresses the nervous system. The higher cerebral functions are affected first, leading to lethargy, reduced muscular activity and loss of reflexes. Since the nervous system is concerned with temperature regulation, all other systems are directly affected.

Respiratory system. The depression of the central nervous system leads to a depression of the respir-

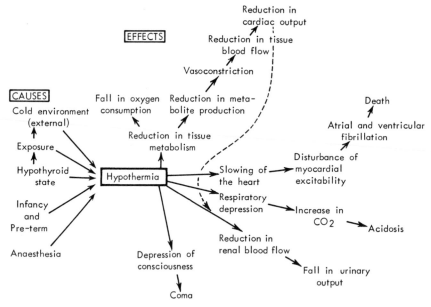

Fig. 6.5 Effects of hypothermia.

atory centre. Breathing is slow and shallow with a prolonged expiratory phase. This leads to carbon dioxide retention and results in acidosis. The lung tissue is also affected by the increased pressure in the pulmonary vessels, leading to pulmonary oedema. Small blood vessels may rupture and blood may be coughed up (haemoptysis).

Cardiovascular system. The heart rate is slowed, partly due to the direct action of the blood temperature on the sino-atrial node. Muscular inactivity prevents adequate venous return, leading to a reduction to cardiac output. There is also a shift of fluid from the blood to the tissues resulting in oedema, haemoconcentration and an increase in blood viscosity. Severe hypothermia also affects the rhythm of the cardiac action producing atrial and ventricular fibrillation.

Renal system. The output of urine is low. This is probably due to a reduction in renal blood flow.

Clinical features

Newborn infant. In mild hypothermia, the feet are cold, but the abdomen is warm, to the touch. In more severe hypothermia both feet and abdomen feel cold. If the hypothermia is secondary to some other condition, there is a sudden fall in body temperature and the infant usually becomes pale and lethargic.

Cold injury. The face and extremities of the affected infant are bright pink and the tip of the nose may be red. The infant refuses his feeds, is lethargic and fails to gain weight. The cry is feeble and whimpering. The skin feels cold to touch and the rectal temperature is often below 34 °C. If the condition is not treated, there is oedema or hardening of subcutaneous fat (sclerema). Breathing is shallow and as the condition deteriorates, the heart rate slows. Pulmonary haemorrhage occurs in the terminal stage.

Principles of treatment and nursing management
1. *Newborn infant.* The infant is placed in an incubator heated to between 29 and 30 °C.
2. *Neonate.*
   a. Rewarming should be gradual, i.e. the environmental temperature should be about 1 or 2 °C above his body temperature, and gradually raised.
   b. Naso-gastric feeds with additional glucose.
   c. Intravenous infusion.
3. *Cold injury.*
   a. Slow warming, i.e. the environmental

temperature should be carefully controlled at 0.5 °C above the rectal temperature and gradually raised by 0.5 °C every hour until a safe environmental temperature has been attained.

   b. Intravenous infusion of 10 per cent glucose may be given if convulsions occur during the rewarming stage. This is due to hypoglycaemia.

   c. Naso-gastric feeds (p. 512).

   d. Antibiotics are given after throat and nasal swabs and blood cultures have been obtained. The choice of antibiotic is important because renal function is often impaired.

4. Routine nursing care.

5. Support for parents. This includes guidance with regard to prevention of hypothermia, e.g. warm environment for the infant; suitable clothes for outdoor wear and recognition of the dangers of exposing a young infant to a cold environment.

Newborn infants, and particularly pre-term infants, tend to have subnormal temperatures because of the poor heat production and increased heat loss. Less heat is produced because of sluggish circulation, weak respiratory movement with poor oxygen consumption, relatively poor muscular activity and, particularly in the pre-term infant, low intake of food. Heat loss is increased because of the relatively greater body surface area and the lack of subcutaneous fat (poor insulation).

Temperature levels

Collapsed state (hypothermia)	below 25 °C
Subnormal	35 °C and below
Normal limits	35.8 °C–37.3 °C
Pyrexia	37.8 °C–(low)–39.5 °C (high)
Hyperpyrexia	39.5 °C and above

Areas where temperature may be measured

1. *Rectum.* This area is suitable for infants and young children or for continuous monitoring.
2. *Axilla.* This area is useful for older children.
3. *Mouth.* This area is not recommended for children, though it may be suitable for children over 12 years of age, or when a thermistor is used.

Types of thermometers in use

1. Glass thermometer (clinical) (Fig. 6.6).
   a. Long bulb thermometer is used for axillary recording.
   b. Short bulb thermometer is used for rectal recording; this is safer than using one with a long bulb.
2. Electronic thermometer (dial reading, with thermistor).
3. Electronic digital reading (with thermistor).
4. Monitors.
5. Disposable thermometers (Temtake).

Times of taking temperature

During the intial stage of illness, this may be 4 hourly. It is then reduced to twice a day, i.e.

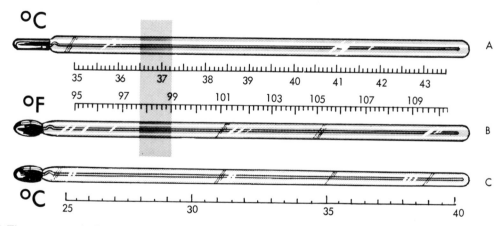

Fig. 6.6 Thermometers. A, For axillary recording. B, For rectal recording (bulb rounded). C, Low registering (rectal).

morning and evening, provided the body temperature has remained relatively normal and steady. If more frequent readings are required, monitoring equipment should be used. This prevents frequent disturbance of the child.

METHOD OF TAKING TEMPERATURE

Axillary (glass thermometer)

Requirements
Thermometer, swabs, antiseptic, e.g. chlorhexidine, Kardex, disposal bag.

An explanation should be given to the child. The young child who is not used to this, may be frightened and may cry. Since this is not a painful procedure, it can be explained to him. He should be asked to hold his arm close to his side or across his chest. Glass thermometers take about 1½ to 2 minutes to register and this is quite a long time (for a small child) to hold still.

The glass thermometer is shaken down to below 35 °C or 25 °C if it is a low registering thermometer. The skin is dried and the thermometer is inserted. The bulb of the thermometer must be between two skin surfaces, i.e. the skin surfaces must be in contact with the bulb. It is held there for the time stated on the thermometer or 1½ to 2 minutes. The thermometer is then removed and the temperature is read and recorded.

The bulb should not be held between the fingers of the operator when reading the thermometer, as this may affect the mercury level and therefore will not give the true temperature of the patient. The thermometer is then washed and replaced in the child's container.

Electronic thermometer
Rectal and oral recordings can be made. To identify each probe the following code is used:

Red — for rectal insertion.
White — for oral or axillary insertion.

Each child should have his own in a container beside his bed (probe only).

The equipment consists of a battery circuit and gauge with an attachment for the probe. There are different types on the market, but the principle is much the same for all. The circuit should be tested (see instructions on the device). The pointer should move to 'test-line'. If it fails to do so it could be due to either battery failure or failure of the system.

Method
Oral measurement. The probe is placed under the tongue.
Axillary measurement. As for glass thermometer.

The lead part is inserted into the instrument and the probe placed in the part to be used. It is left in for 45 seconds; during that time the switch is pressed and held until the pointer stops. The probe is removed and the plug is removed from the meter. The probe is then cleaned with a disinfectant and replaced in its container.

Recording temperature of ambulant children
Excessive exercise increases heat output. It is therefore advisable to let him rest for a little while before taking his temperature. The child should be seated during the procedure and the same method used as described above.

Disposable thermometer
This is a single use chemical thermometer, based on the principle which uses a series of precise temperature sensitive dots. These turn blue to give a reading. It contains no mercury but uses 0.003 g of proprietary chemicals sandwiched in non-sensitising unbreakable plastic layers (non-toxic).

Requirements
Thermometers, disposal bag, Kardex.

Method
This type of thermometer can be used on young children, provided the nurse holds it in position. When there is any doubt, it is safer to use a conventional one rectally.

The Temtake is ready for use by peeling off the polystyrene outer cover. It is then placed in the child's mouth, left in position for 1 minute, withdrawn and read. The last dot coloured is the temperature to be recorded. It is discarded after use.

Rectal method
Whether a *clinical glass thermometer* or an *electronic probe* is used, the method is the same. A trolley

should be available to change the infant's nappy and cleanse the buttocks. During the procedure, the infant should be kept covered and not exposed to public gaze.

The glass thermometer is shaken down to the lowest point. Both types of thermometers are lubricated lightly and the thermometer is inserted into the rectum for an inch (2.5 cm). The child's legs should be supported but not held raised, alternatively he can be placed on his side for this procedure. Each type is left in position for the required time, read, recorded and cleansed as previously described.

Toddler and older child
If the toddler or older child is incontinent, the method is the same as for the infant, except that an explanation should be given. It may also be necessary to have someone assisting, particularly if the child is very unhappy about it. Privacy is also important, even if the child does not require to be cleaned. The thermometer or probe is inserted for 1½ inches (3.7 cm).

Contra-indications
1. Rectum loaded with faeces.
2. Diseases affecting the rectum, e.g. imperforate anus.

Monitor
Temperature may be recorded by skin, oesophagus or rectum.

Method
   Skin. The thermistor is attached with adhesive to any point of dry skin. Cotton wool is placed between the thermistor and the adhesive to ensure effective insulation from outside temperature.
   Oesophagus. The thermistor is lubricated with KY jelly and passed to a midpoint between the nape of the nose and the distal part of the xiphisternum. The flex is attached to the face (cheek) with adhesive tape.
   Rectum. The thermistor is lubricated and passed 1 to 1½ inches (2.5 to 3.7 cm) into the rectum. It is held in position with adhesive tape.
   The flex is then attached to the monitor and constant readings are available.

Measuring and observing the pulse

The pulse is a pressure change which is transmitted as a wave through the arterial wall. When the aorta is full or distended, the wave passes along the walls of the arteries and can be felt at any point where the artery can be pressed against a bone.

These areas are as follows:

1. Radial artery — at the anterior aspect of the wrist.
2. Temporal artery — at the front of the ear or at the temple.
3. Carotid artery — in the neck.
4. Femoral artery — in the groin.

In the infant, where the anterior fontanelle is patent, the pulse can be seen to pulsate. Under certain conditions, nurses are asked to take the apical heart beat.

Points to note about the pulse

Rate
This varies with age, sex, position and activity. In the new-born child and during infancy, the rate may change from 70 beats/min in sleep to 150 beats/min when awake and to 180 beats/min when crying. In older children emotional states have also a marked effect on the pulse rate.

The following table gives approximate values.

Age	Number of beats
Newborn	120–130 beats/min
1 year	110 beats/min
2–5 years	115–100 beats/min
5–10 years	110–90 beats/min

As the child gets older, the pulse rate reaches adult levels, i.e.
   Males — 72 beats/min.
   Females — 84 beats/min.

Rhythm
This determines the regularity with which the heart beat occurs.

Volume — strength
It should be possible to obliterate the pulse with moderate pressure.

Tension
The pulse should feel pliant and soft.

Abnormal variations

Rate
The rate may be increased. This is termed *tachycardia* and is related to the age, sex and activity of the individual. Increase in rate may be found in infections, anaemia and cardiac abnormality. It may be continuous or paroxysmal.

Bradycardia is the term applied to an abnormally slow pulse, e.g. 30 to 40 beats per minute. This is found in head injuries, cerebral tumour and jaundice. It is also associated with drug therapy, e.g. digitalis.

Dicrotic pulse. The beat seems to be followed by a weaker one almost immediately.

Rhythm
Sinus arrhythmia. The pulse is regular, but there is a slight acceleration during inspiration and slight deceleration during expiration. It is more marked in children but is not considered an important deviation and is said to be due to respiratory arrhythmia.

Regular arrhythmia. The interval is not the same, but the rhythm can be grouped. This may occur in heart block.

Irregular arrhythmia. Complete irregularity occurs in atrial fibrillation due to impulses of contractions not being transmitted to the ventricles.

Volume
Changes in volumes are indicated by the following:

1. Thready pulse. This is usually a rapid weak pulse which is easily stopped by pressure. It is found in haemorrhage and exhaustion.
2. Corrigan's or Waterhammer pulse. This is found in aortic valve incompetence; the first half is normal but after reaching its peak, it suddenly recedes under the finger.

Method of feeling the pulse
The child should be at rest either sitting on a chair or bed. It is pointless to attempt to count a pulse when a child has been running about or is distressed by crying.

The radial pulse is felt on the anterior aspect of the wrist, the arm should be supported and relaxed, the nurse feeling for the pulse with her first two fingers. It is recorded for 1 minute, noting its character and any abnormality. It is also important that the nurse's hands are warm.

Distraction for the toddler is essential and usually he can be fascinated by a ticking watch. It is easier to measure the pulse of an infant or toddler while he is asleep; cot sides should therefore not be lowered and the child should be disturbed as little as possible during this procedure. Measurements of the pulse and breathing should therefore be taken before that of the temperature.

Measuring the apical heart beat
Listening to the apical heart beat is more accurate than feeling the pulse. It is the method recommended in cardiac abnormalities. The point of maximum cardiac impulse varies considerably. In a normal sized heart the apex beat could be heard at the different positions of the various age groups as follows:

Infant	The 3rd and 4th intercostal space just outside the nipple line.
From 2 to 5 years	The 4th intercostal space at the nipple line.
Over 5 years	The 5th intercostal space, at or within the nipple line.

The child should be at rest. To listen to the apical heart beat, a stethoscope should be used. The diaphragm of the stethoscope should be warmed by rubbing it with the hand. It is then placed over the point of maximum cardiac impulse and the beats are counted for 1 minute.

Observing and measuring breathing

The act of breathing includes inspiration and expiration and a short period of rest. It is controlled by a collection of cells which are found in the medulla oblongata. Normal breathing should be rhythmical, quiet and regular. The normal rate varies with age, sex, position and activity. During exercise and excitement, for example, the rate will be increased. The following table gives the average rates for different age groups:

Newborn infants	30–35 per min
12 months old	25–30 per min
2 to 5 years old	20–25 per min
Older children	18–20 per min
Adults	16–20 per min

Types of breathing

1. *Shallow*. This type of breathing is associated with rapid breathing. It is found in the following conditions:
   a. Diseases of the lungs and air passages.
   b. Febrile states.
   c. Heart disease.
   d. Haemorrhage and shock.
2. *Deep breathing*. This is associated with a slower rate and may be found in conditions affecting the brain.
3. *Dyspnoea*. This term denotes difficulty in breathing and is found in heart and respiratory diseases. The child is observed to have difficulty with inspiration and expiration. In an effort to overcome this difficulty, he uses his accessory muscles of breathing.
4. *Orthopnoea*. A term applied when the patient is only able to breathe when sitting upright. This is found in severe heart conditions and asthma.
5. *Stertorous breathing*. This describes loud, snoring sounds which accompany breathing. It may be found in unconscious patients.
6. *Sighing breathing*. This is also termed air hunger and is recognised by short inspiration — rapid expiration, and is believed to be due to insufficient supply of oxygen to the respiratory centre of the brain.
7. *Apnoea*. Means cessation of breathing. A transitory form is seen in Cheyne-Stokes breathing, when it is characterised by a gradual quickening and deepening of breathing until a certain pitch is reached. It gradually subsides until

breathing ceases altogether. After a brief pause (a few seconds) the same pattern is repeated.

Method of measuring breathing

1. *Infants*. If the infant is crying, it is impossible to count the rate of breathing. When he is quiet or sleeping, the movements of the chest are observed. Each inspiration and expiration is counted as one.
2. *Toddlers*. The same problems are encountered as in infants. Play during the observation is a useful way to prevent crying.
3. *Older children* present few problems. The chest movements are generally easy to observe and count.

If breathing is shallow and difficult to observe, a hand may be placed gently on the chest and the movements counted. The breathing rate is counted for 1 minute and during that time observations are made of the type and rhythm of breathing.

Respiration monitor

This will record the breathing rate up to 90 per minute. The transducer is attached to the patient's chest with adhesive tape.

Apnoea monitor (Fig. 6.7)

This instrument is valuable as an early warning system both in hospital and at home. Apnoea attacks are believed to be responsible for Sudden Infant Death Syndrome (SIDS). Babies and sometimes young children are found dead in their cots, the cause of which has still not been identified. It is suggested that there may be some fault in the respiratory centre but, in some cases, autopsies have shown the presence of diseases such as pneumonia or meningitis. Where a history of SIDS has been established, apnoea monitors have been issued to parents for subsequent children.

The monitor provides constant surveillance of the small infant. It operates at a pre-selected time interval during which the baby has not taken a breath.

Method. The instrument is pre-checked to ensure that it is in working order. The infant is placed on a small inflated cellular pad. The thermistor is attached to the monitor which is set to the pre-selected time lapse. If the apnoeaic period reaches that level, an alarm is set off.

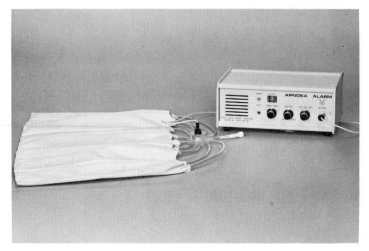

Fig. 6.7 Apnoea monitor, for surveillance of the breathing of infants.

In other types, the transducer is attached to the baby's chest with adhesive tape. The chest movements cause audible signals and if there is no breathing during the pre-selected time interval then the monitor will sound an alarm.

Care of the child receiving radiotherapy

Radiation therapy employs various sources of radiation, e.g. cobalt, caesium and X-ray. In children, radiation therapy is applied externally. The dose and type of radioactive element being used depends on the structure involved. Tissues which are most likely to respond to exposure are those originating from reticulo-endothelial tissues (leukaemia) and those from embryonal tissues (teratoma). Tissues which do not respond so readily are bone and muscle. Rapidly dividing cells like lymphocytes and germ cells are more susceptible than non-dividing cells and highly-differentiated cells such as nerve or muscle cells.

Radiotherapy is used in conjunction with cytotoxic drugs or surgery. The aim of the treatment is to destroy abnormal tissue or interfere with mitosis. The treatment is given in carefully controlled doses for a prescribed period.

Preparation of the child
Although this is not a painful treatment, it is frightening for the child. If he is old enough the physical set-up of the treatment unit should be explained and in some cases it may be advisable to sedate him.

The radiotherapist will mark the area to be irradiated and instructions will be given as to the care of the skin and avoiding removal of the mark. Parents often accompany the child which is reassuring for him, and the treatment can also be given on an outpatient basis. Opaque objects such as pins, buttons and hairgrips are removed and the child is dressed in a cotton gown.

General effects and management
During radiation therapy, a skin reaction may develop but this is usually quite mild. However, skin breakdown may occur due to destruction of normal cells. Washing may be allowed unless instructions to the contrary are given. Initially the skin will be red and this will progressively become brownish. Dry peeling of the skin follows and it then returns to normal. The treated skin should be kept dry and a fine talcum powder should be used.

Rubbing by clothing should be prevented and thought should be given to the type of material worn, e.g. cotton is less irritating than nylon or wool and is to be preferred next to the skin.

It is also recommended that the treated area should not be exposed to strong sunlight, rain or wind.

General malaise and headache may occur as early side-effects and this may be accompanied by nausea and vomiting. Another disturbing effect is the loss of hair. To overcome the trauma of this, the child can be fitted with a wig. Reassurance is essential, in particular, that the loss of hair will not be permanent.

Disposal of radioactive material

Children receiving radioactive isotopes will pass urine and faeces containing these isotopes. Each hospital will issue instructions regarding disposal of contaminated linen and excreta.

Nurses are advised to wear disposable gloves when removing contaminated linen, which is then put into a plastic bag, segregated and disposed of according to the instructions given by the Radiological Protection Adviser. Should the floor or any other area become contaminated, the nurse should wear disposable gloves and mop up the excess liquid with paper towels or tissues and wash the areas with plenty of water. The materials used for mopping up should be placed in a plastic bag and disposed of according to instructions.

Care of the acutely ill child

An acute illness is a state which either occurs suddenly or where a disorder has progressed to the point where the child requires extensive care. It can manifest itself in a variety of ways from a sudden rise in body temperature to difficulty in breathing or convulsions; from a sudden or gradual change from consciousness to the unconscious state.

In an effort to care for a child who exhibits any form of acute change in state it is essential to assess the general state and presenting features and then identify priorities of care. The type of care required will therefore be influenced by the general state of the child and also by his age.

The previous section discussed the importance of observations. Indeed, it is these observations that form the basis on which care must be instituted. It is in relation to the observations that the concept of systematic nursing care can be understood, since the implementation of nursing actions and the ability to respond to changes makes comprehensive nursing both possible and desirable.

It is possible to identify a number of elements which form an integral part of this process. The first part is that of *awareness* of a situation which requires action. This aspect has been fully discussed at the beginning of the chapter and has been followed by a detailed discussion on observation. The next question that arises is what to do with the information obtained. This implies *assessing* the situation to determine the child's problems. It should be stated that the assessment is an ongoing process which begins with the first contact with the child and his parents. This point has also been fully discussed with respect to interviewing both child and parents. However, it is the assessment of changing situation which is demanding and requires a depth of knowledge in an effort to arrive at a suitable decision.

Planning patient care

In response to the observable, i.e. any features exhibited by the patient which constitute either a changing situation or a static one, planning of action is required:

1. It is useful to set goals (either short- or long-term ones) which can be achieved with or without modification.
2. In order to achieve these goals it is necessary to establish priorities. This will also enhance systematic nursing care.
3. To find the most useful methods by which the patient can be helped. These methods will vary in principle but modifications will be required for any given situation. Throughout the book, detailed descriptions are given of various procedures which can be included when required.

Any plan, however, must be flexible to accommodate changing circumstances.

Implementation

This involves the performing of actual nursing care. Any nursing action required must be relevant to the presenting problems and give expression to the goals set. It is the delivery of the patient care which requires a good level of knowledge of the recognised procedures and competence in their performance. Part of the planned care should also include a logical sequence of care which will cause the least disturbance and maximum effect. It is during implementation that the greatest control is between nurse and patient, and throughout this phase the nurse should be able to modify the care according to the prevailing conditions and the age of the child.

Evaluation

Throughout implementation the patient's state must be evaluated, though overall evaluation is undertaken at the completion of the nursing action. It is a means of establishing the result of any action taken so that subsequent planning of care can be instituted. An important aspect of this process is the need for accurate recording: (a) of the problems isolated; (b) the action taken; and (c) the response to that action.

This serves not only as a record but ensures that any decision taken is based on the ability of the patient to respond in his particular way.

There are many nursing actions which are of a routine nature while others must be specific for the moment. It is this aspect of individualised care that requires to be cultivated.

Care systems

There are a variety of care systems used, each with some element of success. The care system which is probably more satisfactory than others is the primary care. The idea is not new and has been used off and on for many years. The major element is in patient assignment where a nurse takes overall responsibility for the nursing management of a child. It is this nurse who assesses and plans and ensures continuity of care by others. It may fall down if it is too inflexible or where lack of communication fails to provide continuity of care.

Team nursing follows much the same line except that communication is primarily within a team and the leader of the team acts as the co-ordinator of care.

Whatever system is used it must be primarily to benefit the patient; full discussions must take place and each member be allowed to contribute.

CARE OF THE CHILD WITH INCREASED BODY TEMPERATURE (PYREXIA)

A rise in body temperature can be due to a variety of causes (see p. 98), but there is also fever of unknown origin which can present with difficulties. Whatever the reason of the temperature increase, the basic management will be similar.

Physiological effect of pyrexia

1. With a rise in body temperature there is a rise in basal metabolic rate. If it is accompanied by decreased food intake due to anorexia the carbohydrate stores fall and protein and fat are metabolised for energy. Muscle and fat in the body tend to be broken down and there is increased urinary excretion of nitrogen. There is also incomplete oxidation of fat and this may lead to ketosis (see p. 230).
2. There is also interference with normal functioning of the central nervous system. In the young child it can cause convulsions and is believed to be due to damage to cells in the brain which are particularly sensitive to change in homeothermy. As the temperature rises, the normal powers of concentration and logical thought are lost and, if it is maintained, the child will become confused, speech may become incoherent and eventually stupor and coma may supervene (see p. 303).

In view of the adverse physiological effects it is important to reduce the pyrexic state to as near normal as possible. A number of actions can be taken:

1. Ensure that the child's environment is comfortably cool, either by decreasing heat output (radiation) or opening a window without causing a draught.
2. Remove excess clothing from the child, either personal or bedclothes.
3. Give extra fluids. Water is important in helping to cool the body and also dilute toxins, if they are the cause.
4. Provide a cool immediate environment with the aid of a fan. Care must be taken to keep it well away from the child and not directed towards the child. A moving fan is preferred to cool the environment rather than a static one which tends to cool one area only.

5. Anti-pyretic drugs may be prescribed, e.g. paracetamol.

Child up to 1 year   60–120 mg
      1–5 years   120–150 mg
      6–12 years 250–500 mg

Paracetamol can cause liver damage if given in excessive amounts.

6. If the temperature fails to decrease appreciably, then a tepid sponge of the body can be given (p. 92).

Rest in bed is generally preferred.

Careful observation of the child and support is necessary, particularly since behavioural changes can occur. If the cause of the pyrexia is an infection then a suitable antibiotic will be given. Fluid intake is important and generally speaking the child will drink eagerly. However, if vomiting and diarrhoea are also features then an intravenous infusion of the fluid and electrolytes will be given. General nursing management will be based on the age of the child. The older the child the greater the chances of excessive sweating. In this case frequent change of clothes/bedclothes and a sponge down will ensure comfort for the child. Although it is possible to monitor the effectiveness of the various actions taken by observations of change in behaviour, colour of skin and decreased restlessness, measurement of the body temperature will give a numerical value which will assist in further planning of care.

CARE OF THE CHILD WITH RESPIRATORY PROBLEMS

Disturbed respiratory functions occur frequently in infants and children, acute infection of the respiratory tract being the most common cause. A common feature in all types of respiratory disorder is difficulty in breathing and this can be due to obstruction along the respiratory tract. Other features accompanying respiratory infections, in particular, include vomiting, diarrhoea and pyrexia. Nursing management will obviously depend on the degree of difficulty and presenting features accompanying the basic problem.

There are a number of principles which can be followed:

1. Rest in bed if the child feels more comfortable. In the acute state the child will probably be inclined to sleep for most of the time.

2. Position the child in such a way that breathing is easier. For example: the sitting or semi-recumbent position is found to be suitable. The problem here is of the infant slipping down. This can be prevented by placing a pillow beneath his legs and supporting his back with a number of pillows. In some units an infant chair is used. This has disadvantages such as the hand bar at the front which tends to cause pressure on the legs leading to swelling of lower limbs and possible damage to the back of the legs. Another disadvantage is that the child tends to fall to the side and cannot maintain his posture. This leads to overcompensation and possible damage to vertebral muscles. Both of these disadvantages could be limited by padding of the bar or by placing a pillow from the bar on to the bed so that the child's legs can rest on it. Sliding to the side is probably difficult to prevent except by using small pillows on either side of the body.

3. Reduce fever (see p. 108).

4. Promote ease of breathing by humidifying the immediate environment (see p. 381). This will help to loosen secretions and allow removal either by coughing in older children or by suction in infants and young children. If difficulty in breathing is due to congestion of nasal passage then decongestion drops can be instilled.

5. Prevent dehydration. Increased breathing rate and pyrexia will lead to some increased water loss. If the child is also vomiting then water and electrolyte loss will be increased. If the child is able to drink then extra fluids should be given in a most suitable form. If the child is unwilling to drink, then fluid must be given by other means, e.g. naso-gastric tube. But if he is unable to drink or unable to retain fluids then an intravenous infusion will be necessary. In all instances an accurate fluid intake and output chart is valuable in assessing the body's ability to cope with fluid.

6. The child with lower respiratory difficulties will require additional intervention: oxygen administration will be called for if there is increased breathing effort with or without cyanosis (p. 382). When distress is apparent, as in

croup, then added humidity should be provided and careful observations made to identify obstruction necessitating intubation or tracheostomy (p. 386).

7. *Support* for the child is important because of the anxiety-inducing state. He should not be left alone at any time and should be comforted or sedated if he is very restless. He must be able to see out of the tent/croupette to limit the sense of isolation.

8. Play at this stage is of lesser importance but a cuddly toy helps to comfort the child. He is usually too preoccupied with effort of breathing that he often has neither strength nor inclination to be concerned with toys, or books (if older).

9. Nutrition. As the child's condition improves the fluid diet is supplemented by easily digested solids. This applies to the older child. The infant will get milk feeds according to his requirements.

CARE OF THE CHILD WITH CARDIOVASCULAR PROBLEMS

There are a number of disorders affecting the heart which can produce situations of crisis nursing. The main condition, however, is that of cardiac failure where the heart fails to pump blood adequately to meet tissue oxygen needs (p. 424).

Nursing management will depend on the presenting feature and where necessary surgical correction will be performed.

1. *Rest.* The aim is to reduce the external workload of the heart. The infant is basically at rest but for the young and older child physical rest is important. Nursing procedures should be arranged logically with the aim of minimising disturbance and movement. Prevent excessive crying by attending to the baby's or young child's immediate needs. Where possible, the mother should be encouraged to hold and cuddle her baby.

2. *Position.* The position adopted by the older child will be one that gives optimum relief and comfort. The cardinal sign of cardiac failure is dyspnoea with tachypnoea. Laboured breathing can be identified by the use of accessory muscles, retraction, flaring of nares and grunting (Fig. 23.9). This will further progress to paroxysmal nocturnal dyspnoea and orthopnoea. Placing the child in the sitting position supported by pillows and allowing him to rest on a padded bedtable will provide help and enable him to rest.

The infant can be nursed in an incubator or cot with the upper part raised.

3. *Alleviation of dyspnoea.* Some relief can be obtained by positioning the child as described above, but in addition oxygen is often given. The methods of administration will vary with the age of the child (see p. 382). The small infant will benefit by being placed in an incubator, without clothes, since clothes increase resistance to chest movement. It is possible to provide relative constancy in oxygen concentration. The older infant and young child can be placed in small tents or croupettes and the older child in a larger tent. Light-weight oxygen masks are useful for children over 5 years and nasal catheters for the older child. During a cyanotic attack the child should be comforted and calmed.

4. *Alleviation of restlessness.* Restlessness increases the workload of the heart and demand for oxygen. Sedation can be achieved by medication, e.g. chloral hydrate. If the restlessness is associated with cyanosis, morphine (0.2 mg/kg) or propranolol (0.1 mg/kg given slowly intravenously) can be prescribed. Administration of oxygen is also useful in relieving restlessness, since this state is often due to hypoxia.

5. *Meeting nutritional needs.* The infant will receive feeds either orally or by naso-gastric tube. Oral feeding should be attempted if the infant is not too weak to suck. The size of the teat should be suitable for the infant's mouth and the milk flow should be such that the infant can obtain milk without too great an effort. It is, however, important that the flow is not too rapid. The infant has tachypnoea and he will have difficulty in breathing and swallowing at the same time. Indeed there is great danger of aspiration of milk. It is also desirable that the amount of milk offered is small and, to ensure that he receives adequate fluid intake and that his caloric needs are met, feeds may be given at more frequent intervals. To prevent too

frequent disturbance, feeds can be given at a controlled rate via a sage pump. The young child and older child initially will be satisfied with fluids only. If the child is on potassium-losing diuretics, foods with high potassium content should be encouraged. Meals should be attractively served and the amounts suitable for the child and his ability to eat. Meals should also be calm without creating fuss at any inability or unwillingness to eat. If oedema is present, a low sodium milk feed is given to the infant, while the child will be given a low sodium diet.

6. Diversion or occupation for the older child must be geared to his state. If he is distressed, reading a story or simply being beside him will satisfy and calm him. Other children, one at a time, will also help him to pass the time. There is no need to create occupation for him if he is distressed. As his condition improves so will his desire to play or read or join other children in suitable games.

CARE OF THE CHILD WITH NEUROLOGICAL PROBLEMS

The care of the child with a neurological disorder begins with an assessment of the presenting feature. This includes examination of the following:

1. Determination of the child's level of consciousness and orientation.
2. Checking the size, equality and reaction of the pupils to light.
3. Noting the strength and type of movement of all four extremities.
4. The presence of convulsion, their onset, duration and type.

There are many conditions which can present in acute form. The nursing management will depend on the presenting features:

1. *Position.* The best position in which to place the child will depend on the presenting features and the cause of the condition. If the child is unconscious then he should be placed in the semiprone position with the head turned to the side, but visible to the nurse at all times.

If he is conscious but there is evidence of increased intracranial pressure then he should be flat or lying with one pillow under his head. In the case of increased pressure due to accumulation of cerebrospinal fluid then relief may be obtained by raising the top of the bed. On the other hand, if there is severe headache due to decrease of fluid, e.g. following an air encephalogram, then lowering the top of the bed may be beneficial. In basilar skull fracture the child may be flat or in high Fowler's position until the otorrhoea or rhinorrhoea stops.

2. *Maintaining an airway.* The aim is to prevent hypoxia. The unconscious position (Fig. 23.9) should be adopted or the most suitable in order to maintain a good airway and prevent inhalation of secretions and vomit. Suction equipment must be available and any secretions aspirated. If the child is unable to maintain his own airway, an endotracheal tube will be passed or artificial ventilation will be required.

3. *Prevention of respiratory complications.* The management is aimed at preventing complications which can arise when the child is in the unconscious state. Removal of secretions, particularly if the cough reflex is depressed, will be an important action. Secretions which cannot be removed will pool in the most gravity-dependent positions of the lungs.

    Physiotherapy will be helpful. Vibration and percussion can be used to loosen secretions which can then be aspirated.

    Oral hygiene is also important as a means of preventing respiratory complications. It may also be necessary to pass a naso-gastric tube and aspirate stomach content to prevent inhalation of vomit.

4. *Prevention of pressure sores.* If the child is unconscious or paralysed, he should be turned every 1 to 2 hours to prevent pressure sores. The child should be handled gently. Daily baths should be given and the skin and bed kept dry and clean. Aids such as sheepskin could be used in an effort to maintain the integrity of the skin.

5. *Protection from injury.* Bed sides could be padded, particularly if the child is restless.

6. *Maintaining normal body temperature*. Pyrexia is often a feature of brain injury. Overheating should be avoided and if pyrexia is present then the actions suggested on page 108 can be attempted. Body temperature should be monitored at a suitable frequency, e.g. 3 to 4 hourly.

7. *Mobility*. A free range of movements should be provided if the child is either unconscious or paralysed. It is also important to maintain the limbs in such a position as to prevent contractures. Splinting may be desirable or necessary. If the child is conscious and not paralysed then he should be encouraged to use his limbs.

8. *Maintaining hydration*.
   a. The conscious child will be able to drink provided his sucking and swallowing reflexes are present. Oral fluids should also be given if he is not vomiting. Indeed the older child may be able to take easily digested foods.
   b. If the child is unconscious, intravenous fluids may be given initially. Thereafter, naso-gastric feeding will replace intravenous feedings and these must be given slowly. Regurgitation and aspiration are particularly dangerous. The head of the bed should be elevated 15 to 20° for feedings. However, it may be preferred to administer the feed by using a slow drip.

The diet should be high in calories and proteins for energy and repair of tissue. This is particularly true since bed-rest and paralysis of one or more limbs will often lead to atrophy of muscles with subsequent weight loss.

In prolonged naso-gastric feeding, the catheter should be changed frequently, e.g. every 24 hours to avoid damage to the nasal mucosa.

9. *Prevention of corneal ulcers*. Absence of the blinking reflex can lead to corneal ulceration. The eyes should be kept closed with eye pads and eye care should be given by bathing the eyes with normal saline. The eye pads can be kept in position with non-allergic tape and the pads changed at least every 3 to 4 hours.

10. *Bowel and bladder care*
    Bowels. While the child is receiving intra-venous fluids only, bowel management does not usually present a problem. As the condition stabilises and feedings are begun either orally or by naso-gastric tube, faecal impaction may occur. To stimulate the bowel, suppositories may be inserted and, as a last resort, enemas may have to be given. Enemas are contra-indicated in the presence of increased intra-cranial pressure as they would further increase the intracranial pressure. Sometimes diarrhoea occurs with a fluid diet and it may be necessary to give binding substances such as kaolin. The anal region must be kept clean and dry to prevent breakdown of skin surrounding the anus.

Bladder. An unconscious patient is usually incontinent and therefore does not require to be catheterised. However, in many units, intermittent catheterisation may be carried out or a uribag and continuous drainage could be used. This serves two purposes: (1) it keeps the bed dry and prevents skin excoriation, and (2) it provides for accurate measurement of urine output. An indwelling catheter is not recommended because of the danger of infection, but if it is required, then regular cleaning of the catheter around the external urethral meatus and surrounding areas is essential.

Psychological care

Understanding and patience is essential whatever the state of the patient. The unconscious child may still be able to hear and it is important not to comment about him, his illness or condition when at his bedside. The conscious, paralysed child will be anxious and unhappy. His questions will need to be answered as honestly and gently as possible. Praise should be given for the effort he makes at rehabilitation. He may be restless, aggressive and uncooperative and the nurse should be firm, but gentle, anticipating his physical and mental needs.

An extension of that care should include the parents who will be most anxious not only of the acute illness but also of what the future will hold. Full explanation will need to be given about the child's illness, treatment, prognosis and progress. While this is usually the responsibility of the doctor in charge of the case, the nurse also has a role to play in clarifying points not understood by the parents.

CARE OF THE CHILD IN CONVULSIONS

Convulsions may be due to a variety of causes — from a focus of irritation within the brain, following trauma, hypoxia, neoplasm, or pyrexia in young children; disturbance of electrolytes, e.g. low serum sodium or ionised calcium and in the neonates, a combination of the latter with hypoglycaemia.

Convulsing muscles consume large amounts of oxygen and this is further increased if there is increased body temperature. Generalised convulsions interfere with respiration, so there is interference with oxygen intake. There is therefore a danger of hypoxia which may lead to cerebral damage. It should also be recognised that the body carries no effective stores of oxygen and there is increased extraction of oxygen from the blood, with the production of a metabolic acidosis from anaerobic metabolism.

Protection of the child

The aim is to prevent injury to the child during convulsion. This can be achieved by padding the bed or cot sides. Care must also be taken to prevent injury to the tongue. This can be achieved by placing a padded object between the teeth, however, this is not always recommended because of the danger of damage to teeth and the possibility of inhaling a tooth.

Maintaining a clear airway

The aim here is to prevent the tongue from obstructing the airway and this can be achieved by placing the child on his side and performing suction when required. Hypoxia must not be allowed to develop as this will increase cerebral irritation and the convulsions.

Relief of convulsions

It is important that the convulsions are controlled as quickly as possible. Medication will be prescribed. Some of the drugs may, however, depress the respiratory centre. Diazepam has been found useful in controlling fits in some cases and does not depress respiration, except in large doses.

Throughout the time careful observations must be made of the convulsions and the vital functions.

CARE OF THE CHILD IN ACUTE RENAL FAILURE

Acute renal failure is an abrupt cessation of the kidney's ability to maintain regulation of the volume and composition of the body fluids. Deterioration proceeds rapidly and urgent treatment is required (see p. 535). Assessment will have to be made to establish the disorder so that treatment can be instituted.

Rest

The child is acutely ill. Hypertension may or may not be present depending on the cause of renal failure and the degree of sodium overload. There may also be pericarditis when uraemia is in an advanced stage. If there is also anaemia, then this will impose an additional strain on the heart. Therefore, rest in bed is essential, the child adopting the most comfortable position.

Nutrition

Adequate carbohydrate and fat must be given to minimise protein catabolism. Various preparations can be given to satisfy caloric requirements, e.g. 'Hycal' or 'Caloreen'. They may be given via a naso-gastric tube in the case of very young children if they have difficulty in taking the feed. A small amount of first-class protein should be given because patients tend to feel better and vomit less than they do on protein-free diet. The protein should be based on egg and milk and given in a quantity of about 0.5 to 1 g/kg body weight per 24 hours. In some cases, e.g. where renal failure is associated with burns or septicaemia, greater amounts of calories and proteins will be required to prevent wasting, and this can be achieved by instituting intravenous feeding.

Correction of biochemical disturbance

This will require an intravenous administration of relevant substance. For example, in acidosis, sodium bicarbonate or lactate. However, severe acidosis is best treated by dialysis. For a detailed description of nursing management during dialysis see page 559.

Uraemic children are prone to infection,

especially of the urinary tract. Antibiotics will be given as prophylactic. Although isolation is not necessary, care should be taken to prevent infecting these children. Anyone working or handling them should be free from infection themselves. If the patient is an infant, then it is advisable that he is nursed in a single room and all necessary precautions taken to protect him from infection.

Daily weighing

Oedema may be a feature and an assessment of its increase or decrease must be made. This can be achieved by daily weighing — an increase in weight in older children and over the accepted increase in infants, would indicate fluid retention, while a reduction in weight would indicate a decrease. Weighing should be done at about the same time each day; a weighing bed would be a great convenience.

CARE OF THE OEDEMATOUS CHILD

Oedema can be found in most parts of the body, e.g. eyelids, limbs, abdomen. When the *eyelids* are affected the child will have difficulty in opening his eyes. This will be distressing for him. To prevent the eyelids from sticking they can be swabbed with normal saline (p. 34). When carrying out any nursing procedure the child should be told in advance (a) that you are coming, and (b) what is going to be done. Sudden appearance without prior warning can make him very anxious.

Oedema of the abdomen will make sitting or lying difficult. The child often finds it more comfortable to be up and about. However, this may not be possible. He should be placed in the position most comfortable to him, usually reclining supported with three or four pillows.

Position changes are very important since fluid will collect in the most dependent parts. When changing his position, he should be lifted gently and not pulled. The skin is already stretched and friction will lead to damage of the skin. The bed should be clean and free from wrinkles or crumbs and a bedcradle will prevent extra weight of bedclothes, which will increase his discomfort.

Input/output recording

It is essential that all fluids taken and excreted must be recorded accurately. Accurate measurement of the urine flow rate is necessary, particularly in pre-renal failure. Urine should be collected by means of plastic bags in either sex, or Paul's tubing in the case of boys, if the child is incontinent. If the renal failure is due to burns then an indwelling catheter is used. This would involve care of the catheter at frequent intervals. The importance of these fluid balance charts is that they allow assessment of renal function and help in the calculation of fluid requirements. It is not only necessary to record the amount of fluids but also the means by which fluid is gained and lost.

Psychological care

Whatever the cause of the renal failure, the child will be acutely ill. The older child may be lethargic and even depressed. He should be allowed to express his anxiety and unhappiness. Some suitable activity should be provided, much depending on his general state and disposition. Every procedure should be explained as fully as possible depending on his level of understanding and where possible he can be actively involved. Parents are suffering too and will need a great deal of understanding and patience. They should be involved in the care of their child as far as that is possible.

CARE OF THE CHILD WITH GASTRO-INTESTINAL DISTURBANCE

There are many conditions involving the gastro-intestinal tract in which the child presents as acutely ill. There are also many disorders which present with some gastro-intestinal disturbance. The main disturbances in the acute phase of many illnesses are vomiting, diarrhoea, obstruction to intestinal outflow with evidence of loss of fluid and electrolyte imbalance.

CARE OF THE CHILD WHO IS VOMITING

Vomiting is a reflex action, co-ordinated in the medulla oblongata, whereby the contents of the stomach are forcibly expelled through the mouth (see p. 484).

Infants commonly bring up small amounts of milk during or soon after a feed. However, vomiting may signal a far more serious condition.

Repeated vomiting of increasing amounts with enough force to project at a distance may indicate pyloric stenosis, upper small bowel obstruction (from duodenal bands, duodenal stenosis or volvulus) the latter producing bile-stained vomitus. Metabolic disorders and infections are accompanied by vomiting.

Support

It is important that the nurse is present during vomiting. In the case of the infant to prevent inhalation of vomitus, while for the young and older child, to relieve the anxiety which vomiting produces. The anxiety is due to the unpleasantness of the event itself and to the fear of making a mess, so reassurance and understanding of the event is important. It is also helpful simply to have someone nearby to help when required.

Privacy

This should be provided whenever possible, not only to limit embarrassment for the child but also to prevent other children witnessing the event which can be disturbing for them.

Positioning

The aim here is to prevent inhalation of vomitus in the infant, and to minimise contamination. The infant can be placed on his side with his head lowered, removing the vomitus as quickly as possible. If he shows signs of choking, suction should be used to clear the mouth and nose.

The older child should, where possible, be encouraged to vomit into a receptacle. The nurse should be with him, holding and comforting him. The position to adopt will obviously vary with the condition but if he cannot lift his head then the same precautions must be taken as for the infant.

Cleanliness

Vomitus has an unpleasant odour, whether freshly expelled or dried in. It is, therefore, essential that the child is washed and his clothes changed. The older child should be given a mouthwash, if he is able, or mouth care, if unable to do so. The infant should be given oral care (see p. 96).

Observations

Throughout the event the child should be observed closely and indeed vomiting can be anticipated. The infant will swallow frequently and may be retching. The older child will say that he is feeling uncomfortable or that he is going to vomit.

Continuous vomiting causes dehydration and therefore accurate reporting of vomiting, amount, type and content, will be very important (see p. 89).

Diarrhoea

Frequent loose stools may occur in all infants, but if these are associated with vomiting, weight loss and abnormal constituents like blood, then they should be considered serious. Many infections are accompanied by diarrhoea and many disorders have as their manifestation, diarrhoea with stools having characteristic appearance. For example, coeliac disease, cystic fibrosis and sugar mal-absorption.

Support

This is particularly important for the older child who will experience anxiety regarding loss of bowel control. He will require reassurance, and a bedpan must be readily available.

Privacy

Privacy is important even for young children and the nurse should remain with the child.

Care of the buttocks

Excoriation of the buttocks can occur rapidly the more frequent the stools are and the longer the infant is left lying in his soiled nappy. As soon as a stool has been passed it must be removed, and the buttocks and anal region cleaned and left dry. A water repellent substance/ointment can be applied to give protection to the skin (see p. 36). For the care of the older child, cleaning of the anal region can be with cotton wool or very soft toilet paper. The area should be dried well and may also be protected with a suitable ointment.

Observations

This involves anticipation of a stool to be passed. The infant or child may be crying, particularly if it is associated with colic. Observations include frequency, effort and contents of stools (see p. 89).

As already stated, any condition can have an acute phase. The method of care and the means used depend on the cause and presenting features. It can involve any or all of the symptoms and the nurse must be able to extrapolate that which is relevant and apply the most suitable nursing care to the situation. With this in mind, it is possible to apply systematic nursing care beginning with awareness of a problem, assessing it, designing nursing care, implementing and finally evaluating.

Nursing a child with cancer

Cancer is the name applied to a group of neoplasms. A neoplasm or tumour is an area of tissue whose growth has outstripped and become independent of the adjoining tissue. Tumours are classified according to tissue of origin and whether they are benign or malignant.

The difference between benign and malignant lies in the fact that a benign tumour is slow growing, well demarcated from the surrounding tissue, is composed of cells from which it is derived, does not infiltrate into adjacent tissues or spread to distant organs and does not threaten life unless it happens to interfere with some function essential for survival.

The malignant tumour differs from a benign one in that it is fast growing; is poorly demarcated from surrounding tissues and is composed of cells which are often markedly different from the cells of origin. It infiltrates adjacent tissues and spreads to distant organs. These tumours sooner or later invariable cause death if untreated.

Cancer in children differs from cancer in adults not only in types and histologies but also in the location of tumours. These include the leukaemias (p. 443), Hodgkin's disease, Wilms' tumour (p. 538), neuroblastoma (p. 538), Rhabdomyosarcoma (a rare soft tissue sarcoma), malignant bone tumour (as primary malignant tumours these are uncommon in children), retinoblastoma (p. 334) and tumours of the central nervous system, i.e. astrocytomas and medulloblastomas. There are also more unusual malignant tumours of the liver and non-malignant ones of tissues such as thyroid and smooth muscle.

Causes of cancer

In man, the only known causes of spontaneous cancer are chemicals and radiation. Controversy surrounds any discussion of virus as a cancer agent though in animals, viruses which can cause cancer can be transmitted from animal to animal, like other infections. In man, the only tumour-producing virus is the papilloma virus that causes warts, which are small benign tumours. Other viruses have been implicated with cancer of specific tissues, e.g. it is suggested that there is an association between carcinoma of the cervix and herpes simplex II virus or that the leukaemias are associated with virus activity.

Chemicals are, however, known to induce cancer. Some of these occur naturally, but most are synthetic. As far as children are concerned, the importance of chemical carcinogens in the development of cancer has still to be studied. Cumulative dose effects are important and, regarding natural cancers, it requires 10 to 40 years exposure before the tumour becomes clinically apparent.

Other causes of cancer include ionising radiation. There is very strong evidence that electromagnetic radiation, e.g. ultraviolet light and X-rays, and particulate radiation, i.e. electrons, neutrons and particles, cause cancer in man. While skin cancer is not found in children, the exposure to the sun's radiation begins in childhood. It is commoner in sunny countries in light-skinned people but is rare in dark-skinned people. It is believed that ultraviolet irradiation forms bonds between adjacent bases in nuclear DNA with formation of abnormal thymine dimers.

Host factors

Many people are exposed to carcinogens but only some actually develop clinical cancer. This implies an individual susceptibility or resistance to environmental carcinogens. Genetic host factors have been demonstrated to be important for several conditions. The association between selected chromosomal disorders and clinical cancer has been established. The relationship between Down's syndrome and leukaemia is one example, while some retinoblastomas, Wilms' tumours and neuroblastomas also have a genetic basis.

Nursing management
While any ill child requires a high level of skilful nursing, the child with cancer presents additional challenge.

Careful observations are important for a thorough and precise assessment since the situation may change rapidly. A number of objectives can be identified when formulating systematic nursing care and these include:

1. Promoting and achieving optimal health.
2. Prevention of complications.
3. Early recognition of recurrent or new symptoms.
4. Recognising anxiety and unhappiness.
5. Providing psychological support.

Promoting and achieving optimal health
Infections are a significant cause of morbidity and mortality in children with cancer. The risk of infection is increased not only by the disease process but also by the chemotherapy, radiotherapy and the intensity of anti-cancer therapy.

Prevention of infection is therefore essential but the methods used may vary. The child is at greatest risk of infection while hospitalised and it may be desirable to isolate him either in a cubicle or under laminar flow and maintain a strict reverse barrier nursing regime (p. 250).

Nutrition
Providing adequate nutrition can present a challenge. The child's likes and dislikes should be ascertained, taking into consideration the need of supplying foods which will promote healing and increase the child's ability to deal with his illness. Some foods may be treated by irradiation, affecting the taste of the food. Soft food should be given in cases of leukaemia, when there is a danger of damage to soft tissue and bleeding. The method of feeding and eating will depend on his general condition and his ability to eat and tolerate food.

Nausea and vomiting tend to be troublesome due to the damaging effect of chemotherapy on the rapidly dividing cells of the gastro-intestinal tract. While nausea and vomiting are severe, fluids and foods should not be forced. It may be necessary to give fluids intravenously.

Anorexia often accompanies chemotherapy but may also be due to the cancer or any other complication such as stomatitis or oesophagitis.

PREVENTION OF COMPLICATIONS AND RECOGNITION OF NEW SYMPTOMS

Diarrhoea
Diarrhoea presents a problem, especially if the abdomen has been irradiated causing cellular damage. Abdominal pain may accompany the diarrhoea. A bland or low-residue diet should be given and the painful spasm may be relieved with an anti-spasmodic drug.

Constipation and ulceration of the lower gastro-intestinal tract
The vinca alkaloids may cause nerve damage which affects intestinal mobility and may lead to paralytic ileus. Observation of stools is very important and if constipation is present then a stool softener should be given. Suppositories might be better avoided particularly if rectal fissures are present. Care of the anus and perineal area will be required and if rectal fissures are present a warm bath may be helpful.

Care of the mouth and teeth
Many chemotherapeutic drugs cause stomatitis. To minimise the effect of this complication, gentle oral care should be given. Toothbrushing is often contra-indicated, but mouthwashes may be given (p. 96). If the use of a toothbrush is permitted, it should be soft and this can be achieved by placing the toothbrush in warm water.

The disease causes problems in almost all the body's systems and as the symptoms indicate further involvement, each must be treated in the most suitable way. For example, involvement of the skeleto-muscular system due to infiltration of malignant cells will produce pain and, where osteoporosis is present, hair-line fractures may result. Movement and touch will cause pain and therefore the child must be handled as gently as possible. The central nervous system may be infiltrated and symptoms such as nausea, vomiting, headache, blurred vision, drowsiness, pain and convulsions will be very distressing.

Pain is a cardinal feature particularly when the

disease is in its final stages. Each child's response to pain varies and it is often difficult to assess the intensity of pain (p. 304). Control of pain is an important aspect of care. No child should be left to suffer pain. There are a number of different ways of controlling pain but if these fail then drugs should not be withheld.

Heat and massage may be beneficial; distraction (where possible) and relaxation techniques may also be useful.

Any combination of drugs that provide relief from pain may be used. Analgesics are useful in modifying the perception of pain; tranquillisers are useful where the anxiety level is high and anti-depressants can be used for depression.

Providing emotional support
Cancer in a child imposes stress on the child as well as on his family. The parents must be fully involved in the care of the child. Communication must be freely available and discussions with the family should be on the basis of equality. The parents need to know not only that the child is suffering from a cancer but also every plan of care decided on.

Reassuring the child is important and can take many forms, from talking to him to touching and holding. The daily routine should be as normal as possible and the child should take part in any activity in which he feels able to participate. All procedures should be clearly explained and for any invasive procedure support and comfort should be available.

Remissions occur and during that time the child should be encouraged to lead as normal a life as possible. All treatment is usually continued for a prescribed period and once treatment is stopped then parents are often frightened of a recurrence or relapse. This may make them over-protective and make life restrictive for the child. They should be encouraged to give free expression to these fears, and free access to medical and nursing advice will do much to minimise their anxiety.

Resuscitation

Death may occur suddenly as a result of cardiac arrest or of respiratory arrest, but since the two are

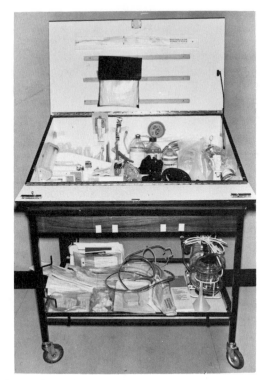

Fig. 6.8 Resuscitation trolley.

closely interrelated, it is usually described as cardio-respiratory arrest. Whatever the cause, it is essential to institute measures quickly to prevent irreversible damage to the central nervous system. In some cases it is possible to anticipate some catastrophe and to prepare for the event, in others, the measures to be taken depend on the situation, e.g. asphyxiation due to inhalation of a foreign body.

It is desirable that each ward should have a resuscitation trolley ventilator, and monitor (Figs. 6.8, 6.9 and 6.10) and that each member of the medical and nursing staff is familiar with the equipment. Generally it is the nursing staff who are responsible for the maintenance of the trolley which should be checked daily. Table 6.2 shows what type of equipment may be necessary, though each hospital will have its own policy. Table 6.3 gives a list of drugs used during resuscitation procedures.

Resuscitative measures involve respiratory and cardiac functions and when both these functions

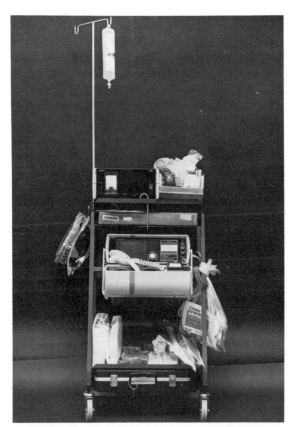

Fig. 6.9 Resuscitation trolley incorporating a defibrillator.

fail, respiratory resuscitation should be applied first, because without adequate oxygenation, the treatment of concurrent impairment of cardiac function will not be successful.

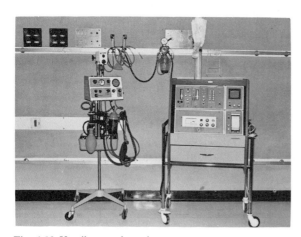

Fig. 6.10 Ventilator and monitor.

Table 6.2 Equipment for resuscitation trolley (see Fig. 6.8)

Suction machine
Ambu Bag; valve; child's mask; infant's mask
Laryngoscopes (a) child, (b) infant, (c) adult. Blades
Spare batteries
Spare bulb
Everseal face masks — sizes 0, 1, 2, 3, 4
Curved face mask mount with expiratory valve and gas inlet
Corrugated extension pieces with mount
500 ml bags with tap
Feeding tube and mount
Rendell Baker face mask size 1
Inglis expiratory valve (metal to rubber)
Gilton face mask adaptor
Guedel airways sizes 000, 1, 2, 3, 4
Small corrugated tubing
Portex endotracheal connectors
Knights' straight connectors 3.5 mm, 4.0 mm, 4.5 mm, 5.0 mm
Knights' curved connectors
Assorted sizes of (flexometallic) endotracheal tubes (6, 5.5, 5, 4.5, 4, 3.5, 3.0)
Warne's neonatal resuscitation tubes
Tracheostomy tubes and tapes sizes 18 EG, 24 FG
Stethoscope
Stopwatch
Ackland's mouth gag
Tongue-holding forceps
Artery forceps
Magill forceps (child's)
Tracheal dilator

Signs of increased respiratory embarrassment and impending obstruction

1. *Accessory breath sounds*
   a. *Development of stertorous breathing* when a rattle is heard at the back of the throat. This occurs on inspiration and expiration as air is forced through accumulated secretions in the pharynx.
   b. *Expiratory stridor.* The classical picture is that of the asthmatic when there is a forced expiratory effort in an endeavour to relieve the build-up of pressure caused by spasm in the bronchioles. Partial obstruction in either bronchus will give the same picture.
   c. *Laryngeal stridor.* This is an inspiratory stridor and occurs when obstruction is at the level of the vocal cords. The inspiration is long and drawn out in an effort to get adequate air past the obstruction.
2. *Paradoxical respiration with increased respiratory rate.* The accessory muscles of respiration are used forcefully when the main muscles of

Table 6.3 Drugs used during resuscitation

Drug	Use
Adrenalin	Cardiac stimulant, acting through the B-receptors increases the strength of ventricular contraction and the heart rate, and dilating the coronary vessels
Calcium gluconate 10% Dextrose 50%	Improves myocardial contractility
Lethidrone neonatal 1 mg in 1 ml	Analgesic; acts as narcotic antagonist and can counteract the respiratory depressant effects of most narcotic drugs
Naloxone 400 μg in 1 ml	(see Lethidrone)
Mannitol 10%	Improves renal perfusion osmotic diuretic
Sodium bicarbonate 8.4%	To correct metabolic acidosis resulting from inadequate peripheral circulation during cardiac arrest
Sodium chloride 0.225%	To correct acid-base disturbance
Diazepam 10 mg in 2 ml	Tranquiliser
Aminophylline 250 mg in 10 ml	Bronchodilator
Dexamethazone 8 mg in 2 ml	Glucocorticoid

respiration, the diaphragm and the external intercostal muscles, fail to provide an adequate exchange of gases. On inspiration, there is a noticeable indrawing above the manubrium sterni, the abdominal muscles are relaxed and the abdomen appears blown out. There is forced expiration when the abdominal muscles contract, thus increasing the intra-abdominal pressure in an effort to aid in the ascent of the diaphragm.

3. *Increased pulse rate*. This will occur when some degree of anoxia is present. The heart is endeavouring to maintain the requirement of the body by circulating blood more rapidly.
4. *Cyanosis*. This will occur gradually or rapidly depending on the severity of the respiratory difficulty. It is not a warning as such, but rather an indication of the degree of obstruction.

Clearing a blocked or partially blocked airway
Requirements
1. Suction apparatus giving from 25 to 38 cm Hg or from 10 to 15 inches Hg vacuum.
2. Supply of sterile suction catheters, whistle tipped with two side holes.
3. Pressure tubing and connection.
4. Water to clear the catheter.
5. Paper tissues.

6. Endotracheal tubes and laryngoscopes should be available.

Pharyngeal suction
The child is placed in the lateral position, or on his back with his head extended (Fig. 6.11). If necessary, the oral cavity is cleared of debris using paper tissues. The catheter is connected, suction commenced, and the oropharynx aspirated, using gentle movements. The catheter is cleared. The pressure is occluded as the catheter is passed to the posterior pharynx; it should not be passed beyond the laryngopharynx. The pressure is released and the catheter is withdrawn gently as secretions are aspirated. The catheter is cleared and the procedure is repeated. If secretions are not being obtained and there is no improvement in the patient's condition, tracheal or bronchial suction will be required. Trauma to the posterior pharyngeal wall can occur when repeated suction is carried out and suction is applied to the tissues. This can lead to haemorrhage or oedema and further increase the obstruction.

Tracheal or bronchial suction
This should be performed under direct vision using a laryngoscope or a bronchoscope, but can be carried out without direct vision by an experi-

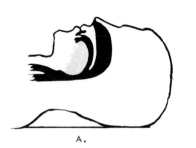 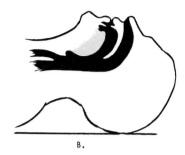

Fig. 6.11 Resuscitation. A, Obstructed airway. B, Maximum airway achieved by extension of the head.

enced person. The dangers are trauma and collapse of lung through excessive use of suction without adequate ventilation of the lungs. After every third attempt to clear the airway, ventilation is necessary. As with pharyngeal suction, the catheter is inserted with the pressure occluded and suction only commenced once the catheter is in position; the catheter is gently withdrawn as soon as suction is commenced.

Respiratory arrest

Causes
Breathing may fail due to the following conditions:

1. Lack of inspired oxygen.
2. Depression of the respiratory centre due to:
   a. Drug overdosage.
   b. Infection, such as poliomyelitis.
   c. Trauma, e.g. spinal injury in the cervical region.
   d. Cerebral oedema.
3. Interference with ventilation due to:
   a. External compression of the airway.
   b. Obstructed airway, e.g. vomit, foreign bodies.
   c. Disease processes, e.g. pneumothorax, muscular paralysis.
4. Inadequate gaseous exchange, e.g. in pulmonary oedema.
5. Inadequate oxygen transport, e.g. cardiac arrest and shock.
6. Inadequate cellular respiration, e.g. in cyanide poisoning.

Signs
Whatever the cause of the respiratory inadequacy, the most important consequence is loss of con-

sciousness due to hypoxia and hypercapnia or hypercarbia (excess carbon dioxide in the blood). This can have secondary effects such as acute respiratory obstruction from the tongue falling back, or absent cough reflexes may lead to inhalation of vomit. When breathing stops cyanosis and convulsions will be present within 1 minute. The pulse rate will be rapid initially but slows down considerably. Within 3 minutes all respiratory efforts will have stopped, and within 5 minutes, the blood pressure will have fallen to a level which is incompatible with survival.

Cardiac arrest

Causes
Cardiac arrest may be due to:

1. Acute hypoxia, due to, e.g. inhalation of vomit.
2. Drug overdosage, e.g. potassium chloride given intravenously too quickly and in high concentrations.
3. Vagal slowing of the heart, e.g. stimulation of the pharyngeal plexus can occur in intubation, laryngoscopy and bronchoscopy.
4. Anaphylactic shock due to some allergy.
5. Cardiac arrhythmias.

Signs
1. Loss of consciousness due to anoxia.
2. Pallor with cyanotic appearance.
3. Absence of peripheral pulses; this can be best estimated by feeling the carotid artery and if it is absent, indicates a grossly inadequate heart or no ejection by the heart.
4. Dilated pupils, which do not react to light; this implies cerebral ischaemia.

Action which can be taken by the nurse
1. Ensure that the upper airway is clear (p. 119).
2. Commence artificial ventilation by using a face mask and rebreathing bag receiving 100 per cent oxygen, or give mouth-to-mouth resuscitation.

Method for mouth-to-mouth resuscitation
Two people will be required to carry out mouth-to-mouth breathing and external cardiac massage. It may not be obvious how expired air can be adequate to produce oxygenation but if Table 6.4 is studied, it will be seen that expired air contains between 14 and 18 per cent oxygen.

The patient's oxygen saturation will be lower than normal, i.e. normally it is 95 per cent, but if effective expired air resuscitation is carried out, an oxygen saturation of 80 per cent may be achieved. In addition, carbon dioxide in the patient's lungs will be effectively removed and blown off into the atmosphere. At the same time,

it appears that satisfactorily low levels of carbon dioxide can be maintained for at least a half hour.

1. The patient is placed on his back.
2. The head is tilted back by extending the neck; the airway is cleared of mucus and the lower jaw is supported with the right hand to keep the tongue forward (Fig. 6.12).
3. The operator's mouth is placed over the patient's mouth and with the left hand the patient's nose is pinched to prevent escape of air. In the case of the child under 3 years old, the operator's mouth will cover the child's mouth and nostrils.
4. Using sufficient pressure to cause the patient's chest to rise, the operator blows into the patient. If the stomach fills with air, the child is turned on to his side and pressure is applied to the epigastrium to empty the stomach of air. If regurgitation occurs along with expulsion of air, the gastric contents must be cleared before continuing. The patient is returned to the supine position and the head position is then adjusted to produce a good airway.
5. The procedure is repeated at a rate of 15 to 20 times per minute until the child is breathing adequately, or until the patient can be intubated.

Table 6.4

Gas	Atmospheric air %	Expired air %
Oxygen	21	14–18
Carbon dioxide	0.04	4.5

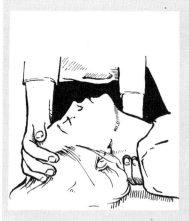 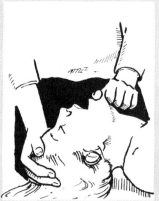 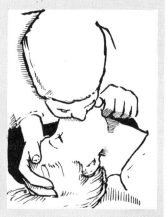

Gradual Extension Of Head

Full Extension – Lift Jaw Up – Open Mouth

Surround The Nose And Mouth Of An Infant Or Mouth Only Of An Adult

Fig. 6.12 Resuscitation — sequence of mouth-to-mouth breathing.

6. In mouth-to-nose resuscitation, the right hand not only supports the lower jaw but seals the lips, and the operator blows down the nose.

The disadvantages of expired air resuscitation all lie with the person carrying out the technique. Many will find the method aesthetically repugnant, but it should be remembered that it is a life-saving method. Infection may be a hazard in some cases but these are probably in the minority so that the risk of infection is probably minimal. The technique requires no apparatus, but training is necessary. It can be easily learned on a model such as the AMBU Manikin. It is also important to learn how to use appliances such as the Brook airway, the Ambu bag and the Cardiff bellows.

External cardiac massage

Although it is said that brain damage is irreversible following cessation of cerebral blood flow for a period of 3 minutes, it is important to recognise that brain damage begins as soon as that organ is deprived of oxygenated blood.

Principles involved

The heart lies within the pericardial sac. This fibroserous sac is continuous with the external coats of the great vessels superiorly and is attached inferiorly to the central tendon of the diaphragm. The heart lies, therefore, in the mediastinum, behind the body of the sternum and the cartilages of the ribs from the second to the sixth inclusive, and in front of the thoracic vertebrae.

The heart is suspended within, but between the attachments of the pericardium, and cannot be displaced from side to side in the chest. Therefore, when the sternum is depressed forcibly, the heart is squeezed between the sternum and the thoracic vertebral bodies. Since the valves of the heart allow blood flow to occur in one direction, the blood in the left ventricles will be ejected into the aorta and therefore produce arterial flow.

Method

1. *Small children and infants.* With a baby, effective massage can be achieved by placing one hand behind the thorax and compressing the sternum backwards with the fingers of the other hand, in a rhythmical manner (Fig. 6.13). In small chil-

dren, a firm surface behind the thorax is essential and a small board can be placed beneath the chest. The heel of the hand is placed over the lower third of the sternum (Fig. 6.14).

2. *Older children.* The child is placed on a firm

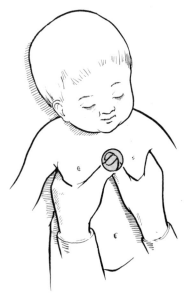

Fig. 6.13 External cardiac massage. (Infant — thumbs only used to transmit pressure.)

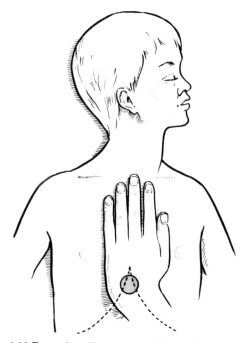

Fig. 6.14 External cardiac massage. (Older child.)

surface; a small board can be placed beneath the chest. The heel of one hand is placed over the lower third of the sternum and the other hand is placed on top (Fig. 6.14).

The chest wall is compressed with a thrusting motion at a rate of approximately 60 to 70 compressions per minute. (Note the time the emergency started.)

Respirations must be supported if they are not present, otherwise cardiac massage will not be effective. This should be carried out by another person at the same time as the cardiac massage. There should be four sternal compressions, then a pause to allow the lungs to be inflated.

Signs of effective cardiac massage
These signs are the reverse of the signs of cardiac arrest:

1. Improvement of colour; the lips may remain cyanosed until rubbed.
2. Palpable pulse in a major vessel; this may be difficult to determine in a small child with the vibrations of the massage.
3. Pupils are contracting to a smaller size. This is the most favourable sign as it indicates adequate perfusion of the brain.

Cardiac arrest may occur in two forms:
1. Asystole.
2. Ventricular fibrillation.

Massage is continued in both states. Sodium bicarbonate is given to counter the metabolic acidosis associated with hypoxia of arrest.

Asystole
Cardiac massage is continued for at least 10 minutes before further measures are contemplated. During this time, the heart may begin to beat unaided when it will be possible to stop the massage.

If the contractions are weak, then it may be necessary to give an injection of adrenalin into the left ventricle. If the blood pressure remains low (below 80 mmHg) it will be necessary to give a slow noradrenaline infusion intravenously. If the heart remains in asystole, the muscle tone of the heart can be improved by injecting calcium chloride either directly into the heart or intra-venously. If asystole persists, massage is continued until the heart fails to fill in diastole or until signs of permanent brain damage are present. The final decision when to stop cardiac massage, rests with the medical officer.

Defibrillation of ventricular fibrillation
In the normal heart, the contraction wave passes over the cardiac muscle in a co-ordinated manner, starting at the sino-atrial node and causing first atrial contraction and then ventricular contraction.

In the fibrillating heart the co-ordinate contraction wave is lost and instead, there are numerous localised areas in the atria and ventricles which contract and relax out of phase with each other to produce a 'trembling heart' which is incapable of ejecting blood into the great vessels. When an electric current of sufficient magnitude is passed on such a heart, it overrides the multiple-irritable foci of contractions and causes a more co-ordinated action, i.e. the muscle fibres contract together.

When an electric current is passed through the chest to the heart muscle is causes it to contract. Following this induced contraction the heart invariably pauses and then starts either beating rhythmically or else develops incoordinated ventricular fibrillation. When a further electric current is applied to the fibrillating heart, it leads to a more regular contraction, followed by a pause and then normal rhythm is resumed.

Internal D.C. defibrillation requires a lower discharge of electrical energy for one-hundredth of the duration of an A.C. current.

External defibrillation. If external cardiac compression has successfully produced a circulation of oxygenated blood, without reversing the ventricular fibrillation, then external defibrillation may be attempted. Because of the high electrical resistance of the chest wall, higher voltages are required to effect electrical defibrillation. An A.C. defibrillator which generates 400 to 500 volts for 0.2 seconds is used. If a longer pulse is used, there is a danger of burning the patient. A D.C. external defibrillator utilises a pulse of 2 to 4 milliseconds and produces 200 to 400 Joules of electrical energy. The amount of electrical energy used can be varied and it is best to start with energy of 20 Joules and increase it if necessary to a maximum of 200 Joules.

It is essential to insulate the patient from the operator. Rubber gloves are recommended and the operator should stand on a dry surface.

There should not be any contact with a metal bed or table and the operator should stand well away from such equipment while the current is applied.

The plates must be moistened with electrode jelly.

Position of plates
1. One plate should lie over the cardiac apex. This will vary with the age and size of the child (p. 104).
2. The other plate should lie over the base of the heart just to the right of the manubrium sterni.

The passage of the electrical current through the patient causes violent contraction of his skeletal muscles resulting in a convulsive movement.

Care of the dying

The approach of death, be it over a short or long period, is always an anxious and unhappy time for the patient and his relatives. For the nurse too it represents, in a sense, failure, and the inevitability of death provokes a feeling of helplessness. For the child it is a puzzling time. Some may feel that death is approaching and the feeling of helplessness will be increased. This will depend on the age of the child, the level of understanding, the degree of illness and the length of illness. In a ward, other children too will be conscious of something happening and they will need to be reassured as well. However, they also tend to be drawn to very ill children and are indeed a source of comfort to them.

CHILD'S REACTION TO DEATH AND DYING
The child's understanding of death will vary with age, intelligence and experience. The younger the child the more difficult it will be for him to understand the concept of death. It will have no significance for the infant, and the young child who is able to talk will repeat definitions of death without any true understanding. Although not under-standing what death means, the young child may perceive the seriousness of his illness from the reactions and changed behaviour of his parents, relatives and nurses. He may react by being anxious and disturbed himself.

Between the ages of 3 and 5 years, children will have heard the word death and will possibly have given it some meaning, but they have difficulty in conceptualising the event. They may show awareness of something serious happening and will exhibit anxiety. They sometimes seek an explanation, and the difficulty lies in finding a suitable one which will not increase their anxiety. Some believe that the child sees it as a punishment, but this applies also to hospitalisation in general. If they stress that they are 'good', or if being 'good' is stressed excessively, then the child may well believe that what is happening is indeed a punishment. Although at this age the child may have experienced loss of some kind, e.g. a pet, he will have great difficulty in applying this experience to himself. It is not desirable to use the euphamism for death as 'gone to sleep'. This will only increase the anxiety and will prevent the child from going to sleep.

As the child grows older there is also increased ability to comprehend the consequences of disease. He will be more able to recognise the meaning of death but he will have great difficulty in coping with the concept of death. The young adolescent will have difficulty in accepting cessation of life and will tend to reject the concept and the fact of death, at least as it applies to himself.

Children will often talk about separation and loneliness. Another means of expressing their anxiety and fear about death is by play. Play can involve many forms and it is important to evaluate both play and drawings, in particular, in an effort to recognise any behavioural changes and respond to these in a positive way. Dreams are also useful as they reveal the child's inner and repressed thoughts. It is possible to use dream references in a way that is perhaps acceptable to the child.

The dilemma whether or what to tell a child
Children are very perceptive to changes in mood, behaviour and attitudes. They can detect the hidden tears and the feeling of hopelessness in others, particularly their parents. They are also

aware that adults do not like to talk about death and dying and therefore tend not to ask any questions or talk about it themselves. Other children, however, may reveal the true nature of the illness to the child, on the basis of what they have heard, and thus cause a lot of pain and anxiety.

When explaining events it is necessary to ascertain the age of the child and the level of knowledge he has first and then follow on questions with other questions determining the meaning of what is asked. Children tend to avoid asking painful questions but ask around a question. It is difficult for them to accept and cope with the truth. What they tend to emphasise is the fact of their loneliness and they need to be reassured that someone will be with them. If the child mentions dying then it is possible to talk about it in general terms. Whatever answer is given it should contain an element of hope.

Stages of dying

Five stages have been identified by E. Kübler-Ross in terms of expected death. While it is possible to recognise these in older children and adolescents, it is doubtful that the young child goes through these stages. Much of this relates more to parents and siblings.

Denial

An awareness of impending death is generally suppressed by denial. It is too difficult to accept and the individual attempts to rationalise and find reasons which are acceptable to him. There may be a desire to seek professional advice or to behave in a way as if nothing has happened. During this stage it is important to listen to what the parent or child has to say and provide active support.

Anger

This stage is often difficult to identify and may not occur in children but in parents; what children seem to experience is more akin to impatience. It is in a sense an expression of desire, almost like looking forward to something. For example, next' birthday or some other pleasant event.

Bargaining

The stage of bargaining is said to be present when the child bargains with himself, with God and others by giving a promise in exchange for improvement or for a lengthening of his life. As he begins to acknowledge what is happening he will enter the stage of depression.

Depression

Depression occurs readily in children of all ages and can be due to many causes, e.g. the child who is subjected to haemodialysis or frequent operations, or frequent readmissions in conditions such as leukaemia. It is a time for listening, if indeed the child can talk about his feelings, and being with him as much as possible. However, it is the parents that the children really want and an effort should be made to enable them to stay with their child. Siblings visiting will also help to relieve the monotony and ease the pain of loneliness.

Acceptance

This is considered to be the final stage of dying. The child appears to be calmer and perhaps takes little interest in what goes on around him. The older child and adolescent will prefer quietness and solitude, with only parents near them. Every possible care should be directed at keeping the child as comfortable as possible.

Nursing skill

The aim is to provide the best possible nursing care within as calm and normal an atmosphere as possible under the circumstances.

Relief from pain. No human being should be allowed to suffer pain, be it physical or mental. Anxiety, fear, loneliness and depression are conditions found in children too. If the child is old enough and asks questions about death or the possibility of dying, then it is important to reassure him, to stay with him and comfort him. Time should be found to stay with him, and opportunity should be given to voice his fears. His parents are extremely important and if they wish to stay with him, care for him and comfort him then they should be given every opportunity to do so.

Provision of an *environment* where the child can maintain his integrity as a person is important. This means that privacy should be available, if it is in the interest of the child, or that of the other children. If he wishes to be part of the ward, and if this is not too distressing either for him or for the other children, then he should be allowed to remain part of the ward.

Great skill and tact is essential to ensure that life is as comfortable as possible. Compassion and understanding of the child's needs should be the nurse's greatest concern. It is not necessary to appear gloomy or depressed and it is important to maintain as normal a relationship as possible under the circumstances. The attitudes adopted will vary according to the conditiions presented, for example: (1) the alert but weak child does not want a great deal of excitement, but may wish to take part in some ward activity. (2) The comatosed child might be better in a cubicle, if available. Conversation should be guarded, since it is difficult to assess level of hearing and understanding. One must assume that his mental faculties are unimpaired. (3) Gentle handling is important and all nursing care such as bathing, change of position, feeding, care of the mouth and hair and all prescribed medical care should be carried out to the end. The child should always look neat and tidy.

Care of relatives

The pain and suffering that parents experience must be great. The nurse should be aware of the emotional state of the parents and should show understanding of their behaviour. People behave differently under differing circumstances. Some are overcome by grief, others may be aggressive. The strain of watching and waiting must find expression somehow and they have a need to express their feeling of helplessness. If they feel like crying, this too should be recognised.

Ministerial care

The parents may wish to have the services of a minister of religion. This may be one of their own choice or one attached to the hospital. It should, however, be recognised that there are many different beliefs and each should be respected and catered for. The nurses should be aware of the child's religious persuasion and should be careful not to impose their own beliefs at the time of approaching death. This is particularly relevant when comfort is expressed in religious terms.

As the time draws near, greater privacy is necessary, leaving the parents with the child as much as possible, while keeping him under constant surveillance and being there when needed.

Last offices

This is a sad task to perform for any nurse. It is emotionally distressing and many nurses find it difficult to accept. Once death has been established by the medical officer, the necessary preparations can be made.

If a cubicle is available, this is desirable to carry out the last offices. If the ward has to be used, the bed should be screened (this should have been done already in the last stages of life). Each hospital will have its own policy and ritual which should be followed. The basic principle is the same, i.e. the body is washed and prepared for the mortuary. If a wound is present, it is redressed, making sure that there is no discharge seeping through. The body must have the name tied on the ankles and it is dressed in a special gown before being taken to the mortuary. All the belongings are collected, listed and placed in a bag and, if the parents are present, these are handed over and should be signed for.

Care of the parents

The death of the child is a tragic event for parents and they should be allowed to express their grief. Privacy is essential. Senior nursing staff generally interview them and give them comfort. It is often difficult to find the right words and it is perhaps better not to say anything. To talk in religious terms is also difficult, particularly if the religious views are not known or are different. Some may be unable to find any comfort in religious explanations. It is better to play it by ear — if religious sentiments are expressed, some comment may be made which coincides with the religious beliefs expressed by the mourners. The rituals of each religious group may be different and each make their own arrangements or specify their needs.

A cup of tea or coffee is often welcome as a means of gaining control. The nurse too is experiencing emotional distress which must find an outlet. Crying is one way of gaining relief but it may have to be controlled until such time as is convenient. Until that time is reached, the nurse must be sufficiently strong to give support to those who are in greatest need.

Chapter 7
General surgical nursing principles

This chapter discusses aspects of nursing related to conditions requiring surgical intervention. The routine nursing is basically the same as previously discussed. The emphasis will therefore be on general pre-operative preparation, specific immediate and continued post-operative management.

Pre-operative preparation

Principles of pre-operative management
Pre-operative management aims to achieve or maintain the best possible physical and mental state which will ensure that the child is able to overcome the trauma of surgical intervention. Further aims are to eliminate or minimise complications during or after surgery by careful anticipation, assessment and treatment.

Types of surgery
Surgery may be either *planned*, where preparation for the operation is possible and the child's general condition is satisfactory, or *emergency*, where the intervention is immediate to prevent serious disability, complications or death. The time for preparation is minimal.

Whether the surgery is planned or emergency there are certain procedures which are necessary to fulfil the above aims:

1. Maintenance of body fluids and electrolyte balance.
2. Replacement of body fluids and electrolytes.
3. Providing a suitable environment. This has to be looked at in relation to the age of the child and his physical state, e.g. neonates have needs different from those of infants and children.
4. Psychological aspect. The recognition that fear and anxiety can interfere with the body's ability to cope with stress.

5. Physical preparation, e.g. skin preparation, rectal lavage, gastric lavage or gastric aspiration.
6. Pre-medication.
7. Preparation for the return of the child from theatre.

Pre-medication
This is based on the child's weight. The choice of drug depends on the anaesthetist and the condition of the child. Atropine, given intramuscularly, is a common choice. Its effects are as follows:

1. Dilatation of pupils due to blockage of cholinergic tone on the pupillary sphincter.
2. Small doses slow the heart and initially there may be disturbance of atrio-ventricular conduction.
3. Salivary secretions are inhibited producing dryness of the mouth. There is also a reduction in intestinal motility.
4. Secretions of the nose, mouth, pharynx and bronchi lead to drying of the respiratory mucous membranes.

Atropine is given as pre-medication for the reasons (3) and (4) above.

INFANTS UP TO 1 YEAR

Pre-operative care
  1. *Cleanliness*. This includes care of the nostrils as well as bodily cleanliness. The umbilicus should have healed, by the tenth day after birth, and should be clean in all children.
  2. *Clothing*. The young infant may be nursed in an incubator and the general care is the same as for the neonate. The older infant should wear loose-fitting clothing which is easily removed and replaced. A jacket made of turkish towelling, tying at the back, is satisfactory. It is also warm and

does not cause fluff in the theatre precincts. The ties of the gown should be loosened while in the anaesthetic room, and the jacket slipped off in theatre without any difficulty or disturbance to the infant.

3. *Hydration.* Fluid and electrolyte imbalance should be corrected according to the needs of the child and as ordered by the medical officer.

If hydration is satisfactory, the last drink should be given 4 to 5 hours prior to the operation. Each hospital has its own policy, for example, nothing being given orally after 5 a.m. if the child goes to theatre in the forenoon; for the afternoon list, he may have a light snack or feed at 10 a.m. The young child cannot understand why he is not given food while other children eat. A crying child will evoke sympathy from other children or visitors and he may be given food by them, despite the 'nothing by mouth' or 'for theatre' notice on the bed. It is essential, therefore, that there is constant supervision and should food or drink be given to the child, this must be reported to the anaesthetist.

4. *Identification.* It is essential that all infants undergoing operation should have identification bracelets, giving name, age, ward and hospital number. Case notes, charts and X-rays are taken to theatre with the child, but these are not proof of identity. The nurse accompanying the infant must be confident that she has the correct child, knows his name, age and diagnosis and that all the necessary pre-operative care has been carried out.

5. *Weight of child.* The weight of the child should also be checked and recorded on the anaesthetic form. This is important so that the correct dose can be calculated.

6. *Pre-medication.* The type of pre-medication will vary with each hospital and with each child. For infants and young children, rectal Pentothal may be given. Unconsciousness usually occurs in 8 to 10 minutes; the child must therefore be handled like any unconscious child (p. 303). Any pre-medication must be given at the time stated by the anaesthetist. Other drugs which may be given include atropine and vitamin K.

CHILDREN

Pre-operative care

1. *Psychological aspect.* The child will hopefully have been prepared for admission and some explanation given for the reason of the admission. Surgical intervention is always frightening for both children and parents. The doctor should have explained to the parents what he intends to do and also what to expect. The mother of the young child may be resident in the ward and this will limit some of the anxiety. However, it is important that parents know what to expect when the child returns from theatre.

The older child should have his questions answered as truthfully as possible and it should be explained to him what to expect so that he is not too upset, particularly if for example intravenous infusion is given. He should also be encouraged to talk about his fears. Admission to hospital should be 1 to 2 days prior to the operation, but this will depend of the condition and the operative measures necessary.

2. *Investigations.* This will also depend on the condition. In most cases, the necessary information will be available from the clinic visit. On admission, all children have a full clinical examination of heart, abdomen and chest. Blood and urine analysis are also carried out routinely. These are necessary because many children have been on the waiting list for some time, and immediate assessment is essential in case other symptoms have now presented and these may lead to complications during or after surgery.

3. *Cleanliness.* This applies to the body, umbilicus, nails and head. A verminous head must be treated before the child goes to theatre. Talcum powder should not be used as it is not sterile, is difficult to remove and is considered a cause of wound infection.

4. *Bowel preparation.* This is only required when operation on the bowel is anticipated, e.g. colostomy, or where bowel movements are irregular. Accurate recording should indicate if a rectal wash out is necessary.

5. *Emptying of bladder.* This is essential in all cases. The toilet-trained child should be given a potty or bedpan/bed bottle for the older child. A full bladder constitutes a danger, as it may be damaged during abdominal incision. Voiding urine during induction of anaesthesia is of nuisance value and involves excessive handling of the child while being anaesthetised.

6. *Hydration and nutrition.* This will depend on the condition of the child. Toddlers and older children may have milk or juice at 5 a.m. (if awake). Nothing should be given after 5 a.m. if he is due to go to theatre in the morning. For the afternoon list, he may have a light snack at 10 a.m.

7. *Clothing.* Warm, loose clothes should be worn. A gown, tying at the back, is useful since it is easy to remove and replace. Turkish towelling is satisfactory as it causes least fluff. If the extremities are cold or cool, socks should be worn; this is to prevent loss of body heat.

8. *Identification.* The danger of operating on the wrong child is an event the nurse must be constantly aware of. The theatre staff are strangers to the child and cannot possibly determine whether he is the one next on the list. Every child must have an identity bracelet containing his name, age, ward and diagnosis. The correct documents should also accompany him. The nurse from the ward should identify the child to the staff in theatre before returning to the ward.

9. *Pre-medication.* The weight of the child must be recorded on the anaesthetic form. Pre-medication is given for the following reasons:

a. To prepare the individual for anaesthetic and thereby help the operative process. Sedation is given to calm the child, as it is easier to anaesthetise a child who is already in a relaxed state. Depressant drugs are best avoided because of the effect on the respiratory centre.

b. Atropine sulphate may be given intramuscularly or subcutaneously (p. 128). It is not a sedative. Omnopon and Scopolamine are also often given as pre-medication.

The drug should be given at the stated time and recorded on the anaesthetic form. The times of administration for older children should be not more than $1\frac{1}{2}$ hours before and not less than 30 minutes before the anaesthetic.

Preparation for emergency operation
Although the time available to prepare the child for operation is limited, it is nevertheless essential to consider all the points mentioned previously. There are however, some additional factors which should be considered.

The stomach usually empties in about $2\frac{1}{2}$ hours if the meal has been light, e.g. gruel, but it may take up to 6 hours for a heavier meal. Studies on healthy individuals show that the stomach responds to changes in the emotional state, for example, sudden fear was attended by marked vasoconstriction and a decrease in acid secretions. Different emotions show different effects. Shock and fright will delay emptying of the stomach. It is, therefore, important to know the time of the accident in relation to the intake of food.

If the accident occurred 2 or 3 hours after taking a meal, it must be presumed that food is still in the stomach. If in any doubt at all, it is safer to pass a large stomach tube size 21 FG or 12 EG for a small child, and size 24 FG or 14 EG for an older child. This may cause vomiting and is perhaps the best way of ensuring that particles of foods are removed, as even large tubes will not allow large particles to pass through the side opening and lumen of the tube. A gastric lavage may also be given. If in any doubt about the emptiness of the stomach, it is safer to delay the operation. The decision to do so rests with the anaesthetist and the degree of urgency for the operation.

For the ill child with an intestinal obstruction, an oesophageal tube No. 11–14 FG or 6–8 EG is passed or No. 9 FG or 4 EG for the infant in the neonatal period. Gastric content is aspirated by syringe and the tube is left open, or attached to the suction apparatus at 5 in Hg or 12 cm Hg (15 kPa) vacuum prior to operation. These tubes are not clamped and act as an escape for gas as well as fluid. This is important in that it prevents abdominal distension which can lead to respiratory difficulties. There is also a great danger that the ill or weak infant or child may inhale vomitus, and this can be avoided by keeping the stomach clear of content.

Psychological aspect. The shock of admission is probably equal to the shock of the reason for admission. The child tends to be more subdued, almost numbed, but this depends on the condition and age of the child and the extent of his injury. Parents will be in a state of shock and this may necessitate a different approach to both admission and pre-operative preparation. Both child and parents should be handled with patience and understanding. Explanations should be given about the routine or pre-operative care and the part the parents can play in preparing the child for the ordeal of the operation.

Preparation for the return from theatre

Part of the pre-operative preparation is the preparation for the return of the child from theatre. The first factor to be considered is *anticipation*. The reason for the operation has been agreed upon by clinical assessment. Though the original assessment may not be the final one, it is still possible to anticipate and prepare for most possibilities. For example, the child who is suffering from a suspected appendicitis may have a closed wound or drainage. He may require an infusion and may also be in need of oxygen. This implies that the equipment for these eventualities should be available. In modern hospitals piped oxygen is available but must be accompanied by the necessary fitments. This includes suction and special resuscitation equipment. The point is that the equipment must be fully working at all times so that an emergency does not arise.

Post-operative nursing care

The immediate post-operative period is spent in the recovery room. The child may still be sedated, but he is able to respond to stimuli. The most essential features during this period are the early recognition of respiratory obstruction and any changes in the child's general condition.

Nursing staff should be detailed to look after any child returning from theatre. Observations are an essential aspect of care and the ability to act is dependent on an understanding of the dangers and problems which may arise. Apart from the routine nursing actions, the following points should be emphasised:

1. Careful handling.
2. Maintenance of clear airway.
3. Maintenance of body temperature.
4. Maintenance of correct fluid and electrolyte balance.
5. Adequate sedation.
6. Observation of the wound.

Careful handling

Transfer from the theatre to the recovery room should be done with care as the child is still unconscious. The head is kept to the side, care being taken to prevent the tongue from falling backward, causing respiratory obstruction. Handling should be gentle and movement of the child limited to those which are absolutely essential.

Once the child is in bed he is placed on his side and his face must be clearly visible at all times. Observations should be constantly made and the slightest change should be recognised and reported.

Maintenance of a clear airway

Observations of breathing should be constant as any change in rhythm, rate, sound and depth may indicate difficulties and any secretions should be sucked out. Change of position should also be considered, particularly if the period of unconsciousness is prolonged. Generally by the time the child has arrived in the ward he has recovered consciousness and is able to move about. Modern anaesthetic techniques also reduce the problem of postanaesthetic vomiting. However, it is only safe to leave him when he is fully awake and is breathing normally. (For signs of obstructed airway and clearing of airway see p. 119.)

Maintenance of body temperature

The aim is to prevent loss of heat when body temperature is normal or below normal, but allow heat loss if the body temperature is high.

Prevention of heat loss

This is a problem affecting pre-term babies, neonates, or children in whom peripheral circulatory failure is present. The child should be returned to a warmed cot in a warm environment, but overheating should be avoided as this increases the metabolic rate and therefore the oxygen requirement. Additional heat by means of an electric blanket and heavy bed clothes should be avoided. The former may cause overheating and the latter may restrict chest movement.

The incubator is ideal for the neonate or small infant. Temperature and humidity can be controlled and kept constant and there is also no need for clothing. This is true of all types of incubators. Various ones are pictured in Figures 10.1–10.5 page 182.

In the pyrexial child, the body temperature should be reduced gradually, depending on the reason for the high temperature. In all cases, the medical officer should be notified who will advise on the action to be taken. A cool fan is useful with the child lying exposed. It is, however, important to keep a check on the body temperature to prevent a too rapid loss of body heat.

Maintenance of fluid and electrolyte balance
Postanaesthetic vomiting is not usual, but should it occur, accurate recording of the frequency and amount is essential.

Minor non-abdominal operations
Children recover quickly from anaesthesia and soon ask for a drink. The time when oral fluids can be given depends on the nature of the operation and the condition of the child. A few sips of water may be given when he is fully conscious, with cough and swallowing reflexes present. This may be followed by a glucose drink and depending on the type of operation and condition, a very light meal may be given. Should vomiting occur, fluids are discontinued temporarily until there is no further vomiting. If it continues, fluid and electrolytes are given parenterally.

The infant who has undergone a minor operation may be given a half-strength milk feed or glucose water about 3 hours after the operation. If he does not vomit, normal feeds can be resumed.

An accurate fluid intake and output chart should be maintained. This should include all fluids taken both orally and parenterally as well as any urine passed and fluid lost by other means, such as vomiting and drainage.

Major operations including abdominal operations
The naso-gastric tube is usually left in position and allowed to drain or the contents may be aspirated at regular intervals. The amount aspirated must be recorded accurately so that this can be added to the assessment of fluid and electrolyte replacement. Fluids and electrolytes are replaced intravenously. This requires additional care to ensure that the stated amount is given over a specified period (p. 451). As the fluid and electrolyte levels become satisfactory and as the child's ability to tolerate oral fluids improves, the intravenous fluid intake is gradually decreased until it can be discontinued.

Sedation
It is unwise and unkind to leave children of any age group without sedation if they show signs of restlessness, distress and pain. The medical officer should be notified as soon as possible. Pain and restlessness quickly exhaust the child and there is a greater demand for oxygen.

Inspection of the wound
On return from theatre frequent inspections of the wound will be essential to determine:

1. *Staining*, which may be either blood (haemorrhage) or serous fluid. In either case loss of extravascular fluid will affect blood volume and may be related to a fall in blood pressure.
2. *Drainage.* Many operations involve some system of drainage. For example, a simple rubber drainage tube which drains on to the dressing, or a drainage tube which has to be attached to a drainage bottle or bag.

   In the simpler form, excessive drainage of matter requires frequent changes of dressing. Drainage tubes must be fitted correctly to the drainage bottle or bag. The extension tubing must not be kinked, as this would interfere with free drainage. In some cases, for example, deep abscess, drainage may be achieved by using a low vacuum suction pump. This avoids soiling of dressing which might be a source of wound infection (p. 138).
3. *Excessive tension of stitches.* This causes severe pain and would also interfere with breathing and movement in general. Both situations should be avoided, the former affecting lung expansion and oxygen intake, the latter causing thrombosis with attendant complications, e.g. pressure sores.
4. *Ruptured stitch line.* This condition should be anticipated where excessive skin tension is present, the condition of the skin is poor or both conditions prevail. The action to be taken

depends on the area involved, for example, a ruptured stitch line not involving other organs but due to infection of the area could probably be treated with saline or sodium hypochlorite. If the stitch line is abdominal then abdominal content may protrude. In this case, the doctor must be notified, but meanwhile the structures should be protected with warm saline packs until a repair can be carried out.

Part of the immediate post-operative nursing care includes observation of temperature, pulse respiration and blood pressure. A rise or fall in any of these must be reported and the necessary actions should be taken or prepared for.

ROUTINE POST-OPERATIVE CARE

Wound care
Dressings are changed according to the type of operation and dressing applied. For example, a closed wound may not have a dressing as such, but stitches are removed on the recommended day, about 8 to 10 days after insertion. There are no doubt variations in different hospitals and in different units in the same hospital. However, the principle of least interference, where closed wounds are concerned, is one that is widely followed. Some surgeons may wish to have the wound inspected every second or third day. A wound which is drained should be dressed every day (p. 138).

Bowels
Bowel action may not be re-established until the second post-operative day. This is largely dependent on the type of operation and the form of nutrition given. Each unit or hospital has its own policy — some may give an aperient on the third operative day, though generally this is not necessary.

Abdominal surgery presents its own problems and complications, e.g. paralytic ileus, but fear of bursting the stitch line may also be a reason, interfering with normal bowel action. Constipation should be avoided since this would lead to excessive straining which would increase intra-abdominal pressure and pain.

Abdominal distension, if due to flatus, can be relieved by introducing a flatus tube (p. 521) and sometimes a small enema may be helpful.

Diet
This depends on the condition of the child and the reason and type of operation, for example:

1. Non-abdominal: a light diet may be given 12 to 24 hours after the operation.
2. Abdominal: initially, fluids are given orally or parenterally. Oral fluids are followed by light diet and if well tolerated, this is followed by a full normal diet.

The nutritional needs of the child have to be assessed carefully. Where there has been excessive tissue destruction as in burns, then the diet should be a high protein one (p. 148).

Nutritional needs of the child after surgery
The nutritional needs of the child undergoing surgery have in part been dealt with in relation to fluid and electrolyte balance. The majority of children in surgical wards have the same feeding problems as those in other wards. In all cases there will be a period of reduced intake within the constraints of the disease from which they are suffering. Those who have sustained injury or have undergone surgery will have a period of reduced intake too, but it is seldom prolonged and any deficit can be readily made up during convalescence. When the period of reduced intake is prolonged, it is vitally important to assess the situation and institute treatment.

There are four situations which will interfere with an adequate intake of food.

1. *Reduction in intake*
   a. Anorexia or lack of appetite. This may be due to the associated condition and is an important cause of inadequate food intake. It is often not recognised by nurses and is indeed one of the greatest problems in hospital. It can only be assessed by careful recording of the actual food eaten. This may involve weighing and measuring of all intake. Parents are also a good guide in determining the food habits prior to the illness and may be of assistance in feeding children.

b. The condition itself may be responsible for the reduction in intake, for example, a lesion of the mouth or of the upper gastro-intestinal tract may prevent transportation of food to the stomach.

c. Repeated surgical intervention which requires anaesthesia. Repeated pre- and post-operative periods of starvation can reduce the intake to unsatisfactory levels. Careful records of the periods involved and the food eaten give an indication that dietary adjustments have to be made.

All dietary constituents are involved and when the intake is dangerously low, the protein taken will be used as a source of heat and energy rather than as its normal function of tissue building and replacement.

2. *Excessive loss of tissue fluids*

Loss of any substance must be replaced. The normal means of replacement is through intake of food. If it is not replaced by food, the body has to draw on its reserves. These reserves are in many instances small in amount so that depletion occurs rapidly. Any disease process, injury or surgical intervention, is followed by a period of breakdown of body protein. The severity and duration of this breakdown (postcatabolic phase) depends on the extent of the injury and surgery, ranging from a few days after an uncomplicated appendicectomy to several weeks in an extensive burn. In the former, the loss is replaced during early convalescence, in the latter, it constitutes a severe drain on body reserves.

Loss of exudate is further increased where skin destruction is extensive. Such loss, consisting mainly of protein and electrolytes, will continue until healing is achieved.

3. *Diminished absorption*

Absorption of broken down food substances occurs in the small intestines. Intestinal injury, disease and extensive resection of the small bowel will lead to loss of important substances. This is due to failure to absorb almost all constituents of the diet, e.g. proteins, fat with fat-soluble vitamins, carbohydrate, minerals, water-soluble vitamins and water.

4. *Increased requirement*

Children and others who have had a reduced intake, increased loss of nutrients or diminished absorption will have an increased need for food to replace the losses. Increased body temperature will also increase the demand for food. If the child is pyrexial, the metabolic rate will be raised and calories are used faster.

There are therefore, many reasons for nutritional inadequacy and the child presents special problems because of the smaller reserves and the greater needs for growth and development. To estimate the needs of the sick child in the situations outlined, it is important to understand the requirements for healthy children in varying age groups. By utilising tables (see for example Table 7.1) it is possible to assess the requirements, though modifications have to be made because the ill child is at bed-rest, and the basic energy needs will therefore not be as in the active child.

Table 7.1 Approximate daily needs

Age (years)	Fluids (ml/kg)	kcal (MJ) per kg	Protein (g/kg)	Thiamine (mg)	Riboflavine (mg)	Ascorbic acid (mg)	Vitamin D (μg)	Vitamin A (μg)	Na (mmol/kg)	K (mmol/kg)
0–1	150	100–120 (0.4–0.48)	3.0–3.5	0.3	0.4	15	10	450	2.5	2.5
1–3	100	90–110 (0.36–0.44)	2.6–3.0	0.5	0.6	20	10	300	2.5	2.5
3–6	90	90–100 (0.36–0.4)	2.0	0.6	0.8	20	10	300	2.0	2.0
7–12	70	80 (0.32)	2.0	0.8	1.0	20	2.5	400	1.5	1.5
Adult	50	40–50 (0.16–0.2)	1.2	1.1	1.7	30	2.5	750	1.5	1.5

However, because of the reasons outlined, the intake must be in excess of normal requirements.

The ill child does not readily accept a high calorie and high protein *solid* diet and therefore, to ensure an adequate intake of food, other methods will have to be found. Two alternative methods will be considered.

1. *Oral fluid supplement*
This supplement is given in addition to normal diet. It is usually in the form of milk shake, providing additional protein and calories in small bulk. The supplement should not interfere with the appetite for main meals and is given in small quantities of about 30 to 60 ml throughout the waking hours. The supplement should meet the following criteria:

a. It should be acceptable and palatable to the child and capable of variation in flavours. Since it may be continued over long periods of time this is an important consideration.
b. It should be stored in the refrigerator and served cold, which makes it more acceptable to the child.
c. It should be of suitable consistency.
d. The composition must be known, so that the intake can be readily calculated. The amount taken varies with the age and weight of the child. Young children will accept up to 300 ml daily, older children 600 to 800 ml, while the 12-year-old will take 1 litre.

2. *Naso-gastric tube feeding*
The feed can be given as interrupted feeding with the tube left in position. It may be given either 3 or 4 hourly with a break through the night so that the hours of sleep are not disturbed (p. 513).

A further discussion on the nutritional needs of the child will be found on page 148 in relation to burns and scald injuries and the information given is also relevant to other forms of injuries.

Physiotherapy
Active physiotherapy may be instituted in some cases. This is to encourage deep-breathing in the postanaesthetic state. Special exercises are used to restore function of damaged joints and muscles after fractures and soft tissue injuries.

Ambulation

Principle involved
Muscular activity prevents the formation of a thrombus and ensures good venous return. This is particularly important when patients tend to remain in one position.

Application of the principle
This requires intelligent assessment of the condition of the child. The principle of ambulation seems to be little understood causing a great deal of distress to the child.

1. The process should be gradual, for example, initially the legs are placed over the side of the bed, allowing gentle movement. The child should not be left alone and if he feels faint or dizzy he should be allowed to rest.
2. As he becomes stronger, walking for short distances should be encouraged. He should be accompanied and the time spent walking should be graded and related to the overall condition of the child.
3. Throughout the immediate post-operative phase, there should be constant assessment and reappraisal of the decisions made. Allowing the child to move about, must, at all times, be according to the condition and the ability to do so without causing needless discomfort and distress.

Rehabilitation
Children tend to recuperate and rehabilitate fairly quickly. Problems may be encountered where amputation has been performed or where long periods of immobilisation were necessary, e.g. orthopaedic cases.

The physiotherapist and occupational therapist as well as nurses play an active part. Limb movement, including muscular and manipulative activity, and schooling are factors involved in the process of rehabilitation.

Convalescence of children depends on the following factors:

1. The condition of the child before, during and after the operation.
2. The child's recuperative powers.
3. Social and economic state of the child's family.

Convalescence can take place in any suitable environment. The child's home may well be the ideal place, particularly from the psychological point of view. There are, however, special convalescent centres catering for this period and arrangements are made in consultation with the medical officer in charge of the child.

Wound care and dressings

Wound care and dressing of wounds is an important nursing function. To be able to do so efficiently requires some knowledge and understanding of the different types of wounds and the healing process.

Types of wounds
A wound is defined as a breach of the body structure either external or internal, produced by some external force. It includes the following types:

1. *Incised wound*. This is produced by sharp-cutting instruments. The wound edges are clean. Bleeding may be profuse and there is usually no bruising surrounding the incised skin, e.g. operation wound.

2. *Punctured wound*. This is produced by a sharp-pointed instrument, e.g. dagger. The skin wound is small and the edges tend to be turned in slightly. Although the puncture may look small externally, it may penetrate quite a distance, injuring soft tissue and organs.

3. *Contused wound*. This is due to tearing and crushing of tissue and may be produced by blunt instruments. Accident wounds tend to be of this type.

4. *Lacerated wound*. This can be of the contused or gunshot varieties. Like the above type, the tissue is torn and crushed.

Healing of wounds
When a body tissue has been damaged or destroyed, the adjacent tissues set to work to repair the damage. The ability to repair the tissue or fill the gap depends on factors such as the extent of the gap and the presence or absence of bacteria. For example, a clean surgical incision where the gap is narrow, will heal quickly if the wound remains free from bacteria; an abscess will take

longer to heal because a relatively large area of tissue has been dissolved and the gap is much larger. There will also be excessive bacterial activity interfering with the healing process.

The healing power of the body is influenced by factors such as:

1. Adequate supply of oxygen to the tissue.
2. Good blood supply carrying nutrients to the area, e.g. vitamin C, protein and iron.
3. Age: babies and children repair their tissues much more quickly than old people.
4. Ability to combat infection.
5. Resting the area affected, e.g. splint for limbs and reduced food intake, i.e. carefully arranged diet, if the alimentary system is affected.

Wounds are said to heal by first intention, second intention and third intention.

First intention healing (primary union)
Wounds which are of the clean incised type (aseptic surgery) heal by first intention.
Course of events. When bleeding stops, the fibrin clot which is formed in the exudate from the injured tissue forms a thin layer which causes the opposing wound margins to adhere lightly together. The connective tissue cells now form fibroblasts which invade the clot. These are accompanied by leucocytes. Capillary buds grow into the clot to nourish the cells and these in turn digest the clot and lay down fibrils which contract to form the repair by scar tissue. The epithelial cells at the edge of the wound multiply to grow over and cover the defect.

The healing process takes about 10 days. During the first few days the tensile strength is low, but increases over the following days until the healing process is complete. The rate of healing varies with different tissue, for example, tendons have a scanty blood supply and healing is slower.

Second intention healing
Healing is by granulation. The initial process is the same as in healing by first intention, but since there is a greater gap and a lack of covering epithelium, there is an exuberant growth until the cavity is filled. The epithelium gradually grows across the surface of the granulation tissue which is gradually converted into fibrous tissue. Granulation tissue is

very vascular and rich to leucocytes and is able to resist infection. If, however, the leucocytes are unable to destroy the bacteria, they form pus. When granulation fails to occupy the wound, it is termed 'indolent'.

Third intention healing
This is the mode of healing of an abscess, involving evacuation or absorption of pus. It allows the abscess walls to collapse and the granulation tissue to fuse.

Delayed healing of wounds
Wounds may take longer to heal when certain conditions, relative to the individual or disease, prevail. The following list summarises some of the causes:

1. Infected wounds:
   a. The organisms may be resistant to drugs.
   b. There is inadequate drainage.
   c. Presence of foreign bodies.
   d. Fistula from an internal organ.
2. Surgical incisions:
   a. The wound is sutured under tension, e.g. stitches may burst.
   b. Haematoma formation preventing or delaying healing.
   c. Sutures which irritate the tissues.
3. Contused wounds:
   a. Damage to skin edges with skin loss.
   b. Burnt tissue.
4. General condition of the child:
   a. Poor nutritional state; proteins and vitamin C in particular are essential for the healing process.
   b. Jaundice; interferes with blood clotting mechanism.
   c. Renal insufficiency; an increased blood urea level also interferes with the healing process.
   d. Corticosteroid therapy; affects healing process by its immuno-suppressive action.

Wound dressing

Wound healing is a natural process of damaged tissue. Normal healing of simple abrasions, scratches and superficial burns, is much more rapid if the wound is left exposed to the air than if covered with a dressing, since dressings tend to keep the wound moist. Nevertheless, many wounds are covered by some type of dressing and it is therefore relevant to discuss the purposes of a dressing which are as follows:

1. It should act as protection of the wound from contamination and subsequent infection.
2. It should protect the wound from friction which could damage the new tissue.
3. It should limit movement of the skin and underlying tissue. Excessive movement could damage tissue, cause bleeding and delay healing.
4. It should provide comfort for the child and prevent pain due to drag.
5. It should absorb any discharge or exudate from a wound, but should not impede its escape from the wound.

Materials used for dressings
Skin does not tolerate constant moisture. Many wounds are left uncovered or are given a protective spray after being sutured. If a dressing is used it should provide ventilation to the underlying skin.
   Gauze. This is made of cotton or rayon. It is soft, absorbent and pliable. It is supplied in varying sizes to suit any wound. The gauze layer in a dressing provides a sterile porous barrier between the wound itself and the overlying dressing.
   Ribbon gauze. Gauze in narrow folded rolls of varying width is used for temporary packing. In the operating theatre it may be used to control bleeding or as packing for the abdominal cavity during the operation.
   Cotton wool. This material is used essentially for padding and absorption. Pure cotton wool is preferred for greater absorption. Cotton wool and rayon mixture is not as absorbent.
   Prepared non-adherent dressings. Cotton impregnated with petroleum jelly (soft paraffin) is used for surface application to raw areas. This is commercially produced and has the advantage in that it prevents the gauze adhering to the wound. Because it is an open-mesh gauze, it allows escape of exudate through its mesh.

Ward dressings
Care of the wound is a routine part of nursing which is mainly carried out in a surgical ward, but

also to some extent on other wards. However careful and expert the nurse may be, it still is a procedure which causes a great deal of anxiety and unhappiness. A wound is more likely to become contaminated if the child is frightened, restless and struggles. The procedure will take much longer, thereby increasing the level of anxiety and making subsequent dressings more difficult to perform. Before discussing the technique itself, it is therefore important to consider several factors which are relevant.

1. Trust

Trust is not something that comes automatically. It requires work on the part of the nurse to establish trust between herself and the child. Where pain is already present this will increase the fear of additional pain. It is therefore important not to present a false picture of the event. It is pointless to say something will not be painful when it is known that it may be painful. The child may not accept the procedure any more readily but at least he will recognise that he is given reasonably honest information.

2. Distraction

The approach to each child varies. The small child should have his attention diverted with a story or a toy. This will help to maintain a calm atmosphere. The older child is interested in the proceedings (this depends on the type of the wound) and likes to watch and ask questions, while others prefer to see as little as possible.

3. Good technique

It is important to study what causes the child pain or discomfort and endeavour to find some means of avoiding it. The technique which is used should be one suitable for the child and the wound. If it causes excessive pain or the child is very distressed, it is wiser to give suitable sedation and change the dressing when the child is calmer. The technique itself should obey the principles of aseptic technique which can be modified to suit the needs of the child and the wound, e.g. using forceps or sterile gloves for cleaning the wound.

4. Observations

Wound care does not simply mean changing the dressing. Every time the procedure is carried out, the wound is assessed and any special or changing features noted. Progress or deterioration of the wound should be reported to the surgeon and the necessary action taken — for example, are the stitches fulfilling their function, or would the wound heal better without them?

5. Reward

This is very important to a child and praise should be given freely. Sweets (if permissible) should also be given as a reward, even if the child has not been co-operative. He should not be made to feel 'bad', but feel that his difficulties have been recognised. Encouragement and understanding are usually effective means of allaying fear and achieving a measure of co-operation.

Dressing technique

The reader is referred to Chapter 13 where the problems and dangers of ward infection are discussed. The problem of infection is even greater during wound care and an understanding of the transmission of infection is an essential prerequisite to an efficient technique based on the principles of asepsis.

Choice of treatment area

A treatment room is probably a better area to treat a wound. It allows for greater privacy, the sound of crying is more muted and therefore other children are not so much affected and are perhaps a little less fearful. Provided the treatment room is well designed with an exhaust-ventilated airlock (Control of Hospital Infection, 1981), which has been shown to reduce infection, then a special room may increase the risk of infection. In wards, which have cubicles, uninfected wounds may be dressed at the bedside. However, if the child is too ill to be moved, bedside wound care would have to be carried out. Some dressings may also be changed in the operating theatre, particularly where large areas of tissue are involved.

When it is necessary to use the ward, it is important to reduce the traffic to a minimum. Cleaning the ward and the treatment room should cease at least 30 minutes before a dressing is commenced, and curtain or screens should, if possible, be drawn at least 10 minutes before the dressing is commenced.

Aseptic technique (see Ch. 13)

Preparation for dressing procedure

A minimum of two nurses will be required, one to act as operator, the other as assistant, but when a small child is to be treated, a third nurse might be necessary.

Trolley. The nurse washes and dries her hands. Masks may be worn according to the policy of the ward or hospital (p. 247). The trolley is washed at the beginning of each dressing round and between each dressing. The top of the trolley is wiped with 70 per cent alcohol (or a phenolic disinfectant) and allowed to dry.

The dressing pack, additional packs, lotions and non-sterile equipment such as adhesive tape, bandages and dressing scissors are placed on the lower shelf of the trolley, which is then taken into the treatment room or to the bedside.

Patient. The child, if old enough, should be given an explanation about the procedure. The assistant should remove the child's clothes and/or bedclothes (if the bedside is used), and the dressed wound site is exposed with the child lying in a suitable position.

Technique

Both operator and assistant wash and dry their hands. If the patient is an infant or small child, a nurse will have to stay with him, give him support and prevent him from falling. Operator and assistant should put on a gown. The operator then opens the pack (the outer bag can be clipped to the side of the trolley for disposables) and flattens the inner paper sheet, using forceps. This provides the sterile field. The gallipot is filled with lotion, sufficient for one dressing.

While the operator prepares the trolley, the assistant removes the outer layer of the dressing. Forceps or sterile plastic gloves can be used. The dressing is placed in the disposal bag.

When the operator is ready, the dressing immediate to the wound is gently removed. Cleaning around the wound is not considered necessary if it is a clean wound, but sterile saline can be used. A clean, stitched wound should not

be moistened but first a fresh, dry, sterile gauze swab may be applied. In some instances, it may be left uncovered 24 hours after the operation. If the dressing adheres to the wound it should be soaked with warm sterile normal saline, to facilitate its removal without damage to the stitch line.

Drained wounds

These wounds should be washed after the immediate dressing has been removed. Chlorhexidine 0.2 to 0.5 per cent aqueous solution is considered suitable or a calcium hypochlorite solution with boric acid (Eusol) may be used for cleaning septic wounds.

The moist swab should be used once only, cleaning from the wound outward. Drained wounds should be covered with a dressing, until the wound is dry and healed. When a closed drainage system such as Redivac is used it may not be necessary to cover it until the drain is removed. Drains should only be used if absolutely necessary and should be removed as soon as possible. All discharging wounds should be adequately covered and the dressing should be changed as soon as it looks moist, since organisms readily penetrate wet dressings.

When the dressing is completed, the child should be comforted, rewarded and returned to his bed or the play area.

Sequence of dressings

When organising a dressing list, clean wounds and those for stitch removal should be attended to at the beginning of the list, while septic and contaminated wounds should be dressed at the end of the list. Each dressing should be considered a separate procedure and the nurse should change her gown between each case. As already stated, the trolley should be cleaned and reset before the next dressing.

Use of forceps for wound dressing

The principle here is to use a non-touch-technique. Three forceps may be required but additional forceps may be necessary. The first forceps is used to remove the dressing and is discarded. The second forceps is used for dipping the sterile swab in the lotion and passing the swab to the third forceps. The third forceps is used for cleaning the wound.

To apply a clean sterile dressing either the second or a new forceps is used. It may be convenient to keep the right (left)-hand forceps for cleaning the wound and the left (right) hand-forceps for dipping and passing.

On completion, all disposable equipment is placed in the bag provided. Equipment to be returned to the central sterile supply department should be discarded into a covered container with disinfectant-detergent solution. The instruments should soak overnight to remove any deposits and allow the disinfectant to act. This method is considered more effective than storing the contaminated instruments in a dry state. Deposits are more difficult to remove and the danger of infection is increased.

Some specific dressing techniques

Removal of sutures
The length of time the sutures remain in position is dependent upon the location and tension. It may vary from 2 to 14 days. Facial sutures are removed in the shortest possible time to lessen the possibility of a scar.

Requirements are as for the dressing trolley, i.e. dressing pack, plus stitch scissors or cutters (Figs. 7.1 & 7.2).

Technique for cleansing the wound is as indicated on page 139 but it is recommended that the wound should not be moistened before the stitches are removed. A dry area is less likely to become infected than a moist one. The principles to be observed in removing sutures are:

1. A relaxed, quiet child is necessary to prevent injury due to movement.

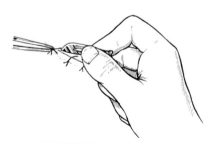

Fig. 7.1 Removal of stitches using a cutter.

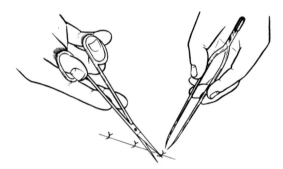

Fig. 7.2 Removal of stitches.

2. To prevent infection of the stitch insertion and underlying tissue, any part of the suture which has been exposed should not be pulled through the underlying tissue.
3. The suture should be cut in one part only to ensure that no suture material is left under the skin. The exception to this rule is the mattress suture.

Method. The removal of sutures should never be a painful operation unless the sutures have become deeply embedded. It is wise to remove first those stitches which are loose and are easily removed. These are probably also least uncomfortable or painful. This gains the child's confidence and makes the procedure much easier. The knot should not be grasped with the dissecting forceps and lifted up as this causes pain and any movement at this point makes the operation more difficult. The scissors or cutter is slipped under the stitch (the blade flat as in Fig. 7.2) and cut where the suture enters the skin. The knot is then held with the forceps and the underlying suture is gently pulled out.

Corset dressing (Fig. 7.3)
This type of dressing may be used when support is required in an effort to unite a wound. It may also be used when frequent dressings are required and a binder is not satisfactory, or when adhesive tape would have to be applied frequently to an abdominal wound.

It is made with Elastoplast (5 cm wide), two pieces of which are cut to the required length. One end of each piece is folded underneath, to form a non-adhesive cover for the dressing. Two or three

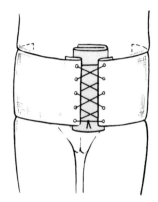

Fig. 7.3 Corset dressing.

eyelets are made by cutting holes about 1 cm from the edge of each non-adhesive piece, and narrow tape is threaded through these and tied. Only the tape then needs to be undone when changing the dressing. If the dressing is applied to give support, the Elastoplast is attached far enough behind to give adequate purchase.

Watershed dressing (Fig. 7.4)
This type of dressing is useful where there is a closed wound adjoining a fistula, colostomy, or a discharging wound. It is made of waterproof adhesive tape.

Two equal lengths of 10 cm are cut from broad adhesive tape. About 7 to 7.5 cm are stuck together, leaving about 2.5 cm free. This forms the base and is attached to the skin between the wound and the fistula. It is essential that the skin is dry and the adhesive tape is applied smoothly

without any wrinkles, which would prevent a proper seal and exudate from the wound could penetrate.

Use of Elastoplast or adhesive tape
Bandages or binders do not always stay in position if a child is ambulant and for this reason Elastoplast is ideal. However, the removal of an adhesive is often the most painful part of a dressing and if this has to be done frequently, the skin may become sore. If this can be anticipated, a piece of Elastoplast, cut to fit the surrounding area of the wound, will overcome this problem. It only needs to be changed when it becomes soiled. The adhesive covering the dressing should be cut to adhere to the surrounding adhesive. Removal will be easier and little or no discomfort should be felt (Figs. 7.5 and 7.6).

Removal of Elastoplast or adhesive. It is painful and unkind to remove adhesive tape from the skin without first loosening it with some solvent. Methylated ether or 'Zoff' (solvent) are effective. The former feels cold to the skin and some children find the vapour unpleasant the latter, however, tends to make the skin red.

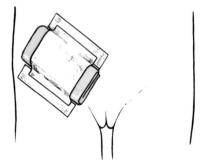

Fig. 7.5 Technique of fixing dressing to an underlay of adhesive tape which does not require to be removed each time the dressing is changed.

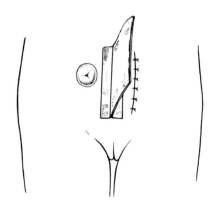

Fig. 7.4 Watershed dressing.

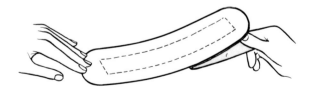

Fig. 7.6 Airstrip ward dressing.

Shortening of peritoneal drainage tube

This is not a pleasant task, but need not be painful. A large sterile safety pin clamped in a strong pair of artery forceps should be ready. The drain is held by the dressing forceps and the suture, if present, is cut. It is then levered gently upwards for about 2.5 to 3 cm depending on the surgeon's instructions. The amount of shortening depends on the type of wound and the amount of drainage expected. The drain is held firmly with the forceps at the level of the skin and the pin is inserted through the drain just above the forceps. The safety pin is closed with forceps and excess drain is cut off. It is important to remember that the drain must not be cut until the safety pin is securely fastened and placed horizontally across the wound line. This is to prevent the drain slipping into the wound. Routine dressing procedure is then followed to complete the wound care.

Burns and scalds

Nursing care of burns and scalds

A burn is a tissue injury caused by thermal (heat), electrical, chemical or radioactive agents. A scald is caused by moist heat. Although a distinction is made between the two types of injuries, the overall effect on the tissues is much the same. However, a burn tends to be more destructive to tissue than a scald.

Causes

In infants and young children scalds are more common than burns and are usually caused by hot water, soup or tea. Burns are caused by clothes catching fire, the child handling hot coals or touching the hot bar of an electric fire. Most of these types of injury occur in the home and many are preventable.

Scalds can occur under the following circumstances:

1. An electric kettle placed on the floor near a plug; the child can be scalded by either pulling at the cord, handling the kettle while it is boiling or merely being in the path of the escaping steam.
2. The handle of a pan projecting over the cooker and the inquisitive child pulling it down or accidentally knocking it down.
3. Teapot being pulled off the table when the child pulls the tablecloth down.
4. Child falling or being put into a bath of very hot water.

Burns are due to the following circumstances:

1. *Flames.* Children playing with matches or standing too close to an open fire. The problem of flammable nightwear in particular must be looked at carefully, since this is one of the most common reasons of burning accidents in children. A mirror placed over an open fire attracts childen and this too leads to burning accidents. Free-standing oil stoves are also a hazard. Greater thought should be given to both design and use of appliances. Safety guards should be provided and used so that accidents of this type can be prevented. These burns are usually deep.
2. *Electrical burns.* These may arise from faulty plugs and wiring or may be due to the use of unguarded electric fires. These burns are usually deep.

The above examples are the most common causes of burns and scalds in children. However, corrosives and radiation burns also occur, the former can be serious if quick action is not taken. The latter type of burn is usually deep and is slow to heal.

Pathophysiology

The common mechanism is changing protein, resulting in cell injury or death. The effect is in accordance with the type, duration and intensity of action of the causative agent. It may vary from mild erythema without any tissue destruction to complete destruction of skin and subjacent tissue, involving muscle and bone. If a large area of the body is involved, it may have both local and general effects.

Initially, there is dilatation of capillaries and small vessels, with an increase in capillary permeability. This leads to plasma loss under the epidermis, producing oedema. This is followed by cellular injury with coagulation of cytoplasm. Loss of protein is from both extra- and intracellular compartments and there is also loss of potassium and magnesium. In full thickness burns, capillaries in the area may be destroyed as well as a substantial number of red cells. The supply of blood in the area will be altered by the damaged capillaries. Loss of skin leads to increased loss of fluid by evaporation of exudation from the surface.

Apart from the local effects, there are also cardinal systemic effects. These are related to haemoconcentration where there is a rise in the viscosity of the blood due to loss of fluid and hypovolaemia (low blood volume) leading to decreased tissue and organ perfusion. This in turn leads to a low glomerular filtration rate and oliguria (small urinary output) and eventually to acute renal failure by the inability of the nephron to deal with the hypoxic state, the accumulation of the products of metabolism and tissue destruction.

Principles of treatment and nursing management
The management depends on the severity and type of burn. The general principles for all burns are:

1. Adequate pulmonary ventilation.
2. Relief of pain.
3. Replacement of fluid loss.
4. Strict asepsis and care of the wound — control of infection.
5. Maintenance of nutrition.

On admission the child should be weighed. This is important in calculating fluid replacement and drug therapy. If necessary, the child is weighed in the nurse's arms. To obtain the child's weight, the nurse's weight is subtracted from the total weight.

Ensuring adequate ventilation. If the burns involve the lips and nares, oedema of the upper respiratory tract can lead to respiratory obstruction. Inhalation of smoke can also lead to damage of the lower respiratory tract. This can be relieved either by a tracheostomy or by passing an endotracheal tube. It may also be necessary to provide assisted ventilation to ensure effective oxygenation (p. 395). A naso-gastric tube is passed to drain gastric contents to prevent regurgitation and aspiration.

Replacement therapy of fluids lost is started to prevent and combat shock. The amount is calculated on the basis of the child's weight and the

extent of the burn. With *extensive* deep burns, whole blood may have to be given in place of plasma for one or more periods. Each time period is calculated from the time the burn occurred, not the admission of the child. For example:

First period	4 hours (from time of burn)
Second period	4 hours
Third period	4 hours
Fourth period	6 hours
Fifth period	6 hours
Sixth period	12 hours = total 36 hours

This is based on the recognition that the loss of fluid occurs in the first 36 hours. Amount is related to the extent and type of burn. A burn chart (Fig. 7.7) is used to assess the amount and extent of injury. The rate of loss is fast in the first 8 hours and gradually decreases in the next 12 to 16 hours.

The body's means of dealing with such loss is by vasoconstriction in the undamaged vessels of the skin and splanchnic area, increasing flow of blood to the vital organs. Some fluid may return from undamaged extracellular spaces and also be absorbed from the intestines.

Replacement fluid may be blood, plasma, Ringer's lactate or isotonic saline (if plasma is not available). Maintenance requirements are met by intravenous dextrose 5 per cent (50 to 70 ml/kg). During this period, careful assessment is essential. An accurate fluid intake and output chart must be maintained. The urine specific gravity must be measured. It may be necessary to insert a catheter into the bladder (a) to measure output accurately and (b) to prevent urine contaminating the wound. Urinary output should be maintained above 10 ml/h for infants and above 20 to 30 ml/h for older children.

The medical officer will also assess the haemoglobin level and red blood cell volume. Blood pressure readings may be difficult to obtain from severely burned children.

Sedation
Distress and apprehension is a common feature. Pain will be severe in mild or moderate burns, but not in deep burns. If pain is severe in extensive superficial burns or partial thickness burns, seda-

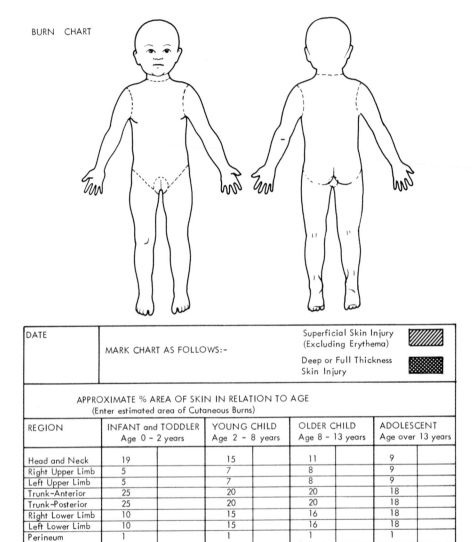

BURN CHART

DATE	MARK CHART AS FOLLOWS:-		Superficial Skin Injury (Excluding Erythema)				
			Deep or Full Thickness Skin Injury				

APPROXIMATE % AREA OF SKIN IN RELATION TO AGE (Enter estimated area of Cutaneous Burns)							
REGION	INFANT and TODDLER Age 0 - 2 years		YOUNG CHILD Age 2 - 8 years		OLDER CHILD Age 8 - 13 years		ADOLESCENT Age over 13 years
Head and Neck	19		15		11		9
Right Upper Limb	5		7		8		9
Left Upper Limb	5		7		8		9
Trunk–Anterior	25		20		20		18
Trunk–Posterior	25		20		20		18
Right Lower Limb	10		15		16		18
Left Lower Limb	10		15		16		18
Perineum	1		1		1		1
Total	100%		100%		100%		100%

Fig. 7.7 Burn chart — approximate percentage area of skin in relation to age.

tion may be given intravenously, e.g. morphine 0.2 mg/kg.

Nursing management

A child suffering from a burn or scald is an extremely frightened one. He should not be left on his own, particularly during the shock phase. In some units, parents are not allowed to stay with the child. They too are in a state of shock and cannot be expected to comfort their child while in such emotional distress.

Isolation

The aim is to protect the child from infection. On admission, throat and nose swabs are taken to detect the haemolytic streptococcus. It is also usual to swab various parts of the wound. If a cubicle is used, it should ideally have plenum ventilation and an exhaust-ventilated airlock. Good barrier nursing techniques (p. 250) are of special importance for these children. Staphylococci are commonly transferred by air but most Gram-negative burn infections when not acquired from the patient's own intestinal flora, are acquired by contact. Cross-infection should therefore be reduced by limiting the number of people entering the isolation area.

Prevention of infection

This is not only achieved by isolating the child, but by ensuring that the techniques used are such that cross-infection is minimised. All members of staff should be aware of their responsibility. Gowns and masks should be worn by all who are in contact with the child. This is particularly important during the early stages while healing has not yet started. Hand washing by all who handle the child is essential and anyone with a nose or throat infection should not come in contact with the child.

Sterile linen should be used on the bed and the burned areas should be placed on sterile towels. Blankets should be boilable and changed as necessary or at least once a week.

Renal assessment

One of the cardinal systemic effects is poor organ perfusion, leading to a low glomerular filtration rate and oliguria and eventually to renal failure (p. 535). To assess renal function, urine tests are carried out to identify abnormal substances. The urine should be tested for blood, which may be present as a result of massive red cell or muscle destruction; protein, as a result of kidney failure; ketones, when the body metabolises protein or fats in the absence of carbohydrates; sugar, which may be present as a result of increased turnover of glucose-producing hyperglycaemia, and creatinine levels as an indication of renal damage.

General nursing care

This involves all nursing procedures such as oral hygiene, care of the hair, perineal and skin care.

Oral care depends on the extent of the incapacity, whether the mouth is burned and whether the child is conscious. The child's mouth and teeth must be kept moist and clean. Care of the hair should be as for any other patient, however, the method used must depend on the condition of the child and the areas involved.

Care of the skin

All unburned areas are washed at least once a day.

This is to maintain normal habits, keep the child clean and to reduce bacterial spread from these areas to the burned ones.

Care of pressure areas

This is particularly important in these children where movement is limited and there is continuous pressure over one or more areas which are subject to pressure sore formation. Frequent position change is essential and any position which provides comfort should be tried. Unburned areas can be treated and protected by silicone cream. Special beds are useful both in treating the burns and preventing pressure sores, e.g. Stryker bed.

Nutrition

The nutritional needs of a burned child will be greater than those of a healthy child. This is because of the extensive destruction of tissue which must be replaced. The greatest need is for protein foods, but iron is also necessary to combat anaemia. Appetite tends to be poor and naso-gastric feeding may have to be instituted.

Initially, the main requirement is for fluids which can be given in the form of orange juice and milk, if the child is able to swallow and if there is no vomiting. Additional protein can be given in the form of Complan (p. 148) with the addition of vitamins A, D and C.

Treatment

Local treatment of burns depends on the extent, type and area involved.

Two methods may be used (1) exposure and (2) dressed, but the aims of each are much the same and include the following:

1. To clean the wound.
2. To prevent infection.
3. To promote healing by providing a suitable environment.
4. If grafting is necessary, to provide a suitable surface.
5. To maintain function in the affected part.

Cleaning of wound

The wound is cleansed under full aseptic conditions. Warm 1 per cent Cetrimide solution is used, blisters are punctured and loose skin is removed.

The area is then dried, in some units this is done with sterile towels or a hairdrier. The burned area may be left exposed or covered with a dressing.

Exposure

The burn is left exposed to the air, which should be at a temperature of 24 to 27 °C. Restraint will be needed and the child should be positioned in such a way as to reduce oedema and cracking of the crust which forms within 48 hours. Exposure method has several advantages over the dressed method:

1. Coagulation of exudate in the presence of air produces a hard, dry, impervious layer which is more resistant to external infection.
2. The burned areas can be observed more readily.
3. It permits heat loss by evaporation and radiation. Dressings reduce desirable heat loss and there will be a rise in body temperature. The wound surfaces tend to become moist and any moisture leaking through the dressing encourages bacterial activity leading to infection of the wound.

Not all cases are considered suitable for exposure treatment. For example, if the burn is circumferential, i.e. trunk, neck or limbs, air flow can be increased by using special devices and beds, e.g. nylon mesh frames and Stryker frames.

Each area has to be treated specifically to prevent complications, e.g. *eyelids* — crusting should be prevented by moistening them with liquid paraffin. Crusting may prevent the eyelids from closing, resulting in corneal ulceration.

Eyes. When the eyes can be opened, the cornea can be protected from infection by irrigation with normal saline and by inserting a substance like Albucid.

Perineum. Gallows traction may be used in infants. Cleanliness of the area is essential particularly after defaecation and urination. To prevent soiling and wetting, a bedpan can be placed under the frame.

Hands and feet. Burns of the hands or feet can be treated by enclosing them in a polythene bag containing silver sulphadiazine and holding the bag in position with a bandage. The limb is then elevated.

Dressings

After cleaning and drying, the burned areas are covered with a single layer of open mesh tulle gras, covered with gauze and cotton wool to absorb any exudate. The dressing should not be disturbed for 10 to 14 days, unless it becomes moist, slips or where pressure is excessive. Superficial burns may have healed within that time, while deep burns will be forming sloughs. The sloughs have to be removed before skin grafts can be performed.

Separation of sloughs can be hastened by the use of soaks of sodium hypochlorite solution (Milton), by the application of digestive enzymes, e.g. trypsin, or by surgical excision.

When removing dressings, the outer dressing is removed carefully to avoid excessive movement. The inner dressing may stick and to prevent damage to the healing surface, the dressing may be soaked off. Hand sprays are useful in that they can be applied to local areas and prevent infection of uninfected parts.

Care of healed areas

Healed areas, whether grafted or not, are massaged with lanoline cream. Greasing of grafted or scarred areas should be continued until the areas are soft and supple. This takes some months. It is also important to keep the areas clean; soap and water should be used for that purpose. Physiotherapy plays an important part in maintaining limb movements and preventing contractures.

Play and occupational therapy should be considered an essential aspect of nursing care. The child of whatever age must find some means of expression of a very traumatic event. Love and understanding, not pity, are the essential ingredients so that he can learn to accept the often disfiguring result of his injuries. School work will also help him to keep abreast with the children at school, as there is often a long period of absence from school following extensive burns.

The older severely burned child may well feel guilty about the accident and may be frightened of the consequences, for example, anger of loved ones or even loss of love from parents. If parents find it difficult to hold the child (if bandaged), then a mother substitute, preferably a close relation, should be available to take over that function. Scarring can produce a feeling of helplessness and rejection. Even successful surgery may fail to satisfy this feeling. Although other children do show compassion and understanding, there may be some who make him feel different. The child will require a great deal of support, just as the parents will need support, so that each will gradually learn to accept the disfigurement and adjust to it and the change in their lives brought about by this traumatic event.

Skin grafts

The purpose of skin grafts is to replace lost or damaged skin. They are used in reconstructive surgery (plastic surgery) to repair defects and malformation, both congenital and acquired; and in cosmetic surgery to reconstruct tissues around the neck and face, to restore function and correct defects.

The basis of skin grafts is that living skin is moved from one area to another where it is able to obtain fresh blood supply and become incorporated as living tissue. Table 7.2 shows the types of skin graft used and the areas to which they can be grafted.

Pre-operative care

The aim is to prepare the child so that the graft will be satisfactorily incorporated into the defective tissue. This involves:

1. Optimal physical state, this can be achieved by ensuring adequate nutrition (pp. 148–150).
2. Good haemoglobin level.
3. Preparation of donor and recipient sites.
4. Where possible, the nature of the operation should be explained to child and his parents.

Post-operative care

The main risk in any skin graft operation is death of the grafted tissue. This can occur if the graft is deprived of blood from the receiving area and this can happen if there is infection, movement and interference with the blood supply. The following nursing functions should be observed:

1. Ensure that the bandage is securely applied and adequate splintage is used.
2. Leave the graft undisturbed for the time specified by the surgeon, e.g. split-skin or full thick-

Table 7.2 Skin grafts

Type of graft	Donor site	Thickness
Free graft		
Split skin (Thiersch) The skin is completely detached from the donor site and embedded on the prepared tissue of the recipient	Thigh, arm, abdominal wall, etc.	Epidermis and part of dermis
Full thickness The graft is usually sutured in position to ensure continuous contact with the recipient's tissue	Back of the pinna of the ear, mastoid area	Epidermis; dermis
Pinch (1 cm discs) These are applied to raw areas, where they become incorporated in the granulation tissue. They heal with scarring	Upper thigh or arm	Epidermis at edges with dermis, subcutaneous fat and blood vessels
Pedicle A large part of thicker skin is detached at one end and fixed on a new site		
Flap	Calf for cross-leg flap, abdominal wall for hand or forearm	Epidermis, dermis subcutaneous fat and blood vessels
Tube (not so often used)	Chest for arm or neck, forehead for face, etc.	Epidermis, dermis subcutaneous fat and blood vessels

ness graft should not be disturbed for 7 to 10 days.

3. Change dressings gently and take care not to remove the graft; the area should be dabbed gently and strong antiseptic solutions should not be applied.
4. Prevent the child from disturbing the dressing; this may necessitate immobilisation of his arms.
5. Care of the donor site for prevention of infection and to encourage healing, e.g. adequate nutrition, etc. A dressing is usually applied for the first 24 to 48 hours when the area may be left exposed. Care should be taken not to injure the site by friction from bedclothes or clothing.
6. Routine nursing care.

Nutritional needs of children with burns or scalds injuries

After any injury, there is a period when the body breaks down its own protein and when the child is unable to satisfy his basic nutritional needs. It is therefore essential to replace this protein loss and to ensure that the basic nutritional needs are met. There is also a need to provide adequate amounts of calories to prevent the use of the body's fat and protein in order to provide the necessary calories. To meet these extra needs the following measures can be used to supply the necessary nutrients:

1. Where possible, children eat ordinary ward diet, including milk with their meals. In addition they are provided with high protein and high calorie supplements from the diet kitchen.
2. If a child cannot, or will not, eat and drink enough to meet the nutritional needs, a tube feed can be given. This can be given during the night only, or throughout the 24 hours.

An example of an inadequate diet after injury is clearly illustrated in Figures 7.8 and 7.9. These graphs are derived from an actual case

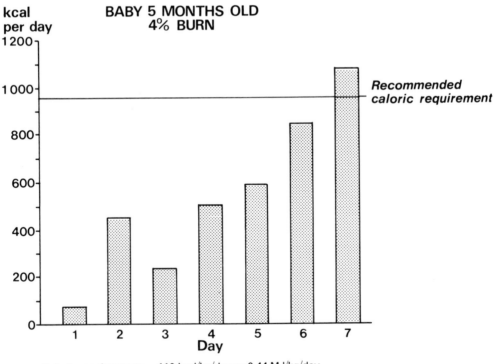

Calorie requirements = 110 kcal/kg/day or 0.44 MJ/kg/day
Infant's weight = 8 kg
= 880 kcal/day or 3.52 MJ/day

Fig. 7.8 Actual caloric intake of baby 5 months old with a 4 per cent burn. (Seven-day period.) The horizontal line shows the recommended caloric intake.

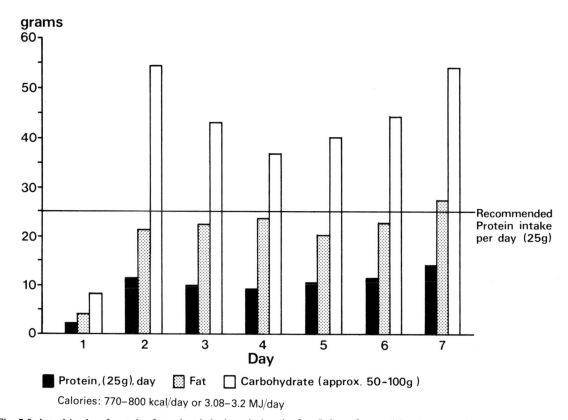

Fig. 7.9 Actual intake of protein, fat and carbohydrate during the first 7 days after receiving 4 per cent burn.

and show that the child was receiving inadequate amounts of protein, fats, carbohydrates and caloric intake while he was kept on his regular diet.

Food supplements

These are foods prepared according to the individual child's needs:

1. *Milk shake.* This is made with milk and Carnation build-up. It contains 18 g protein, 320 kcal (1.28 MJ) per 300 ml approximately (½ pint). It can also be made with milk, Complan, ice-cream, Gastro-caloreen. This contains 16 g protein, 500 kcal (2 MJ) per 300 ml (½ pint).
2. Orange juice with added Gastro-caloreen (100 g per 570 ml); this will provide 670 kcal (2.68 MJ).
3. Fresh cow's milk with added Gastro-caloreen (50 g per 600 ml will contain 17 g protein and

provide 530 kcal (2.12 MJ). (Milk without supplements contains 20 g protein and provides 380 kcal (1.52 MJ).) To increase the caloric value of milk, 100 ml of Gastro-caloreen is added to 500 ml of fresh milk (50 g of the powder is dissolved in 50 ml of water).

Normally each child is given 300 ml of milk shake and 600 ml of orange juice per day, giving an extra 16 to 18 g protein and 1000 to 1170 kcal (4 to 4.68 MJ) per day. A young child can be given half this amount.

If children are reluctant to take the milk shake, they may take it more readily in the form of hot chocolate or hot coffee. These drinks are made with milk and caloreen. Lime, lemon juice and Coca-Cola can be given instead of orange juice.

Naso-gastric feeds

Each feed is calculated individually and is based

on the child's weight, age and severity of the injury. The following points have to be considered:

1. *Protein.* Ideally about 15 per cent of the calories should come from protein. If more than 20 per cent is provided, then some will be broken down and used to provide calories instead of being used to repair tissues.
2. *Calorie value.* 1 kcal (0.004 MJ)/per 1 ml of feed is usually well tolerated and is the maximum desired concentration. Too concentrated a feed gives a high osmotic load and may cause diarrhoea. If the calorie intake is too low, weight loss will result.
3. *Fat.* Too much fat is not easily tolerated and may lead to diarrhoea. Not more than 30 per cent of the calories should come from fat, and preferably less than that amount.
4. *Electrolytes.* Blood analysis will monitor the electrolyte state and adjustments are made according to the analysis.
5. *Bacteria.* It is important to prevent contamination of milk feeds and for this reason it is safer to use prepacked powders rather than milk-based feeds or liquidised meals. It is also more accurate in determining the nutritional components. A liquidised food will have suffered some nutritional loss during cooking and it is difficult to assess the nutritional content. An additional disadvantage is the need to add water to liquidised food so that it can pass through a fine tube. This decreases the nutrient value of the feed.

Products commonly used in supplementary feeds
1. Complan contains 20 g protein, 16 g fat and provides 444 kcal per 100 g (1.77 MJ).
2. Casilan contains 90 g protein per 100 g and does not contain electrolytes. It is therefore useful where increased protein is desirable without increasing the electrolyte and fat content of the feed.
3. Caloreen is electrolyte free, and 'Gastro-caloreen' contains the electrolytes sodium and potassium. Both products are glucose-polymers which do not have the osmotic load of glucose and do not taste sweet. Their energy value is the same as that of glucose and sugar, i.e.

4 kcal per gram (0.01 MJ). Gastro-caloreen is dissolved in hot, sterile water, before adding it to the feed (it does not mix well in cold fluid).
4. Abidec contains vitamins A, D, C, and B groups, the dose varying according to the age of the child, usually from 0.3 to 0.6 ml.

The mixture is dissolved in 1200 ml of sterile water and the child is given either 170 ml × 12, i.e. 2 hourly; or 85 ml × 24, i.e. hourly.

Table 7.3 gives an example of a supplementary feed.

The treatment of severely catabolic patients varies. Current practices in the USA and Europe advocate giving additional amino acids to all severely catabolic patients routinely, whilst others use them only for exceptionally severe burns or slow healing wounds. They are useful in reversing the catabolic process and getting the patient back into positive nitrogen balance more rapidly.

Colostomy

Anatomy and physiology
The large bowel is divided into the right colon, upper left colon, sigmoid colon, rectum and anal canal. For purposes of colostomy, the right colon is not generally used but the transverse colon has a mesentery and is often used for a transverse colostomy. The descending colon has no mesentery and is not used for loop colostomies.

The sigmoid colon is the common site for end colostomies after excision of the rectum. It has a mesentery. The rectum is 6 to 8 cm long in children; it leads into the pelvis below the peritoneal reflection and into the anal canal and anus.

Omentum
The greater omentum is attached to the transverse colon. When the transverse colostomy is to be constructed, part of the omentum is removed from the transverse colon.

Blood supply of the large bowel
A good blood supply is essential for a colostomy to be successful. Two main arteries supply the large bowel and each has an accompanying vein. The superior mesenteric artery supplies the right

Table 7.3 Example of supplementary feed

8-year-old child weighing 25 kg
Normal daily requirement:

70 ml per kg of body weight	= 1750 ml
2 g protein per kg of body weight	= 50 g protein
80 kcal (0.32 MJ) per kg of body weight	= 2000 kcal (8 MJ)
2 mmol sodium per kg of body weight	= 50 mmol Na
2 mmol potassium per kg of body weight	= 50 mmol K

These daily requirements can be met by giving the following:

	Protein	*kcal*	*Sodium*	*Potassium*
230 g Complan	77.5 g	2027	46.5 mmol	50.4 mmol
35 g Casilan	(this provides	(8.1 MJ)		
220 g Gastro-caloreen	15% of the			
0.6 ml Abidec	calories.)			

colon and transverse colon. The inferior artery gives a well-defined left colic branch and a series of sigmoid arteries. When the inferior mesenteric artery passes into the pelvis the name changes to superior rectal artery.

The arteries branch and these branches run parallel to each other in the mesentery of the bowel towards the bowel wall. Close to the bowel wall they join together to form a marginal artery and short vessels run from the marginal artery into the bowel.

Physiology of a colostomy
The normal large bowel acts as a reservoir for faecal material. From the terminal ileum, intestinal juice is poured into the caecum. The juice is an odourless brown fluid and is full of tiny air bubbles. After reaching the caecum, it becomes solid and the air bubbles coalesce to form gas in the large bowel. Bacterial action produces the characteristic odour of faeces.

The faecal material is conveyed along the large bowel by means of peristaltic action. This activity can be seen on sigmoidoscopy during X-ray examination and at operation. It has been studied experimentally. The peristaltic activity consists of small segmental waves and of well-developed progressive waves which push the faeces along the lumen of the colon.

After operation there is diminution of peristaltic activity for a few days with little movement of faecal matter. It is unusual for a new colostomy to

work for a period of 2 to 3 days after operation.

Flatus moves more freely than faecal matter and the first sign of returning activity is the passage of flatus. Faeces follow. The actions may be quite vigorous and irregular. After a week, function begins to settle down, motions tend to become firmer and some form of regularity develops.

Sphincter action and colostomies
The normal anal orifice is guarded by the anal sphincter muscles which open and close as necessary. The sphincter preserves continence. Rectal distension produces a sensation identified by the individual as the need to defaecate.

A colostomy has no sphincter. Patients develop a sensation but they have no control of bowel action.

Definition of colostomy
A colostomy is a hole in the large bowel and opening on to the skin, thereby creating an artificial anus.

Types of colostomy (Fig. 7.10)
1. *Terminal or end colostomy*: in this form of colostomy, the bowel is divided and the end is brought through the abdominal wall (as an end colostomy).
2. *Loop colostomy*: a loop of bowel is brought out of the abdomen. There are two openings, a proximal and a distal one. A transverse colostomy is commonly a loop colostomy.

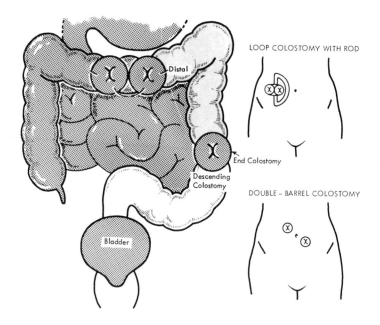

Fig. 7.10 Types of colostomy.

FAECAL STOMAS IN CHILDREN

These include ileostomies and colostomies. They are usually created for the following reasons:

Hirschsprung's disease

This is a congenital malformation in which the nerves of the distal end of the bowel are missing. The length of the bowel affected varies greatly, but the defect always extends to include the anus. The abnormal bowel produces a partial obstruction which may become apparent either in infancy or childhood. The usual treatment is to remove most of the abnormal bowel and to bring the normal bowel down through the sphincters of the anus to the skin. This is satisfactory in an older child, but the infant has a colostomy performed until he is old enough for corrective treatment.

The colostomy may be situated either at the junction of the normal and abnormal bowel (in which case the colostomy is closed at the time of corrective operation) or alternatively, the colostomy may be placed further up the bowel (in which case the colostomy is closed as a separate procedure after the corrective operation has healed). The latter is usually a right transverse colostomy whereas the former will depend entirely

on where the transition between the normal and abnormal bowel occurs.

When the abnormal bowel extends up to include part of the small bowel, an ileostomy is required at the site of transition. Difficulties with nutrition and electrolyte balance commonly occur at this early age and it is usual to perform the corrective surgery at as early an age as possible. Apart from this group, most of the Hirschsprung's babies have their corrective operation and colostomy closure between 10 and 20 months of age.

Imperforate anus

Many babies with imperforate anus can have corrective surgery performed soon after birth and may never require colostomy. In others, the bowel ends high in the pelvis above the level of the sphincter muscles and corrective surgery is usually delayed until the child is older. A temporary colostomy is constructed in the transverse colon, although sometimes in the sigmoid.

Some of these children (about one in five) have defects in the nerve supply to their bladder and bowel, and may require a permanent colostomy and permanent urinary diversion.

Ileostomy

Ileostomy may be performed in an infant suffering from conditions such as Hirschsprung's disease, affecting the long segment, gangrene of the colon, or meconium ileus.

An ileostomy (Fig. 7.11) is an opening into the ileum which is the longest part of the small intestine. A small part of the ileum, about $1\frac{1}{2}$ to 2 cm, is brought out through the abdominal wall and sewn back on itself. It is usually situated in the lower right section of the abdomen and provides a new outlet for faeces to replace the colon and rectum. The lower part of the small intestine is used so that the digestive processes, which take place in the upper part, are not involved. However, since absorption of water and salts normally takes place in the colon, the excretion will be more fluid, i.e. at least initially, until the ileum takes over some of the functions. The normal excretion will then become more semi-solid. Another important point to consider in relation to care of the stoma, is that the discharge contains enzymes which will break down the surrounding skin, which must therefore be kept free from excretion. The discharge tends to flow during the day and also during the night, as there is no controlling sphincter.

Nursing management
The baby with an ileostomy may lose excessive quantities of fluid post-operatively. This loss has to be replaced by intravenous infusion. Stools tend to be loose and this leads to loss of electrolytes, e.g. magnesium, which could lead to convulsions. Fluid replacement should therefore also contain essential electrolytes. Frequent monitoring of serum electrolyte levels will be necessary and the type of milk to be chosen should supply the recommended nutrients and electrolytes to produce a more formed ileostomy action.

Care of the ileostomy and colostomy stoma
Stoma and skin care is extremely important. The opening of the colon requires special care to prevent ulceration of the skin around the ileostomy/colostomy. In the immediate post-operative period, dressing and cleaning of the area should be with full aseptic technique. Prevention of infection is essential, so that healing can take place around the stoma. There are different schools of thought regarding stoma care, e.g.:

1. Applying a layer of tulle gras to the protruding stoma and wrapping a napkin around the abdomen. Faeces are discharged on to the dressing and napkin. Should bleeding from the

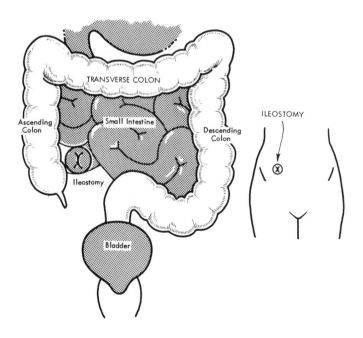

Fig. 7.11 Ileostomy.

mucosa of the bowel occur, this can be arrested by applying a pad soaked in 1:10 000 adrenalin.

2. Applying an ileostomy/colostomy bag immediately after operation. This method is considered better than the previous one, since any faecal discharge will cause damage to the skin, particularly in an ileostomy.

In both methods the following routine has been found satisfactory:

1. The skin should be cleaned with warm water and dried gently; a bath can be given, since soap and water do not harm the stoma.
2. The skin is painted with tincture benzoin compound up to the margin of the stoma. It should be applied to the area to which the stomahesive is applied.
3. A Karaya gum ring is dipped in cold water (it dissolves in water) and is applied to the skin around the stoma. Karaya is a skin-protecting substance which, when formed into a ring provides a snug, leak-proof fit around the stoma.
4. The ileostomy/colostomy bag is applied on to the ring and fixed carefully in position. Care should be taken to ensure that air is removed, so that a smooth, even fit is achieved. In infants, the bag can be supported by a Netaplast belt. The bag is brought through an opening cut in the Netaplast.

   The bag is left in position for some days and is emptied as required, following the above routine. The same bag can be used again, after it has been washed. The bags, which have either a spout or a sleeve-like opening at the bottom so they can be drained without removal after each bowel action, are disposable.
5. Removal of the seal should be by gently peeling it from the skin, or the seal can be loosened with warm water and then removing the Karaya.

Stomahesive is another substance which can be used as a base to which appliances may be attached. The seal can be cut to fit the stoma. The skin should be cleaned in the usual way before applying the stomahesive. The flange is then attached to the polythene surface of the stomahesive by means of a double-sided plaster.

Colostomy wash-out

If the distal loop still contains meconium or faeces, there is a danger of prolapse of the colostomy. To prevent this, the distal loop is washed out, using small quantities of warm, normal saline, introduced through a soft rubber catheter. The catheter should be inserted for about 2.5 cm before the fluid is allowed to flow in. If there is no obstruction, the catheter can be advanced to about 8 to 10 cm with the fluid flowing. The funnel and tubing are then inverted to syphon the fluid back.

Urinary diversion (Ileal conduit) (Fig. 7.12)

A segment of the ileum is converted into a conduit or pipeline, for urinary drainage. The segment is isolated from the intestinal tract and the two separated portions are anastomosed and continue to function normally.

The ureters are spliced into one end of the ileal segment and the other end is brought out through the abdominal wall to form a stoma. There is no voluntary control and the stoma discharges a few drops of urine every 10 to 20 seconds.

Care of the stoma is the same as for ileostomy and colostomy. The important point is that of achieving a leak-proof situation so that the skin is not damaged. Skin cleanliness is vital to prevent excoriation. Various types of bags are available, all are lightweight and disposable. A small valve at the bottom permits drainage of the contents and for night-time, it can be converted into a continuous drainage system.

Permanent urinary diversion

This has to be considered in children with spina bifida and other gross malformations of the urinary tract, including ectopic vesicae and urethral abnormalities. The aim of urinary diversion is to improve renal function, minimise the possibility of recurrent urinary infection and to collect urine in such a way as to cause minimum inconvenience to the child and yet provide a reliable system which will allow the individual to lead a satisfactory life. There are various techniques which can be used in children, one of which is the cutaneous ureterostomy, which involves the formation of a skin stoma and which is useful in very ill children.

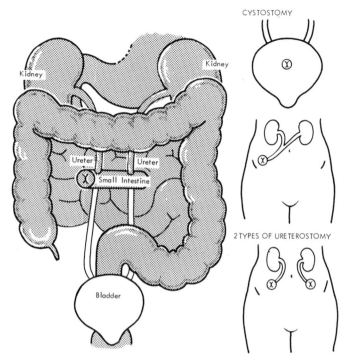

Fig. 7.12 Ureterostomy (urinary diversion).

Support and guidance for the child and parents
The older child needs constant support in learning to accept and manage his stoma. For him, even a minor abnormality can create problems in his relationship with his peers. Children can be tactless and there is a tendency to make fun of him. It also means that the stoma care should be such, that it causes least inconvenience and that the bag can be changed easily.

Parents too will have to be shown how to care for the stoma, and should be able to do so under supervision. However, they should be introduced to this treatment gradually when they are emotionally ready to take over the care of their child. They will require information on how to obtain bags and any equipment necessary.

Chapter 8
Neonatal surgical nursing principles

Surgery for the newborn infant may be necessary if there is an anomaly present. The presentation of the infant varies widely.

Many infants born with a congenital anomaly also have to cope with being pre-term. Thanks to an awareness of their needs, and to improved facilities and care, many of these babies can now survive surgical treatment.

Neonates with certain surgical conditions such as left diaphragmatic hernia and gastroschisis must be transferred for surgery with minimum delay, while others can survive for varying periods without surgical intervention. However, certain aspects must be considered in order that any baby with a surgical problem be in optimum condition for surgery, thus increasing his chance of survival. This is particularly important for those infants who may have to travel considerable distances to a neonatal surgical centre.

A newborn ill infant will have to be transferred from either another hospital or from home, and it is important to discuss the means and the condition of transfer. This transfer is normally organised by the relevant authority and may require special equipment, such as a portable incubator (Figs. 8.1 and 8.2). Also, to ensure that the infant's condition is satisfactory the following factors will have to be considered.

Temperature
The baby should be placed in an incubator or radiant warmer or, if immediate transfer is arranged, a portable incubator may be used. His temperature must be monitored carefully, but handling kept to a minimum, therefore temperature monitoring may be done by the use of temperature probes attached to the skin (p. 103).

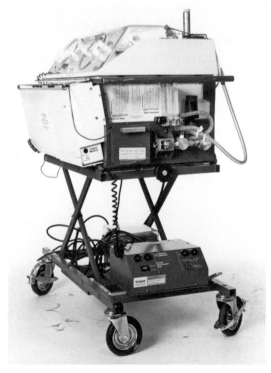

Fig. 8.1 Portable incubator (side view).

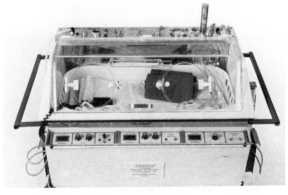

Fig. 8.2 Portable incubator (showing controls and oxygen sensor).

Maintaining pulmonary ventilation

If it is thought that the baby requires oxygen, blood gas analysis will determine the amount necessary. The simplest method of delivering oxygen to an infant is via a perspex head box. It is sometimes necessary to assist the infant's breathing. If, for example, he is pre-term and suffering from a severe degree of respiratory distress syndrome (RDS) he may require intermittent positive pressure ventilation (IPPV) (p. 395) which would necessitate intubation via the nasal or oral route. A less severe degree of respiratory distress syndrome may be treated by constant positive airway pressure (CPAP) (p. 395). This can be administered by one of two methods:

1. A short nasal tube is inserted and attached to a mechanical ventilator.
2. An endotracheal tube is passed and attached to the ventilator. It is possible to give a combination of air and oxygen via the ventilator.

When oxygen is given via a head box a probe should be left in position close to the baby's airway, so that the amount of oxygen being given can be closely monitored. Similarly, oxygen given via a ventilator should be monitored. Whether oxygen, air or a mixture of both are given, warmed humidity should be used to bring them to body temperature and to prevent drying of secretions.

Maintaining fluid balance

An intravenous infusion should be established before transfer, if it is considered necessary. This is useful for the following reasons:

1. Normally, early feeding is recommended to assist in the prevention of hypoglycaemia, which is a possible cause of brain damage if untreated. The infant proceeding to surgery is unable to have alimentary feeding due to the need for general anaesthesia, and perhaps also due to an alimentary tract problem; therefore intravenous fluids are an alternative.
2. It may become necessary to correct a disturbance of the infant's acid-base balance. Although improving ventilation will correct respiratory acidosis, metabolic acidosis or a combination of both may require the administration of 8.4 per cent sodium bicarbonate intravenously.

3. Immediate access to a vein is valuable, should it become necessary to administer other drugs in an emergency situation.

The intravenous infusion can be administered via a peripheral vein, but the umbilical vein is sometimes used. This is perhaps less disturbing to the infant but it can be hazardous as the canula may enter the portal vein, interrupting the blood supply. Some centres now have the ability to use ultrasound equipment to determine the position of the catheter.

SUPPORT FOR THE PARENTS

Just as important as the clinical well-being of the infant is consideration for the parents. Some parents will have learned during the pregnancy that their baby is likely to have an abnormality, while others will have anticipated the birth of a healthy infant. All will suffer to some degree when the baby requires surgery. In the anxiety and business of preparing a baby with a surgical emergency for transfer, the parents must not be 'forgotten' and should be treated with considerable tact, honesty and understanding. They should be kept informed of events and must be made aware of any anxiety for the baby's complete recovery. As an example, the parents of a baby with myelomeningocele should not be led to believe that surgery to the baby's back (normally the initial reason for transfer to a surgical unit) will cure the condition when, depending on the severity of the condition, the child will be permanently handicapped to some degree.

It is known that some infants who are separated from their mothers at a very early stage go on to suffer some emotional problems as developing children; therefore it is vitally important that parents be given the opportunity to see and touch their newborn baby before he is taken away. This helps to create a bond which, subsequently, should develop normally. If the infant has to travel some distance, making it absolutely impossible for a parent to be with him, a photograph may help. Many units now take 'instant' photographs in an effort to reduce the gulf of separation.

The parents should be given as much information as possible about the unit where their baby is being admitted and should be encouraged to telephone the staff when neither of them can accompany him.

DOCUMENTATION

It is important that the unit to which the infant is being transferred is given notification so that preparation can be made to receive him. Case notes and X-rays should be sent with the baby to give the receiving staff as much information as is known of the infant and his family.

Any treatment given, observations and laboratory results should be recorded in writing and given to the receiving unit as this helps in preventing delay in taking an ill infant to theatre. The baby should be identified with a wrist or ankle band.

It is useful for the receiving unit to be told whether the religious needs of the parents have been met.

Written parental consent for operation or treatment must accompany the infant and it is important that a telephone number is available for use in an emergency.

TRANSFER

An experienced nurse and, if necessary, a doctor should escort the infant to the referral hospital so that they can act efficiently and quickly in any emergency.

The transport used should be heated and have good lighting. The temperature of the incubator will be maintained by battery during a short journey, but on a more prolonged journey the ambulance must be able to produce a source from which it can be heated.

During the journey the following aims should be met:

1. *Maintenance of body temperature.*
2. *Maintenance of a clear airway.* Suction equipment must be available.
3. *Good oxygenation.* If the infant's colour deteriorates it may be necessary to increase the oxygen concentration without knowing current gas measurements.
4. *Adequate ventilation.* If a portable ventilator is not available hand-bagging may help abnormal respiratory rates.
5. *Treatment of apnoea.* It may only be necessary for the infant to have the soles of his feet gently

flicked or his abdomen stroked should he become apnoeic. If this does not stimulate him satisfactorily a brief period of nasal/oral suction may be necessary prior to ventilation with a bag and mask.

6. *Maintenance of fluid balance.* It is essential that intravenous systems be checked regularly throughout the journey in order that the correct amount of fluid be given and that the site remains patent.
7. *Prevention of aspiration.* A naso-gastric tube may be passed, and the stomach emptied, prior to any journey being undertaken. The movement of the ambulance may cause aspiration of stomach contents.

ADMISSION AND GENERAL CARE

The infant should be admitted to the unit as swiftly as possible and be weighed before being placed in an incubator or radiant heater as it is important not to disturb him more than is necessary.

The receiving nurse should check his identification and obtain relevant information from the escorting nurse. The nursing care plan will be established.

The intravenous system and any catheters in place should be checked for patency and if a ventilator is used the baby must be attached to the system without delay.

In some units, swabs from axilla, rectum, nose, throat and umbilicus may be sent for bacterial culture and sensitivity. If anything is grown, a guide to the appropriate antibiotic will be given, should the baby show signs of early infection.

The following care is given and observations made:

1. *Breathing.* If the baby is not being ventilated by mechanical means any abnormality in his breathing pattern should be noted, for example whether it is irregular, shallow or grunting. An apnoea monitor may be used (p. 159, Fig. 8.3). To help lung expansion and circulation, the baby's position will be changed and recorded regularly, particularly if he is inactive.
2. *Colour.* Any change in the infant's colour, for example pallor or cyanosis, could be an early indication of significant problems.

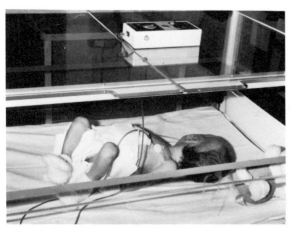

Fig. 8.3 Infant with apnoea monitor attachment.

3. *Apical heart beat.* A cardiac monitor may be used. This will give a recording of the baby's apical heart beat and may also indicate certain abnormalities. Although this is used, the nurse should also listen 2-hourly to the baby's apical heart beat through a stethoscope.

4. *Temperature.* The neonate will require nursing in either an incubator or a radiant heater (Fig. 8.4). If his temperature is not maintained one of the following methods may also be used:

   a. As the surface area of the infant's head is large, heat loss can be excessive. Covering the head can conserve heat.

   b. Use of a soft blanket or a piece of gamgee. This has the disadvantage of making it more difficult to observe colour and breathing.

   c. Aluminium foil wrapped around the baby, leaving his face clear, can be effective but observation of the infant is difficult. It can also cause heat retention, leading to a rapid increase in body temperature.

   d. Clear polythene film wrapped round the infant's body, leaving his head clear, acts as insulation. Good observation is not impaired.

   e. Bubble polythene packing material wrapped round the outside of the incubator acts as insulation.

   f. A perspex heat shield placed in the incubator will conserve heat. This can be rather

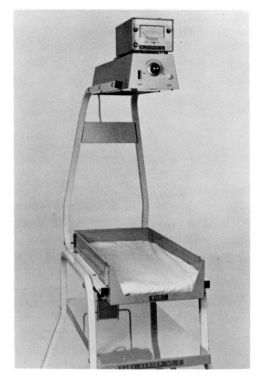

Fig. 8.4 Baby warmer. (Useful in maintaining a warm environment while a procedure is performed on the baby.)

cumbersome, therefore, if the infant is very tiny, a perspex oxygen head box placed over his trunk and limbs is an excellent substitute.

Any additional form of heating must be recorded along with the infant's body temperature. The temperature of the incubator or radiant heater is also noted (Table 8.1).

5. *Oxygen.* Blood gas recordings can be obtained by using a PO_2 monitor (Fig. 8.5) which will indicate trends in the gases. A lead is applied to the skin over a convex area, such as the abdomen, and must reach a temperature of 42 to 43 °C before recording with any accuracy;

Table 8.1 Recommended temperature of incubator in relation to size of infant

Under 1000 g	35–36 °C
1000–1500 g	34–35 °C
1500–2000 g	33–34 °C
2000–3000 g	32–33 °C
Over 3000 g	31–33 °C

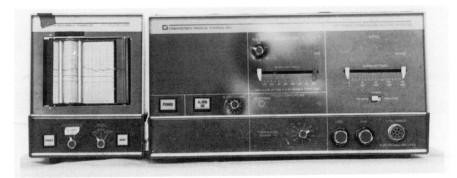

Fig. 8.5 Transcutaneous blood gas monitor.

therefore it is essential that the site is changed 2 to 4-hourly to prevent burning of the skin. If oxygen therapy is administered it should be analysed constantly and the amount being given recorded hourly. The oxygen analyser should be checked for accuracy in air and in 100 per cent oxygen 4-hourly and any necessary adjustments made. The battery must also be checked.

The humidity given along with the oxygen must be heated to body temperature. This should be checked hourly and any fluid which has collected in the delivery tubing should be emptied out so that the flow of oxygen is not impeded.

6. *Assisted ventilation*. If assisted ventilation is necessary the following observations are made:
   a. Regular inspection of the endotracheal tube at its entry site to ensure maintenance of its position. Air entering each lung may be heard through a stethoscope and any changes must be reported immediately.
   b. Ventilator settings are maintained as ordered and are recorded hourly.
   c. The fluid, giving humidity, should be checked hourly so that the correct level is maintained. It is necessary to keep it at the correct temperature. The collection chamber on the humidity circuit is emptied hourly, as is the tubing.
   d. Regular maintenance of the ventilator by a trained technician ascertains that all parts are working efficiently.
7. *Suction of mucoid secretions*.
   a. *Oral and nasal*. It may be necessary to use gentle suction at intervals to clear the

baby's pharynx. The catheter used should be round-ended and large enough for any thickened secretions but, if too large, it may cause damage to the infant's delicate mucosa. The catheter is attached, via bubble tubing, to vacuum at approximately 100 cm of water. It is gently inserted nasally or orally and, when in position, a small hole on the side of the tubing is covered by the nurse's finger and the tube slowly withdrawn. Suctioning should not be a prolonged procedure as this may cause apnoea. The tubing is cleared with water and a clean catheter is attached to it, ready for use when required.

   b. *Endotracheal*. If the infant has an endotracheal tube in position it must be kept unblocked. After disconnecting it from the ventilator tubing, 0.5 ml sterile water is inserted down the endotracheal tube. The operator will normally wear sterile gloves as it is vitally important to prevent infection. A second endotracheal tube cut to the identical length of the one used will indicate how far the suction catheter should now be inserted to reach the tip of the tube. Suction is carried out as above.

   Sterile water is used to clear the tubing when the airway has been cleared of secretions.

   The amount, consistency and colour of secretions should be recorded.

8. *Intravenous fluid intake* (see p. 448). Intravenous fluid intake must be closely monitored as it is essential that the correct amount be administered, thus avoiding either overloading

of the cardiovascular system or infusion of an inadequate amount. A mechanical regulator such as an infusion pump, gravity regulator or syringe pump will normally ensure that the correct amounts of fluid are delivered. These machines have a sounding alarm to alert the nurse to problems. However, it is not wise practice to rely entirely on machinery and hourly recordings of the amount of fluid given and the type used should be made. The site must also be examined and recorded hourly so that any extravasation of fluid into the tissues, not detected by the mechanical regulator, will be observed by the nurse and dealt with promptly. This could prevent harmful damage to deep tissues. The type of fluid being administered, any additives such as potassium chloride, and the rate of flow must be prescribed in writing by a doctor.

While the infant is receiving intravenous fluids his blood sugar may be monitored regularly. This can be done from a subcutaneous blood sample.

9. *Urinary output.* It is essential to establish whether a newborn infant is passing urine and the nurse should observe when it is first passed, how often, and whether it comes in a steady stream or in a trickle. It is also important to record whether relatively small, moderate or large amounts are passed. If it is thought that the child has a urinary tract problem or if there is another reason why the urinary output may be abnormal it is necessary to measure the amounts voided. Some infants do not pass urine for up to 48 hours after birth so it is probably unnecessary to show concern before that period unless the baby is considered to have some related problem.

10. *Faeces.* For a short time after birth black, sticky meconium will be passed. Within approximately 3 days from birth, the infant will normally pass 'changing' stools which are beginning to resemble the normal soft, yellow stools of infancy.

Stools are observed for frequency, colour and consistency and are recorded. Any abnormality must be reported without delay. Blood in a stool can be the first indication of potentially dangerous intestinal problems.

11. *Gastric secretions/vomit.* A normal baby should not vomit and will certainly not be expected to vomit bile, so the presence of this yellow or green substance can be an indication of some type of gastro-intestinal problem.

A vomiting baby should have a naso-gastric tube passed. This is left open-ended and secretions can be drained into a small urine drainage bag to allow easy observation. Stomach contents are aspirated through the naso-gastric tube hourly and the contents of the bag measured. The colour and amount of gastric contents obtained are recorded.

The fluid should be checked with litmus paper at regular intervals to determine that its position in the stomach is maintained. Red litmus paper will change to a blue colour with acid gastric aspirate.

12. *Protection of catheters.* Some infants are very active and it is worthwhile using mittens to prevent them pulling at catheters as to replace them unnecessarily may cause the baby great distress. The mittens should be removed 4-hourly so that the infant's hands can be inspected and cleaned and it can be ascertained that there are no loose threads which may wind themselves around his fingers.

13. *Umbilical cleaning.* Regular cleansing and drying of the umbilicus will protect it from infection.

14. *Oral toilet.* The infant who is unable to suck feeds should have its mouth cleaned with a solution such as glycothymoline every 4 hours.

ROUTINE PRE-OPERATIVE CARE

Depending on the surgical problem present, specific pre-operative care may be required but the following points should be noted:

1. *Cleanliness.* Except in an extreme emergency, the baby should be clean, with particular emphasis being paid to his umbilicus and to the site of operation.

2. *Identification.* Some form of identification is necessary and should be attached to the baby's wrist or ankle, giving his name, date of birth and hospital number if known.

His case notes, any X-rays, charts and the most recent laboratory results should be taken to theatre. His identification is checked against the information in theatre as a safeguard against the wrong procedure being performed.

3. *Drugs.*

a. Babies less than 1 week old may be given 500 μg of vitamin K_1 intramuscularly before operation. Vitamin K is manufactured in the large intestine by bacteria. Newborn infants do not have sufficient intestinal bacteria and, therefore, vitamin K is often deficient in neonates. This could lead to bleeding, since vitamin K is a necessary factor in the clotting mechanism. Due to liver immaturity the administration of vitamin K_1 is not so effective in the pre-term baby, but is nevertheless thought to be of value.

b. Pre-medication of atropine is normally given 30 minutes pre-operatively. Its effects are as follows:

1. Dilatation of pupils due to blockage of cholinergic tone on the pupillary sphincter.

2. Small doses slow the heart and initially there may be disturbance of atrio-ventricular conduction.

3. Salivary secretions are inhibited, producing dryness of the mouth. There is also a reduction in intestinal motility.

4. Secretions of the nose, mouth, pharynx and bronchi lead to drying of the respiratory mucous membrane. Atropine is given as pre-medication for the reasons 3 and 4 above. The dosage may vary considerably, depending on the wishes of the anaesthetist, but is likely to be in the region of 15 μg/kg.

c. Other drugs. Other medication prescribed, for example antibiotics, should be given and their administration recorded, as with all drugs.

4. *Fluids.* The infant should be given nothing per alimentary tract for 4 hours prior to operation. Intravenous therapy may be established pre-operatively. All fluids given must be recorded and the chart sent to theatre. This will also show recordings of output; urine, gastric secretions/vomit and faeces.

5. *Temperature.* The baby should be sent to theatre in an incubator or radiant heater. If additional methods of maintaining his temperature are not used pre-operatively he should have a swaddler, some gamgee or a small blanket sent to theatre with him as they may be required following operation.

His body temperature should be recorded as close to the time of operation as possible without handling and exposing him too often: for example, it can be taken and recorded along with respiratory and apical heart beat when the pre-medication is being given.

He should also have a nappy change at this time and any linen which requires changing can also be dealt with.

6. *Blood urea and electrolytes.* These may be analysed so that any necessary adjustments can be made to intravenous therapy.

7. *Blood grouping and cross-matching.* This will be done before major surgery as it may be necessary to replace blood lost at operation.

8. *Consent.* The medical staff must obtain written consent of any surgery. If the infant has been admitted from a maternity unit and is not accompanied by a parent, the consent will have been sent with him. If the parents are present the surgeon will discuss the problem, explaining the operation and other treatment necessary, before obtaining permission.

It is useful for a nurse to be present at this interview so that the parents can discuss with her what they have been told, as questions often arise when they have had some time to think about the information and explanations given by the surgeon.

ROUTINE POST-OPERATIVE CARE

The general care which the neonate receives prior to operation will probably be continued for a short time after operation, until he is beginning to recover.

The essential routine post-operative principles which apply to a child of any age (p. 131) will also apply following neonatal surgery. A detailed description of the post-operative care of the more common conditions is given in the relevant sections.

Chapter 9
Administration of drugs

Weight and measures

Since 1975 the SI (Système Internationale) has been used in the UK, and since nurses administer drugs and manipulate various units of measurements, it is essential that they should be familiar with these units. The metric system on which the SI system is based is relatively easy to manipulate. In this system, whether measuring weight, volume or length, the multiples are always 10.

Metric weight
The standard unit for weight is the gram (g).

10 milligram	= 1 centigram
10 centigram	= 1 gram
10 gram	= 1 decagram
10 decagram	= 1 hectagram
10 hectagram	= 1 kilogram

In practice, only three of these stages are used:

milligram (mg)	1000 mg	= 1 gram (g)
gram (g)	1000 g	= 1 kg
kilogram (kg)		

In addition, for very small doses the term microgram (μg) is used, i.e. 1/1000 part of a milligram. For quantities less than 1 gram, a nought should be used before the decimal point, e.g. 0.5 g.

500 gram	= $\frac{1}{2}$ kilogram	= 0.5 kg
500 mg	= $\frac{1}{2}$ gram	= 0.5 g
250 mg	= $\frac{1}{4}$ gram	= 0.25 g
125 mg	= $\frac{1}{8}$ g	= 0.125 g
1 mg	= 1/1000 g	= 0.001 g
10 mg	= 10/1000 g	= 0.010 g

Volumes
The standard unit for measuring by volume is the litre:

10 millilitres	= 1 centilitre
10 centilitres	= 1 decilitre
10 decilitres	= 1 litre

Only two stages are used — millitre and litre:
1000 millilitres (ml) = 1 litre (1)

Nurses may see the term 'cc' = cubic centimetre. This is arrived at because 1 litre of water at 4°C weighs 1 kg and occupies a volume of almost exactly 1000 cubic centimetres, therefore 1 cc = 1 ml at 4°C.

Unit of length
Standard unit for length is the metre.

10 millimetres	= 1 centimetre
100 centimetres	= 1 metre
1000 metres	= 1 kilometre

In hospital practice, three units are used:

millimetres (mm)
centimetres (cm)
metre (m)

Concentrations
The litre is accepted as the volume unit in medicine, therefore concentration of mass will be in kg/l (kg per litre) and concentrations of substances relate to their molecular weight and are measured in moles per litre (mol/l). Since we are not likely to come across the pure kg/l concentration, the unit more frequently used will be g/l. The same applies to the mole, the mmol/l being the unit most used for measuring glucose, uric acid and cholestrol concentration. Occasionally, the μmol/l is used.

Units of activity
Normally a medicine is presented as a given weight per tablet, e.g. aspirin 300 mg, or in the case of

a solution so much weight in a given volume, e.g. 10 mg in 1 ml. Other products are expressed as units, e.g. insulin is prescribed in untis, e.g. 32 units, and the range of units used varies widely. In insulin it ranges from 20 to 80 units per ml, though recently this has been changed to 100 units per ml. On the other hand, penicillin and other antibiotics have their strengths measured in hundreds of thousands of units. In order to avoid a great number of noughts, the term *mega unit* is used: 1 mega unit = 1 million units. Each product has its own scale of units of strength. There is no overall unit which applies to all preparations.

Solutions and their dilution

A solution can be defined as a liquid, known as the *solvent*, in which is dissolved another substance called the *solute*. The solute can be:

1. A solid such as salt or sugar.
2. Another liquid such as glycerine.
3. A gas, such as formaldehyde or ammonia.

Water is the most usual solvent in hospitals but alcohol is also used. Where the solute is only soluble in oil then oil is the solvent, e.g. vitamins A and D.

When describing the strength of a solution, it is the proportion of solute present in a given quantity of solvent. This is expressed as a proportion, i.e. 1 in 4 solution, or as a percentage which is the amount present in 100 parts of solution.

1 in 4 becomes 25 in 100 or   25%
1 in 10 = 100 ml in 1 litre   = 10%
1 in 40 = 25 ml in 1 litre   = 2½%
1 in 100 = 10 ml in 1 litre   = 1%
1 in 1000 = 1 ml in 1 litre   = 0.1%

Weight in volume (w/v) solutions

When a solid such as common salt is dissolved in a liquid, it is weighed and dissolved in a volume of water and the final volume of water added, for example, 1 gram of salt dissolved in water, the whole made up to a final volume, e. g. 1 in 500 (w/v). One gram of salt is not added to 500 ml of water, since the 1 gram occupies a certain volume and the final solution would be more than 500 ml.

Whatever the unit used to express the amount by weight initially, this must be converted to grams in order to express the strength, whether as a percentage or as a proportion or ratio.

Volume in volume (v/v) solutions

Here 2 liquids are mixed and the measured volume of each is taken, e.g. 25 per cent solution (v/v) of glycerine in water = 25 ml of glycerine and sufficient water to make up to 100 ml total. Whatever unit is used, each solute and solvent must be in the same unit, e.g. ml in ml.

Example: 25 ml of glycerine to be made up to 100 litres solution 25 ml in 100 litres

= 25 ml in 100 000 ml
   (since 1 litre = 1000 ml)
= 0.025 ml in 100 ml
= 0.025% (v/v)

Molar solutions

The molecular weight of a compound is the sum of the atomic weights of its constituent elements. Water (H_2O) has a molecular weight of 18 made up of 2 atoms of hydrogen (atomic weight of 1 atom of hydrogen is 1), H_2 = 2 and 1 of oxygen (atomic weight is 16); total weight is 18. The molecular weight of any substance in grams is called a *mole* and a molar solution contains 1 mole per litre of the particular substance, i.e. molecular weight of sodium lactate is 112, a one-sixth molar solution would contain 112/6 = 18.7 g of sodium lactate per litre of solution.

Dilution of lotions

The nurse may be called upon to prepare a weak lotion from a more concentrated one:

1. Ensure that the strength required and the strength available are expressed in the same system, i.e. either as proportion or as percentage.
2. Divide the strength required by the strength available and multiply the volume to be prepared. This gives the amount of concentrate required to make up the final solution.

$$\frac{\text{Strength required}}{\text{Strength available}} \times \text{Final solution}$$

Example: Prepare 100 ml of 2% solution using a concentrate of 1 in 5

Strength required = 2%
Strength available = 1 in 5 = 20%

$$\frac{2}{20} \times 100 = 10 \text{ ml}$$

Take 10 ml of concentrate and dilute to 100 ml with water.

Calculations of drug dosage
A child's dosage is based on the surface area and is probably a more accurate method.

1. Child's dose =

$$\frac{surface\ area\ of\ child\ in\ sq\ m \times adult\ dose}{1.75}$$

or

surface area in sq m $\times$ 60 = percentage of adult dose.

Calculation of approximate surface area:

$$\text{Surface area (m}^2) = \frac{4\ w + 7}{w + 90}$$

Where w is weight in kg.

Another method is:

2. Based on the weight of the child in relation to that of the adults. Dose in mg/kg if adult dose is 1 mg/kg.

Equivalents — Imperial and Metric
Height
2.5 cm = 1 inch

To convert inches to centimetres
Example
  1 inch   = 2.5 cm
  12 inches   = 2.5 $\times$ 12 = 30.00 cm
To convert centimetres to inches
Example

24 cm = ? inch

$$2.5 \text{ cm} = 1 \text{ inch} \therefore 1 \text{ cm} = \frac{1}{2.5} \text{ inch}$$

$$\therefore 24 \text{ cm} = \frac{1 \times 24}{2.5} = \frac{24 \times 2}{5} = \frac{48}{5} = 9.6 \text{ in}$$

Weight
2.2 lb = 1 kg

To convert lb to kg
Example
  16 lb = ? kg
  2.2 lb = 1 kg

$$16 \text{ lb} = \frac{16 \times 1}{2.2} = \frac{160}{22} = 7.2 \text{ kg}$$

To convert kg to lb
  Example
    4.5 kg= ? lb
    1 kg= 2.2 lb
    4.5 kg= 2.2 $\times$ 4.5 = 9.90 lb

Volume
1 minim (drop)	= 0.06 ml
17 minims	= 1 ml
1 fluid ounce	= 28.4 ml
20 fluid ounces	= 368 ml
35 fluid ounces	= 1 litre
1 gallon	= 4.5 litres

Administration of medicines

The nurse's role and responsibility
Medicines are *only* given on the written instruction of the medical officer, therefore nurses are not asked or expected to prescribe, nor are they allowed to dispense drugs of any kind without the permission of a qualified medical practitioner. The nurse's responsibility is then more easily identified as:

1. The handling of the child and skill in giving the drug.
2. Knowledge of the drug to be given (Tables 9.1 and 9.2).
3. Knowledge and recognition of idiosyncrasies or intolerance, e.g. allergic response to penicillin.
4. Responsibility relating to giving drugs at stated times.
5. Ensuring that the drug is available and in suitable form for the age group and condition.
6. Reporting of inability or unwillingness to take the drug, and also of vomiting of the drug.
7. Signature of the Kardex indicating that the drug has been given.

Handling of the child
This can present a great challenge to the nurse and

Table 9.1 Drugs commonly used

Drug	Type	Route	Conditions
Acetazolamide	Diuretic	Oral	Nephrotic syndrome
Actinomycin D	Antibiotic	i.v.	Treatment of Wilm's tumour and neuroblastoma
Adrenaline 1:1000	Adrenergic	s.c.	Status asthmaticus, urticaria
Aminophylline	Bronchodilator	Oral i.m. i.v.	Bronchial asthma
Aspirin, soluble	Analgesic	Oral	Anti-pyretic, relief of pain
Atropine sulphate	Parasympathetic inhibitor	Oral s.c	Mydriasis, slows heart rate, inhibits salivary, nose, mouth and bronchial secretions
Bendrofluazide	Diuretic	Oral	Retention of sodium in steroid therapy
Bephenium hydroxynaphthoate	Anthelmintic	Oral	Hookworm and roundworm infestation
Calciferol (vitamin D_2)		Oral	Rickets
Calcium chloride	Electrolyte	Oral	Hypocalcaemic tetany (mild) cardiac stimulant
Calcium gluconate	Electrolyte	Oral i.v.	In severe hypocalcaemic tetany
Calcium lactate	Electrolyte	Oral	Rickets
Carbamazepine (tegretol)	Anticonvulsant	Oral	Grand mal epilepsy
Chloral hydrate	Hypnotic	Oral	Convulsions
Chlorothiazide	Diuretic	Oral	Hypertension, oedema
Chlorpromazine	Sedative, antiemetic (cerebral action)	Oral i.m.	Vomiting
Cyclophosphamide	Alkylating agent (linking molecules)	Oral i.v	Malignant disease
Desferrioxamine mesylate	Chelating agent (binding)		Iron poisoning
Diazepam	Minor tranquilliser	Oral i.m. i.v.	Anti-spasmodic in convulsions and as pre-medication
Diazoxide	Adrenergic blocking agent	Oral i.v.	Hypoglycaemia Hypertension
Digoxin	Myocardial stimulant	Oral,	Cardiac failure
Ephedrine	Symphathomimetic	Oral	Bronchospasm
Ferrous gluconate		Oral	Anaemia
Ferrous sulphate		Oral	Anaemia
Folic acid	Nucleic acid catalyst	Oral	Anaemia
Frusemide	Diuretic	Oral	Oedema
Glucagon	Releasing agent for insulin, growth hormone, etc	i.m. i.v.	Hypoglycaemia; as a diagnostic test in glycogen storage disease
Heparin	Anti-coagulant	i.v.	Thrombosis, post-operatively
Hyoscine hydrobromide	Sedative	Oral s.c.	Pre-medication

Table 9.1 (*cont'd*)

Magnesium chloride	Electrolyte	Oral	Neonatal hypomagnesaemia
Mepacrine HCL	Antiparasitic	Oral	Giardiasis
Mercaptopurine	Antimetabolite	Oral	Leukaemia
Methotrexate	Antimetabolite	Oral	Leukaemia
Nitrazepam	Hypnotic	Oral	Convulsions
Orciprenaline	Bronchodilator	Oral	Asthma
Pancreatin BP	Digestive enzyme	Oral	Fibrocystic disease of the pancreas
Paraveratum	Narcotic analgesic	s.c. i.m.	Pre-and post-operative analgesic
Paracetamol	Analgesic	Oral	Pyrexia and pain
Paraldehyde	Anticonvulsant	Oral i.m.	Status epilepticus
Pethidine	Narcotic, analgesic	Oral s.c.	Muscle relaxant, relief of pain
Phenobarbitone	Sedative, anticonvulsant	Oral, i.m., i.v.	Grand mal
Phenytoin	Anticonvulsant	Oral i.v. i.m.	Status epilepticus
Phytomenadione (vitamin K$_1$)		Oral i.m.	Haemorrhagic disease of the newborn
Piperazine hydrate	Anthelmintic	Oral	Threadworm and roundworm
Salbutamol (Ventolin)	Bronchodilator	Oral	Bronchial asthma
Senna	Irritant purgative	Oral at night	Encopresis Constipation
Spironolactone	Synthetic steroid diuretic	Oral	Nephrotic syndrome
Thiopentone sod.	Short-acting barbiturate	Rectal	Basal anaesthesia
Thyroxine	Hormone	Oral	Hypothyroidism
Trimeprazine tart. (Vallergan)	Antihistamine sedative	Oral	Pruritis
Vincristine	Antimetabolite	i.v.	Acute lymphoblastic leukaemia
Warfarin	Anticoagulant	Oral	Post-operative cardiothoracic

depends on the route of administration. All human beings tend to be suspicious and perhaps frightened of drugs, and children in particular need careful handling. Indeed, the first time that medicines are given is crucial in determining subsequent behaviour related to taking medicine. There are many situations over which nurses have little or no control, e.g. the taste of the drug, but it is nevertheless incumbent on them to find the form most acceptable to the child.

Psychological preparation
However young the child, it is vital to prepare him for the procedure in order to achieve a measure of co-operation.

Infant. It is important to talk to him, to pick him up while giving the medicine, and to cuddle him if he is frightened or upset.

Toddler. This is a difficult group to manage. It might help to play with him or to use a doll, etc. with which he can play out the situation, e.g.

Table 9.2 Chemotherapeutic agents and antibiotics in common use

Drug	Route	Sensitivity	Effective in (condition)
Amphotericin B	Oral i.v.	Filamentous and yeast-like fungi	Histoplasmosis
Ampicillin	Oral i.m. i.v.	Staphyl. pyogenes Strepto. pyogenes E. coli	Meningitis
Cephalexin	Oral	Broad spectrum	Urinary and respiratory infections
Cephaloridine	i.m.	Broad spectrum	Urinary and respiratory infections
Chloramphenicol	Oral i.m. i.v.	Gram-positive	Meningitis, chronic bronchitis, pertussis
Cloxacillin and flucloxallin	Oral i.m. i.v	Broad spectrum Staph. aureus	
Colistin sulphate (polymyxin E)	Oral	Gram-negative	Gastroenteritis
Colistin sulphomethate (polymyxin E)	i.m. i.v.	Gram-negative	
Erythromycin	Oral i.v.	Hospital Staphyl. Staphylococcus Streptococcus	Endocarditis
Gentamicin	i.m.	Broad spectrum	
Isoniazid (I.N.A.H.)	Oral	Tubercle	Tuberculosis
Kanamycin	i.m.	Gram-negative	Septicaemia
Nalidixic acid	Oral	E. coli	Renal infections
Neomycin	Oral	Broad spectrum	
Nitrofuradantoin	Oral		Renal infection
Nystatin	Oral	Monialiasis	Thrush
Oxytetracycline	Oral i.v. i.m.	Virus	Bronchitis
P.A.S.	Oral	Tubercle	Tuberculosis
Penicillin G	i.m.	Staphyl. Strepto. Cl. Welchii Pneumococcus	Meningitis
Penicillin prolonged action	i.m.	Staphyl. Strepto. Cl. Welchii Pneumococcus	
Penicillin V	Oral	Staphyl. Strepto. Cl. Welchii Pneumococcus	Respiratory infection, Tonsillitis
Phthalylsulphathiazole	Oral		Intestinal infection (antibacterial)
Streptomycin	Oral i.m.	Staph; strept; Pneumoc; E. coli	

Table 9.2 (*cont'd*)

Sulphadimidine	Oral i.m.	Pneumococcus Staphyl.	Systemic, urinary tract infection
Sulphadiazine	i.v.	E. coli	
Sulphafurazole	Oral	Pneumococcus staphyl. E. coli	Systemic, urinary tract infection
Sulphamethizole	Oral	E. coli	Gastroenteritis
Sulphaselazine	Oral	E. coli	Gastroenteritis
Tetracycline HCL	Oral i.m. i.v.	Broad spectrum	Systemic-generalised infections

giving medicine to the doll. He should be lifted out and held securely, yet lovingly. It is not easy to carry out this procedure alone and it is therefore essential to have at least one other nurse to help. Parents either visiting or resident can be of help here.

Older children. Their response varies with the illness and their level of understanding. Generally, they are helpful and tend to be proud to be able to take medicines without fuss. However, some difficulties may still be encountered. Force should be avoided and some means should be found to make it possible and easier for them to take the medicine. Whenever possible, children should be sitting up to take medicine.

Methods of administration

Drugs may be given by the following routes:

1. Local

The drug is brought into direct contact with the tissue to be treated, e.g. gentian violet or benzyl benzoate, applied to the skin or mucous membrane. Local applications are easy to apply, generally painless, but may be messy.

2. Oral

This is the most common method. It is painless but may be unpleasant to taste, or may be difficult to swallow. Absorption into the bloodstream is through the oral mucous membrane, stomach or jejunum. The drug circulates in the bloodstream and is carried to the part of the body where it is to act.

If the drug is to act through the oral mucous membrane, it is important that the patient does not swallow it, as this would render it ineffective.

Stomach. Few drugs are absorbed here and some may cause local irritation to the gastric mucosa. Alcohol, which is rapidly absorbed, can be detected in the bloodstream within 5 minutes of ingestion, however, the rate of absorption is decreased if it is taken with food. Drugs such as aspirin or ferrous sulphate may cause irritation which can be prevented by giving them with milk. It is also important to recognise that some drugs may be affected when given with an acid substance such as rose hip syrup.

Jejunum and ileum. Most drugs are absorbed into the bloodstream through the jejunum, although some are absorbed in the distal part of the ileum. Some substances are not absorbed because they are inactivated by enzymes in the small intestine, e.g. insulin is inactivated when given orally, and vitamin B_{12} is not absorbed due to lack of the intrinsic factor.

3. Rectal administration

The rectal mucous membrane is able to absorb substances in relatively small quantities. Absorption takes place if the drug is administered as suppositories, or if given in fluid form it may have a local action, e.g. corticosteroids, used in ulcerative colitis.

4. Injection

Drugs may be given by this means if the child is unable to take drugs orally. There is increased certainty of absorption, though the rate varies with the type of injection, and it is also more rapid in effect than oral administrations. Injections are given by the following routes:

a. Subcutaneous or hypodermic.
b. Intramuscular.
c. Intravenous.
d. Intrathecal.

Control of drugs

The types of drugs which can be administered by nurses and doctors are strictly regulated by laws enacted by Parliament. These laws regulate the supply, storage and administration of drugs. The statues concerned are the *Pharmacy Act*: 1933 and subsequent orders and regulations; *Dangerous Drugs Act*, (1920) now the Controlled Drugs Act and the Therapeutic Substances Act (1967). The *Misuse of Drugs Act* came into force in 1973. This Act combines and extends the Dangerous Drugs Acts 1965 and 1967.

Principles of the Act

Addiction to drugs presents a serious problem to any society. In order to achieve some control and to protect both the individual and society, certain laws have been enacted. These include the following:

That the import, export, production, supply and possession of controlled drugs are unlawful except as provided by the regulations, or, in the case of import and export, by any licences issued by the Home Secretary.

Controlled drugs are classified in two ways:

1. As 'classes' for the purpose of maximum penalties which may be applied for offences on the basis of the drug's potential harmfulness when misued.
2. As 'groups' so that controls may be applied to their use for legitimate purposes.

This classification is further broken down into four schedules:

Schedule 1. These include: codeine, pholcodeine, cocaine, morphine or any combination in such *small* amounts which will not cause harm or lead to dependence. They can be sold over the counter without prescription, but an invoice or a copy must be kept for 2 years.

Schedule 2. These include opiates (heroin, morphine, methadone, amphetamines). A licence is required to export or import these and they may only be supplied on the authority of a prescription. The regulations as to safe custody, destruction, marking of containers and keeping of records, must be observed.

Schedule 3. These include a small number of minor stimulant drugs, e.g. benzphetamine and other drugs which are not thought to be harmful if misused.

Schedule 4. These include the hallucinogenic drugs, e.g. LSD and cannabis which have virtually no therapeutic use and for which a licence from the Home Office is needed.

Advice on the use of drugs is given by an Advisory Council to the Home Secretary on the misuse of drugs. If the Home Secretary considers that a social problem exists in any area caused by the extensive misuse a dangerous or otherwise harmful drugs, the Act empowers him to require doctors and pharmacists to give particulars for a specified period regarding the amounts of these drugs prescribed, administered or supplied. This information is mandatory.

Legislation also covers the requisition of drugs, possession and supply of drugs, i.e. persons who are legally permitted to possess and supply Schedules 2, 3 and 4 drugs. These include, general practitioner, pharmacist, licence holder, constable when acting in the course of his duties, nursing personnel in charge of a ward, theatre or department in hospital or nursing home.

Registers

Records must be kept of all drugs in Schedule 2 and 4. The register contains the following and must be maintained according to the regulations.

1. The class of drug must be specified at the head of each page.
2. Entries must be made on the day of transaction (in hospitals) or on the next day (in businesses).
3. No cancellation, obliteration or alteration may be made, any correction must be dated and entered as a marginal note or footnote.
4. Entries must be in ink or otherwise indelible.
5. The register must not be used for other purposes.

6. Each department must have its own register and these must be kept for 2 years from the last date of entry.

Marking of bottles and other containers
1. Bottles, etc. must be clearly marked with the amount of drug contained.
2. If the drug is a preparation made up from various drugs, cachets or other dosage units, the container must be marked with the amount of controlled drugs in each dosage unit and the number of dosage units in it.

Regulations applying to hospitals
These regulations relate to the procedures for ordering controlled drugs and for the safe custody of these drugs. These include the following:

1. Drugs must be kept in a locked safe, cabinet or room, and no unauthorised person may have access to them. The keys must be kept by the nurse in charge.
2. Drugs can only be given on the written instruction of the medical officer.
3. The drug must only be given to the patient for whom it has been prescribed.
4. The drug and its details must be written up in the controlled drugs book and signed by the nurse who administers the drug and by the person checking the drug and dose.
5. Any drug wasted must be recorded with the signature of a witness.
6. Regular inspection of 'controlled drugs' by the pharmacist.

Storage of drugs outside the Controlled Drugs Act
Regulations concerning the use and control of the drug cupboard are laid down by each hospital authority. These regulations are based on the rules stated by Act of Parliament.

1. Only drugs, etc. outside 'control' can be kept in this cupboard.
2. The cupboard must be kept locked at all times except for the removal, replacement and checking of drugs.
3. The medicine cupboard should be checked daily and only those medicines kept which are required for the patients present in the ward.

Any medicines not required should be returned to the pharmacy.
4. Bottles should be kept clean and the label must be readable.
5. Medicines which require cool storage should be stored in a special refrigerator, i.e. one which contains only drugs.

Guidelines for the administration of medicines
In an effort to prevent errors in drug administration and their consequences, guidelines are issued by each hospital authority.
The following points should be considered:

1. The greatest care and concentration is required. This means that the nurse who is administering medicines must not be interrupted or distracted by other matters.
2. The prescription is read carefully. If there is any doubt about the name or dose of the drug, it should not be given until someone in authority has been consulted.
3. The child's identification bracelet must always be checked before the medicine is administered.
4. The drug should be checked against the prescription preferably by a second nurse, immediately before administering the drug.
5. When giving a drug like Digitalis, it is important to check the apex heart-beat (p. 104) of the patient before and after the drug has been given. Digitalis slows the heart beat, and should it reach a level below that permitted, the drug may have to be omitted. It is also necessary to observe any allergic reaction, such as urticaria. This must be reported and recorded before the causative drug is repeated.
6. Recognition of adverse effects. These are often unrecognised and under-reported in children and particularly in the newborn. The nurse should be aware of the possibility of reactions and, should they occur, report them to the medical officer. For example, most drugs affect the gastro-intestinal system causing nausea and vomiting, or diarrhoea and monilial infection; while some drugs may depress bone marrow function, others may affect the nervous system causing drowsiness, ataxia, dyskinesia and hyperkinesis. Examples of drugs affecting the nervous system are phenobarbitone, which can

cause drowsiness and hyperkinesis, and phenytoin causing ataxia. Literature is usually available and the nurse should study these in order to become aware of possible adverse effects.

7. Where possible, the medicine must be examined to make sure that no deterioration has taken place or that the expiry date has not been passed.

8. To ensure that the label is readable, the labelled side of the bottle should be uppermost when pouring out liquid medicine. Should the label become soiled, the bottle or container must be returned to the pharmacy.

9. As soon as the drug has been given to the child, the fact should be recorded on the Kardex. This will prevent double administration of the drug.

Oral administration of drugs

Principles involved

1. Patience to find the simplest and most pleasant way of giving the medicine to the child.
2. Knowledge of the action and reaction of drugs.
3. Understanding of the methods of absorption.
4. Accuracy to ensure that the correct drug and amount is given to the correct patient in the correct time.
5. Recognition of allergic response and observation of the patient to whom the drug is administered.

Reasons
It is the simplest and most convenient method, provided that the child can swallow and that the action of the drug is not diminished by gastric juices.

Requirements
Medicine trolley, containing the required number of medicine glasses, teaspoons (preferably graduated), graduated pipettes or a medicine syringe; drugs to be administered; sterile water; tissues; prescription sheets or Kardex; sweets (Fig. 9.1).

Methods for infants
Two nurses will be required, one to hold and comfort the child, the other to give the medicine.

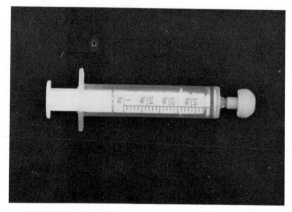

Fig. 9.1 Medicine syringe for oral administration of medicine to infants.

A bib or tissue should be placed round the baby's neck.

Two nurses wash and dry their hands. The nurse holding the baby puts on a gown and lifts him out of the cot (if possible). The infant should be held firmly with the outer arm of the baby restrained and the inner arm tucked well out of the way. The infant is allowed to suck the medicine from a spoon or from a special dropper. It must not be forced into the baby's mouth as this may lead to spluttering, spitting or inhalation. If a large quantity of medicine has to be given, one quarter of a teaspoonful is given at a time and the spoon is held in readiness to collect any medicine which might be ejected; it is then given again. The use of the medicine syringe will ensure that the baby receives his medicine without spluttering. A small amount is placed on his tongue and repeated until the full amount has been given. Water given afterwards helps to rinse the baby's mouth, removes the strange taste and ensures that the drug has been swallowed.

Method for toddlers and older children
The guidelines of administering medicines should be carefully followed. The method will vary with the type of drug, e.g. whether in liquid or solid form. Some children may not be able to swallow tablets whole and these may be crushed between two spoons but care should be taken not to lose any part of the tablet in the crushing process.

A sweet or drink should be given if this is permissible and care should be taken to ensure that all the drug has been swallowed. Medicines should not be given at meal times (if this is possible) unless specially ordered. It is recommended that generally medicines are given when the stomach is empty. However, some drugs are known to cause gastric irritation, and these may be given with milk.

As each new drug comes on the market, literature is provided by the drug manufacturers and it is important that these leaflets are read by the nursing staff. They will give information as to the most effective way the drug can be given, e.g. some drugs should not be given with any other liquid as a chemical change may occur, altering the active principle. They may also contain information about possible drug interactions.

Knowledge of drugs, the dose for different age groups, their action and possible side-effects and reactions are important. Much can be learned from a medicine round and it is essential to learn about new drugs as they come into use.

When the medicine round has been completed, bottles are cleaned and all medicines are returned to their respective places. The amount of drugs left should be noted to ensure an adequate supply for 24 hours. Drugs must be kept out of the reach of children at all times and trolleys should never be left in the ward unattended. The advantage of using a specially designed trolley is that it can be locked. This is of particular importance when the nurse is required to attend to some emergency during the medicine round, thereby ensuring that children will not touch the trolley or take any drugs from it.

After-care of the child

1. Recognition and reporting of any side-effects of the medicine is of paramount importance.
2. The toddler or child should be left with a clean mouth.
3. If the child has been unhappy during the procedure, he should be comforted. A reward such as a sweet should be given (if permissible) in recognition of his attempt to overcome his fear or reluctance to take the medicine.

Rectal administration

Reasons

1. As an alternative to the oral route in the following circumstances:
   a. To give a drug which would be unpleasant to take orally.
   b. To give a drug to an unconscious or uncooperative patient.
2. To obtain a local response, as with laxative suppositories.
3. For rectal anaesthetic administration.

Preparation and care of the child

This is dependent on the type of drug to be administered. If possible, adequate explanation should be given. The child should have voided urine and the rectum must be empty of faeces before injecting the drug, if anything other than a laxative suppository is to be given.

It is important to remember that if the drug to be given is a basal narcotic anaesthetic, permission must be obtained from the parents and the child should be prepared as for a general anaesthetic. The dose of such drugs is calculated according to the body weight, therefore an accurate weight of the child must be obtained.

Requirements for rectal administration of a drug in fluid form

1. Medicine glass with measured and checked amount of drug, standing in a gallipot of warm water.
2. 20 ml syringe, or funnel and tubing and disposable catheter size 12 FG or 6 EG.
3. Swabs.
4. Lubricant, e.g. KY jelly.
5. Water-repellent sheet.

Method

The drug is checked at the bedside with the chart. If a controlled drug is being given, the necessary rules apply.

The bed should be protected with the water-repellent sheet and the child kept adequately covered. If the nurse is right-handed, it is easier to place the patient in the left lateral position; if left-handed, vice versa. One nurse should distract the child's attention with a book or toy while the second nurse assembles the apparatus, lightly lubricates the catheter and fills the apparatus with fluid to expel air. The catheter is introduced into the rectum for 8 to 10 centimetres in an upward and slightly forward direction. The funnel should be held just about the level of the buttocks and the fluid allowed to run in very slowly. When all the drug has been given (it may take 3 to 5 minutes to give 30 ml) the catheter is left in for 1 minute while the buttocks are compressed. The catheter is then gently removed. To maintain compression of the buttocks and prevent reflux of the substance, adhesive strapping can be applied across the buttocks.

After-care of the child
If the substance given is a basal narcotic, the anaesthetising effect is very rapid. The child must never be left alone and should be nursed as any child who has been given a general anesthetic.

Care should be taken to ensure that the substance is retained, except when a local response is desired. The foot of the bed can be elevated when 60 ml or more of a substance have been given.

Introduction of a suppository
A suppository consists of gelantinous material which melts when in contact with body heat and releases the drug. Various drugs may be given by this method. The introduction of laxative suppository has largely taken the place of enemata.

Requirements
1. Lubricant, e.g. KY jelly.
2. Finger cots or disposable gloves.
3. Suppository.
4. Receptacle for disposable items.
5. Water-repellent sheet, where necessary.

Method
Suppositories are painless to introduce and, therefore, should hold no terror for the child. An explanation should be given so that the child will understand the procedure and will co-operate. The child is placed comfortably on his side, the suppository is lubricated and is then inserted into the rectum with the protected finger until it is no longer in contact.

After-care of the child
The child should not be left without means of going to the toilet, or obtaining a bedpan quickly when required. The suppository is normally effective about half an hour after insertion. The resultant bowel action should be inspected and reported, and the child's toilet completed.

Hypodermic or subcutaneous injection
A hypodermic injection is an injection into the hypoderm, i.e. the layer of tissue below the epidermis. Drugs may be administered by this method when:

1. Vomiting is present.
2. A rapid action is desired.
3. The drug may be rendered ineffective by the action of the digestive juices.

Principles involved

1. Knowledge of the anatomy of the site, e.g. the hypoderm is rich in lymph derived from the dermis, but does not contain blood vessels or nerve endings which are present in the dermis. The more superficial the injection, the slower the rate of absorption which occurs through the lymphatic system.
2. The reason for inserting the needle at an angle of 25°. This is to ensure that the injection is not given deeper than hypodermic tissue.
3. Knowledge of aseptic technique.
4. Knowledge of drugs. Certain drugs, because of their chemical effect on the tissues, must never be given hypodermically, due to the danger of necrosis of the tissues, e.g. paraldehyde.
5. Importance of aiding dispersal of the injected fluid by massage.

Requirements

1. Mediswabs and sterile dry swabs.
2. Disposable syringe (1 or 2 ml) and suitable needles, e.g. No. 25 on a sterile tray.
3. Drug to be injected.
4. File and Kardex.

Preparation of the child

Adequate explanation and truthfulness are essential. Two nurses will be required, one to prepare and comfort the child, expose the appropriate site and hold him still, and the other to give the drug. Charging the syringe before arrival at the bedside reduces tension as the child is less likely to be afraid if he cannot see the syringe and needle.

Method

The nurse washes and dries her hands. The needle is then connected to the syringe, keeping the needle point sheathed until the syringe is ready to be charged. The rubber top of the bottle is cleaned with a mediswab; alternatively, the vial containing the drug is opened.

When the glass vial is to be opened, care is required to keep the fingers well way from the neck of the vial. A swab may be wrapped round the neck of the vial as a precaution.

When the syringe is charged and all the air excluded, the drug is checked and taken to the bedside. The drug is checked again with the Kardex and the child's nameband. The syringe should be kept out of sight as long as possible.

The assistant exposes the upper outer aspect of the arm, or any other suitable site, e.g. upper anterior aspect of the thigh. The skin is cleansed and held taut with one hand, while the syringe is held in the other hand, with the bevel of the needle uppermost.

The needle is then introduced through the skin at an angle of 25° to the skin (Fig. 9.2). It should penetrate into the subcutaneous tissue for approxi-

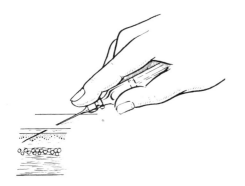

Fig. 9.2 Hypodermic injection. Demonstrating the angle of the needle in relation to the skin.

mately 0.5 cm. The piston is withdrawn slightly to make sure the needle is not in a blood vessel and the drug is gently injected. The swab is then placed over the site of the insertion of the needle and the needle is withdrawn. The area is gently massaged in an upward direction to aid dispersal of the drug. The administration of the drug is then recorded on the Kardex and the used equipment is disposed of. Needles and syringes are placed in a special container for disposal.

After-care of the child

Most small children will cry, either just as the needle is inserted or while the drug is injected. As soon as the proceedings are completed, the child should be picked up and given some comfort. He should never be left to cry himself to sleep. Praise should be given to an older child for co-operation.

Intramuscular injection

In this method the drug is injected into the muscular tissue and then enters the capillaries. Since muscle tissue is highly vascular, absorption into the blood stream is faster than via the lymphatics. However, absorption may be delayed when poorly soluble acids or bases are injected by this route, e.g. parenteral phenytoin. This is due to the action of the tissue fluids on the drug forming more of the poorly soluble acid which precipitates and is absorbed very slowly. Drugs are given by this route for the same reasons as those given for hypodermic injection. However, the amount injected may be larger and the substance may be more readily absorbed causing less irritation to the tissue.

Principles involved

1. Knowledge of anatomy of the sites and the risks involved. The upper outer quadrant of the buttock provides a good muscle and an area where large blood vessels and nerves are least likely to be involved. However, in the small child there is danger of damage to the sciatic nerve and this site should only be used as an alternative one when frequent and prolonged treatment is necessary (Fig. 9.3). The lateral aspect of the thigh is considered a safer area for injection.

2. Recognition that this type of injection may

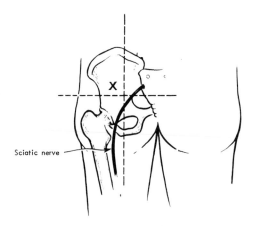

Fig. 9.3 This demonstrates the anatomical position of the sciatic nerve and the method of determining the point at which an intramuscular injection is safest. The longitudinal line is taken as being from the ischial tuberosity to the iliac crest and the transverse line as midway between the fold of the buttocks below the ischial tuberosity and the upper limit of the iliac crest.

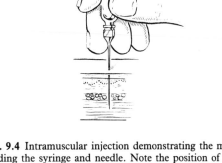

Fig. 9.4 Intramuscular injection demonstrating the method of holding the syringe and needle. Note the position of the middle finger to prevent the needle being introduced up to the hilt.

cause pain and that there is greater danger of injury to the child if he struggles.
3. Understanding of the method of absorption of drugs, e.g. via the capillaries.
4. Knowledge of aseptic technique. This is particularly important when the patient is an infant or small child wearing a napkin.

Requirements
As for hypodermic injection except that larger needles are required, e.g. No. 21 or 23 gauge.

Preparation of the child
Adequate explanation and absolute truthfulness are essential. The child should be told that the injection will cause some discomfort, if not some pain, but that the injection will be much less painful if he lies still and is quite limp and relaxed.

Two nurses will be required, one to prepare and comfort the child, expose the appropriate site and hold him still, the other to administer the drug. If the patient is an infant or small child wearing a napkin, then it is important to remove the wet or soiled napkin and cleanse the napkin area, before the injection is given.

Method
The method is the same as for hypodermic injec-

tion with the important difference that the needle is inserted at right angles to the skin (Fig. 9.4).

Principles of techniques

1. The needle is not inserted up to the hilt because of the danger of breaking, if the child moves suddenly. In this eventuality it could not be recovered without operation. This must be remembered when selecting the size of the needle to be used.
2. The needle is inserted quickly as this reduces pain to the minimum.
3. The piston is withdrawn slightly after insertion of the needle to ensure that it has not penetrated a blood vessel.
4. The air bubble in the syringe will enter the needle after the injection has been given, thus ensuring that there will be minimal leakage of the drug into the subcutaneous tissues as the needle is withdrawn.
5. The skin is pulled downwards before the insertion of the needle. When the skin is released, the path taken by the needle is no longer straight and, therefore, leakage of the drug along this channel cannot occur. Leakage might cause considerable discomfort if the drug is irritating to the subcutaneous tissue.

An iron preparation could cause staining of the skin.

6. Slow injection of the drug permits dispersal of the fluid with less pain and massaging after the injection aids dispersal.

7. A needle 38 mm long will penetrate muscle if injected for two-thirds of its length. Such a needle has also an adequate bore to enable drugs to be given with less force and thus reduces pain. The use of a smaller needle is dangerous as it is more easily broken and less likely to penetrate the muscle deeply enough for the absorption of the drug. Considerable pain and reaction in the subcutaneous tissue is caused by certain drugs, if not given correctly.

8. The recommended amount and type of fluid must be used for dissolving the drug to be given. If less fluid is used, the material injected is more concentrated and, therefore, more irritating to the tissues. It ceases to be an isotonic solution and will cause considerable pain and may lead to tissue necrosis.

9. When a course of injections is given, the sites must be chosen in rotation to prevent injury to the tissue.

10. Injections of over 2 ml in infants and 3 ml in the older child should be given in divided doses using two sites.

Chapter 10
Care of pre-term and low-weight babies

The definitions of the 'pre-term' and 'low-weight' infant are based on the decision reached at the Second European Congress of Perinatal Medicine (1970), which states:

Live born infants, delivered before 37 weeks from the first day of the last menstrual period, are considered to have a short-ened gestational period and are said to be premature or pre-term.

Infants who weigh 2500 g or less at birth are considered to have had either a shortened gestational period, a less than expected rate of intra-uterine growth, or both. These are termed infants of low birth weight.

Prematurity and low weight are usually concomitant, particularly among infants weighing 1500 g or less at birth. Both are associated with increased neonatal morbidity and mortality.

Incidence
The incidence of true prematurity in Great Britain is said to be about 7 per cent of all births. There is considerable variation in incidence throughout the country and within different districts. The rates are higher in big industrial cities and among social class IV and V.

Maternal factors
Toxaemia, hypertension, malnutrition or chronic ill health, for example diabetes mellitus. In general, premature birth is associated with conditions in which the uterus is unable to retain the fetus, for example premature separation, separation of the placenta and infarction of placenta.

Fetal factors
Chromosomal abnormalities (e.g. autosomal trisomics), multiple fetus, radiation injury, etc. — gross fetal deformity.

Characteristics of pre-term babies
The characteristics vary and are most marked in babies with the shortest gestational age.

Length
Measurement of length of the infant from the vertex (crown of the head) to the heel is considered the most reliable method of estimating the gestational age of a healthy pre-term baby. This is calculated on the basis that after the 28th week the infant measures $1\frac{1}{4}$ × weeks of gestational age (cm), e.g. $1\frac{1}{4}$ × 28 = 28 + 7 = 35 cm. Length appears to be relatively constant and is little affected by factors such as sex, multiple birth, etc.

Weight
There are wide variations in the mean birth-weight in different countries and in different regions within a country. Birth-weight is influenced by factors such as congenital abnormalities, multiple pregnancies, biological factors, etc. The mean birth-weights recorded by Butler and Alberman (1969) of babies, both male and female, born in England, Scotland and Wales during 1 week, were at 28 weeks (1130 g), 32 weeks (1890 g), 36 weeks (2790 g) and 40 weeks (3415 g).

During the first few days of life there is a decrease in weight. This loss is generally not regained until the 3rd week of life. Once the birth-weight is reached there is a relatively rapid weight increase which is greater than that of term babies.

General proportions
The pre-term baby has a large head in proportion to the size of his body. Average head circumference at various gestational ages have been found to be as follows (Crosse, 1971): 28 weeks (25 cm), 32 weeks (29 cm), 36 weeks (32 cm) and 40 weeks (35 cm).

The chest is relatively small, while the abdomen is relatively large and the limbs are thin in comparison with the rest of the body.

Activity

The lower the gestational age of the infant, the less active he will be. Provided the general condition is good, even the smallest infant will show periods of muscular activity, particularly if not restricted by clothing.

Temperature control

The pre-term infant tends to have a subnormal body temperature. This is due to poor heat production and increased heat loss. Failure to produce adequate heat is due to lack of brown adipose tissue (which has high metabolic activity), feeble respiration with poor oxygen combustion, poor muscular activity and low food intake. Loss of heat is increased because of the relatively greater body surface and lack of subcutaneous fat. The infant's lack of heat regulation is partly due to immaturity of the heat regulating centre and partly due to failure to respond to external stimuli. This is said to be partly due to defective sweat mechanism as well as lack of subcutaneous fat.

In the first week of life the pre-term infant shows marked fluctuations in temperature and this is related to fluctuations in environmental temperatures.

Respiratory system

The shorter the gestational period the less well developed will be the lungs. The alveoli tend to be small with few blood vessels surrounding the cellular stroma in an infant weighing 900 g. The more mature the infant and the greater his weight, the larger will be the alveoli, the walls of which are virtually formed by capillaries.

The respiratory muscles are weak and the respiratory centre is poorly developed. There is also lack of pulmonary lipoprotein, i.e. a surfactant which reduces surface tension in the lungs. Surfactant is believed to act by stabilising the smaller alveoli, thereby preventing their collapse in expiration.

Respiration tends to be irregular in rhythm and depth; there are often periods of apnoea, during which cyanosis develops. When recording respiratory rate it must be counted for 1 minute for accurate estimation.

The cough reflex is absent in the smallest pre-term infant. This can lead to inhalation of regurgitated fluids with serious consequences.

The nasal passages are very narrow and injury to nasal mucosa can easily occur. This is important to remember when passing naso-gastric tubes or endotracheal tubes via the nose.

Respiratory rate varies with all new-born and pre-term infants. In the resting new-born infant, the rate may be 60 to 80 per minute; this gradually decreases to a more usual rate of 34 to 36 per minute.

Circulatory system

The heart is relatively large at birth; its action is slow and feeble in some pre-term babies. Extra-systoles occur and murmurs may be heard at or shortly after birth. These disappear when the fetal cardiac openings gradually close. Peripheral circulation is often poor and the walls of the blood vessels are also weak. This is particularly the case in the intracranial vessels. This may account for the tendency to intracranial haemorrhage which is shown by the pre-term infant. Blood pressure is lower than that of full-term infants, the level decreasing with decreasing birth-weight. The systolic pressure of a full-term baby is about 80 mmHg and that of a pre-term baby 45 to 60 mmHg. The diastolic pressure is proportionally low, varying from 30 to 45 mmHg. The pulse rate varies between 100 and 160/min. Arrhythmia tends to be present and, to obtain an accurate sound, it is advisable to listen to the apex beat with a stethoscope (p. 104).

Digestive system

The lower the gestational age, the more feeble are the sucking and swallowing reflexes, the smallest infant being unable to feed effectively. Regurgitation is a common feature. This is due to a poorly developed mechanism for closure of the cardiac sphincter and a relatively strong pyloric sphincter.

Digestion depends on the development of the digestive apparatus. The stomach of an infant weighing 900 g shows little mucosal folding; the secretory glands, as well as muscle, are poorly developed. Poorly developed musculature of the intestines leads to distension and retention of digested material.

The liver is relatively large but poorly developed, particularly in the smaller infants. This predisposes the infant to jaundice, due to the inability to conjugate bilirubin, i.e it is insoluble and excretion into the bile is not possible.

Digestion. Protein digestion appears to be well developed even in the smallest pre-term infant. Protein, either of human or animal type, appears to be tolerated and absorbed.

Fats. Absorption of fats appears to be a problem even though fat-splitting enzymes are present. This may be related to poorly developed lacteals.

Carbohydrates. In the form of glucose, these are readily absorbed.

Urinary system

At the time of birth, kidney function has to adjust to the changed environment. Renal function is less efficient with a lowered rate of glomerular filtration, low clearance of solutes and urea. This results in decreased ability to concentrate urine and urination is scanty. Disturbance of water and electrolyte balance occurs readily. This is due to poorly developed tubules.

Nervous system

The development of the nervous system depends largely on the degree of maturity. The centres controlling the vital functions, e.g. respiration, body temperature and reflex centres, are poorly developed. Reflexes, such as the Moro and tonic neck reflexes are present in normal premature infants, but tendon reflexes are variable. Because of the poor development of the nervous system, the smallest infants in particular, are more lethargic, more difficult to rouse and many have a feeble cry.

Genital systems

The genitals are small; in the female the labia minora are not covered by the labia majora until full term. In the male, the testicles may be in the abdomen, inguinal canal or scrotum.

Eyes

Maturity of the fundus occurs by about 34 weeks' gestation. There are two recognised stages of development, i.e. immature and transitional, which take place between 24 and 33 to 34 weeks. During these stages the infant is liable to become blind if oxygen is given in high concentration over a prolonged period.

General appearance

The skin is usually thin, red and wrinkled. Little subcutaneous fat is present. The nails are soft and lanugo is prominent but there is little or no vernix caseosa. The hair is short and scanty and eyebrows are often absent.

Care of the infant

The importance of special care for these infants has long been recognised and special units exists where specialist nursing and medical care can be instituted. The Report of the Expert Group on Special Care for Babies (1971) recommends the establishment of special care units where the infants can be given this care. It bases its recommendation on the evidence that neonatal mortality can be reduced if the newborn baby can receive effective care. The specialised unit should also be able to provide simple care so that the transition from specialised care to home care can be readily achieved.

Although the report deals mainly with care of the low-weight infant in maternity hospitals, many of the problems are found in neonatal units of a paediatric hospital. The care of these infants is very specialised and since it also often involves congenital abnormalities, it is important that the sick children's nurse should be able to perform this specialised function.

Preparation for the care of the infant should be made before labour begins, if premature labour is expected. The preparation will also depend on the degree of prematurity.

The care of the infant is considered primarily in relation to both the healthy and the sick premature infant in a paediatric unit.

The following aspects of care will be considered:

1. Handling.
2. Preservation of body temperature.
3. The incubator.
4. Prevention of infection.
5. Administration of oxygen.

6. Bathing.

7. Feeding of infant.

Handling of the infant

The more premature the infant, the greater the care required when handling him. There is a greater possibility of precipitating a cyanotic attack. This occurs to a greater extent after feeding, when regurgitation of feed occurs resulting in inhalation of feed. All nursing care should be carried out with the infant in the incubator. However, some handling must take place; to change the infant's napkin, change his position or to cleanse him. It is essential that any handling or holding and lifting should be done gently. The nurse's hands should be warm and any equipment used cause the least discomfort to the baby. Solutions and water should be warm and not used excessively. The incubator or cot should be adjustable, thus avoiding excessive handling.

Preservation of body temperature

The pre-term infant has difficulty in maintaining relatively constant temperature and variations readily occur. An infant will progress satisfactorily provided his rectal temperature is maintained between 35.5 and 37°C. The smaller the infant, the lower the rectal temperature, but as he gains weight and his general condition improves, there is also greater stability of his temperature.

It is neither desirable nor necessary to increase the body temperature rapidly. This may lead to hyperpyrexia which is associated with an increased metabolic rate and increased oxygen requirement.

The low-weight infant should be nursed in an environmental temperature where a normal body temperature is maintained with minimal metabolic effort. This is highest for the smallest and youngest sick infants. Investigations such as Scopes and Ahmed (1966) suggest that the environmental temperature (thermoneutral range) lies between 31 and 35°C. Heat loss is not affected by changes in relative humidity within the thermoneutral range, but heat loss can be reduced when the temperature is lower and the relative humidity is increased.

Other methods can be used, e.g. servo-controlled incubators which provide a more sensitive temperature regulation. The thermistor probe is taped to the infant's skin so that any changes in skin temperature will require adjustment to incubator temperature.

The low-weight infant who is nursed in an open cot also requires careful environmental control. The nursery temperature should be over 25°C for infants weighing about 2000 g and up to 30°C for those weighing less than 2000 g (see Table 8.1).

The incubator (Figs. 10.1–10.5)

This is basically a box, designed to maintain a constant internal temperature by the use of a thermostat. There are many different types available and all have the same function but some are more complex than others; for example, there are attachments for oxygen administration, a water container to provide humidity, an air filter, an ice compartment and an attachment for a nebuliser. There is easy access to controls and it is possible to change the fan filter (where applicable). Most incubators have an internal thermometer which can be easily read.

Nursing procedures can be carried out through 'windows' or 'sleeves' on one or both sides of the incubator, or through the open lid. In the latter type a warm environment can be maintained by a heating canopy placed at a short distance above the incubator.

Before receiving the infant into the incubator, it is pre-warmed to approximately 29.4°C for infants of 1.7 kg and 32.2°C for the smaller infant.

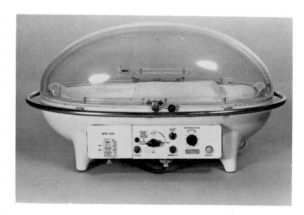

Fig. 10.1

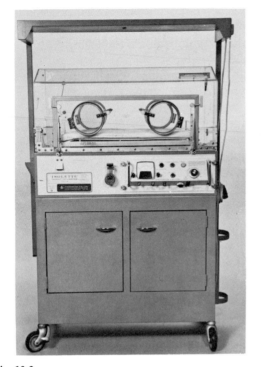

Fig. 10.2

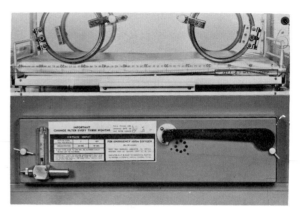

Fig. 10.3

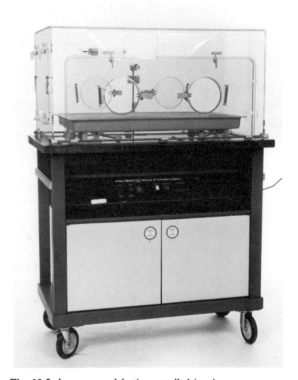

Fig. 10.5 A newer model; air-controlled incubator.

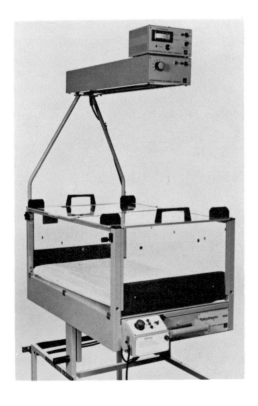

Fig. 10.4

The tank is filled with distilled or sterile water and a napkin is placed on the foam mattress. The infant is nursed naked.

This has the following advantages:

1. Allows unimpeded breathing.
2. Enables the infant to move about unrestricted by clothing.
3. Allows easy observation of breathing.
4. Avoids excessive handling of infant which clothing him would require.

Humidity
A relative humidity of 70 to 80 per cent prevents dehydration and the irritant action of oxygen (if oxygen is administered).

Care of the incubator
The outside of the incubator is cleaned daily. Any vomitus, urine or faecal matter must be removed without delay. A disinfectant such as Savlon 1–100 can be used to wipe the inside plastic windows.

The tank is filled daily with fresh distilled or sterile water (if humidity is required). If exudate penetrates the interior of the incubator and cannot be removed, another incubator should be prepared and the infant transferred.

When the infant is able to leave the incubator, thorough cleaning and disinfection are carried out. The incubator is dismantled and can be treated in a special tank or it can be fumigated as follows:

The tank is drained of water leaving the current on at control 1. The tank is then filled with 600 ml of 1–100 formaldehyde in water. The humidifier control is turned to 'humid'. It is left running for 30 minutes and allowed to steam up. The humidifier is drained and the incubator lid is opened. The current is left on until all traces of formaldehyde have been dispersed. The current is then switched off.

Oxygen administration to pre-term infant

Poor lung expansion presents a serious problem for the pre-term infant, due to poorly developed lung tissue, i.e. lack of alveoli and surfactant.

Administration of oxygen for these infants must be carefully controlled, since high concentration over a prolonged period causes damage to the infant's retinal tissue leading to blindness.

The recommended concentration of oxygen is about 30 to 35 per cent and to ensure that this is maintained, regular tests should be carried out. To ensure that the greatest concentration of oxygen is near the infant's nose, a plastic hood is placed over the baby's head. When testing oxygen concentration, the sample should be from the air within the plastic hood. As an additional safeguard, a warning disc is placed on the incubator when high concentrations are given over a prolonged period.

Prevention of infection

Caring for such small infants calls for skill and an understanding of the difficulties which may be encountered. These are closely related to the lack of maturity of the body systems. Whatever nursing function is involved, it must have as its basic aim the protection of the infant from infection.

The pre-term, low-weight infant has a poorly developed immunological system. He has little or no resistance to infection. No one with a cold, sore throat, skin lesions or other forms of infection should work with these infants. In some units, it is policy to wear a mask and gown while attending to the infant. The principles of prevention of infection apply here as elsewhere in the hospital field and any infection occurring in an infant must be considered a failure of the application of these principles.

Weighing
In order to avoid unnecessary handling, weighing should not be frequent, perhaps twice a week. The smallest infant can be weighed while in the incubator, placing the infant on to a sling which is attached to a hook through a hole in the incubator. This is attached to a spring balance. There are incubators available which have a scale incorporated. The older and heavier infant can be weighed on communal scales. These must be cleaned between weighing and each infant is placed on a clean paper.

Provided the infant feeds well and has normal bowel movements, daily weighing is not necessary. Individual scales are ideal of course. However, these are not always available and provided the necessary care is taken, there is no reason why communal scales cannot be used safely.

Bathing

This will depend on the policy of each unit. Some advocate oiling, others the use of hexachlorophane 3 per cent or sterile water.

The principal aims are:

1. Preventing loss of body heat.
2. Prevention of excessive handling.
3. Avoiding mechanical irritation of the skin.

The newborn pre-term infant will be allowed to recover from the ordeal of birth. Blood and debris can be gently removed with a warm solution of hexachlorophane 3 per cent or Cetrimide 1:500. Sterile swabs or cotton wool balls should be used. Thereafter the skin folds, i.e. neck, axillae, groins and back of the ears are treated daily in a similar way. The napkin area is cleaned at each 'napkin change'. Handling during napkin change should be minimal, the infant preferably being turned on his side rather than having his legs lifted.

The older healthy infant can be given a bath every second or third day. The temperature of the water should be about 40.5 to 43.5°C, the latter temperature being more suitable for washing the infant on the nurse's knee.

Care of the eyes

The closed eyelids should be cleaned daily with sterile warm water, using a cotton wool roll. A separate piece of cotton wool should be used for each eye and each movement.

Care of the nose

The nostrils should be left untouched if clear. The outer nares only may be cleaned, if necessary, with a swab wrung out in warm sterile water. Obstructed nasal passages can be cleared by the following means:

1. If one nostril is obstructed, stimulating the clear nostril will cause sneezing and clear the obstruction.
2. Both nostrils blocked presents a bigger problem. If sneezing can be produced without interfering with the nostrils, this is to be recommended; but it may not be possible to do so and the mucus plug can be eased out gently, using a fine roll of cotton wool. It is important not to push the mucus plug up into the nostril.

This could led to inhalation of the material with serious consequences.

Care of the mouth

A healthy mouth does not require cleaning, as the mucous membrane is very easily injured, encouraging bacterial invasion. The mouth should; however, be inspected at each feeding time, so that the presence of thrush is recognised early and treatment instituted as quickly as possible.

Care of the cord (See p. 36)

Feeding

A good knowledge of infant feeding and an understanding of the cause of feeding difficulties is essential to be able to handle these infants.

Feeding difficulties are related to the weak tongue and palate muscles as well as the incomplete development of the nervous system, i.e. weak sucking and swallowing reflexes (p. 9).

Principles of feeding

In the first week of life, the metabolic requirements of the premature baby are low since, while other adjustments to postnatal life are taking place, glycogen stores are utilised as the main source of energy. During the second week, however, there is a rapid increase in the demand for food. Individual babies vary somewhat in their maximal caloric requirements so that amounts of 90 to 165 kcal (0.36 to 0.66 MJ)/kg/d are recommended. As a general rule weight gain is inadequate unless the daily intake is 130 kcal (0.52 MJ)/kg/d, although 90 kcal (0.36 MJ)/kg is considered sufficient by some paediatricians.

The type of milk influences the caloric requirements since the poor ability of the pre-term infant to absorb fat is probably the most important factor in influencing the total caloric needs.

Feeding is always a difficult problem in premature infants who require a high protein intake, over 5 g per kg of body weight, and a high intake of carbohydrate (as cane sugar or lactose) if they are to gain weight adequately after the initial loss during the first week of life. On the other hand they tolerate fat poorly.

Early feeding is recommended to help in preventing hypoglycaemia and hyperbilirubinaemia. These conditions, among others, cause brain damage in newborn pre-term babies. The feeding regime depends on the gestational period and the weight of the infant.

1. *Pre-term infants under 32 weeks and weighing under 1500 g. Week 1* The infant is fed hourly from 2 hours old. A naso-gastric tube is passed (p. 510) and the gastric contents are aspirated 4-hourly just before a feed. The aspirate is measured and returned via the tube. If the volume exceeds a third of the last feed, the amount to be given is reduced by that amount. This is to prevent gastric distension and regurgitation of feed. *Week 2* The infant is fed 2-hourly and this is continued until he reaches 36 weeks, when 3-hourly feeds are given.

2. *Pre-term infants of 32 to 34 weeks' gestation weighing 1500 to 2200 g.* The infant is fed 2-hourly from 2 hours old. A naso-gastric tube is passed and the gastric contents aspirated as described above. The amount of feed given depends on the amount aspirated. Feeds are given 2-hourly until the infant reaches 36 weeks, when the feeds are given 3-hourly.

3. *Pre-term infants of 34 to 37 weeks' gestation.* Feeding may be delayed until the baby is 12 hours old or until he is hungry. The first feed consists of Dextrose, the amount depending on his weight. If he is well enough and can suck, the feed can be given by bottle and teat. The first milk feed may be either breast milk or Ostermilk complete formula and this is repeated at 4-hourly intervals.

The following table is a guide to the volume of milk required by the pre-term infant up to 34 weeks' gestation:

Day	Amount ml/kg of body weight
1	50–65
2	75
3	100
4	125
5	150
6	160
7	175
14	200
21	225
28	175
60	150
90	130

The light-for-dates babies require relatively more calories than pre-term babies. The extra calories required are calculated on their expected birth weights.

Method of feeding

Whichever method of feeding is followed, special precautions should be taken. These are related to the poor development, particularly of the infant whose gestational period is very short. The head should be raised to reduce the possibility of regurgitation and to prevent air passing quickly out of the stomach into the intestines. If the infant is nursed in an incubator or cot with minimal handling, the cot or incubator mattress should be raised and the baby turned on his right side. In this position, there is less pressure on the heart by the dilating stomach and the stomach empties more easily into the duodenum. Should regurgitation occur, the fluid can run out of the corner of the mouth, thereby decreasing the danger of inhalation.

Breast feeding. This should be the first choice if the baby is capable of sucking. Breast milk can also be expressed and given to the infant if he is not strong or fit enough to suck from the breast. There are human milk banks which supply milk to institutions. The milk has to be pasteurised and is stored after cooling in a refrigerator at 4 to 5°C. It can also be deep frozen at −12 to −14°C. Laboratory tests for bacteria should be carried out on all pooled milk, particularly if the source is suspect. (See method of breast feeding, p. 38.)

Bottle feeding. An ordinary small feeding bottle can be used. The teat should not be too hard and the hole should be large enough to allow a rapid flow of milk, but not a stream, when the bottle is inverted.

When inserting the teat, it is important to check that the tongue does not stick to the roof of the mouth. Unless the teat is placed on the tongue, the infant cannot suck effectively. Twisting of the teat in the infant's mouth should be avoided, as this may injure the mucous membrane. Suction can be stimulated by pressing the teat down on the tongue or applying gentle upward pressure under the chin. Winding should be done after the feed, with the infant supported in the sitting position for a short time.

After the feed he is left lying on his right side,

but should be changed to his left side about half way through the feeding interval. The smaller infant should be left in his cot, but the larger infant (if well enough) can be lifted out and fed on the nurse's knee.

Catheter feeding. (See naso-gastric and naso-duodenal/jejunal feeding, p. 38.) The reasons for this type of feeding are mainly the inability of the weak, small infant to suck and swallow or the infant becomes cyanosed when fed by bottle. The method is basically the same as for full term, normal weight infants, but there are dangers and problems which are more specific to the pre-term, low-weight infant.

Since the nasal passages are very narrow, there is a danger that even a fine polyvinyl catheter may damage nasal mucous membrane. If an indwelling catheter cannot be tolerated by the infant it may be better to use interrupted catheter feeding. Oesophageal feeding is considered safer than stomach feeding by preventing gastric irritation and there is less likelihood of vomiting. The feed should be given slowly and care should be taken that the feed does not overflow into the air passages.

Preparation for home

As the infant grows and develops, his temperature controlling mechanism will also be more efficient. The temperature in the incubator will be gradually decreased and he will adjust to the room environment. He will also be clothed now and handling will be more extensive. If feeding is satisfactory, temperature is stable and his weight gain satisfactory, he can be transferred to an open cot.

The mother can now be guided in handling her child. She may be apprehensive to do so but with supervision and help, she will be able to cope with her infant. The liaison health visitor has a role here. She can assess the home conditions and provide means of support when the child returns home. Adequate follow-up and after-care is an essential feature in ensuring that the pre-term and low-weight infant has the best possible opportunity to develop to his full potential.

Part 4
The biochemical and physiological environment
(normal and abnormal)

Chapter 11
Nutrition in infancy and childhood

It has long been recognised that nutrition is an important factor in development of the young. Without adequate nutrition the fetus will fail to develop satisfactorily nor can bodily functions be maintained effectively.

Nutrition is the science of the foods, the nutrients and other components, their action and interaction: a balance in relationships to health and disease. It also requires an understanding of the processes by which food is ingested, digested, absorbed, transported, utilised and eliminated.

Nutrients are the constituents in food. These include water, protein, and the amino-acids of which they are composed, fats and fatty acids, carbohydrates, minerals and vitamins.

Failure to obtain adequate nourishment is known as *undernutrition* and an excess of one or more nutrients and usually of calories is known as *overnutrition*. Both these terms, under and over-nutrition can cause impairment of health and are collectively known as malnutrition.

Nutrition and physical growth

Growth is defined as an increase in the physical size of the body as a whole or as an increase in any of its parts, associated with an increase in the number and/or size of cells. Development is defined as the acquisition of function associated with cell differentiation and maturation of individual organ systems. Growth and development are influenced by a number of factors (see p. 4), one of which is nutrition not only post-natally but also pre-and perinatally.

Many factors influence an infant's birth-weight, e.g. maternal nutrition, smoking, drinking and placental efficiency. Immediately after birth there is weight loss, but by the 10th day this loss will have been regained. Thereafter, weight increase is rapid so that by the 4th month of age most babies will have doubled their birth-weight and by 12 months it is three times that of the birth-weight. After the first year weight increase proceeds at a slower but constant rate, averaging 2.3 kg/year until the 9th or 10th year when the rate of weight gain increases. This continues until adolescence when a rapid increase in the rate occurs.

There is also an increase in height, the increments decreasing from birth until adolescence, when a spurt in growth occurs. Length increases by 50 per cent in the first year, doubles by 4 years, and by 13 years it is usually three times the birth height. There is a growth spurt during adolescence, though it varies in age of onset, rate and duration. Increase in height shows after adolescence until the epiphyseal line closes, when it ceases.

There are racial variations in rate and pattern of growth. Some of these are genetically controlled whereas others depend on nutritional factors. Negroes tend to be ahead of whites in skeletal ossification at birth; their permanent teeth tend to erupt earlier. The Negro child tends to maintain his advancement for about 2 to 3 years; after that there is little difference between European whites and African Negroes. Asian children tend to be smaller than Negro and white children.

Social factors in child nutrition
Nutrition is closely related to the cultural practices of communities. In many communities food has assumed symbolic meaning and value. The food chosen is often not related to nutritional needs but satisfies some other function, be it as part of festivity, worship or mourning. Problems arise when there is little or no alternative food available. However, economic pressures and alien influence cause changes in dietary habit. Where the change

is not accepted or where economic conditions are limited, then malnutrition is a manifestation. Malnutrition itself creates a vicious cycle of failure since children who grow up in such conditions are severely disadvantaged. It is not only poverty which creates problems but, in many areas, over-population. Malnutrition as a result of poor mother-ing must also be considered, particularly in the light of fatigue due to poor living conditions. In many underdeveloped countries scarcity of food is a big problem but so is ignorance. There is also malnutrition in advanced countries, though this is less severe than in underdeveloped countries. However, cause and effect are much the same. Poor malnourished mothers produce low-weight babies and the physical and intellectual growth of these children is liable to be impaired.

After-effects of malnutrition

There is a great deal of evidence that malnutrition leads to permanent growth retardation, and growth recovery has social implications. The degree of recovery depends partly on the age of insult but largely on the environment to which the children return.

The gravest risk is the possible effect on brain growth and it is suggested that brain growth and intellectual development are most impaired if the deprivation occurred at the period of maximum growth. Recovery would not occur even with good feeding once the normal growing period has passed. Malnutrition can prevent the attainment of full physical potential and thus has a direct effect on the adult type.

Other areas which can be influenced are the personality, abilities and modes of behaviour not only of the child but also of the adult. Metabolic adjustments underlie the characteristic apathy and listlessness of the child who has reduced muscle mass. Development will be retarded as he spends much of his time static and lacking in curiosity. He has to conserve his energy and does not evoke stimulation. In the advanced stages there are de-ficiencies of intracellular electrolytes and his weak-ness is such that he cannot walk or sit up. Whether he can 'catch up' in sensory-motor development may be in doubt and he is ill prepared for future learning.

Lack of physical development is also associated with poor psychological development. It is recog-nised that the malnourished child has difficulty in interpersonal relationship and this may originate in very early infancy. The social setting he is born into may affect subsequent development, e.g. if he is born into an unwanted, unresponsive environ-ment his situation will be poor and his chances of a healthy emotional development will be limited. This will also affect the child's social acceptability. If he stimulates no interest it will add to increasing failure in his interaction with other adults or lead to rejection by others and this can lead to feelings of inadequacy with subsequent truancy and other anti-social behaviour.

There are some common primary nutritional disorders in Great Britain affecting children, for example, obesity and rickets. The latter is found more frequently in Asian children; however, rickets can also be due to anticonvulsant therapy, malabsorption, renal glomerular and tubular disease.

Iron deficiency anaemia can occur in pre-term babies, twins and older infants in whom weaning has been delayed; other causes may be dislike of meat or vegetables by toddlers and the possibility of blood loss, particularly from the gastro-intestinal tract, should be considered.

THE NUTRIENTS: THEIR CHARACTERISTICS AND FUNCTIONS

Nutrition may be defined as the process by which the organism utilises food. Foods are organic substances classified into three groups — proteins, carbohydrates and fats — all of which may occur in animal or vegetables substances. However, nutrients include any substance which provides nutrition or which can be utilised by the body, for example, water, mineral salts and vitamins.

PROTEIN AND AMINO-ACIDS

Proteins are extremely complex, nitrogenous organic compounds in which amino-acids are the units of structure. They contain the elements carbon, hydrogen, oxygen, nitrogen and, with few exceptions, sulphur. Most proteins also contain phosphorus, and some specialised proteins contain very small amounts of iron, copper and other inorganic elements. Twenty-two amino-acids are widely distributed in protein and others have been identified in one or more proteins.

Studies on rats have shown that they failed to grow or survive if some amino-acids were omitted from the diet, but that the elimination of other amino-acids had no such harmful effects. The same appears to be the case for human beings. Amino-acids, therefore, were classified as *essential* and *non-essential*. Strictly speaking all amino-acids are essential units for the synthesis of the protein molecule. However, the body can manufacture many amino-acids if it has an adequate nitrogen source, but it cannot produce certain others in adequate amounts to meet the body's needs. Those amino-acids which cannot be synthesised in sufficient amounts by the body, and which must be provided by the diet, are essential. Growing children require about nine or 10, while adults require eight amino-acids. Table 11.1 shows essential and non-essential amino-acids.

Depending on their ability to maintain life and promote growth, proteins have been classified as *complete*, *partially complete* and *totally incomplete proteins*.

Complete proteins

These contain enough of the essential amino-acids to promote a normal rate of growth. These proteins are said to have *high biological* value. Egg, milk, meat (including poultry and fish) are all complete but not necessarily identical in quality. Wheat germ and dried yeast have a biological value approaching that of animal sources.

Table 11.1 Essential and non-essential amino-acids

Essential amino-acids	Non-essential amino-acids	
Threonine	Glycine	Aspartic acid
Valine	Alanine	Glutamic acid
Leucine	Serine	
Isoleucine	Tyrosine	
Phenylalanine	Proline	
Tryptophan	Hydroxyproline	
Histidine	Cystine	
Methionine	Cysteine	
Lysine	Arginine	
	Hydroxylysine	

Partially complete proteins

These proteins will maintain life but they lack some of the amino-acids necessary for growth. Certain cereals and legumes are included in this group.

Totally incomplete proteins

These proteins are incapable of replacing or building new tissue. Zein, one of the proteins found in corn, and gelatin are examples of proteins.

Functions of proteins

1. Maintenance and growth

Proteins constitute the chief solid matter of muscles, organs and endocrine glands. They are the major constituents of the matrix of bones and teeth, skin, nails, hair, blood cells and serum.

2. Regulation of body processes

Body proteins have highly specialised functions in the regulation of body processes. For example, haemoglobin performs a vital role as oxygen carrier to the tissues. Plasma proteins regulate osmotic pressure and maintain water balance. They maintain normal, slightly alkaline reaction of the blood and maintain resistance to invading micro-organisms, since antibodies are protein in nature. Enzymes which are specific catalysts for metabolic processes are protein in nature. Hormones which influence and control many body processes are also protein in nature.

Individual amino-acids have specific functions. For example, tryptophan serves as a precursor for niacin (one of the B-complex vitamins). Glycine contributes to the formation of haemoglobin and is also an important constituent of the purines and pyrimidines in nucleic acid.

3. Energy

Proteins are a potential source of energy, each gram yielding approximately 4 kcal (0. 01 MJ). When proteins are used for energy they will be lost for synthesis purposes.

Dietary protein

Proteins, particularly animal proteins which are of

high biological value, are expensive forms of food. The amount of protein taken must be within safe levels. Although the total requirement increases during early childhood, the amount required for each kg of body weight decreases rapidly in the first year but remains constant at about 1.5 g/kg until school age. For example, at birth the minimal protein requirement is 2.8 g/kg/day decreasing to 1.5 g/kg/day by 1 year. From 1 year to 5 years the minimal requirement is 1.5 g/kg/day and decreasing slowly until by the age of 18 years it is 0.8 g/kg/day.

Food sources
Protein content is *high* in dry milk, meat, fish, poultry, cheese, nuts; *intermediate* in eggs, legumes, flour, cereals, liquid milk and *low* in most fruits and vegetables.

Digestion and absorption

Digestion
The purpose of digestion is to hydrolyse proteins to amino-acids so that they can be absorbed and utilised by the body. In addition to foods ingested, the mixture to be digested includes a sizeable amount of protein released from worn out cells of the mucosa and the digestive enzymes themselves.

Saliva contains no proteolytic enzyme and thus the action of saliva and the mouth acts as an increase in the surface area of the food mass resulting from chewing of food.

Most of the hydrolysis of protein occurs in the stomach, duodenum and jejunum. Specific enzymes act on specific linkages. For example, pepsinogen, produced in the stomach, is activated by hydrochloric acid and converted into pepsin. It then acts on the peptide chains, splitting them and resulting in shorter fragments. Another enzyme, trypsinogen (produced by the pancreas), is activated to trypsin by enterokinase (produced in the intestinal wall) which splits peptic linkage at points where lysine or arginine provide the carboxyl group.

Absorption
Amino-acids are absorbed from the proximal intestine into the portal circulation. The rate of absorption appears to be controlled by the levels existing in the blood. Amino-acids are rapidly removed from the circulation and the concentration in the blood tends to be relatively low. They are absorbed by active transport but some diffusion of amino-acids also occur.

Metabolism
Each cell within the body utilises the available amino-acids to synthesise all the numerous proteins required for its own functions and also uses amino-acids to supply energy.

Nitrogen balance
Nitrogen balance = nitrogen intake − nitrogen excretion (faeces + urine + skin). Nitrogen balance studies are based on the fact that protein, on average, contains 16 per cent nitrogen; therefore, 1 g nitrogen will be found in 6.25 g protein.

Nitrogen equilibrium is that state of balance when the intake of nitrogen is equal to that which is excreted. This is the normal state.

Positive nitrogen balance is that state in which the intake of nitrogen exceeds the excretion. It indicates that new protein tissues are being synthesised, as in children and pregnancy. It can also occur when tissues *depleted* of protein during illness or injury are being *replaced*.

Negative nitrogen balance is that in which the excretion of nitrogen exceeds the intake. It occurs in illness or physiological stress at any age when:

1. The calorie content of the diet is inadequate and therefore tissues are being broken down to supply energy.
2. The quality of protein is poor.
3. Injury, immobilisation and disease are causing excessive breakdown of tissues.

In times of stress there is increased adrenocortical activity and anorexia and it will be further exaggerated by increased faecal loss which frequently accompanies diarrhoea. This nitrogen balance can occur in even the mildest of infections and requires replacement after the infective episode is over. Failure to do so is a common cause of clinical malnutrition.

Synthesis of proteins
Each cell is capable of synthesising all the proteins for its own function. This synthesis is governed by

the genetic code that exists in each cell. It takes place in the cytoplasm and when completed the protein is set free from the ribosomes to perform its function in the cell. Amino-acids enter the cell by active transport from the metabolic pool. Some of the non-essential amino-acids may be synthesised within the cell itself, but most of the material for synthesis of non-essential amino-acids are keto-acids formed in the metabolism of carbohydrates and ammonia that is released through deamination of amino-acids.

Dietary proteins

Protein is a source not only of energy but also of nitrogen. The amino group ($-NH_2$) cannot be synthesised in man and therefore must be obtained from the diet, although skeletal muscle acts as a protein store. About one-third of the protein comes from plant sources and two-thirds from animal sources. These include foods such as meat, fish, cheese, nuts, dried peas, beans and cereals. When legumes are soaked in water the proportion of protein is diluted.

Excessive intakes

Protein intakes greater than 20 per cent of total calories during infancy increase solutes and, as a result, increase the requirement for water. Dehydration may result. Older children can generally cope physiologically with excessive intakes of protein.

Deficient intakes

Nutritional disorders in general tend to be protein in their manifestations. There are variations from one part of the world to another, due primarily to the great variation in the nutrient value of the diet. Protein energy malnutrition (PEM) includes a range of pathological conditions due to a lack, in various proportions, of proteins and calories. This occurs most frequently in infants and young children and is also associated with infections. The conditions can be mild, moderate or severe. The clinical presentation of protein *protein energy malnutrition* PEM varies with the degrees, duration of protein and energy depletion, the age of the individual and the modifications produced by associated vitamin, mineral and trace element deficiencies.

Mild PEM is most common in the post-weaning period from 9 months to 2 years, but it can occur at any age. The main features are: growth failure, infection (due to altered immunity and greater susceptibility to infection), anaemia (due to lack of iron, folic acid and other vitamins), decreased activity, listlessness, retardation of physical and mental development (these can be reversed with treatment) and skin and hair changes (found in moderate to severe forms of PEM).

Forms of PEM include:

1. *Kwashiorkor*. The *presenting features* include: failure to thrive, oedema, apathy, anorexia, vomiting and diarrhoea, changes in skin, hair and mucous membranes.

2. *Marasmus*. Marasmus can occur at any age but is becoming particularly common in early infancy assicated with a failure of breast-feeding and the development of gastro-enteritis. It can be caused and complicated by a wide variety of illnesses, e.g. infections, anomalies of the gastro-intestinal tract, malabsorption, chronic renal disease and central nervous system disturbances. Psychological factors may also contribute, e.g. maternal deprivation and neglect associated with anorexia, vomiting and rumination.

   The *presenting features* include: failure to thrive, irritable crying or apathy. Chronic diarrhoea with or without vomiting are common and sometimes the children are ravenously hungry.

   General appearance is of shrunken, wasted infant due to diminished subcutaneous fat. There are growth and musculo-skeletal changes. In pure marasmus there are no skin, hair and mucous membrane changes and oedema is not present.

   When the characteristics of both marasmus and kwashiorkor are present this is termed marasmic kwashiorkor.

Pathophysiology

There is a change in the amount of distribution of body water, body fat, minerals and total body protein, particularly muscle.

Cessation or slowing of growth is associated with a gradual increase of total body water as a percentage of body weight. This is mainly due to disappearances of fat stores and wasting muscle and other tissues.

Associated with the increase in total body water there is a proportionate rise in ECP (extracellular fluid) leading to oedema. Organs such as the liver, pancreas, gastro-intestinal tract and the endocrine systems are affected producing changes such as fatty liver, atrophy of acinar cells of the pancreas and atrophy of intestinal mucosa. Other systems and organs involved include the haemopoietic system and the brain (apathy and irritability).

Principles of treatment and nursing management

1. *Mild protein energy malnutrition*
   a. Can be treated as an outpatient.
   b. Nutritional guidance: for example,
      protein   2 to 3 g/kg/day
      energy   100 to 150 kcal (0.4 to 0.6 MJ)/kg/day
      vitamin A   5000 μg/day
      vitamin D   10 μg/day
2. *Severe protein energy malnutrition*
   a. Hospitalisation.
   b. Treatment of dehydration: intravenous infusion (see p. 448); plasma in hypovolaemia; Darrow's solution.
   c. Electrolyte disturbance.
   d. Correction of hypoglycaemia.
   e. Treatment of infection: antibiotics (penicillin, kanamycin).
   f. Rectal swabs.
   g. Dietary management:
      (i) Initially small feeds (frequently). Half-strength Darrow's solution 90 ml/kg/day for 24 hours; then full-strength milk (90 ml/kg/day) increasing to 150 ml/kg/day over 2 to 3 days.
      (ii) Once improved, add cereals and other foods.
      (iii) Vitamins A and D daily. Vitamin K once on admission.
      (iv) Iron and folic acid.
   h. General nursing management:
      (i) Buttocks' care.
      (ii) Oral hygiene.
      (iii) Skin care.
      (iv) Gentle handling (particularly if oedematous).
      (v) General cleanliness.
      (i) Parental support and guidance. The parents will require support and guidance. The condition should be explained to them and the advice given should be realistic with regard to availability of staple foods and the cost of food. If changes are suggested they should be acceptable to the parents and suit their cultural requirements. Guidance in infant care and management should be provided and where possible the mother should take part in the care of her infant while in hospital. On return home supporting services should be available either as home visits or clinic attendance.

CARBOHYDRATES

Carbohydrates are the most abundant organic compounds in the universe. They include the structural parts of plants in the form of cellulose as well as stores of starches and sugars. Sugars and starches are a major source of man's food energy.

Composition

Carbohydrates are simple sugars or polymers such as starch, that can be hydrolysed to simple sugars by the action of digestive enzymes or by heating with dilute acids. They contain carbon (C), hydrogen (H) and oxygen (O). Generally, but not always, the hydrogen and oxygen are present in the proportion to form water.

Classification of carbohydrates

Carbohydrates are classified as monosaccharides (simple sugars), disaccharides (double sugars) and polysaccharides, which include many molecules of simple sugars.

Monosaccharides

These are compounds which cannot be hydrolysed to simpler compounds. Glucose, galactose, fructose and mannose have the same empiric formula ($C_6H_{12}O_6$) but they differ in the arrangement of the groupings about the carbon atoms and are distinctive in their physical properties such as solubility and sweetness.

Glucose Also known as dextrose, grape sugar is found in sweet fruits such as grapes, cherries, oranges and some vegetables such as sweet corn and carrots. Glucose is the chief end-product of the digestion of the disaccharides and polysaccharides. It is the form of carbohydrate circulating in the blood and is utilised by the cell for energy.

Fructose This occurs naturally in some fruits and vegetables and especially in honey. It is the sweetest sugar known.

Galactose This is not free in nature, its only source being from hydrolysis of lactose.

Mannose This is of limited distribution in foods and of little consequence in nutrition.

Disaccharides

These result when two hexoses are combined with the loss of 1 molecule of water ($C_{12}H_{22}O_{11}$). They are water soluble, diffusable and form crystals They vary in sweetness and are split into simple sugars by acid hydrolysis or by digestive enzymes.

Sucrose

This is the table sugar, found in cane or beet sugar and brown sugar. Many fruits and some vegetables contain small amounts of sucrose.

Lactose

Lactose or milk sugar is produced by mammals and occurs only in milk. It is less sweet than sucrose and is a combination of glucose and galactose.

Maltose

Maltose or malt sugar is formed during the breakdown of starch by digestion. Maltose is produced in the malting and fermentation of grains and is present in beer and malted breakfast cereals. It is a combination of two glucose units.

Polysaccharides ($C_6H_{10}O_5$)

These are complex compounds with a relatively high molecular weight. They are not sweet and are insoluble in water. They are digested with varying degrees of completeness. Starches, dextrins, glycogen and several indigestible carbohydrates, i.e. cellulose, are of nutritional interest.

Functions of carbohydrates

Almost all of the dietary carbohydrate is eventually utilised to meet the energy needs of the body. Some of the available carbohydrate is used for the synthesis of a number of regulatory compounds.

1. Energy

Each gram of carbohydrate when oxidised yields on average four calories. Some of the carbohydrate, in the form of glucose, will be used directly to meet immediate tissue energy needs. A small amount will be stored as glycogen in the liver and muscles, and some will be stored as adipose tissue for later conversion to energy.

Glucose is the sole form of energy for the brain and nervous tissue and must be readily available. Any failure to supply glucose or the oxygen for its oxidation will rapidly lead to damage to the brain, particularly in the newborn period. Brain growth occurs very rapidly in the last weeks of intrauterine life. It is, therefore, important that babies born before term should not be deprived of glucose, so that brain growth can proceed. Small-for-dates babies are liable to develop hypoglycaemia and are, therefore, at risk.

2. Protein-sparing action

The body will use carbohydrate as its main source of energy, thereby sparing protein for tissue building. However, if there is deficiency of calories in the diet, then adipose and protein tissues will be used.

3. Regulation of fat metabolism

Some carbohydrate is necessary in the diet so that oxidation of fats can proceed normally. When carbohydrate is restricted in the diet, fats will be metabolised faster than the body can deal with its products. When fats are incompletely oxidised ketones are formed.

4. Role in gastro-intestinal function

It is believed that lactose promotes growth of

desirable bacteria in the small intestine. Some of these bacteria are useful for the synthesis of vitamin B complex and vitamin K. Lactose also enhances the absorption of calcium. While cellulose, hemicellulose and pectins yield no nutrients to the body, they aid in the stimulation of peristaltic action of the gastro-intestinal tract and by absorbing water give bulk to the intestinal contents.

Carbohydrates, particularly monosaccharides, are very important constituents of many compounds which regulate metabolism. For example, heparin (a monopolysaccharide) prevents the clotting of blood; immunopolysaccharides form part of the immune mechanism.

Digestion and absorption

The purpose of carbohydrate digestion is to hydrolyse the di- and polysaccharides of the diet to their constituent simple sugars. Hydrolysis is the chemical *decomposition* of a substance by water, the water itself being also decomposed. This hydrolysis is accomplished by the digestive enzymes. Some hydrolysis of starch to maltose takes place in the mouth by the action of salivary amylase and continues in the stomach until the food mass is acidified. However, the principal site of digestion is in the small intestine where the pancreatic enzymes convert them into disaccharides. The disaccharides are further broken down into monosaccharides which are then actively transported into the portal system.

Maltose, isomaltose and sucrose activity reach adult levels by 28 to 32 weeks' gestation, while lactose is present at low levels at 28 weeks' gestation increasing near term and reaching adult levels at birth. Salivary and pancreatic amylase are low during the first months after birth, but there is a gradual increase in pancreatic amylase during the first 5 years of life.

Glucose, fructose and galactose are absorbed into the portal system and carried to the liver. Most absorption occurs in the jejunum. When the concentration of sugar in the intestine is great, the need for carriers to ferry sugars across the epithelial cells may exceed the numbers present; therefore, some sugars will move along the tract to carrier sites in the ileum.

Metabolism of carbohydrate is essentially concerned with glucose. It consists of an interrelated series of biochemical reactions that are facilitated by enzyme activity. Glucose metabolism cannot be completely separated from the metabolism of fats and proteins. For example, proteins and fats are potential sources of glucose, and glucose can be converted to fatty acids, glycerol and certain amino-acids.

When the glucose reaches the liver, a number of changes take place which are concerned with the regulation of the level of glucose in the blood and with synthesising certain essential compounds from glucose. The liver is under the influence of hormones secreted by the pancreas (insulin, glucagon) adrenal glands (cortisol, adrenalin), pituitary gland (ACTH, growth hormone) and the thyroid gland (throxine).

The blood glucose

The normal blood glucose level is maintained within a narrow range by a balance between storage of substrate in the fed state as glycogen, amino-acids and triglycerides, and mobilisation of these energy stores in the fasting state. The normal values for the first 72 hours are 20 to 80 mg/dl (1.1 to 4.4 mmol/l) and for older age groups, 60 to 100 mg/dl (3.3 to 5.5 mmol/l). Insulin is the simple, most important hormone regulating blood glucose and is the only hormone to reduce it. The functions of insulin are as follows:

1. Increases the role of removal of glucose from the circulation by increasing the entry of glucose into cells.
2. Converts glucose into glycogen.
3. Depresses release of glucose from fuel stores.
4. Inhibits glycogenolysis (liberation of glucose from glycogen).
5. Inhibits gluconeogenesis (formation of glucose from non-carbohydrate sources).
6. Inhibits breakdown of proteins into amino-acids.
7. Inhibits lipolysis (hydrolysis of fats).

There are at least four important hormones which oppose the effect of insulin. These are: cortisol, glucagon, adrenalin and growth hormone.

They increase blood glucose in different ways which include:

1. Reducing glucose uptake into muscle cells.
2. Increasing glycogenolysis and gluconeogenesis.
3. Intensifying the breakdown of muscle protein to amino-acids.
4. Increasing lipolysis.

Dietary carbohydrate

Dietary carbohydrate helps to provide energy requirements and acts as a store of energy of glucogen. Sugars also play an important part in detoxication of ammonia and combating acidosis. The detoxicating process is by conjugation with glucuronic acid which is formed either from glucose or galactose; the latter is more rapid in the newborn. It is, therefore, suggested that galactose as well as glucose should be given in the newborn period in order to conjugate bilirubin, steroids and drugs such as chloramphenicol. In oral feeding, lactose is a ready source of both glucose and galactose.

Recommended intakes

Since carbohhydrate can be synthesised from amino-acids and fats, there is no specific recommendation, but a minimum intake of 50 to 100 g/d is suggested by some.

Food sources

In the young infant's diet, lactose is the predominant carbohydrate found in both human and cow's milk. As the child grows older, cereals, bread and other foods, such as potatoes, are added.

Deficient intakes

If intakes of carbohydrate are low, amino-acids and fats are metabolised for energy and converted to glycogen. When this happens there is a possibility of ketosis developing from the breakdown of fats. When protein is broken down urea will be formed and this will necessitate additional water for excretion. If carbohydrates have been completely eliminated from the diet then symptoms, such as dehydration, ketosis, loss of body protein, fatigue and loss of energy, can soon occur.

Excessive intakes

Excessive intakes of sugar, cakes, etc. will prevent the intake of other essential nutrients resulting in nutritional deficiencies as well as problems of overweight. It can lead to irritation of the gastro-intestinal mucosa and load the enzyme system. In certain disorders it can favour increased fermentation and gas production and may be associated with diarrhoea. It may lead to increased levels of serum triglycerides which may be responsible for cardiovascular disease in adults.

Disorders of carbohydrate metabolism

There are a number of disorders due to defective carbohydrate metabolism. Most of these are discussed in the chapter dealing with metabolism disorders (see Ch. 15). These include: diabetes, mellitus, galactosaemia, glycogen storage disease and hypoglycaemia.

LIPIDS (FATS)

Like carbohydrates, fats are compounds of carbon, hydrogen and oxygen, but the proportion of oxygen is lower. Fats include oils and fat-like substances that have a greasy feel and insoluble in water but soluble in certain organic solvents such as ether, alcohol and benzene. Chemically, food fats consist mainly of mixtures of triglycerides. Each triglyceride is a combination of three fatty acids with a unit of glycerol. The differences between one fat and another are mainly due to the different fatty acids in each.

There are many fatty acids found in nature which differ in the number of carbon atoms and 'double bonds' they contain. There are: saturated, polyunsaturated and monounsaturated fatty acids.

Saturated fatty acids are stable and have no double bonds. Examples of these are: palmitic and stearic acids, which are major constituents of lard, suet and cocoa butter; butyric acid which is present in small amounts in milk fat and butter but makes an important contribution to their taste.

Unsaturated fatty acids have two or more double bonds which react gradually with air and make the fat rancid. These include oleic acid, linoleic acid, linolenic acid and arachidonic acid. The last three are considered 'essential fatty acids' because they are required in small quantities for normal health, but cannot be made within the body. Deficiency of these essential fatty acids leads to growth retardation, skin changes with hair loss, increase in metabolic rate and early death.

Functions of fats
The primary function of fat is to supply energy; each gram of fat when oxidised yields approximately nine calories. This energy is continuously available from the stores of adipose tissue. Adipose tissue is stored in the subcutaneous tissues and in the abdominal cavity. It also surrounds the organs and is laced throughout muscle tissue. Fats serve as carriers of the fat-soluble vitamins A, D, E and K, give a pleasant taste of food and provide satiety because the rate at which a meal is emptied from the stomach is related to its fat content.

Phospholipids are important components of membrane structure and consitutents of all cells and are involved in the absorption and transport of fat.

Digestion and absorption
Fats are hydrolysed primarily in the small intestine. Although gastric lipase may bring about some hydrolysis of finely divided fats from foods such as egg yolk and cream, the action is not considered very important.

As the chyme enters the duodenum the presence of fat stimulates the intestinal wall to secrete *cholecystokinin*, a hormone that stimulates release of bile from the gall-bladder.

Bile has several important functions in fat digestion and absorption:

1. It stimulates peristalsis.
2. It neutralises the acid chyme so as to provide the optimum hydrogen ion concentration for enzyme activity.
3. It emulsifies fats thereby increasing the surface area exposed to enzyme action.
4. It lowers the surface tension so that intimate contact between the fat droplets and the enzymes is possible.

The triglycerides are hydrolysed by lipase, and the end-products of lipid hydrolysis that are presented for absorption include fatty acids, glycerols, monoglycerides and also some di- and triglycerides. Absorption of triglycerides occurs by two distinct processes, depending upon the length of the fatty acid chain. Long chain fatty acids have 12 to 18 carbon atoms and short chain have eight to 10. Most dietary fatty acids are long chain, so that failure of their absorption is the commonest cause of steatorrhoea.

Long-chain trigylcerides
Although some lipolysis occurs in the stomach, long chain trigylcerides are mainly hydrolysed by pancreatic lipase. The triglycerides are finally split to monoglycerides. Bile salts are not essential for this but accelerate it by emulsifying the triglycerides and lowering the optimal pH of the enzyme to the slightly acid conditions found in the intestine normally. The fatty acids and monoglycerides enter the mucosal cell passively. It requires the presence of normal microvilli, which increase the absorptive area enormously, and a good functioning enterohepatic circulation.

Medium chain triglycerides
Medium chain triglycerides contain fatty acids with six to 10 atoms of carbon and contribute about 4 per cent of the fat in normal diets. They are liquid at room temperature and have considerable water solubility. They are more readily and more completely hydrolysed by pancreatic lipase and are also hydrolysed in the stomach and colon. They can be absorbed directly into mucosal cell where hydrolysis takes place. Once in the mucosal cells the medium chain fatty acids are passed directly into the portal circulation and are metabolised in the liver. Ketones and acetates represent other water-soluble hepatic metabolites of medium chain fatty acids, and medium chain triglycerides (MCT) have been used to induce ketosis for the treatment of intractable epilepsy (see p. 307). Medium chain triglycerides play a valuable part in the correction of energy deficiency caused by the malabsorption of long chain triglycerides. Besides aiding nutrition, MCT will diminish the flow of chyle in the thoracic duct and, in association with reduction in the dietary long chain triglycerides, can avoid the unpleasant aspects of steatorrhoea such as flatus, abdominal distension and discomfort as well as offensive stools.

New-born infants absorb approximately 85 to 90 per cent of the fat provided by human milk. Many infants absorb less than 70 per cent of cow's milk fat. Absorption of fat begins to reach adult levels between the ages of 6 to 9 months.

The amount of fat in the stomach controls the emptying rate. The more fat in the food, the longer it remains. It enters the duodenum in regulated amounts where it unites with bile and pancreatic juice. When it interacts with bile, an emulsion is formed which produces mixed micelles which are both fat and water soluble. They are then acted on by pancreatic and intestinal lipase. Pancreatic lipase activity is low in newborn infants, especially in the premature infant. The bile acid pool is also reduced in the new-born.

Lipids are absorbed in the jejunum but bile salts are not absorbed with the lipids. They re-enter the intestine and are transported to the liver where they are resecreted.

Recommended intakes

No recommendations for intakes of fat have been made. However, if less than 30 per cent of energy intakes are derived from fat, a dry and unpalatable diet may result. As little as 1 per cent of the calories from linoleic acid is sufficient to prevent symptoms of essential fatty acid deficiency in infants.

Food sources

Milk, either human or cow's, provides approximately 50 per cent of the calories as fat. Approximately 4 per cent of the total calories in human milk and 1 per cent of the total calories in cow's milk are provided by linoleic acid. Other food sources are oils, lard, butter, margarine, bacon and salad dressing, which are the most concentrated sources of fat.

Deficient intakes

The only clinical symptoms that result from diets deficient in fats are those of linoleic acid deficiency or essential fatty acid deficiency (EFAD). This results in dry, thickened skin with desquamation.

Excessive intakes

Excessive intakes of fat satiate children and limit their appetite for other foods. Very high fat intakes may produce ketosis.

VITAMINS

A vitamin is a chemical compound which occurs naturally in food and is essential in small amounts for health. They are essential for normal metabolism of amino-acids, fats and carbohydrate to produce energy and synthesise tissue, enzymes, hormones and other vital compounds.

Vitamins have been classified into two groups.

The first supply active groups for enzymes. These are called 'pro enzymes'. They are *water* soluble, are not stored or toxic, are excreted in the urine and are required because the body cannot synthesise them. Included in this group are the B group vitamins thiamin, riboflavin, nicotinic acid, pyridoxine, folic acid, biotin, pantothenic acid, vitamin B_{12} (cobalamine) and vitamin C (ascorbic acid).

The second group are *fat soluble* and include vitamins A, D, E and K. These vitamins alter the conformation of complex molecules and membranes but do not supply active sites. They are stored, may be toxic, and the need for them may have arisen from requirements of some highly-specialised tissue.

Deficiency of a vitamin may be:

1. *Primary* or *exogenous* when the diet provides less than the requirements.
2. *Secondary* or *endogenous* when deficiency may arise when the diet is adequate but one or more aspects of vitamin utilisation by the body is defective, e.g. digestion, absorption, transport or intracellular metabolism.

Vitamins can also have a toxic effect, but the toxicity is confined, as far as is known, to the fat-soluble vitamins A, D and K.

There is also evidence of vitamin dependency. It refers to disorders of metabolism of genetic origin which respond to high doses of a vitamin. An abnormal gene product, arising in one of several possible ways, prevents the optimal action of a coenzyme-apoenzyme complex. The cells might fail (1) to take up the vitamins; or (2) to convert them to the coenzyme form; or (3) the apoenzyme might be altered so that it does not bind to the coenzyme. The first two are *biosynthetic* and could depress the activity of many apoenzymes and the third is *binding* involving only a single apoenzyme. Treatment would depend on the type of disorder.

Vitamin A (Retinol)

Several biologically-active compounds are collectively known as vitamin A. Retinol and 3-dehydroretinols are alcohols. Retinol is an aldehyde while retinoic acid is the vitamin A acid.

Foods supply vitamin A in the form of carotenes, as vitamin A esters and as free vitamin A. Retinol is found only in animal foods, but milk and some vegetable foods also contain the deep yellow or orange carotenes which can be converted in the body to retinol. The most important of these is the beta (β)-carotene. The absorption of vitamin A and the carotenes is facilitated by bile and thyroxin. The presence of mineral oil in the intestinal tract reduces absorption of vitamin A. Mineral oil is not absorbed and since it holds carotenes and vitamin A in solution, the vitamins are lost in excretion. Retinyl esters, retinol and retinoic acid are transported in the chylomicrons, through the lymph circulation to the thoracic duct and then enter the bloodstream to be carried to the liver for storage. Significant amounts of vitamin A are also absorbed directly into the portal circulation. Liver reserves are low in new-born infants.

Functions of vitamin A

Retinol is essential for visual adaptation to changes in light. Rhodopsin (visual purple), the light-sensitive pigment of the rods of the retina, is a compound that contains retinol coupled to a protein opsin. When light hits the retina, retinol is isomerised and rhodopsin splits into opsin and retinene. In darkness retinene is isomerised to the original retinol and again combines with opsin to regenerate rhodopsin, preventing night-blindness. In epithelial tissue vitamin A is necessary for normal mucociliary function. It also affects the stability of lysosome membranes and, when deficient, cell-mediated immunity is impaired. It influences synthesis of protein, thereby affecting growth of the skeleton and soft tissue. It interacts metabolically with other vitamins, including D and E and hormones. Vitamin E appears to spare vitamin A by protecting it from oxidation and increasing absorption, utilisation and storage.

Recommended intakes

The recommended allowance of vitamin A for infants is based on the average retinol content of human milk:

Under 6 months	420 μg
6 to 12 months	400 μg
1 to 3 years	400 μg
4 to 6 years	500 μg
7 to 10 years	700 μg
11 to 18 years (M)	1000 μg
11 to 18 years (F)	800 μg

Deficient intakes

Xerophthalmia, due to severe vitamin A deficiency, can lead to blindness. Other conditions due to deficient intakes are night-blindness and keratomalacia where there is deformity and loss of corneal substance with some permanent damage.

Excessive intakes

Hypervitaminosis A is a well-defined clinical entity due to excessive intakes of vitamin A.

Acute poisoning has resulted from single large doses (about 100 000 μg). The child becomes restless and symptoms of raised intracranial pressure with headache and vomiting develop. Recovery is spontaneous on cessation of intake of the vitamin.

Chronic poisoning takes several weeks or several years to appear depending upon the level of dosage and the age of the child.

Clinical features include sparse, coarse hair, dry and rough skin; cracked lips and enlarged spleen; and bony changes with stunted growth can also be seen. Prognosis is usually very good with the withdrawal of vitamin A and the symptoms disappear over several weeks.

Vitamin D

This is a fat-soluble vitamin which occurs in two forms: ergocalciferol (activated ergosterol, calciferol, vitamin D_2) found in irradiated yeast and cholecalciferol formed in human skin by exposure to sunlight (ultraviolet radiation) and found chiefly in fish-liver oils and egg yolks.

Vitamin D is absorbed from the intestine together with fats and transported to the liver on vitamin D-binding protein. It is changed there to $25(OH)D_3$ and is then transported to the kidney where it undergoes one of two hydroxylations. If there is a need for *calcium* or *phosphate*, the kidney is stimulated (by the action of parathyroid hormone) to produce $1.25(OH)_2D_3$ which acts as a calcium and phosphorus-mobilising hormone. Vitamin D also controls phosphorus and calcium absorption.

Food sources
Few foods contain vitamin D and all those which do so are animal products. They contain vitamin D_3 (cholecalciferol) which is derived from the action of sunlight on the animal's skin or from its own food. The amount present varies with the seasons. Main sources are margarine (includes added vitamin D), fatty fish, eggs and butter.

Deficient intakes
Vitamin D deficiency results in low levels of serum inorganic phosphorus and plasma calcium, and elevated levels of alkaline phosphatase. The disease caused by dietary deficiency is *rickets* (see p. 586).

Excessive intakes
Large doses of vitamin D consumed over long periods of time result in symptoms of toxicity. The toxic effects are generally associated with hypercalcaemia, although those effects can be present in the absence of hypercalcaemia. The child, usually between 3 and 6 months, becomes irritable, anorexic and constipated; he develops vomiting, polyuria and weight loss. Prolonged hypercalcaemia may lead to nephrocalcinosis and renal failure. The treatment aims at lowering serum calcium rapidly by induction of sodium diuresis which promotes calciuria.

Principles of treatment and nursing management
1. Intravenous infusion of saline to ensure adequate expansion of extracellular volume before starting frusemide (see p. 448 for care of the child during intravenous infusion.)
2. *Drugs*
   a. Frusemide to induce sodium diuresis.
   b. If diuresis fails: corticosteroids, mithramycin and calcitonin may be used.

3. *Dietary measures.* A low calcium diet is given. Intake should be restricted to 150 mg calcium daily in infants and to 300 to 400 mg daily in older children. Vitamin D intake should be minimal. All milk products are forbidden and a special low calcium milk (Locasol) is used for drinking and cooking. Since proprietary baby foods are fortified with vitamin D, extra caution will be necessary. Foods which are rich in calcium, i.e. fish like sardines and herrings, are usually forbidden. Most flours are fortified with calcium, therefore only unfortified flour is allowed. Calcium is present in eggs, cereals, some fruits and vegetables and these may have to be restricted. Water too contains calcium and where a high fluid intake is required, boiled water may be used.
4. Routine nursing care.
5. *Parental support.* This involves interviewing of parents and an explanation of the character of the illness. Nutritional guidance by the medical officer and dietician regarding suitable foods to be given.

Vitamin E (Tocopherol)
The vitamin E group includes four tocopherols, 'a' being the most active. Vitamin E is an intracellular antioxidant which appears to act by maintaining the stability of membranes complexed with polyunsaturated phospholipids. It may also inhibit the oxidation of selemide and sulphide-containing proteins in mitochondria and smooth endoplasmic reticulum.

Food sources
Tocopherol is widely distributed in food and occurs in highest concentration in cereal grain oils. Other foods include vegetable oils, milk, eggs, fish, meat, leafy vegetables and cereal. Human milk contains more tocopherol than cow's milk and colostrum is a richer source than later human milk.

Deficient intakes
Primary deficiency may occur in early infancy especially in low-birth-weight infants and if the milk formula is high in polyunsaturated fat. Secondary deficiency may occur in malabsorption

from any cause, especially if there is steatorrhoea, as in coeliac disease, cystic fibrosis and biliary atresia. Anaemia, haemolytic in type, is the only disorder in children due to this deficiency and it has been found that in premature infants it was made worse by large doses of iron.

Laboratory tests show that the red blood cells are abnormally fragile when exposed to hydrogen peroxide.

Excessive intakes
Vitamin E appears to be the least toxic of the fat-soluble vitamins.

Vitamin K
Vitamin K consists of a number of related compounds known as quinones. Phyeloquinone (vitamine K_1) and farnoquinone (vitamin K_2) occur naturally. Menadione (vitamin K_3) is a synthetic compound. Vitamin K controls the formation in the liver of prothrombin (Factor II), Factor VIII (proconvertin), IX (Christmas factor), and X (Stuart factor) as well as a fifth, recently identified, coagulation factor.

Food sources
Green leafy vegetables are the richest food source. Lesser amounts are found in meat and dairy products. Human milk contains 15 $\mu g/l$ and cow's milk, 60 $\mu g/l$.

Deficient intakes
Vitamin K is usually obtained mainly from intestinal bacterial synthesis. Lack of bacterial flora probably explains the hypoprothrombinaemia which occurs during the first 5 days of life. The coagulation factors are large proteins which do not cross the placental barrier to the fetus. They have to be produced by the fetal liver and, if this is immature, as it is in premature babies or low-weight babies, deficient production is common and whole blood will be required.

Non-absorbable sulphonamides or oral antibiotics may also interfere and cause deficiency. Coumarin anticoagulants are antimetabolites of vitamin K.

Vitamin K deficiency is treated by intramuscular injection of Phytonadione 1 to 2 mg.

Excessive intakes
Menadione and its water-soluble analogues have induced haemolysis if given in large doses. Children suffering from G6PO deficiency are especially susceptible. Large doses in the new-born have produced anaemia, hyperbilirubinaemia and kernicterus in the premature infant.

Water-soluble vitamins
While the fat-soluble vitamins can be stored, water-soluble vitamins are stored in small amounts and therefore deficiencies may occur in a relatively short period of time if the nutrient is absent from the diet. The water-soluble vitamins include those of the B complex and vitamin C (ascorbic acid). Many, but not all, of the B-complex vitamins have been described. Their chemical and physical properties are fairly well understood and many have now been synthesised.

Vitamin B complex
These are water-soluble substances each of which has a different chemical structure but which have several features in common. They act as 'co-factors' in different enzyme systems in the body. Principally these vitamins combine with specific proteins to function as parts of the various oxidative enzyme systems which are concerned with the breakdown of carbohydrate, proteins and fat in the body. They are intimately involved in the mechanism which releases energy, carbon dioxide and water as the end-products of metabolism.

Thiamine (Vitamin B_1)
Thiamine takes part in a number of different reactions, playing a role in glycolysis and the glycolytic pathways, the citric acid cycle and others. Consequently, it is necessary for the steady and continuous release of energy from carbohydrate. Phosphoric esters of thiamine are involved in metabolism and function of excitable membranes. It is therefore believed to have a role in neurophysiology.

Recommended intakes
The requirements for thiamine is determined by the carbohydrate and calorie intake:
Under 6 months 0.3 mg
6 to 12 months   0.5 mg

1 to 3 years	0.5 mg
4 to 6 years	0.7 mg
7 to 9 years	0.9 mg
Adolescents (M)	1 to 1.2 mg
Adolescents (F)	0.9 to 1 mg

Food sources
Thiamine is widely distributed in both animal and vegetable foods. For example, milk, eggs, pork, vegetables, fruit, whole grain cereals and fortified breakfast cereals. Cooking results in considerable losses from these foods.

Thiamine deficiency (Beriberi)
The disease is virtually confined to breast-fed infants of thiamine-deficient mothers with very low content of thiamine in their breast milk. It occurs in South-East Asia where mothers eat a polished rice diet.

Clinical features
The infantile form of beriberi is always a serious disease. Three main syndromes have been described (Jelliffe, 1968).

1. *Acute cardiac*. The onset is sudden between 2 and 4 months with restlessness, bouts of screaming and breathlessness. The infant is pale but cyanosed. Physical signs of acute cardic failure are present and death may occur rapidly.
2. *Aphonic*. Coughing and choking commencing between 5 and 7 months. Hoarseness, dysphonia and aphonia give rise to the characteristic noiseless cry with laryngeal nerve paralysis or oedema of the larynx.
3. *Pseudomeningeal*. The disease simulates meningitis in the older infant from 8 to 10 months of age. There is apathy, drowsiness, head retraction and signs of raised intracranial pressure.

Beriberi is rare after the age of 1 year. When it occurs in older children, the manifestations are similar to those seen in adults.

Principles of treatment and nursing management

1. Intravenous thiamine hydrochloride 25 mg or Intramuscular injection of 100 mg. In the cardiac form a diuresis within a few hours following the injection is diagnostic as well as therapeutic.
2. Maintenance therapy of 25 mg intramuscularly for 3 days and followed by 10 mg orally twice a day. The mother should be treated at the same time.
3. Oxygen therapy.
4. Accurate fluid intake and output measurement.
5. Daily weighing.
6. Satisfying nutritional needs for age of infant.
   a. Oral.
   b. Naso-gastric feeding.
7. Observations of neurological functions.
8. Routine care.
9. Support and guidance for parents. Education with regard to diet is important. Where possible the diet should be more diverse particularly when overdependence on rice is the rule. Enrichment of rice with thiamine has been shown to be effective.

Nicotinic acid (Niacin)
The amino-acid tryptophan can be converted to niacin but in man it is insufficient to meet requirements. Niacin functions as an essential component of the coenzymes (NADO) and (NAD) which are necessary for many biochemical reactions. They are essential for the transfer of hydrogen in the intercellular respiratory mechanisms of all cells. They are also essential for cellular biosynthesis of fatty acids and function in energy release and in amino-acid metabolism.

Recommended intakes

Under 6 months	5 mg
6 to 12 months	8 mg
1 to 3 years	9 mg
4 to 6 years	12.1 mg
7 to 9 years	14.5 mg
10 to 12 years (M)	17.2 mg
10 to 12 years (F)	15.5 mg
13 to 15 years (M)	19.1 mg
13 to 15 years (F)	16.5 mg
16 to 19 years (M)	20.3 mg
16 to 19 years (F)	15.2 mg

Food sources
Meat, poultry, liver, legumes, dairy products and eggs.

Deficient intakes

Deficiency of niacin leads to pellagra. The disease typically occurs in adults but as whole communities tend to be affected some cases will appear among children of all ages. The manifestations are similar to those in adults.

Diets based on maize give rise to endemic pellagra in parts of the Middle East (Egypt and Syria), Africa and South-East Europe. Although maize contains nicotinic acid it is present in a bound form. Since tryptophan gives rise to nicotinic acid in the body, but because it is present in very low amounts in maize, it contributes to its pellagragenic effect.

Cases can also occur secondary to other disorders. For example, patients treated with isoniazid for tuberculosis for a prolonged period may develop pellagra. Similar manifestations occur in Hartnup disease (a rare genetic metabolic defect in which the basic defect involves the intestinal and renal transport of many amino-acids; the clinical manifestations relate to tryptophan).

Clinical features

Skin changes are usually first noted. They occur in parts which are exposed to sunlight and trauma. Sores and fissures appear on the outer canthus of the eye, the edge of the alae nasi, the lips, anus and genitalia. The tongue is described as 'raw beef' in appearance; it is, red, swollen and painful. Similar changes occur in the gastro-intestinal tract leading to diarrhoea and malabsorption.

Principles of treatment and nursing management

1. Medication. Oral nicotinamide 50 mg three times a day. In severe anorexia and diarrhoea, the drug may be given intravenously (3 mg).
2. Provision of adequate tryptophan in the form of high quality protein from milk, eggs and meat.
3. Routine nursing care.
4. Oral care.
5. Guidance for parents. Education in dietary needs. Less dependence on maize and incorporation of better protein and vitamin sources may be learned. However, this may only come about with social and economic changes in countries where this condition occurs.

Vitamin C (Ascorbic acid)

Ascorbic acid is a white crystalline compound of relatively simple structure. It is closely related to the monosaccharide sugars. It is synthesised from glucose and other simple sugars by plants and by most animal species. Vitamin C is active in two forms, L-ascorbic acid (the reduced form) and L-dehydroascorbic acid (the oxidised form). The latter is oxidised further with complete loss of activity.

Physiology

Ascorbic acid is rapidly absorbed from the gastro-intestinal tract and distributed to the various tissues of the body. The adrenal gland contains an especially high concentration of vitamin C. Other tissues such as the pancreas, thymus, spleen, liver, pituitary and kidney also contain appreciable amounts. Since tissues can only hold a limited amount of vitamin C, any excess is excreted. A blood plasma concentration of 0.4 to 1.0 mg per 100 ml is satisfactory.

Function of vitamin C

Vitamin C has many functions, some of which are not yet clearly understood. It is a reactant in a number of enzyme systems and is involved in cell respiration. However, the principal function of ascorbic acid is in the formation of collagenous intracellular substances. Collagen is a protein widely distributed in fibrous tissue structures such as cartilage, bone matrices, dentine and the vascular endothelium. Ascorbic acid is essential for the hydroxylation of two amino-acids, proline and lysine to hydroxyproline and hydroxylysine which are important constituents of collagen. Maintaining the integrity of collagen is an important function of vitamin C and this helps to explain the role of vitamin C in wound healing and the body's ability to withstand the stresses of injury and infection.

Other functions include:

1. Oxidation of phenylalanine to tyrosine.
2. Reduction of ferric iron to ferrous iron in the gastro-intestinal tract so that it is more readily absorbed.
3. Release of iron from transferrin in the plasma for incorporation into tissue ferritin.

4. Conversion of folic acid to its active form, folinic acid.

The last three are of importance in preventing anaemia.

It appears the ascorbic acid may be involved in the synthesis of steroid hormones from cholesterol, because as adrenocortical activity increases, the concentration of ascorbic acid and of cholesterol in the adrenal gland decreases.

Food sources

Vitamin C is not widely distributed in foods. Small amounts occur in milk, especially breast milk, and in liver, but the main sources are from fruit and vegetables, e.g. blackcurrants 200 mg/100 g, oranges 50 mg/100 g, brussels sprouts 87 mg/100 g, potatoes (varies with season), e.g. new potatoes 30 mg/100 g, autumn 20 mg/100 g, winter 10 mg/100 g and spring 8 mg/100 g.

Since many fruits and vegetables are difficult to store and are also relatively expensive when out of season, this vitamin is often deficient in a British diet. In addition vitamin C is readily lost during storage, preparation and cooking which further decreases its availability.

Effects of deficient intakes

Pathology

A deficiency of ascorbic acid results in defective formation of the intercellular cement substance in connective tissues, bones and dentine resulting in weakening of capillaries with subsequent haemorrhage and defects in bone and related structures. Wounds heal poorly and tend to break down easily. Bone lesions form due to cessation of endochondrol growth which is as a result of failure of the osteoblasts to form osteoid tissue. Instead, a fibrous union is formed between the diaphysis and the epiphysis, and costochondrol junctions enlarge.

Prophylaxis

Prevention of this condition can be achieved by giving infants unboiled orange juice daily, beginning with 5 ml in the 2nd to 4th week of life, with progressive increases until at 5 months the intake is 60 to 90 ml. If the infant reacts unfavourably, ascorbic acid 25 to 30 mg/d should be given.

Principles of treatment and nursing management

1. Medication. Ascorbic acid 50 mg four times a day orally for one week then decrease to 50 mg three times a day for one month. Thereafter, prophylactic doses are given. If there is vomiting or diarrhoea, one half of the oral dose can be given intramuscularly or intravenously as sodium ascorbate. Correction of anaemia.
2. Bed cradle to prevent pressure of bedclothes on limbs.
3. Gentle handling since bones are swollen and painful.
4. Oral care; cleanliness of mouth must be maintained. Since gums tend to bleed gingivitis can occur if teeth have erupted.
5. Routine nursing.
6. Support for parents. Since the cause has been identified, guidance regarding diet and vitamin C intake should be given.

Minerals (Elements)

The bulk of living matter is made up to 11 elements: Hydrogen (H), Carbon (C), Nitrogen (N), Oxygen (O), Sodium (Na), Magnesium (Mg), phosphorus (P), sulphur (S), chloride (CI), potassium (K), and calcium (Ca). Some of these are constituents of protein, carbohydrates and fats; others are regarded as electrolytes especially concerned in the maintenance of fluid and acid-base balance. All these elements can be regarded as *essential macroelements*.

There are also essential trace elements (microelements) which are necessary. These include: iron, iodine, copper, manganese, zinc, cobalt, molybdenum, selenium, chromium, tin, vanadium, fluorine, silicon, nickel and arsenic. These elements are both poorly absorbed and excreted and may, therefore, accumulate in toxic amounts.

With the exception of iron, it is uncommon for element deficiency to occur spontaneously in man. However, with the introduction of synthetic diets as treatment for inborn error of metabolism, development of intravenous feeding and the need for renal dialysis, there is a recognition of the nutritional importance of the elements.

Minerals are inorganic nutrients that remain as ash when plant or animal tissues are burned.

Although they contribute only 3 or 4 per cent of the body weight, they play important roles in the regulation of body fluids, acid-base balance and metabolic processes, where they function as catalysts and are found as constituents of enzymes and hormones. Calcium and phosphorus account for three-quarters of the universal elements in the body and five other elements account for most of the rest. Many of the elements are present in such minute amounts that they are generally referred to as trace elements or micronutrients.

Functions of minerals

Mineral elements are present in organic compounds and as phosphoproteins, phospholipids, haemoglobin and thyroxine. They are also present as inorganic compounds such as sodium chloride and calcium phosphate and as free ions. They enter the structure of every cell of the body. Hard skeletal structures contain the greater proportions of some elements such as calcium, phosphorus and magnesium, while soft tissues contain relatively higher proportions of potassium.

Dynamic equilibrium

Generally a balance exists between the intake of an element and its excretion. There is, however, a constant adjustment between absorption and excretion to prevent overload which might produce toxic effects. Precise mechanisms ensure that homeostasis is maintained even though there is a continuous flow of nutrients into and away from the cell. This state of dynamic equilibrium is maintained provided there is an adequate supply of nutrients.

Calcium

Bone contains most of body's calcium and phosphorus and about half of its magnesium. Growth requires deposition of these elements throughout the intra-uterine period until adult life.

Functions of calcium

Both calcium and phosphorus function in the synthesis and remodelling of skeletal tissue. The bones not only provide the rigid framework for the body, but they also act as reserves of calcium to the circulation so that the concentration in the plasma is kept constant. Crystalline protein fibres and collagen form a cellular matrix on which minerals are deposited and are set into a ground-substance of micropolysaccharides.

Calcium also has extraskeletal functions. It acts as a catalyst for the conversion of prothrombin to thrombin which induces clotting by converting fibrinogen to fibrin.

Calcium activates pancreatic lipase, which splits fatty acids from the glycerol molecule, and many enzymes that function in the release of energy. It increases the permeability of cell membranes, and calcium ions are involved in the synthesis of acetylcholine, a neuro-transmitter essential for the transmission of nerve impulses and directly involved with muscle contraction. Low levels of calcium ions lead to muscle spasms. It is also necessary for pancreatic secretion of insulin when stimulated by glucose.

Food sources

Milk and milk products, meat, fish, eggs, beans, fruits and vegetables.

Absorption of calcium

Calcium salts are more soluble in acid solution and therefore most absorption occurs in the duodenum. Once bile and pancreatic juices have united with the chyme, the solubility of the calcium salts and hence the absorption are reduced. There is an increasing rate of accumulation of calcium in the body during growth.

Many dietary factors enhance or interfere with the absorption of calcium. Vitamin D facilitates the entry of calcium into the mucosal cells and also improves the absorption from the duodenum. Calcium absorption is increased with high protein diets. This is believed to be due to the influence of amino-acids such as lysine and serine. Absorption of calcium can be reduced by oxalic acid, phylic acid, excess fat and excess phosphate because they form insoluble complexes with calcium.

Calcium deficiency

Suboptimal intakes of calcium may result in retarded calcification of bones and teeth in the young. Acute deficiency is not usually seen unless there is a concurrent lack of phosphorus and vitamin D.

Steatorrhoea impairs calcium absorption and so does gastro-intestinal hurry, but in both these conditions vitamin D is malabsorbed as well.

As 99 per cent of total body calcium is in the bone, calcium deficiency causes demineralisation of bone, usually without affecting serum levels of calcium, phosphate or alkaline phosphatase. This state is called *osteoporosis* and is characterised by diminished quantity of bone which is normal histologically. It can be produced by failure of formation of bone matrix due to deficiency of vitamin C or protein, and the effects of hormones (parathormone). It can also be due to:

1. Prematurity and prepubertal period.
2. Immobilisation, either local or general.
3. Nutritional deficiencies such as calcium, vitamin C, protein and energy malnutrition (malabsorption, nephrotic syndrome, cirrhosis of the liver).
4. Hormonal, e.g. Turner's syndrome (XO), Cushing's syndrome, steroid therapy.
5. Genetic, e.g. osteogenesis imperfecta.

Treatment is to correct underlying causes of osteoporosis. Increase in oral calcium does not usually affect the process but may increase calcium absorption slightly and retard the skeletal loss. Treatment of the underlying cause will increase nutritional demands for calcium so that calcium salts and physiological doses of vitamin D will be required. Calcium in milk is probably absorbed and 1 litre of milk will provide over 1.37 g calcium.

Osteoporosis can occur in pre-term infants. Breast feeding does not provide the required amount of calcium which they would have received in utero, while the calcium in cow's milk is not available because of impaired absorption. Although osteoporosis is present in the pre-term baby, it does not cause any long-term problems.

Idiopathic juvenile osteoporosis
Prepubertal children aged 8 to 13 years present with fractures or pain in joints and back. The joint pains are often due to impaction fractures of weight-bearing metaphyses due to porosis of newly-formed bone. Some cases are acute and severe, but milder cases may be missed. The cause of this condition is unknown and there is usually spontaneous remission during puberty.

Hypocalcaemia

Blood calcium is present in ionised and protein-bound forms in approximately equal proportions with a small amount of diffusible non-ionised calcium. The serum calcium level can be lowered by alteration in plasma protein levels, particularly albumin. Calcium is a catalyst in many enzyme reactions, including regulation of the permeability of cell membranes, contraction and relaxation of muscle fibres, blood clotting and transmission of nerve impulses. Clinically, a fall in ionised calcium produces tetany.

In newborn infants, tetany is characterised by rhythmic, focal, myoclonic jerks which are sometimes followed by generalised convulsions and cyanosis.

In older infants there are muscular spasms and laryngismus stridulus and in older children paraesthesia, cramps and carpopedal spasms.

Principles of treatment and nursing management

1. Medication. Treatment of hypocalcaemia consists of giving 0.2 ml/kg of a 10 per cent solution of calcium gluconate. This is given slowly intravenously.
2. Management of convulsions.
   a. Magnesium salts are given, e.g. this is given intramuscularly in doses of 0.2 ml/kg of body weight of a 50 per cent solution of magnesium sulphate. If magnesium is given intravenously, it must be given over 10 minutes with electrocardiographic control.
   b. Measurements of vital functions, particularly heart rate since there is a danger of rapidly decreasing heart rate.
   c. Observation of convulsions and nursing management (p. 305).
3. Routine nursing care.
4. Meeting nutritional needs for the age of the child.
5. Support for parents. The condition must be explained to the parents, and where necessary, guidance regarding nutrition should be given.

Hypercalcaemia

Hypercalcaemia is associated with a number of disorders, e.g. it is associated with malignant disease, sarcoidosis, hyperthyroidism, hyperparathyroidism, vitamin D excess, prolonged immobilisation and idiopathic hypercalcaemia in infancy.

Clinical features

Hypercalcaemia from whatever cause, is associated with anorexia, nausea, vomiting and constipation, and sometimes hypotonia, hypertension and stupor occurs. There may be increased calcium in urine and renal concentrating power can be decreased with accompanying polyuria, polydipsia and decreased glomerular filtration. Microscopic haematuria and renal colic may be due to stone formation.

Idiopathic hypercalcaemia occurs in two different forms. *The mild* form is believed to be due to excessive intake of vitamin D. It usually occurs in infants 3 to 6 months old. The infant is irritable, anorexic, constipated, develops vomiting and fails to thrive. The severe form is rare and tends to be part of a syndrome which includes osteosclerosis, hypercalcinuria, nephrocalcinosis, mental retardation, elfin facies, supravalvular aortic stenosis and multiple pulmonary peripheral stenosis.

Principles of treatment and nursing management

1. Serum calcium can be lowered rapidly by inducing sodium diuresis which promotes calciuria. An intravenous saline is given to ensure adequate expansion of the extracellular volume before giving frusemide. For care of the child with an intravenous infusion, see page 448.
2. If diuresis fails, corticosteroids, mithramycin (a cytotoxic antibiotic which can be used as an emergency therapy in severe hypercalcaemia associated with malignant disease) and calcitonin.
3. Nutritional management. A low calcium diet aims to restrict intake to 150 mg calcium daily in infants and to 300 to 400 mg daily in older children. Vitamin intake should be minimal. All milk products are forbidden and a special low calcium milk, e.g. Locasal, is used for drinking and cooking. Proprietary baby cereals and baby foods must be used with caution as many are fortified with skimmed milk powder and vitamin D. Any food which has a high calcium content should be restricted, e.g. fish (where bones are eaten), eggs, some fruits and vegetables, dried fruits and nuts. Since most of the UK flours are fortified, only 100 per cent stone-ground whole wheat flour and unfortified flours are allowed.

In many areas of the world water provides significant amounts of calcium. The use of water softeners, distilled water or at least boiled water is essential. Pharmaceutical substances which contain calcium must be avoided and this includes toothpaste, while vitamin preparations must exclude vitamin D.
4. Routine nursing care.
5. Support and guidance to parents. The condition must be fully explained to the parents. The dietician should provide a list of foods which can and cannot be allowed. If the diet causes economic hardship then help should be provided by the social services.

Iron

Iron is the most abundant trace mineral in the body. Normal newborn infants contain 250 to 300 mg of iron. Before growth ceases at the end of adolescence a further 3 to 4 g must be acquired to avoid iron deficiency. Since growth is not uniform throughout this period but is greater during the late fetal life and early infancy with another growth spurt at puberty, iron requirements will be greatest during these periods of rapid growth.

At birth, the total body iron is dependent on birth-weight, cord haemoglobin and time of cord clamping. Since birth-weight is important, low-birth-weight infants, particularly if pre-term, are very liable to develop iron deficiency later in infancy.

Iron is distributed among a number of different tissues. Haemoglobin iron forms the majority throughout life but it varies with age. For example, during the first 6 to 8 weeks the bone marrow is hyperplastic and haemoglobin iron diminishes while storage iron increases. During the later part of the first year, iron stores are depleted as haemoglobin mass increases. During adolescent growth spurt, storage iron tends to be low.

About 5 per cent of body iron is found in myoglobin, the pigment of muscle and less than 1 per cent in iron-containing intracellular enzymes. Iron is transported in the blood bound to the protein transferrin which both accepts and releases iron. It is stored as ferritin and haemosidirin, both of which can be mobilised for body need.

Iron absorption

Iron absorption regulates total body iron by a mechanism which traps iron in intestinal mucosal cells. When these cells flake off there is some gastro-intestinal iron loss. Iron absorption is increased when iron stores are low and there is increased erythropoiesis. This results in increased absorption at times of physiological needs such as infancy, adolescence and pregnancy.

Concentration of haemoglobin

The concentration of haemoglobin at birth averages 17 to 19 g/100 ml of blood. During the first 6 to 8 weeks of life it decreases to approximately 10 to 11 g/100 ml because of the destruction of fetal cells and decreased erythropoiesis. After this age there is a gradual increase in haemoglobin concentration to 13 g/100 ml at 2 years of age. During adolescence there is a sharp increase in males at the time of the growth spurt.

Functions of iron

Iron in haemoglobin and myoglobin is stabilised in the ferrous state and can be reversibly bonded to oxygen. In this form it carries oxygen to and carbon dioxide from tissues. Iron is also a component of the cytochrome system, which functions in cellular oxidation-reduction reactions. It acts as a co-factor in many other enzyme systems involved in the formation of high-energy phosphate bonds. It catalyses the conversion of β-carotene to vitamin A and plays a role in the synthesis of purines, collagen and antibody production.

Loss of iron due to blood loss

There is about 1 mg of iron in every 2 ml of whole blood, so that small continuing blood loss may lead to iron-deficiency anaemia. This can occur into the gastro-intestinal tract in many infants fed on cow's milk that has not been treated. The mechanism is not understood but it is related to the quantity of dietary milk protein. Hypersensitivity to milk protein leads to exfoliation of mucosal cells. The loss can be stopped if milk proteins are withdrawn

or evaporated milk is given. For this reason pasteurised and homogenised cow's milk is unsuitable for infants feeds.

During menstruation, girls can lose from 4.4 mg to 27 mg of iron at each period. Where the loss is high, it should be replaced.

Sources of iron

Neither breast milk nor cow's milk makes a significant contribution to dietary iron, but many infant foods contain added iron. Many milks for infants are fortified but the iron content varies considerably. The iron contained in breast milk is much better absorbed than that contained in cow's milk. However, if the infant is completely breast-fed, by 6 months he will develop iron deficiency.

After the age of 1 year children usually receive a diet similar to that of adults. European diets contain 6 mg of iron/100 kcal (0.4 MJ). Many countries have much lower iron intakes. This is particularly the case where the diet comes mainly from cereals and very little from animal sources. Foods such as organ meats, dried legumes, shellfish and muscle meats provide the richest and most usable sources. Other sources include nuts, green vegetables and whole wheat flour.

Clinical effects

Pallor is the most common sign in iron deficiency anaemia. About 10 per cent of patients have an enlarged spleen. If the haemoglobin is very low, about 4 g/100 ml, the child becomes lethargic with impaired cardio-respiratory functions. Pica may occur although the relationship is not clearly understood. The child may also be prone to infection. Iron loss is increased in gastroenteritis and iron absorption is reduced in children with pyrexia. Iron deficiency interferes with cell-mediated immunity and the bactericidal effect of phagocytes, and produces depressed lymphocyte responses. (For treatment of iron deficiency anaemia, see p. 435.)

Iron overload

Symptoms due to iron overload in childhood are extremely rare except in high transfusion regimes for chronic anaemia, particularly thalassaemia (see p. 438). Iron accumulation may also occur due to dietary iron overload or to the inborn error of iron metabolism, idiopathic haemochromatosis.

Tissue damage can occur due to iron deposition in the parenchyme of the liver, the pancreas including the islets of Langerhans, the heart muscle and endocrine organs.

Dietary iron overload has been recognised in two areas of the world, in Ethiopia and in South Africa. In Ethiopia, this is due to the high consumption of grain while in South Africa it is derived from pots used in cooking and more importantly from fermenting beer. This beer has a pH of 3 to 3.5 which leaches iron from the pot, and alcohol and iron-complexing ligands such as fructose, promote absorption. The liver becomes cirrhotic and this is correlated with the degree of dietary siderosis. A similar syndrome may be seen in red-wine-drinking areas of the world.

Therapeutic iron overload can occur due to massive doses of iron and to repeated blood transfusions.

Effects of overload include growth retardation, failure of puberty, particularly in boys, hepatic cirrhosis, cardiac failure, diabetes mellitus and renal failure. Treatment consists of desferrioxamine given intramuscularly (see p. 439).

Other elemental deficiencies and toxicity include *copper*, which is essential for erythropoiesis. It facilitates the absorption and transport of iron. Cytochrome oxidase, a copper-containing enzyme, is essential for cell metabolism. Dairy products are poor sources and organ meats, shellfish, nuts and store fruits are rich sources.

Copper deficiency occurs in infancy, usually as a result of exclusive breast or cow's milk diets. Menkes' kinky hair syndrome is a sex-linked abnormality caused by a defect in absorption of copper.

Copper toxicity occurs due to excessive accumulation of copper in many tissues. This is the case in hepatolenticular degeneration (Wilson's disease, an autosomal recessive condition). In erythrocytes, it leads to acute haemolytic anaemia. There is accumulation in nerve cells, especially in putamen and caudate nuclei in the brain as well as the cerebral cortex resulting in tremors, choreoathetoid movements, rigidity, dysarthria and eventually dementia. Kayser–Fleischer ring in the cornea and sunflower cataract are characteristic.

Treatment aims at reducing copper levels. Oral copper binders are given with meals or D-penicillamine 250 mg is given daily orally to start. This is increased every week up to a maintenance dose of 2 to 4 g daily in divided doses. It is given on an empty stomach. When a reduction to normal of plasma-free copper has been achieved, the dose is decreased to 1.5 g daily.

Zinc

Zinc is a constituent of many metalloenzymes and acts as coenzyme in a variety of enzyme systems. It is attached loosely to plasma and much more firmly to globulins. Considerable amounts are found in skin, hair, bones and teeth and testes. Deficiency leads to dwarfism and hypogonadism.

Fluorine

This essential trace element is found mostly in bones and teeth but traces are also present in the thyroid and skin. The main source is drinking water, which, if it contains 1 part per million (considered to be ideal), will provide about 1 to 2 mg daily to adults. Other rich sources are sea fish and tea. Prolonged low intakes of fluorine predispose to dental caries, although other factors are also involved (see p. 96).

Iodine

Seventy to 80 per cent of iodine in the human adult is present in the thyroid gland. Thyroglobulin, the chief constituent of colloid, is the storage form of thyroid hormone and represents normally about 90 per cent of the total iodine in the gland. Iodine content of food varies widely. Marine foods are by far the richest.

Deficiency of iodine results in goitre and should be corrected with iodised salt. Children born to mothers who have a very limited intake of iodine or who have goitre, may have hypothroidism at birth, resulting in cretinism (see p. 274).

Fluid content of the body

The total body water depends on age, sex and the amount of adipose tissue present. Neonates have relatively the greatest body water content, and the more obese the person the less will be the percentage of body water content. Each body cell is bathed in tissue fluid and it is convenient, though strictly speaking incorrect, to consider that body water is separated into two compartments: intracellular and extracellular. This is a simplification of the true situation, since these 'compartments' are further divided into several subcompartments which differ substantially from one another in their water content and in other properties. For example, the extracellular compartment is further divided into interstitial (tissue) fluid and the fluid in the intravascular vessels.

The ratio of extracellular fluid to intracellular fluid changes with growth, especially during the first year, due to the rapid increase in cell numbers and contraction of the interstitial space. During puberty and adolescence further increases in muscle bulk in the male and subcutaneous fat in the female complete the transition to the adult pattern of water distribution. The total body water equals approximately 75 per cent of an infants' body weight at birth and 65 per cent after the neonatal period. The distribution of body water peculiar to the infant accounts for his vulnerability to disturbance of fluid and electrolytes, even during illnesses which are not associated with vomiting and diarrhoea.

The interfaces which separate the various body compartments are permeable to water, which moves freely across them so that the apparent steady state which exists in health is really a dynamic equilibrium. The extracellular fluid and intracellular fluid are separated by the cell membrane, which behaves as a semi-permeable membrane allowing the passage of water and a few substances but not of electrolytes.

The interstitial fluid and the plasma are separated by the capillary wall, which has quite different properties. It acts as a semi-permeable membrane with a much larger 'pore size' than the cell membrane. It, therefore, not only allows water to pass freely but also small molecules of the size of albumin and therefore the large molecules in the plasma exert on osmotic effect between the plasma and the interstitial fluid.

WATER

The body's need for water is second only to that for oxygen. Man can survive for many weeks without food but for only a few days without water.

The functions of water are manifold. It is an essential component of body structure and in its capacity as a solvent, water plays a fundamental role in cellular reactions. Many substances are soluble in water and many others, such as fats and fat-soluble compounds, can be carried in fine emulsions. Water is the medium of all body fluids including the digestive juices, the lymph, the blood, the urine, and sweat. Water is the means by which nutrients are carried to the cells and wastes are removed to the lungs, kidney, intestines, and skin. The metabolic wastes are diluted by water, thereby preventing cellular damage.

Water regulates body temperature by taking up the heat produced in cellular reactions and distributing it throughout the body. About 25 per cent of the heat loss from the body occurs by evaporation from the lungs and skin. Water is essential as a body lubricant, e.g. saliva makes swallowing food possible and the fluids that lubricate the joints.

Sources of water to the body

Water is obtained from liquids, preformed water in foods, and the water resulting from the oxidation of foodstuffs. Water is the principal constituent by weight of almost all foods. For example, milk contains 87 per cent water; eggs, 75 per cent; bread, 35 per cent and meat 40–75 per cent. While oxidation of nutrients results in the release of water. One gram of fat produces 1.07 ml water; 1 gram protein produces 4.1 ml water, and 1 gram of carbohydrate produces 5.5 ml water.

Regulation of water intake

In the child and adult, the intake of water is regulated by a complex mechanism operating through the thirst centre in the hypothalamus, but the infant is not able to act himself in response to thirst. Water intake is intermittent throughout the 24 hour day, but the body is able to control the water loss through various routes, preventing the body being alternatively waterlogged and dehydrated.

To maintain the fluid content at a relatively constant level it is important to ensure that the

Table 11.2 Average water requirements for infants and children

Age	Water requirements (ml/kg/day)
Birth to 10 days	80–100
10 days	125–150
3 months	140–160
6 months	130–155
1 year	120–135
2 years	115–125
6 years	90–100
10 years	70–85
14 years	50–60

infant and child should have adequate fluid intake.

Table 11.2 shows ranges of average water requirements.

Feeding of infants and children of all ages

FEEDING THE NEW-BORN BABY

The purpose of food intake is to provide nutrients for energy and repair of tissue, but in childhood it is also necessary for growth involving an increase in size of all tissues in the body. Provided an infant is born with adequate fetal stores and has ultra-violet irradiation of the skin, human milk can supply all his nutritional needs for optimal growth for at least the first 4 months of life. However, it is also possible to rear infants successfully on a large number of preparations based on cow's milk provided the parents understand the importance of hygiene and correct reconstitution of milk powders.

Production of human milk

During pregnancy the breasts enlarge greatly and structural changes take place. For example, during the first half of pregnancy there is further duct development and many alveoli appear to form lobules. No milk is secreted by the gland cells at this stage. During the second half of pregnancy the epithelial cells swell and there is a gradual initiation of secretory activity with the accumulation of milk.

Lactation consists of two distinct processes:

1. Milk secretion, i.e. the production of milk by the alveolar epithelium and its passage into the lumen of the gland.
2. Milk ejection, i.e. the discharge of milk from the breasts. This depends not only on the suction exerted by the infant but also on a contractile mechanism in the breasts which ejects milk.

Milk

Milk is a naturally balanced food containing about 55 g of first-class protein per litre, mineral salts (especially calcium and phosphorous for bone and tooth formation), practically all the vitamins, fat and soluble carbohydrate.

The fluid secreted during the first 3 days after parturition is called colostrum. It is yellow in colour and rich in protein and salts. It contains large granular bodies called colostrum corpuscles which represent either discharged alveolar cells of the gland or leucocytes loaded with fat. These are abundant in the first few days and disappear at the end of the second week. It is important to look at the differences in composition of colostrum, mature human milk and cow's milk. Indeed the differences between human and cow's milk are quite striking, as Table 2.1 shows.

The protein content of milk, which is made up to lactalbumin and caseinogen, is highest in colostrum (8.5 per cent) and falls during the first few weeks until it reaches a steady level of about 1.25 per cent.

The proportions of lactalbumin and caseinogen are different in human and cow's milk. In human milk there are about two parts of lactalbumin to one of caseinogen whereas in cow's milk the caseinogen is six times in excess of lactalbumin. The caseinogen of cow's milk forms large masses in the stomach which are relatively insoluble.

The quantity and composition of milk is directly related to the mother's diet. For example, if the diet is inadquate the yield of milk is reduced in later lactation.

Drug intake by the mother will also affect the baby, though not all drugs are equally effective. For example, bromides may cause drowsiness, and addiction to morphine has been reported in children of mothers addicted to the drug. Purgatives like phenolphthalein may also affect the baby.

Introduction of solids

Nutritional needs can be entirely met until 4 months of age by milk and sunshine. However, the age at which solids are introduced varies in different communities, from a few weeks until the end of the first year, or even, the second year of life. In Europe and North America solids are introduced quite early but it is recomended that solids should not be introduced before the age of 4 months. This is in order to prevent obesity. It has also been suggested that there is a critical period at which children are developmentally ready to chew solids as distinct from thickened feeds. This is normally when the infant is 6 to 7 months old but depends upon the general development of the child.

The first food to be introduced is usually a cereal. In Western European cultures this is usually a specifically prepared infant cereal made most commonly from wheat, containing added iron and vitamin D. Protein is usually provided today by a great variety of manufactured foodstuffs either tinned or in jars. These are either strained for the younger infant or less finely mixed for the older infant. These foods provide adequate nutrients for infants and are very convenient but very expensive. If the adult diet is adequate, sieving or liquidising foods prepared for the adult family is satisfactory. By the age of 1 year the child is given an adult diet with foods cut up into manageable pieces. The time of weaning is also the time of teething and of an increasing incidence of infections. The child is becoming more independent and often refuses food, takes a long time to eat or is very selective in the foods he will eat. Generally speaking it should not cause concern provided the child is gaining weight. Milk continues to be very important but as more solid food is eaten less milk will be drunk. The amount of food to be given will vary with each child but, to begin with, teaspoons rather than a cupful of solids are more readily accepted until the child has accustomed himself to the new tastes.

Food refusal

All normal infants go through phases, particularly in the second year, in which they will refuse food. It causes a great deal of anxiety in parents who may use a variety of methods to encourage the child to eat. Mealtimes are turned into battlefields. This problem may be short-lived, but in some cases it can persist and develop into emotional problems. A calm approach, without forcing the child to eat, will probably be more successful than bullying or even punishing the child. Appetite varies in children as it does in adults and it is worthwhile to recognise this fact and make allowances. Appetite control appears to be in two areas in the hypothalamus; one acts as the satiety 'centre' and the other is the appetite 'centre' which stimulates food intake. A balance between these two 'centres' controls food intake. There are other factors which influence this balance such as sensory input from the gastro-intestinal tract, including the sense of taste and smell and chemoreceptors in the intestine sensitive to nutrients. Appetite and satiety are also conditioned reflexes and these are influenced by family and environmental factors.

SPECIAL NUTRITIONAL PROBLEMS OF CHILDREN AND ADOLESCENTS

Two problems are particularly associated with children and adolescents and these are anaemia and obesity. Anaemia is discussed fully in Chapter 25.

Obesity

Obesity is found when adequate energy intake is available and therefore seems to be a problem of affluent societies. The more prosperous a country, the more frequently will one find obese children and adolescents.

Although there is little information about obesity some facts are now emerging. It is suggested that juveniles or adults who become obese are not obese at birth. If an infant is overweight at birth then it is due to other problems, such as diabetes mellitus in the mother. There is also indication that the best predictor of juvenile onset of obesity is the weight of the mother during pregnancy or a strong family history of obesity. There is increasing evidence that genetic influences are important in the pathogenesis of early onset juvenile obesity.

During infancy, girls are somewhat fatter than boys, and this difference becomes notably greater during adolescence. There is a gradual increase in body-fat deposition in late childhood and early adolescence. In girls, this deposition of fat accelerates up to the 16th or 17th year of life, at which time normal fat deposits begin to slacken. The opposite takes place for boys, who tend to become leaner during their growth spurt and sexual maturation, when body fat actually decreases to its lowest level in the late teens.

Studies of obesity have indicated that there is an increase in the size of the adipose tissue organ which occurs as part of the growth process. A large amount of fat is deposited in fetal adipose tissue particularly during the last trimester of pregnancy. There is little increase in early childhood but, during puberty, there is a twofold increase in adipose cells. This increased cellularity of the adipose organ which is associated with juvenile obesity is believed to be the most important feature of the current concept of obesity. It may also be the reason why juvenile onset obesity tends to be so resistant to treatment.

Obesity is rarely associated with serious disease in children or adolescents and only occasionally is it associated with endocrine disorders. It is important to identify unusual eating patterns or any evidence of hyperphagia. If hyperphagia is demonstrated then it is necessary to examine the underlying cause, which may be family stresses which are manifested in the child's overeating. A child who feels rejected by parents or peers tends to eat for comfort and thereby perpetuates the obesity. Some are profoundly disturbed by their looks particularly during early adolescence. Some may develop anorexia or apparent anorexia and this must be recognised if any overweight girl shows signs of becoming obsessional about her weight and particularly if she becomes thinner than her ideal weight.

Management of obesity

For success in treatment it is important that the child should want to lose weight. A general examination of the child is carried out and skinfold thickness of subcutaneous fat should be estimated between finger and thumb in at least the triceps and abdominal areas.

Whatever other measures are used in the treatment of obesity, dietary control is essential and this also involves a modification of the child's eating habit.

A free diet for a child consists of ample amounts of natural protein and vitamin-containing foods divided into three meals without snacks. Foods made from sugar and white flour are excluded from the diet and animal fat is reduced in amount. If food is necessary to comfort the child then it should not be denied, as this may increase his anxiety. A favourite item can be allowed daily such as an ice cream, a small bar of chocolate, a piece of cake or a few sweet biscuits. The use of such a food can still be allowed while the child has to give up many other enjoyable items.

Foods such as sugar should not be used and if the child does not enjoy unsweetened drinks then saccharin may be used. Low calorie squash or fizzy drinks can be given and wholemeal bread or low calorie crisp bread can be substituted for white bread. Bread intake should not exceed 90 g/day. Fatty spreads should average a maximum 30 g/day. Milk intake should be 285 to 568 ml ($\frac{1}{2}$ to 1 pint) per day. Whole grain cereals such as Branflakes, All-Bran and Weetabix can be taken without added sugar, but with milk from the daily ration. Grilling should replace frying and potatoes should be baked or boiled.

All dietary control involves modification of eating behaviour. The child should be encouraged to eat slowly and put eating utensils back on the plate between mouthfuls. Food should be eaten only at proper mealtimes and in relaxed pleasant surroundings.

Energy-controlled diets

Energy-controlled diets may be necessary in some seriously obese children or where a rapid weight loss is desirable. A long-term low energy diet may stunt a child's growth even at 1000 kcal (4 MJ) and it is essential that certain minimal daily intakes should be allowed. A balanced diet should be planned with a few hundred calories a day allowed for items which give a child special pleasure. As a rough guideline children should be allowed 25 kcal (0.1 MJ) per lb or up to 60 kcal/kg (0.24 MJ) of ideal body weight per day.

Most obese children who need treatment are at school and this creates problem with dieting. School dinners tend to have a high content of refined carbohydrate. It is therefore desirable if these children could have a packed lunch. Soup can be taken in cold weather in a vacuum flask and a low calorie drink in summer. Sandwiches can be made of wholemeal bread or crisp bread and filled with meat, meat extract, cheese, nuts or salad, and fruit or savoury biscuits can be included. A small sweet item can also be taken to prevent the temptation to buy something sweet.

Drugs

Drugs can be considered if the child has lost some weight and has reached a weight plateau at which hunger prevents him from keeping to a reasonable diet. The drug of choice for children is Diethylpropion. A child of 10 years or older can be given half of a 75 mg long-acting tablet in the morning. A child whose ideal weight is at least 50 kg should be given a whole tablet in the morning. The child should be seen weekly or fortnightly and, if no weight loss has occurred, the drug must be stopped.

Food intolerance

Food intolerance, also often called food allergy, may have an immunological basis. Food intolerances may be mechanical or due to impaired digestion; others may be due to genetically determined enzyme deficiencies such as disaccharidase deficiencies or favisms. In these cases specific foods are involved. Contaminants and additives can have toxic effects and sensitivities of unknown mechanisms as is found in coeliac disease which can be considered as a food intolerance.

Food allergies can be divided into two types. The first is immediate by hypersensitivity medicated by IgE and other circulating antibodies. The second type is when antigens cause tissue damage through cellular immunity. The dramatic symptoms of an immediate allergic reaction vary. There may be a burning sensation of the mouth and lips with localised swelling or erythema or acute systemic reactions with anaphylactic shock, urticaria, angio-oedema, vomiting and diarrhoea, sometimes blood being present, and bronchospasm.

A number of foods can be implicated in these allergic reactions but chocolate, fruit, eggs, nuts, fish, meat, cereals and milk are common.

Cow's milk allergy

There is evidence that some children are allergic to cow's milk. Clinical features vary but have been described to include the following:

1. Symptoms of diarrhoea, vomiting, abdominal pain and failure to thrive in the first year of life particularly if these follow gastroenteritis.
2. A syndrome with clinical features and an abnormal jejunal mucosa similar to coeliac disease, but due to milk sensitivity. This responds both clinically and histologically to a milk-free diet. Milk protein, in this case, acts similarly to wheat gluten in coeliac disease.
3. Young infants frequently have occult blood in their stools. This blood loss can be stopped by withdrawal of milk protein.

Treatment of milk allergy is the avoidance of natural cow's milk protein. Goat's milk is often tolerated, and soya milk can be given but may not be tolerated by some. A hydrolised milk substitute such as Nutramigen or Pregestimil can be used. No tinned and manufactured foods containing milk solids should be given. A diet can be constructed of strained meat, carbohydrate and corn or olive oil, together with calcium, other elements and vitamins. This condition is self-limiting and rarely lasts beyond the age of 3 years. Once the child is thriving, milk is gradually reintroduced.

Diets in disease

The failure to ingest an adequate amount of nutrients, or inability to digest, absorb or metabolise foodstuffs, sooner or later leads to nutritional deficiency. Many illnesses such as infections, injuries and metabolic disturbances lead to deficiencies even where the individual possesses good nutritional status because he is either unable to ingest sufficient food or because the disease process imposes greatly increased demands for most, if not all, of the nutrients. For many patients no dietary modification is required. However, for others modified diets are the principal therapeutic agents in some metabolic diseases such as diabetes mellitus and phenylketonuria.

The purposes of diet therapy are:

1. To maintain good nutritional status.
2. To correct deficiencies that may have occurred.

3. To afford rest to the whole body or to certain organs which may be affected.
4. To adjust the food intake to the body's ability to metabolise the nutrients.

Effect of illness on food acceptance and utilisation

Anorexia in the older child and feeding difficulties in infants commonly complicate any illness, operation or injury. However short the illness there is frequently a temporary reduction in food intake as well as in fluid intake. Vomiting and diarrhoea are common in any infective illness in infancy. Respiration rates are often high and a raised body temperature will further increase fluid requirements. Even if there is no fluid loss, if there is a reduction of intake it may lead to hypertonic dehydration particularly in artificially fed infants under the age of 1.

Generally, there is little to worry about the energy intake at least for the first 2 to 3 days, although ketones are frequently found in the urine in even a mildly ill child. In most acute illnesses, the child begins to eat within 2 to 3 days and provided the protein intake is adequate then generally no permanent harm will result. Carbohydrates or sweetened drinks should be given as soon as possible.

Older children generally adjust to hospitalisation but some may find it difficult to accept food. There is even greater difficulty when a therapeutic diet has to be taken. It is important to determine the likes and dislikes of the child and, as far as it is possible to ensure that these are satisfied. The food should also be presented in such a way that it encourages appetite, and where necessary assistance should be provided either in the cutting up of food and pouring of beverages or in feeding the helpless child.

FOOD REQUIREMENTS OF THE ACUTELY ILL CHILD

Nutritional assessment must be made of the acutely ill child. His requirements are higher than those normal for age, sex and size.

The *basal energy requirements* should be increased in proportion to the severity of the injury or operation (see Ch. 7).

Protein intake should be increased in post-injury catabolism. Normally 1 to 2.5 g/kg/day is recommended. There is a problem that if it is increased too much then a raised blood urea will result.

Carbohydrate and fat usually contribute to energy in almost equal proportions and this should be continued in the sick child unless there is a specific contra-indication. Glucose intolerance can occur after injury or sepsis and this can cause glycosuria. Substances such as Caloreen, Maxijul and Prosparol can be given to increase energy intake.

Methods of feeding

Oral feeding should be encouraged whenever possible but if the child is weak or unable to swallow the volumes required then naso-gastric feeding may be necessary (p. 512). If there is an abnormality of the gastro-intestinal tract, intravenous feeding or elemental diets may be required (p. 455).

Chronic illness

The majority of children will not be immobilised for prolonged periods. However, prolonged bed-rest is usually indicated in children suffering from diseases of bones and joints. Prolonged bed-rest leads to changes in the metabolism of energy, protein and calcium.

Energy metabolism

Energy requirements will be reduced and therefore energy intake needs to be reduced, dependent upon the nutritional status of the child.

Protein metabolism

Prolonged bed-rest leads to muscle wasting due to lack of use of voluntary movement and maintenance of normal postural reflexes. Negative nitrogen balance results, reaching its peak at about 10 days. Prevention of this negative nitrogen balance depends on active movements of those muscles which can be used.

Calcium metabolism

Resorption of bone with loss of mineral and diffuse osteoporosis occur during prolonged bed-rest. When activity is possible again fractures may occur as muscle wasting impairs protective reflexes.

After immobilisation there is increased renal excretion of calcium phosphorus and hydroxyproline (an amino-acid) and this remains high until remineralisation occurs. Osteoporosis is reversed following remobilisation but active exercises in bed have not been successful.

Therapeutic diets

There are many conditions where special diets are recommended. The conditions are discussed in Part 4 and this section primarily discusses the rationale of the diets and the conditions where they are used.

Disorders of the gastro-intestinal tract

Hiatus hernia (p. 482)

Dietary measures consist of small, frequent feeds which are thickened. This can be achieved by using a preparation of carob flour (Lestagel), or if energy is required then Benger's food can be used. This is a preparation of wheat flour predigested with pancreatic enzymes. Hyperacidity can be treated with antacids. Gaviscon, which consists of alginates and antacids, will serve both as an antacid and as a food thickener.

Coeliac disease (p. 500)

In this condition a gluten-free diet is given. All gluten-containing foods such as wheat, oats, rye, barley, semolina, farola, macaroni, spaghetti, cereals made from wheat, meat pies, and any food containing wheat, e.g. potato croquettes, are not allowed.

Food allowed
Gluten-free flour (wheat starch) and foods made with gluten-free flour:
custard, potato flour, cornflour, soya flour.
Cereals: cornflakes, puffed rice, rice krispies, oatmeal.
Protein: meats, fish, poultry, eggs, cheese, milk.
Fats: butter, margarine, oils, salad dressings.
Carbohydrates: fruits, vegetables, puddings and pastries made with corn, rice or potato flour.

A number of foods are available on prescription, e.g. gluten-free bread and bread mix, gluten-free flour, wheat starch, gluten-free biscuits, rusks, and pastas. Most chemists are able to supply tinned gluten-free bread and all other gluten-free products.

Cystic fibrosis (p. 506)

Nutritional therapy is accomplished by replacement of pancreatic enzymes with or without manipulation of the diet. Pancreatic replacement therapy improves both the steatorrhoea and the azotorrhoea (excessive loss of nitrogen in faeces) which occur in this condition but does not always completely abolish them. Preparations of pancreatin are available commercially. These are extracts of hog pancreas containing lipase, amylase and trypsin. The optimum dose varies from patient to patient and is determined by the clinical response. Excessive diarrhoea, abdominal distension or discomfort, and failure to gain weight and height are indications for an increase in dosage. Pancreatic enzymes must be given with all meals and snacks and not only at normal medicine times.

The method of administration varies with age. For small babies it is usually given in powder form either united with feeds or sprinkled on the food. Older children prefer to take the pancreatin in tablet form, since the powder has an unpleasant taste.

Occasionally, dietary restrictions are also required. If the child has abdominal distenson, discomfort and offensive-smelling flatus this can be improved by restricting dietary long-chain fat. Small frequent meals are better tolerated than larger meals and each meal must be accompanied by pancreatic enzymes.

The energy intake should be above the normal for their expected weight and 200 kcal (0.8 MJ) kg/d has been recommended.

Failure of absorption of fat, which may occur even with large doses of pancreatic enzymes, would indicate that fat needs to be restricted. Most older children can manage 40 g daily without too many symptoms. If the fat needs to be restricted further, it may be an advantage to boost energy intake by the use of MCT (medium chain triglycerides) which will also reduce stool bulk and abdominal distension. When starch is the cause of abdominal distension and flatulence and it cannot be controlled by increasing pancreatic enzymes, then it may be necessary to reduce starch intake.

The *protein* intake should be above normal but

excess protein is not well tolerated. When it is necessary to stimulate growth, amino-acid replacement of protein and Pregestimil can be useful. Intra-gastric drip feeds of an elemental diet at night have helped children with growth retardation due to cystic fibrosis.

It is also essential to give supplementary *vitamins* since fat-soluble vitamins may be depleted. Water-soluble preparations such as Abidec are needed to provide about twice the normal requirements. Some authorities recommend vitamin E preparation in a water-soluble base.

Since the sweat electrolytes are high in this condition, supplements of *sodium chloride* 2 to 5 g/d may be needed when there is increased sweating due to high environmental temperature. This is particularly the case in infants on low-solute milks.

Sugar malabsorption

Deficiency of enzymes such as isomaltase, sucrase, maltase and lactase leads to malabsorption of sugar. There are three congenital diseases which appear to have an autosomal recessive inheritance, but there can also be secondary types of sugar malabsorption. The latter are due to damage to mucosal cells and the commonest of these is secondary lactase deficiency. Secondary lactose intolerance tends to be transient.

Children with sugar malabsorption usually present with failure to thrive and watery, explosive diarrhoea, due to fermentation of malabsorbed sugar within the intestine with formation of lactic acid and volatile fatty acids. Acid stools are irritating to the bowel causing gastro-intestinal hurry and secondary generalised malabsorption with steatorrhoea.

Five different diets can be prescribed:

1. *Carbohydrate-free regimen.* This regime may be used if there is intolerance to all carbohydrates. This is usually a temporary state; oral feeds of eggs or Casilan as protein sources and Prosparol in small quantities to provide fat can be used in conjunction with intravenous feeding.
2. *Fructose only.* Fructose Formula Galactomin No. 19 is used with full vitamin and trace element supplement in glucose/galactose intolerance which is a congenital condition. Both in infants and older children substitutes for milk are necessary and a special diet may be required for life. Foods which are allowed include: meat, fish, eggs, a fructose-only milk formula, honey, pure fats and oils, gelatin and vegetables such as sprouts, spinach, green beans and broccoli.
3. *Lactose-free regime.* Lactose is the disaccharide present in milk products and a lactose-free diet in an older child is simple with the exclusion of those foods. For infants a milk substitute will have to be given. There are many lactose-free preparations available. Initially, small volume feeds are given frequently using diluted milk substitute. This is gradually increased as the child's condition improves. Since the feeds will be low in energy, glucose or Caloreen may be given to boost energy intake. As the child grows solids are introduced such as meat, eggs, fish, milk-free cereals and vegetables.
4. *Sucrose-free diet.* This diet is given in sucrose isomaltose, a congential disorder. Sucrose is cane or beet sugar and is present in its natural state in nearly all fruits and, since vitamin C will be low in this diet, it should be given as a supplement.
5. *Starch, lactose and sucrose-free diet.* This diet is given when malabsorption of all disaccharides occurs secondary to some disorder such as gastro-intestinal infection. Glucose and fructose are generally the carbohydrates used in these cases. As the child's condition improves starch and disaccharides are reintroduced. Starch is introduced first, followed by sucrose, and finally lactose is given.

Dietary treatment for diseases of the colon

These include diseases such as ulcerative colitis, Crohn's disease, irritable colon syndrome, functional constipation and various parasitic dysenteries. Nutritional requirements are greater than normal particularly for protein and iron.

Dietary fibre

Dietary fibre has recently assumed great importance in the prevention and management of chronic disease of the colon.

Dietary fibre is defined as the remnants of ingested plant material resistant to hydrolysis by digestive enzymes in man. It consists of four main groups of materials, namely, celluloses, hemi-celluloses, lignins and pectins. The latter comes mainly from fruits, particularly apples.

Fibre-containing foods, such as bran, have been shown to increase faecal bulk, soften the stools and increase the frequency of defaecation and flatus production. When diarrhoea is present it makes the stool more solid, and it has been used to achieve this result in patients with ileostomies. The increase in faecal weight is believed to be due to the absorption of water by cellulose, promotion of colonic peristalsis by the increased bulk and a reduction in transit time. Fibre also promotes intestinal loss of iron and calcium so that deficiency may occur, if intakes of these elements or vitamin D are limited.

High fibre diet
These include the following foods: bread, cakes, pastries made from 100 per cent whole wheat flour; breakfast cereals, particularly All-Bran; and plenty of fruit and vegetables. A high fibre diet is valuable in children with functional constipation.

Low fibre diet
In this diet unabsorbable material is avoided or reduced to a minimum. Therefore, foods such as fruit, vegetables and whole grain cereals are excluded. Cooked sieved fruit and vegetables are allowed, since sieving removes much of the fibre. Vitamin C intake will be minimal in this diet and therefore supplements should be given either as fruit juices or as ascorbic acid tablets.

Diet for ulcerative colitis
The dietary regime consists of a high energy, high protein and low fibre diet with low lactose if needed. Vitamin supplements and iron are given. In some cases, increasing the dietary fibre with unprocessed bran has shown a decrease in diarrhoea. If an elemental diet is used, this can be given by naso-duodenal tube. All the nutrients are absorbed in the upper few metres of the small intestine and produce minimal residue, minimal stimulation of gastro-intestinal secretions, and a reduction in the number of colonic organisms. Elemental diets have also been found useful in Crohn's disease (p. 501). They can be taken orally as a supplement or as a complete feed.

To make them more palatable they are given ice-cold. Some adolescents have preferred to pass an intra-gastric tube themselves, when at home, to allow nocturnal infusion.

Diets in renal disease

Acute nephritis (p. 532)
The aim is to maintain the internal environment until diuresis occurs. In this condition, there is sodium and water retention and this can lead to life-threatening hypertension. If there is mild hypertension then *no salt* is added to food. Generally all that is required is to change to a low-electrolyte milk formula to replace cow's milk. This reduces protein and electrolyte intake and therefore solute load. If more moderate or severe hypertension is present, a low sodium intake with a diuretic and possibly hypertensive drugs may be required.

If oliguria is present then the fluid intake is restricted to the insensible loss (30 ml/kg/day in the infant and 10 ml/kg/day in the older child and adult) plus the previous day's urinary output. Restriction of sodium and potassium intake is required.

An adequate energy intake is required. Diets are calculated individually and should be high in carbohydrate but hyperosmolar diarrhoea may result if solutions are too concentrated. Protein is restricted to 1 to 1.5 g/kg/day in the young child and 0.5 g/kg/day in the older child. This is to prevent a further rise in blood urea. Reduced intake occurs spontaneously due to anorexia.

All diet and fluid restrictions may be lifted as soon as diuresis occurs, which is usually after about 10 days from the onset of oliguria or haematuria. With increase in urine volume, there is weight loss and a decrease in blood pressure and blood urea levels, and therefore sodium, water and protein intakes should be increased.

Diet in nephrotic syndrome
Patients who have proteinuria and a normal serum albumin level do not require a special diet at the time. When the serum albumin level is 2 g/100 ml or less it is advisable to give a calculated protein intake, e.g. in a child 1 to 3 years it is 4.5 to 3 g/kg, and in a child 3 to 6 years, 3.0 g/kg. The

energy intake must be adequate to ensure that protein is not used as an energy source. At least two-thirds of the protein intake should be of high biological value. Fortified foods can be given particularly if the child is unable to eat enough meat, fish, cheese and eggs.

In this condition there is relative sodium and water overload with poor perfusion so plasma aldosterone levels are high. Therefore, salt should not be added to foods, and foods containing added salt such as bacon, ham and cheese should be avoided.

Acute renal failure (p. 535)
The underlying cause of the renal failure is treated first and the chemical environment of the body must be maintained within safe limits until renal functions return. For example, correction of the low blood volume is essential before restoring normal hydration carefully avoiding overhydration. Electrolyte correction is important to avoid neurological complications.

In children with severe oliguria, fluid intake should equal the urinary output plus insensible loss via skin and lungs. In an infant this latter loss amounts to 30 ml/kg/day while in older children it is 15 ml/kg/day. Additional fluid replacement should be to equal losses due to vomiting and diarrhoea.

Raised serum potassium above 7 mmol/l may cause cardiac arrhythmias or arrest. All food and drink given should be low in potassium. If convulsions are present these may be due to decreased levels of calcium and magnesium. It is, therefore, necessary to give these elements.

Energy requirements will be greater and it is suggested that approximately 150 to 200 kcal (0.6 to 0.8 MJ) per kg of body weight is needed. This energy requirement can only be achieved by a concentrated mixture of carbohydrate and fat. This can be achieved by giving glucose polymers such as Hycal (a liquid glucose) or Caloreen and Maxijul. Prosparol is a useful way of providing fat in a water-miscible form and can be mixed with both Hycal and Caloreen. Vitamin and mineral supplements should be given with all diets.

During the recovery phase there is usually diuresis and when this is excessive it can lead to dehydration. In this case, the fluid lost must be replaced. As the blood urea falls, more protein is added to the diet with losses of sodium and potassium which must also be replaced. With increasing renal function it is possible to return to a normal diet.

Chronic renal failure (p. 536)
The aim of dietary treatment is to provide enough nutrients for normal activity and growth but avoid excess requiring renal excretion. Food should be served attractively and be palatable because anorexia and vomiting are features of this condition.

Protein restrictions are rarely required if energy intake is adequate and if the blood urea level is less than 35 mmol/l. The amount of protein recommended varies with age. For infants it is 2 g/kg/day and for children over 1 year, 1 g/kg/day.

In order to meet the high energy requirements and in consideration of the lack of appetite, supplementary drinks should be offered containing up to 4 kcal (0.2 MJ)/ml. Dietary restrictions are only necessary if there is hypertension or gross oedema.

Patients are encouraged to drink as much as possible. Many patients with chronic renal failure pass large volumes of urine of fixed specific gravity because they are unable to concentrate or dilute their glomerular filtrate. Thirst usually controls fluid intake adequately but sometimes increasing fluid intake will increase the excretion of urea and toxic metabolites. In water retention, fluid intake and sodium would be restricted, particularly if weight gain is excessive in the presence of hyponatraemia.

Diets in cardiac disease
Failure to thrive and grow is common in children with congenital heart disease. Growth failure and congenital heart disease may be due to the same genetic or chromosomal abnormality but intrauterine infection cannot be excluded. In these cases it is also likely that growth is not accelerated following surgery to correct the cardiac anomaly. Growth failure is also common in isolated congenital heart disease, particularly in infants and children who are cyanosed, have large left to right shunts, and those in chronic heart failure.

The energy demands may be high because of

increase in cardiac, and more importantly, respiratory work, e.g. dyspnoea. Failure to meet energy requirements is related to infection, which tends to occur frequently, anorexia and difficulty in breathing when lying on the left side while feeding from the right breast.

If bottle or breast feeding is not possible then small, frequent feeds can be given by tube. The feeds should be of high energy value, but sodium free, e.g. Caloreen and Prosparol. Vitamins and folic acid are also required.

In congestive heart failure there is fluid and sodium retention. Vomiting and sweating, as well as hyperventilation, lead to water loss; therefore this must be replaced with high fluid intake which is low in electrolytes. Potassium loss occurs with diuretic therapy and this must be monitored carefully.

Ketogenic diet (p. 307)

Ketogenic diet has now been used for many years to control intractable seizures in childhood. It is most effective in 2 to 5-years-olds with minor seizures, akinetic or myoclonic types of epilepsy.

The basis of this diet is a very high fat, low carbohydrate and adequate protein diet. It consists mainly of butter, cream, oil, bacon and fatty meat. Prosparol can also be given. 80 to 90 per cent of energy will be given as fat.

More recently medium chain triglycerides have been used to supply 60 per cent of total calculated energy requirements. They appear to control seizures and produce a lower cholesterol. They are, however, not very palatable and can cause gastro-intestinal upsets.

Feingold diet

This diet has now been used for a number of years. It is based on the hypothesis that some individuals are genetically predisposed to react to chemicals added to food. In children it is believed to cause a variety of behaviour patterns including restlessness, irritability, and short attention span. These symptoms have been termed 'hyperactivity', 'hyperkinetic' and 'learning disability'. Feingold, an allergist, proposes that the hyperactivity is related to the intake of artificial colours and flavours.

The diet is based on eliminating all foods containing natural salicylates, colouring, flavourings and preservatives. This includes almonds, cucumbers, currants and many other foods.

The diet is said to be effective in some children, but more research is required on the effect of additives on behaviour in children.

Diet and diabetes mellitus (p. 281)

There are a variety of diets being used but the essential point is to achieve good diabetic control and therefore, dietary regulations are necessary. The diet should provide adequate energy for normal growth and development. In general, children's energy requirements are about 1000 kcal (4 MJ)/day for the first year of life with an extra 100 kcal (0.4 MJ)/day for each additional year of life.

Fifty-five per cent of these calories should be as carbohydrate so that an average 5-year-old taking 1400 kcal (5.6 MJ)/day might eat 175 g of carbohydrate a day.

Unless special attention is paid to carbohydrate intake, diabetic children tend to consume a high fat, low carbohydrate diet because of limitations imposed on eating simple carbohydrates such as sugar.

Extra carbohydrate is allowed before and, if necessary, after undertaking exercise, e.g. running for long periods. This may be in the form of additional complex carbohydrate taken at a meal prior to the extended period of exercise. Sucrose or glucose, which are quickly absorbed, can be taken before short bursts of exercise such as swimming.

Distribution of carbohydrate allowance through the day needs to be matched to the insulin regime prescribed. An understanding of the mode of action of insulin is important in order to rationalise carbohydrate distribution (p. 284).

Normally the child has three main meals plus snacks in the mid-morning, mid-afternoon and at bedtime. The size and timing of meals and snacks should be arranged according to each child's daily pattern of activity, varying with school days and weekends, school term and holidays and taking the insulin regime into consideration.

Guidance must be given to the family soon after the diagnosis has been made. The family will be given food tables which list the quantity of each food needed to provide 10 g of carbohydrate. Initially food should be weighed and a small weighing scale can be prescribed.

The majority of dietary carbohydrate should be in the form of polysaccharides, i.e. bread, potatoes, cereals and beans. Sources of rapidly absorbed mono-and disaccharides, e.g. sweets and chocolates, should be excluded except in illness or hypoglycaemic emergency. Refined (fibre-free) starch preparation should be used sparingly. It is also suggested that a reduction in fat intake may be of long-term benefit to the child and that a maximum of 35 per cent of dietary energy should be obtained from fat and a minimum of 55 per cent should be supplied by carbohydrate. All diets should be nutritionally adequate in vitamins and minerals according to normal physiological requirements.

Chapter 12
Fluid and electrolyte balance

The ability of the whole organism to function normally depends upon the maintenance of a stable internal environment. The term 'internal environment' refers primarily to the **fluid** and **electrolyte** content of the body. For any individual to be healthy, the body must contain proper concentrations of fluids and electrolytes. This is particularly important for the new-born infant and during the first year of the child's life, when the young child's loss of fluids is proportionately greater than the adult's and therefore subject to greater irregularity.

Fluid content of the body

The total body water depends on age, sex and the amount of adipose tissue present. Neonates have relatively the greatest body water content, and the more obese the person, the less will be the percentage of body water content. Each body cell is bathed in tissue fluid and it is convenient, though strictly speaking incorrect, to consider that body water is separated into two compartments: intracellular and extracellular. This is a simplification of the true situation, since these 'compartments' are further divided into several subcompartments which differ substantially from one another in their water content and other properties. For example, the extracellular compartment is further divided into interstitial (tissue) fluid and the fluid in the intravascular vessels.

The ratio of extracellular fluid to intracellular fluid changes with growth, especially during the first year, due to the rapid increase in cell numbers and contraction of the interstitial space. During puberty and adolescence further increases in muscle bulk in the male and subcutaneous fat in the female, complete the transition to the adult pattern of water distribution. The total body water equals approximately 75 per cent of an infant's body weight at birth and 65 per cent after the neonatal period. The distribution of body water peculiar to the infant accounts for his vulnerability to disturbance of fluid and electrolytes, even during illness which are not associated with vomiting and diarrhoea.

The interface which separates the various body compartments are permeable to water, which moves freely across them so that the apparent steady state which exists in health is really a dynamic equilibrium. The extracellular fluid and intracellular fluid are separated by the cell membrane, which behaves as a semipermeable membrane allowing the passage of water and a few substances but not of electrolytes.

The interstitial fluid and the plasma are separated by the capillary wall, which has quite different properties. It acts as a semipermeable membrane with a much larger 'pore size' than the cell membrane. It therefore not only allows water to pass freely but also small molecules such as electrolytes. The capillary wall is not permeable to molecules of the size of albumin and therefore the large molecules in the plasma exert an osmotic effect between the plasma and the interstitial fluid.

The concept of balance
The total quantity of water in the body normally remains the same, there being an approximate state of balance between the amount of water taken in from different sources (see p. 211) and the total amount eliminated by various routes, e.g. kidneys, lungs, skin and faeces. During growth a positive water balance is necessary since additional water is required as a constituent of tissue and for

increases in the volume of body fluids. The amount of water required for growth, however, is very small for all ages.

This concept of balance between input and output is not only applicable to water but also to sodium, potassium, chloride, calcium, nitrogenous materials, energy, etc.

Renal water loss
This is partly under hormonal control, i.e. anti-diuretic hormone (ADH), produced in the hypo-thalamus and transported to the posterior lobe of the pituitary gland. It is discharged into the blood-stream in response to nervous impulses which orig-inate in the hypothalamus. For example, increase in the osmolarity of extracellular fluid in a specific area of hypothalamus stimulates ADH secretion. ADH appears to act mainly on the distal convol-uted tubules and collecting ducts of the kidney. When ADH is absent, the epithelial lining of the distal tubules and collecting tubules do not allow water to pass through and there is more urine passed which is hypotonic. When ADH is present, the epithelium becomes permeable to water and the urine is more concentrated.

Water loss from the lungs
The expired air is humidified, but this loss is reduced because the air is cooled as it passes through the nasopharynx. Infants and children have a similar rate of water loss from the lungs, but infants lose more than adults in normal activity.

Water loss through the skin
Insensible water loss from the skin is by diffusion through the outer layers of the skin and partly in the form of sweat. Sweat is a dilute aqueous solution of sodium chloride and sweating therefore involves loss of sodium as well as water.

During febrile illness when hyperventilation occurs the insensible water loss from lungs and skin may be doubled. Unless replacement fluid is given the infant will become dehydrated. When nursed in 100 per cent humidity, the insensible water loss is minimal. When an ultrasonic nebu-liser is used fine water particles can reach the alveoli and absorption of water can take place.

Water loss from the *alimentary tract* accounts for small amounts. Although digestive juices are secreted into the intestinal lumen, most of them are reabsorbed before they reach the pelvic colon. Water loss is increased in diarrhoea and vomiting.

Electrolytes

Chemical compounds in solution may either remain intact, e.g. dextrose, creatinine and urea, or they dissociate (break down) into separate particles. Compounds which give rise to ions in solution are called electrolytes. These ions are elec-trically charged particles, carrying either a positive or negative charge. Water is a good solvent in which dissociation of electrolytes occurs.

In the body, electrolytes consist of *cations*, positively charged ions which include sodium (Na^+), potassium (K^+), calcium (Ca^+) and magne-sium (Mg^{++}), and *anions* or negatively charged ions include chloride (Cl^-), bicarbonate (HCO_3^-), phosphate (HPO_4^-), sulphate (SO_4^-) and ions of organic acids as well as many proteins.

Each body compartment has a different fluid composition. The amount of fluid in the compart-ment is age-dependent but the composition appears to be relatively similar throughout life. Differences in electrolyte composition of blood are most marked in the immediate new-born period, but tend to diminish soon after birth.

Table 12.1 shows that sodium (Na^+ and chloride (Cl^-) are the main extracellular fluid elec-trolytes and potassium, magnesium, phosphate and protein are the main intracellular fluid electrolytes.

The differences in the composition of the intra-cellular and extracellular fluids are important in maintaining cellular function. They result from the activity of a sodium/potassium 'pump' which actively transports these ions across the cell membranes.

In each compartment the sum of the anions and the sum of the cations must balance so as to main-tain electrical neutrality. The chief intracellular cation is potassium which is balanced mainly by protein and phosphate anions. The chief extra-cellular cation is sodium, which is balanced by chloride and bicarbonate anions and, in the blood, protein.

Potassium loss affecting intracellular fluid is

Table 12.1 Electrolyte composition of body compartments

	Plasma	Interstitial	Intracellular
Cation (mEq/L)			
Na^+	140	138	9
K^+	5	8	155
Ca^{++}	5	8	4
Mg^{++}	4	6	32
	154	160	200
Anion (mEq/L)			
Cl^-	100	119	5
HCO_3^-	26	26	10
Protein	19	7	65
Organic acid	6	6	—
HPO_4^{--}	2	1	95
SO_4^{--}	1	1	25
	154	160	200

difficult to determine because any variation is hardly reflected in the composition of extracellular fluid. The latter is normally used for biochemical analysis.

Varieties of disturbance

It is helpful to look at each ion disturbance separately, although not all of these disturbances are of equal importance. Some are much more common than others. Those seen more frequently are the following:

1. Sodium ion depletion.
   Sodium ion retention.
2. Disturbances of the amount of water in the body.
3. Potassium depletion.
   Potassium retention.
4. Magnesium ion disturbances.
5. Calcium disturbance.
6. Disturbances of hydrogen ion concentration.

SODIUM DISTURBANCE
The body is normally in sodium equilibrium. This is achieved by dietary intake and urinary loss and, in warm environments, in sweat.

Abnormalities of sodium balance
Extracellular fluid volume is determined by the amount of sodium it contains. This is achieved by the action of ADH, which maintains the osmolarity of this compartment. The osmolar effect of a substance is determined by the number of particles of that substance present in the solution; and the concentration of the various ions within the body compartments is held at a steady concentration by movement of water across the cell membrane. The movement of water is controlled by the osmotic strength of the intracellular and extracellular fluid.

The concentration of substances in biological fluids is often expressed in millimoles per litre (mmol/l) rather than moles per litre because the quantities in solution are so small.

When thinking about the behaviour of chemicals in solution, it is the number of molecules or ionic charges which are considered, and therefore gram molecular weight and mole are used to 'measure' the chemicals.

Sodium depletion
Sodium can be lost in the following ways: by loss of plasma in haemorrhage and burns, and by sweating, vomiting and diarrhoea. It can also occur when there is renal malfunction, e.g. chronic pyelonephritis. Sodium loss leads to decrease of volume in the extracellular compartment. Depletion of the interstitial fluid compartment gives rise to clinical signs of dehydration. When sodium is lost chloride and water are usually lost as well (Fig. 12.1).

Effect
The skin loses its elasticity and takes on a 'pinched' look. The eyes become 'sunken', the tongue is dry. The circulating blood volume falls and this tends to lead to peripheral circulatory failure. Blood pressure falls and this leads to a reflex increase in heart rate and vasoconstriction. A decrease in the plasma volume without a corresponding decrease in cells makes the blood more viscous. This leads to sluggish blood flow and underperfusion of the tissues with oxygen (hypoxia). However, there is a compensatory mechanism which aims at restoring the blood volume; a fall in the capillary pressure due to

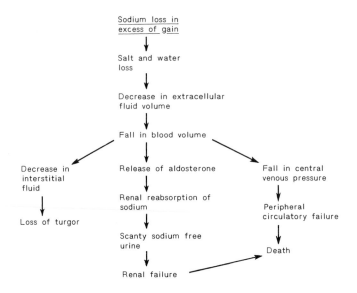

Fig. 12.1 Effects of sodium depletion.

reflex arteriolar vasoconstriction and a rise in the plasma osmotic pressure, allows entrance of interstitial fluid into the blood vessels, thus restoring the blood volume. Urinary output is also decreased and sodium is reabsorbed through the action of aldosterone.

Sodium retention
This leads to expansion of both extracellular compartments, thus causing an increase in cardiac output and a general tendency to oedema. It occurs whenever dietary sodium intake exceeds renal excretory ability. Healthy kidneys have no difficulty in excreting large ions.

Effects (Fig. 12.2)
Sodium is predominantly an extracellular cation. Retention of sodium results in retention of chloride and water. This leads to an expansion of the extracellular fluid compartment resulting in oedema. Healthy kidneys have no difficulty in eliminating very large intake of sodium, but if the kidneys are failing then retention of sodium will occur. Excessive secretion of adrenal cortical hormones also results in excessive reabsorption of sodium.

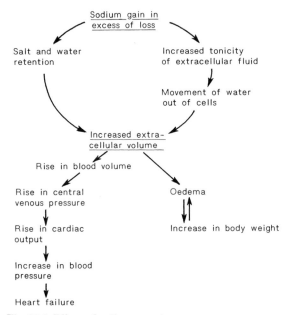

Fig. 12.2 Effects of sodium retention.

DISTURBANCE OF WATER BALANCE

Water depletion
This is the state where the water content of the body is reduced relative to the salt content. The salt concentration in the body fluids tends to be high.

Causes

1. Insufficient water intake. Difficulty in swallowing, e.g. due to some obstruction in the oesophagus, unconsciousness.
2. Excessive water loss. This may occur in children with diabetes insipidus or in conditions where the ability of the kidneys to concentrate urine is diminished. Excessive sweating, vomiting and diarrhoea are also common causes of excessive water loss.

Effects (Fig. 12.3)

Loss of water tends to make the extracellular fluid hypertonic, i.e. greater salt concentration. Water moves from the intracellular to the extracellular compartment and water depletion therefore affects all the body fluid compartments, roughly in proportion to their relative sizes. Hypertonicity of the body fluids elicits the sensation of thirst and this may be intense in water depletion. Hypertonicity also affects the osmoreceptors in the hypothalamus so that the output of anti-diuretic hormone from the posterior pituitary is increased. This leads to increased water reabsorption by the kidneys so that urine volume is mall and highly concentrated. If water depletion is severe it can lead to confusion and disorientation and ultimately coma.

Water retention

The water content of the body is increased relative to its salt content. The tonicity of the body fluids is reduced.

Causes

Water excess may occur when renal excretory function is depressed, as in renal failure or congestive cardiac failure. Excessive secretion of ADH would also lead to reabsorption of water.

Effects (Fig. 12.4)

When water is retained it eventually becomes distributed throughout all the fluid compartments of the body. First the extracellular fluids become hypotonic and then water is drawn by an osmotic gradient into the cells. When this happens in brain cells it can cause disturbance of higher cerebral function. This is known as water intoxication. The symptoms are confusion, irritability, headache and dizziness, eventually leading to convulsions, coma and death.

POTASSIUM DISTURBANCE

Potassium depletion

A low concentration of potassium in the serum is called hypokalaemia. When potassium concentration is low it indicates a fall in the total body potassium stores or in the serum potassium concentrations, or in both. Potassium is the main intracellular cation which is difficult to measure.

Causes

Potassium depletion occurs when the losses exceed intake. Loss may also be via the alimentary tract due to vomiting or diarrhoea. In cases of severe

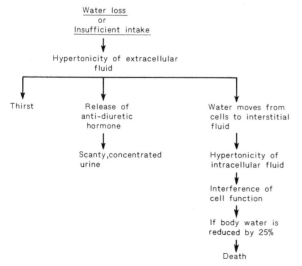

Fig. 12.3 Effects of water depletion.

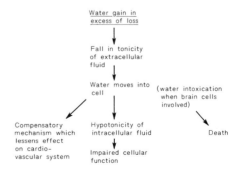

Fig. 12.4 Effects of water retention.

vomiting the cause of potassium loss is more complex, e.g. loss in the volume of extracellular fluid results in secretion of aldosterone which promotes potassium secretion in the distal tubules (nephrons).

There are other causes of urinary loss of potassium including increased secretion of adrenocortical hormones and tissue breakdown.

Effects (Fig. 12.5)
Mild potassium depletion does not show any obvious effect. However, severe depletion will affect many body systems. These include:

1. Mental changes: apathy; confusion; drowsiness leading to coma.
2. Muscular weakness: all types of muscles are involved. Both skeletal and smooth muscle are affected. Paralytic ileus may lead to intestinal öbstruction. Cardiac muscle is also affected — leading to abnormal heart rhythms and characteristic changes in ECG.
3. Disturbance of renal function. The kidney is unable to concentrate or dilute urine. Large

amounts of urine are passed leading to water loss.

Potassium retention
This usually means a rise in the potassium concentration in the extracellular fluid and is also called hyperkalaemia.

Causes

1. Renal failure: potassium is normally excreted by the kidneys.
2. Adrenal failure: insufficient secretion of aldosterone results in loss of sodium and retention of potassium.
3. Intravenous infusions of potassium salts. Rapid i.v. infusion.
4. Cellular damage releases potassium into the plasma.

Effects (Fig. 12.6).
The effects of potassium retention are much the same as those due to potassium depletion. They include:

1. Mental changes.
2. Skeletal muscle weakness. When extreme, it results in a flaccid paralysis.
3. Depression of cardiac muscle. Cardiac muscle becomes weaker, the rate slows and may become irregular. Changes in ECG include peaking of 'T' wave. Very high levels of serum potassium lead to cardiac arrest.

DISTURBANCE OF MAGNESIUM BALANCE
The importance of magnesium has recently been recognised. Magnesium is an essentially intracellu-

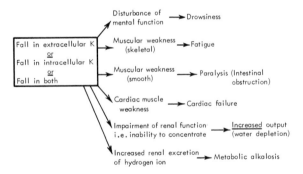

Fig. 12.5 Effects of potassium depletion.

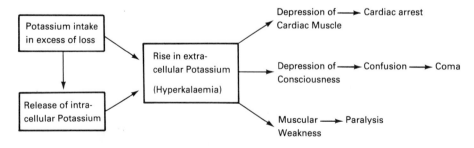

Fig. 12.6 Effects of potassium retention.

lar ion and its function is closely related to certain enzyme systems.

Magnesium depletion

This affects neuromuscular and mental function. The neuromuscular effects are similar to those of tetany caused by a low blood calcium. When potassium is lost, magnesium loss is also likely to occur.

Effects

These include muscular tremor, twitching, convulsions and hallucinations.

Magnesium retention

This may occur if there is dietary excess which is not excreted by the kidneys. The effects are similar to those of increased blood calcium — namely, muscular weakness, mental apathy. They are due to decreased excitability of nerve and muscle membranes.

DISTURBANCE OF CALCIUM BALANCE

Calcium exists in the body in two forms: one as free ions, the other bound to plasma proteins. Calcium imbalance has to be considered as two separate types.

Reduction in total body calcium

This leads to weakness of the skeleton, e.g. spontaneous fractures or deformity (rickets).

Causes

Inadequate absorption of calcium from the intestines, vitamin D deficiency (p. 586).

Reduction in calcium ion concentration

This leads to *increase* in the excitability of muscle and nerve which results in spontaneous contractions of muscles (tetany). In a child, this is characterised by carpo-pedal spasms, laryngismus stridulus and convulsions. Causes are as for 'total body calcium'.

ACID-BASE DISTURBANCE

Acid-base balance is concerned with the concentration of hydrogen ions (H^+) in the body fluids, particularly extracellular fluid, since intracellular fluid and electrolytes are difficult to measure.

Hydrogen ions must be maintained within certain limits so that the body's cells can function efficiently. As with other ions, there are forces or mechanisms at work which tend to shift the hydrogen ions outside the normal range and others which resist these changes.

An acid is defined as a substance which can liberate or donate a hydrogen ion into a solution. A base is a substance which accepts hydrogen ions. Typical acids are hydrochloric acid, carbonic acid and lactic acid; typical bases are bicarbonate ions, chloride ions and ammonia.

Certain ions can act both as acids and as bases. For example, proteins can donate hydrogen ions and can accept hydrogen ions. There are also substances called *buffers* which are only partially dissociated into hydrogen ions. Buffers are solutions which resist major changes of hydrogen ion concentration in a solution when a strong acid or base is added. In biological systems buffers are composed of a mixture of weak acids and their conjugate bases are known as a buffer pair. For example:

$H^+ Cl^-$ and $Na^+ HCO_3^-$
(hydrochloric acid) (sodium bicarbonate)
strong acid conjugate base

Na^+Cl^- and $H^+HCO_3^-$ (carbonic acid)
salt weak acid

Haemoglobin is one of the most important protein buffers in the body. Reduced haemoglobin has an increased tendency to accept hydrogen ions. It becomes a weaker acid and is therefore better able to mop up hydrogen ions produced by tissue metabolism.

The pH of blood is largely dependent on the carbonic acid-bicarbonate buffer pair. pH is defined as $\log_{10} (H^+)$ where (H^+) is the hydrogen ion concentration or hydrogen ion activity. The range of blood pH which is compatible with life is approximately 6.8 to 7.8.

It is usual to separate acid-base disturbances into two categories — *respiratory and metabolic*. Respiratory disturbances are due to abnormalities in the partial pressure (tension) of carbon dioxide in the blood (carbon dioxide combines with water to form carbonic acid, which dissociates to produce hydrogen ions). Metabolic disturbances are due to amounts of other acids.

Respiratory acidosis

This disorder occurs as a result of inadequate alveolar ventilation with retention of CO_2. The common paediatric disorders responsible for respiratory acidosis include: acute airway obstruction such as asthma and laryngotracheitis, cystic fibrosis, depression of the respiratory centre by drugs and trauma, and respiratory distress syndrome in the new-born.

Respiratory alkalosis

The primary problem is a fall in the concentration of carbonic acid in the blood. This is due to increased alveolar ventilation (hyperventilation). It occurs in salicylate poisoning, encephalitis or when emotional factors have a direct effect on the respiratory centre.

Respiratory acid-base changes are accompanied by renal hydrogen ion excretion. These compensatory changes restore the blood pH to or towards, normal. A respiratory acidosis is accompanied by a compensatory metabolic alkalosis, a respiratory alkalosis is accompanied by a compensatory metabolic acidosis.

Metabolic alkalosis

The primary problem is a rise in plasma bicarbonate level. This occurs when there is a decrease in hydrogen ion concentration in plasma. Loss of hydrogen ions from the extracellular fluid occurs by vomiting or by intracellular shift when there is potassium depletion.

Metabolic acidosis

There are several causes, but the more common ones in children are: (1) excessive production of acids; it occurs in diabetes mellitus and starvation where the production of keto acids from excessive fat catabolism causes metabolic acidosis. (2) Inadequate excretion of acids; accumulation of the acid residues of protein metabolism may occur in renal insufficiency. (3) Loss of bicarbonates. This is seen in intestinal obstruction when the digestive juices, rich in bicarbonate, are lost in vomiting and it can also occur in severe diarrhoea.

DEHYDRATION

Dehydration includes both loss of water and loss of solute. Three types of dehydration have been recognised.

1. Isotonic dehydration

In this state the loss of water and electrolytes is equal. It occurs in infants suffering from gastroenteritis where vomiting and diarrhoea cause the dehydration and electrolyte imbalance. It results in: dehydration from loss of water, sodium, potassium, chloride and bicarbonate; using up body stores because of reduced intake; and impairment of renal function leading to metabolic acidosis.

2. Hypertonic dehydration

In this state, the loss of water is greater than the loss of sodium. It occurs under the following circumstances:

1. In gastroenteritis, when increased water is lost in stools.
2. Increased insensible water loss occurring in high fever and hyperventilation as in acute infections.
3. Incorrect feeding formula where the electrolyte and protein content is high.
4. Diabetes insipidus where there is excessive renal loss of water.
5 Low water intake either deliberate or due to damage of the brain.

In hypertonic dehydration the events which lead to this state are believed to be as follows. Water is considered to be the dynamic factor in maintaining the osmolarity of the fluid compartments, while sodium and chloride are the major extracellular electrolytes maintaining the tonicity of plasma. The reason for considering water the dynamic factor is that it is water which moves across the body compartments, increasing or decreasing the concentration of the electrolytes.

Hypertonic dehydration, as found in gastroenteritis and hypernatraemia (increased sodium), is due to fluid loss which is greater than sodium loss. Diarrhoea consists of hypotonic stools and if feeds have a high solute content (such as full-strength milk) then the hypernatraemic state is further increased. This imposes an extra burden on the kidneys which attempt to conserve as much water as possible, but the additional load of sodium pulls water away from the body. There is also the additional water loss through the skin (fever) and increased breathing rate (lungs). All these factors lead to greater loss of water than sodium which leaves the compartments in a hypernatraemic/tonic state. The danger exists where the intracellular compartments are depleted of water due to the osmotic gradient which exists between the ECF and ICF. The effect this can have on cells, particularly brain cells, is extremely dangerous. It is related to the structural and functional changes in the central nervous system, e.g. leading to shrinkage in brain volume, decrease in cerebrospinal fluid pressure and damage to the minute vessels. This will affect its function and accounts for varying behaviour patterns such as irritability, sleepiness and convulsions.

The danger of increased solutes in feeds has now been recognised and changes have been recommended in the constitution of dried milk and in the preparation of feeds (*Present Day Practice in Infant Feeding*, DHSS, 1975).

3. Hyponatraemia and hyponatraemic dehydration

In hyponatraemia without dehydration there is a deficit of extracellular sodium. The following are situations where this can occur, though there are others:

1. Low salt intake — often associated with diuretic therapy.
2. Loss of sodium containing secretions from the gastro-intestinal tract, e.g. drainage or suction of intestinal juice, biliary or pancreatic secretion.
3. Loss of sodium through urine, e.g. in nephrotic syndrome.
4 Loss of sodium through the skin in cystic fibrosis of the pancreas.
5 In adrenocortical disease.

In hyponatraemia with dehydration there is extracellular dilution with water, due to excessive water retention as in nephritis, tubular necrosis and presence of excessive anti-diuretic hormone.

Hyponatraemic dehydration may be present in an infant suffering from gastroenteritis when he is shocked and possibly comatosed.

Replacement therapy

This is based on the assessment of dehydration by physical signs. Each of the dehydration states presents characteristic clinical features. Plasma electrolytes, including plasma bicarbonate and blood urea, should be estimated by biochemical tests. These will include qualitative and quantitative assessment of dehydration, such as:

1. Haemoglobin and packed cell volume.
2. Blood urea.
3. Osmolarity or specific gravity of urine.
4. Plasma protein.
5. Plasma bicarbonate.
6. Plasma sodium and chloride.
7. Plasma potassium.

These tests provide useful information, but in assessing the child's needs the clinical state is also considered. Each dehydration state can be further assessed on the basis of percentage loss of body weight.

In hypotonic dehydration the fluid deficit is replaced by isotonic fluids; in isotonic dehydration by isotonic fluids, while hypertonic dehydration presents greater difficulties and has to be assessed carefully. Initially fluid replacement should be by increasing the blood volume with plasma, blood or normal saline, 20 ml/kg over 1 to 2 hours. Since the sodium loss is less than in other forms of dehydration, fluid replacement should be by hypotonic solutions, e.g. N/5 or N/2 saline. But in gastroenteritis where there will also be sodium loss due to vomiting and diarrhoea, replacement is with 0.3 per cent NaCl and 4.3 per cent dextrose. Replacement should not be too rapid since it may lead to rapid swelling of the brain tissue and convulsions as water re-enters the depleted cells.

Maintenance of fluid is also important when preparing the neonate for surgery. Full assessment and laboratory investigation are necessary so that the best possible conditions prevail. The treatment required will therefore depend on the infant's need, e.g. replacement or maintenance.

Method of fluid administration
This will depend on the condition of the child, and the type of fluid and electrolyte imbalance.

Oral. This method is used where the infant or child is able to take oral fluids, does not vomit and has mild diarrhoea.

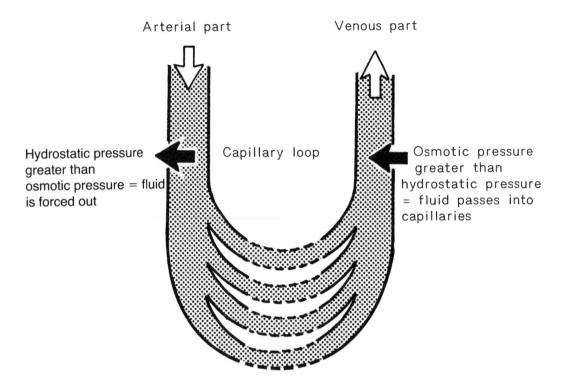

Fig. 12.7 Regulation of passage of water from the capillaries to the tissue spaces.

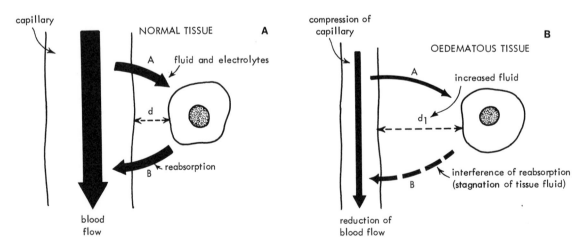

Fig. 12.8 A, Normal tissue. B, changes due to accumulation of fluid (oedema). (d = the distance between the capillary and the cell; d_1 = the increased distance.

Parenteral. Intravenous fluid is the choice when vomiting is a feature and when fluid and electrolytes are rapidly lost by diarrhoea.

Subcutaneous. This method is useful, but only small amounts can be given over a relatively short period (see Cardiovascular system).

Oedema

There is a constant exchange of fluid and crystalloids across the capillary membrane which separates the intravascular compartments. Fluid moves out at the arterial end and back in again at the venous end. The intravascular pressure at the arterial end of a capillary is approximately 30 mmHg. This is greater than the osmotic (oncotic) pressure of the plasma proteins which is approximately 25 mmHg. Therefore fluid is forced out into the interstitial fluid compartment (Fig. 12.7).

At the venous end of the capillary, the intravascular pressure is only about 10 mmHg, while the oncotic (protein) pressure is 25 mmHg, i.e. the same as at the arterial end. Interstitial fluid is able to return to the intravascular compartment leaving only a small amount of fluid to be carried away by the lymphatics.

Oedema occurs under the following conditions:

1. When the intravascular pressure is raised, e.g. heart failure.
2. When the plasma protein concentration is reduced, e.g. nephrotic syndrome.
3. When lymphatic drainage is impeded.
4. When there is increased permeability due to inflammation or allergy.

Oedema is said to occur when the interstitial fluid volume is expanded by more than about 10 per cent of its normal size (Figs. 12.8 and 12.9).

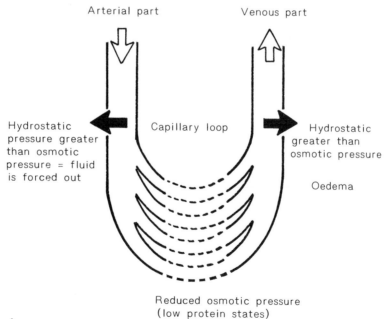

Fig. 12.9 Formation of oedema.

Chapter 13
Micro-biology and the process of disease

GENERAL PATHOLOGY

Pathology is the study of disease, i.e. the inadequate adaptation to changes in the external and internal environment. It is not a single entity but comprises a variety of mechanisms which produce changes in structure and function. Many of the changes are not beneficial and trigger off other processes leading to disease. It is possible to classify pathological change into four broad categories, i.e. inflammation, degeneration, neoplasia and congenital or inherited disease.

HYPERSENSITIVITY

Hypersensitivity or allergy can be defined as any immunological reaction which produces tissue damage in the reacting individual. Diseases due to hypersensitivity take a number of forms and four main categories or types have been identified. Type I accounts for asthma, eczema, urticaria and anaphylaxis (a generalised reaction). These reactions are due to IgE which has the special property of binding cell surfaces, especially mast cells. These cells are found in large numbers in the vicinity of blood vessels. By their action the blood vessels become leaky, causing inflammation (p. 235) in the skin, nose or conjunctivae. They contain chemical substances such as histamine and serotonin which, when released, cause contraction of smooth muscle cells, e.g. in bronchial walls where the bronchi become narrowed, causing asthma. These are local effects. If the antigen is introduced into the circulation, e.g. by injection of anti-tetanus antitoxin, then there may be general circulatory collapse and death. This is termed anaphylaxis or anaphylactic shock.

In Type II hypersensitivity the antigens are an integral part of the surface of the host cells. They are considered to be cytolytic or cytotoxic. Type II reactions involve the combination of antibody with the antigen at the cell surface and usually the fixation and activation of complement. The cells most commonly involved are the red blood corpuscles and platelets. When red cells are involved a haemolytic anaemia results, e.g. haemolytic disease of the newborn. When platelets are involved, as in certain drug sensitivities, bleeding or purpura results. This is because most of the body's platelets may be destroyed. The antibody concerned in Type II reactions is usually IgG and sometimes IgM.

Type III, known as the toxic immune complex, forms in the circulation or on vascular basement membranes composed of antigen, immunoglobin IgG or IgM and complement. An example where this mechanism is active is in serum sickness, following an injection of serum containing antitoxin to diphtheria or tetanus.

Type IV reactions develop readily in response to micro-biological antigens, notably tubercle bacilli. As a result delayed hypersensitivity plays an important part in tissue destruction as seen in tuberculosis. There are other bacteria and viruses which have similar effects. Drugs and chemicals may also cause hypersensitivity in the skin. The mechanism is different and not clearly understood, but the basis is a reaction between the antigen and circulating T cell lymphocytes, which have been previously sensitised to the antigen involved. Destruction of tissue is due to lysosomal enzymes released from the macrophages injured by the reaction.

There are other types of hypersensitivity, one of which is important in auto-immune disease. In this case, IgG or IgM antibodies are formed to some of the body's own secretions, e.g. intrinsic factor, combine with them and neutralise their biological activity, thereby causing diseases such as pernicious anaemia.

Hypersensitivity plays an important role in rejection of organ and tissue transplants. Skin may be grafted from one part of an individual's body to another part of his body and there will be no rejection. This is frequently done in cases of burns. Skin grafted from one individual to another will die and be rejected. The same applies to organ transplants. This failure to accept foreign tissue and organs is due to the recipient's body recognising the grafted tissue as foreign and attacking it, as it will attack invading bacteria. This is now believed to be due to a specific cell-mediated immunity similar to Type IV hypersensitivity. The cells involved are T cells which respond to the foreign tissue by becoming sensitised. They return to the graft site and react again with the antigenic foreign transplant and release lymphokines which attract, immobilise and damage even larger numbers of macrophages thereby leading to graft rejection.

Inflammation

Inflammation is the reaction to injury of the living microcirculation and its contents. The microcirculation consists of arterioles, venules, capillaries and lymphatics with their fluid and cellular blood constituents. This reaction can be due to bacterial invasion, heat, cold, irritant chemicals and trauma. It can be acute or chronic.

Changes in acute inflammation

Immediately after entry of the irritant stimulus there is brief *constriction* of arterioles followed by their prolonged *dilatation*. This leads to flushing of the capillary network with blood and the opening up of dormant capillary channels. There is also dilatation of venules and lymphatics.

Blood flow is *increased* and may remain so or may become sluggish. The white blood cells leave the centre of the stream and move to the periphery. They then form a layer against the inner surface of the cells which line the lumen of the blood vessels. This is known as margination and is a preparation for the leucocytes to migrate through the vessel wall into the adjacent tissue.

There are also changes in the walls of the venules and capillaries. While normally these vessels are permeable to water and small solutes, and only slightly permeable to plasma protein, in inflammation the wall of these vessels loses its impermeability to plasma protein. They pour out through the wall into the tissues. This causes swelling of the tissues known as oedema. The protein which collects outside the vessels will be removed via the lymphatic system. The protein which consists of immunoglobulin and complement provides useful functions such as accelerating the destruction of bacteria lying in the vicinity and taking part, while the fibrinogen is converted to insoluble fibrin, in blood coagulation. Red cells and platelets also leave the vessel together with the leucocytes.

Suppuration

Suppuration occurs as in intermediate stage. The leucocytes are killed by the bacteria present and their bodies are lignefied by their own lysosomal enzymes to form a creamy viscous fluid known as pus. This mass of bacteria, dead, dying and lignefied leucocytes and the remaining inflamed tissue is termed an *abscess*.

Pain

The pain is partly due to pressure on sensory nerve endings by the exuded fluid, especially if the space in which it can expand is limited, and partly due to the release of substances which stimulate these nerves. A number of substances identified include histamin, serotonin, kinins and prostaglandins.

Healing and repair

Any tissue that has survived destruction will heal and repair itself. When a wound occurs there is rupture of blood vessels with escape of blood. Normally bleeding stops fairly quickly but the wounded tissues fill up with partially solidified blood before haemostasis is complete. The wound and the presence of blood produce inflammatory changes in the adjacent intact blood vessels with the migration of leucocytes into the wound area. Many cells will be present, some of which are capable of phagocytic action. It is the presence of macrophages which makes wound healing possible. New blood vessels appear which grow into the wounded area and provide the essential blood supply. Gradually these fine vessels differentiate into arterioles and venules which also acquire a vasomotor nerve supply. Other tissue and lymphatic circulation become re-established by a similar process.

New connective tissue is produced by the action of fibroblasts. The connective tissue becomes progressively denser and the zone of new dense connective tissue is commonly known as a scar. The fibroblasts have the property of contractility. The ability of skin wounds to contract in size is now attributed to the myo-fibroblasts. As the cells contract they pull on the margins of the wound, thereby reducing the size of the wound.

A wound is said to heal quicker if the edges are in close apposition. This is often called primary union. Secondary union means that the healing of a wound takes longer because a substantial tissue defect has to be filled in gradually and is replaced by new connective tissue.

The new tissue looks granular and is known as granulation tissue.

Factors influencing wound healing

Wound healing is generally an efficient process. There are, however, factors which can interfere with any stage of healing. The commonest cause is persistent active inflammation due to bacterial invasion. This provides exudate faster than the macrophages can remove it, or there may be interference by blocking the phagocytic receptor sites on the surface of the macrophages with immuno-globulin plus bacterial antigen.

A reasonably good blood supply is essential for wound healing to supply oxygen and nutrients for energy. New blood vessels must reach the wound from a patent adjacent microcirculation.

Excess movement of the damaged wound edges will also slow the healing and remodelling process. It is, therefore, desirable that there should be limited movement. To encourage synthesis of collagen, vitamin C is necessary. Lack of vitamin C prevents the hydroxylation of proline and thereby makes it impossible to synthesise mature cross-linked collagen. Dietary intake should be satisfactory and trace elements such as zinc may be required in high amounts for optimal healing.

Micro-biology

The study of micro-biology has significant impli-

cations for the nurse because of its close links with *infection*, and in this chapter the particular hazards of hospital infection are examined, but before turning our attention to the hospital, a few basic principles must be established.

Infection

Infection can be defined simply as the adverse effects produced in or on tissue (plant, animal or human) by the invasion and multiplication of micro-organisms.

There are many different types of micro-organisms (microbes) which produce many varying effects. However, not all produce disease and indeed many play an important part in life processes. For example, nitrogen-fixing bacteria of the soil, or the conversion of nitrogenous substances into nitrates (the form in which plants absorb nitrogen) are produced by bacteria, and other bacteria play an important part in processes such as the production of cheese.

Microbes which cause disease are said to be *pathogenic*; those which live on the host but do not cause any ill health are called *commensals*. The latter are believed to have a positive function in that they prevent other microbes from harming the host. Some commensals such as *Staphylococcus pyrogenes* which live in the nose and on the skin, or the *Streptococcus viridans* which live in the mouth and throat, are potentially pathogenic. If the person's (host's) resistance to infection becomes lowered, they may produce disease.

Classification of micro-organisms

Microbes are small objects which can only be seen by the use of microscopes. They are of varying size. The largest is about 1/100 mm (10μm) in length. The smallest is about 0.01 μm.

There are three important groups of disease-producing micro-organisms: bacteria, viruses and fungi.

Bacteria

Bacteria are the largest of the microbes. Three fundamental forms are recognised (Fig. 13.1):

1. Cocci (spheroidal forms).

2. Bacilli (straight rods).
3. Spirilla (spirochaetes) (curved rods).

1. Cocci
a. Staphylococci which grow in culture as clusters looking like bunches of grapes.
b. Streptococci, which form long or short chains.
c. Diplococci (neisseria) which appear as pairs of kidney-shaped bodies.
d. Pneumococci which also appear in pairs.

2. Bacilli
These may be regular and rectangular or irregular and beaded. Examples are: *Escherichia coli* (*E. coli*), anthrax bacillus, diphtheria bacillus.

3. Spirochaetes
These are long slender organisms which are spirally coiled. Examples are the treponema of syphilis and the leptospira of Weil's disease.

Actinomycetes
These are short rod-like structures which may join to become long branching filaments. They are anaerobes causing chronic inflammation in man.

Viruses
These vary greatly in size and shape. Some are round, very irregular, tadpole-like or filamentous. The largest viruses appear to be similar to the smallest bacteria. The smallest ones have a simpler structure and are made up of little more then a few molecules of nucleo-protein, the fundamental substance that makes up living matter. Viruses are classified according to their affinities for different tissues in the body. They can only reproduce within living cells.

Neurotropic viruses attack and destroy nerve cells. e.g. poliomyelitis and rabies; pantropic viruses attack all cells of the body, e.g. yellow fever; viscerotropic viruses attack the abdominal viscera, especially the liver.

Pathogenic fungi
Like other fungi they consist largely of rounded bodies called *spores* and filamentous threads called *hyphae*, which are matted together to form a myselium.

The study of the behaviour of bacteria — one type of microbe — should help the nurse to understand the effects of microbial invasion.

Multiplication of bacteria
Bacteria multiply by cell division. Different types of bacteria have different methods of reproducing themselves. In the laboratory, a large number of different media are used to grow bacteria; the selection of each medium will depend on the suitability for growth on the particular bacterium.

The rate at which bacteria multiply depends on the availability of food supply, the removal of waste products and adequate ventilation. The growth cycle of bacteria indicates that there is a definite pattern.

When the bacteria enter a host they have to adjust to the new environment and then start to multiply. If the infection is overwhelming, this phase continues until the patient dies. In most instances, however, the body defences of the host slow down the rate of multiplication and eventually stop it completely.

Some types of bacteria are capable of developing *spores*. This allows them to remain in a state of suspended animation if conditions for multiplication are unfavourable. When conditions become favourable again, they change into the ordinary vegetative forms. The chief spore-bearing bacteria include some of the most dangerous pathogens, for example, the bacteria of gas gangrene, tetanus and anthrax (Fig. 13.2).

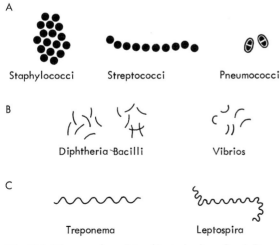

Fig. 13.1 Diagram of a variety of bacteria. A, = Cocci. B, = Bacilli. C, = Spirochaetes.

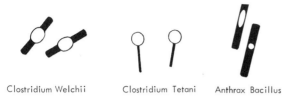

Clostridium Welchii   Clostridium Tetani   Anthrax Bacillus

Fig. 13.2 Diagram of a variety of spores.

Identification of bacteria

Before identification can take place, it is essential to prevent contamination with extraneous organisms. The equipment and method used are specialised. Identification involves cultivation of bacteria using a medium suitable for that particular bacteria, daily examination of incubated plates and further isolation on plates.

Bacteria take appropriate dyes with avidity. The behaviour towards a staining method sometimes supplies the means of identification. The commonest staining is Gram's method, in which the magnesium ribonucleate present in some bacteria is stained a deep purple with a mixture of violet dye and iodine. This purple stain cannot be readily washed out with alcohol. Bacteria which stain in this way are called Gram-positive. Other bacteria do not retain the purple dye, and are stained pink. These are called Gram-negative.

Examples of Gram-positive bacteria are: staphylococci, streptococci, diphtheria bacillus, gas gangrene bacillus. Examples of Gram-negative bacteria are: *Escherichia coli*, proteus, typhoid bacillus.

Other tests may have to be used to confirm the identity of the bacteria. The colityphoid-dysentery group, for example, are all Gram-negative bacilli and look alike under the microscope. They do differ, however, in the way they ferment sugars and whether or not they produce gas during the fermentation process.

Serological tests are also used to identify bacteria. Antisera are used against various bacteria which may have an effect on specific bacteria, for example, agglutination or clumping. A more complicated serological test is used to identify viruses. This is called the *complement fixation test*.

In most tests a microscope is used although there are limits to its power. With the use of the electron microscope, it is possible to obtain photo-

graphs of objects from 1 to 10 nm (0.001 to 0.01 μm) in diameter.

Infection and immunity

When defining infection it was stated that it implies the invasion and multiplication of microorganisms in or on tissue, either animal, plant or human. Microbes are found in all environments in which they can possibly exist, a fact worth bearing in mind by the nurse.

Modes of spread of infection

The principal ways in which infection is spread are:

1. *Respiratory tract.* The microbes are inspired. They are present in droplets of saliva given off by an infected person, i.e. a carrier, by coughing, sneezing or even talking, or from infected dust.

Droplets vary in size. The larger droplets tend to fall to the ground while the smaller droplets rise, the fluid evaporates and the particles become lighter. They are then wafted long distances in air currents. However, the greatest danger is to those nearest to the infected person. Examples of diseases spread by droplet infection are pneumonia, tonsillitis, diphtheria, meningococcal meningitis, etc. Virus infections include colds, influenza, measles, etc.

Bacteria of any kind can be carried in the air in dust particles. Dust lands on the surface of human beings or is inhaled.

2. *Intestinal tract.* The organisms are swallowed with food, water, or dust. Food and water are contaminated when hygiene is poor, i.e. an infected person handles food or food is left uncovered and flies or dust contaminate it. Infections which are spread in this way include the salmonella infection, i.e. typhoid and paratyphoid, dysentery.

3. *The skin and mucous membrane.* The skin is the body's natural barrier to infection. This barrier is only effective if the skin is unbroken; once damage which involves a break in the skin occurs, bacteria have easy access. Any type of wound either surgically produced or accidentally produced

can become infected. Microbes are normally present on skin (commensals) but do not cause any harm. However, when they enter the underlying tissue changes take place which will interfere with the normal function of that tissue.

Animals and insects can also transmit microbes. Some use the paths mentioned, for example, milk from infected cattle can transmit tuberculosis, brucellosis and streptococcal infection to humans via the alimentary tract. Rats can infect man, either by biting or scratching or through the rat flea. Diseases which are transmitted in this way are typhus fever, plague and Weil's disease (infectious jaundice). Cats, dogs, monkeys, tortoises and birds have been recognised as carriers of disease to man. Some of the diseases are transmitted via the respiratory tracts (viral pneumonia, rabies) others via the skin (rabies). Mosquitoes, among other insects, transmit pathogenic microbes to man (viruses which cause encephalitis) and a protozoan bacteria, causing malaria.

Infection can also occur to or via any part of the body which has an external pathway. Two have already been discussed, the respiratory and alimentary tracts, but the genito-urinary tract can also be involved. This is of particular importance where these areas are subjected to nursing interference, such as catheterisation or vaginal douching.

Effect of infection

The effect on the person infected with a pathogenic micro-organism depends on factors such as:

1. The ability of the body to protect itself against the invading microbes.
2. The activity or pathogenicity of the micro-organism.

1. THE BODY'S PROTECTION
The healthy individual is able to protect himself from potentially harmful micro-organisms by a number of very effective mechanisms. These are present from birth and do not depend upon having previous experience of any particular micro-organism. Together they form the *innate immune mechanism*. It is effective against a wide range of

potentially infective agents and, therefore non-specific. It seems to be genetically controlled, varying with the different species (animal and human), but there is little variation between individuals.

Acquired immunity, on the other hand, is not necessarily present from birth but depends upon the development of an immune response to individual micro-organisms and is specific only for the inducing organism.

A. Innate immune mechanism
Listed below are some of the factors contributing to this mechanism:

1. *Heredity*. This has been demonstarted by studies on tuberculosis infection in twins. If one homozygous twin develops tuberculosis, the other twin has a 3:1 chance of developing the disease; for heterozygous twins the chances are 1:3. Another example of genetic control is where the individual has a hereditary abnormality of the red blood cells (sickle-cell) which are less readily parasitised by *Plasmodium falciparum* thus conferring immunity to malaria.

2. *The age of the individual*. Infectious diseases are more severe at the extremes of life. In the young this appears to be associated with immaturity of the immunological mechanisms affecting the ability of the lymphoid system to deal with, and react to, foreign antigens. The elderly are more susceptible to infection because of failing body functions.

3. *Nutritional factors*. Poor nutrition is recognised as having adverse effects on susceptibility to infection, at least where bacterial infections are involved. In the case of viruses, however, malnutrition appears to interfere with proliferation of the agent (since these depend on the normal metabolic function of the host cells). Animal experiments have shown that undernourished animals were less susceptible to a variety of viruses. However, poor diet is also often associated with poor environmental conditions and increased incidence of infection often correlates with poor sanitary conditions.

4. *Hormonal influences*. Deficiency of insulin, thyroxin (thyroid) and adrenal dysfunction are associated with decreased resistance to infection. The relationship is not quite clear, but it is known that the glucocorticoids are anti-inflammatory

agents which decrease the ability of phagocytes to digest ingested material (they are immuno-suppressive).

5. *The intact skin and mucous membrane.* The outer horny layer of the skin and the cilia of respiratory mucous membrane provide mechanical barriers. The secretions of the skin are anti-fungal and antibacterial, while the moist secretions of the mucous membrane are bactericidal and viricidal However, certain areas of the body such as the soles of the feet, are deficient in sebaceous glands which is believed to be a cause of susceptibility to fungal infection (athlete's foot). Micro-organisms which are swallowed are destroyed by the acid gastric juices.

6. *Bactericidal substances of the tissues and body fluids.* These are the lysozymes which are found in high concentration in leucocytes as well as in most tissue fluids except cerebrospinal fluid, sweat and urine. They act as a mucolytic enzyme acting on the cell wall of many Gram-positive bacteria and killing them. There are also a variety of basic proteins which are capable of killing bacteria.

7. *Phagocytosis.* This is the ability of phagocytic cells to engulf micro-organisms or inert particles which enter the tissue fluids or bloodstream. Phagocytic cells contain digestive enzymes which degrade ingested material.

8. *Temperature.* Many micro-organisms are temperature-dependent. For example, the tubercle bacillus which is pathogenic for mammalian species, will not infect cold-blooded animals. Pyrexia follows many different types of infection and it is believed to be a protective response to the infecting micro-organisms.

The complement system

This is an extremely complex group of serum proteins present in low concentration in normal serum. It has the ability to lyse red blood cells and destroy Gram-negative bacteria. Complement action is of some considerable importance because of its ability to neutralise various types of cells after they have interacted with antibodies. Complement appears to render bacteria susceptible to lysozyme and it is also involved in the attraction of phagocytes to sites of antigen-antibody interaction.

Complement fixation tests are applied in diagnosing bacterial and viral infections.

The immunoglobulins

Immunologists distinguish five main classes of immunoglobulins referred to as IgG, IgM, IgA, IgE and IgD. Each has a different structure and properties.

Immunoglobulin G or IgG is the major one and is concerned with complement activation and agglutination; IgM is believed to play an important role in protection against micro-organism.

The new-born baby leaves a protective environment where the immunoglobulins have been transmitted from the mother. These antibodies provide the baby with a passive immunity which tides him over the period until his own immunological system begins to mature. The transference involves the gamma chain of the IgG. In some infants, however, this transference is absent and they suffer from agammaglobulinaemia. These children cannot make antibodies, they suffer from progressive bacterial or viral infection and may die within 2 years of birth.

B. Acquired immunity

Micro-organisms which are able to circumvent the innate non-specific immune mechanisms come up against the host's second line of defence. This form of immunity depends on the effect produced by *antigens* of the invading micro-organisms.

Antigens

Antigens are substances of various chemical types capable of stimulating the immune system of the host animal or human, to produce a response specifically directed at the causative substance only.

The antigens of the invading micro-organisms come in contact with cells of the host (macrophages and lymphocytes) which leads to the initiation of an immune response. The response can be in two forms:

1. *Humoral response.* In this form, immunoglobulins or antibodies appear in the blood and combine with the antigen. The result may be:

   a. Clumping together of the antigen molecules.

b. Neutralisation of their toxicity.

c. Facilitation of uptake and digestion by phagocytes.

2. *Cell-mediated immunity*. Lymphoid cells which have already been exposed to antigen react with the causative antigen by producing a cytotoxic effect on foreign cells. This is of particular importance when a tissue has been grafted.

An acquired immune state may be brought about in an individual in two main ways:

1. Induced by apparent clinical infection or by deliberate artificial immunisation. This is termed *actively acquired immunity*. Some may induce a lifetime immunity, e.g. diphtheria, smallpox, whooping cough and mumps; others confer immunity for only a short time, e.g. common cold, influenza, bacillary dysentery. One reason, among others, for the short-term immunity is the fact that different strains of the same species may be involved and the acquisition of immunity to one strain does not prevent infection by another strain of the same organism.

2. *Passively acquired immunity* is an immunity transferred from an actively immunised individual to a non-immunised individual. Administration of immune sera usually prepared in another species, e.g. the horse, is a therapeutic procedure in diphtheria and in gas gangrene. Passive immunity may also be conferred on the infant by the passage of maternal antibodies across the placenta. Pooled human immunoglobulin is also used as a source of antibodies in a number of situations including measles and infectious hepatitis.

2. PATHOGENICITY OF THE MICRO-ORGANISMS

As already noted the effects of infection are dependent not only on the host but also on the pathogenicity of the micro-organisms. Pathogenicity can be measured in a number of ways:

1. *Infectivity*, i.e. the capacity of the micro-organism to spread from one individual to another.

2. *Toxigenicity*, i.e. the capacity of the micro-organism to produce toxins which damage the tissues of the host. The virulence of bacteria is proportional to their toxin production.

3. *The capacity to invade the tissues of the host, to multiply and spread within them.* Organisms vary in their power to invade tissues, e.g. anthrax bacillus invades the bloodstream rapidly, while the diphtheria bacillus scarcely penetrates the superficial tissue.

Immunisation

The control of infectious diseases — which were both killing and crippling — is mainly due to the immunisation of children.

Immunity may be defined as the power to resist the effects of disease-producing organisms. In the new-born infant immunity transferred from the mother in utero provides resistance to infection for a limited period. The breast-fed baby is further protected by the antibodies received via breast milk. But since the infant and young child's immunological system is still immature, he is more prone to suffer infectious diseases than older children. The body is nevertheless capable of fighting some infection, for example gastric juice will destroy most swallowed bacteria and nasal secretions are also effective against inspired bacteria.

Immunity may also be obtained from an attack of an infectious disease, though not all diseases confer immunity to further attacks, for example the common cold. Immunity is achieved when a person manufactures antibodies; the immunity so obtained may be effective for many years and in some cases for a lifetime. Immunity to a specific disease can also be obtained by the injection of the organism in various forms (see p. 242). Immunisation of children is not compulsory but parents are advised to have their children protected. The majority of children suffer little or no side-effects. However, there is some risk, for example from smallpox and pertussis vaccinations. For this reason, the Department of Health has issued guidelines regarding the methods to be used and the precautions to be taken before the various prophylactics are given. For example, a child with a history of asthma, eczema or convulsions may not be given some of the prophylactics, i.e.

Table 13.1 Vaccination and immunisation schedule

Age	Immunisation
From 3 months	Diphtheria Whooping cough Tetanus Poliomyelitis
5–6 months	Diphtheria Whooping cough Tetanus Poliomyelitis
9–11 months	Diphtheria Whooping cough Tetanus Poliomyelitis
12–24 months	Measles
About 5 years	Diphtheria (booster) Tetanus (booster) Poliomyelitis (booster)
10–14 years (girls only)	Rubella (German measles)
Girls and boys at about 13 years	Tuberculosis
15–19 years (leaving school)	Tetanus Poliomyelitis

pertussis vaccine. It is also recommended that children under 1 year of age should not be given smallpox vaccination. Table 13.1 shows a vaccination schedule, which may vary with different health authorities.

Infectious diseases

Although there has been a decrease in the incidence of infectious diseases, it would be wrong to assume that they have been totally eradicated. A report of the National Child Development Study, sponsored by the National Children's Bureau, shows that the number of children vaccinated and immunised varies with the social class of the family. This means that there are a large number of children who have not been protected and who are therefore at risk.

It is also important to recognise that with greater possibility of travel to other countries, there will be greater opportunity for contact with more exotic diseases, such as typhoid, which are of an infective nature.

Many infectious diseases present with features indicating upper respiratory, digestive and/or cerebral disorders, which may also be found in non-infectious diseases. Infectious diseases are specific in that the spread of infection is often of epidemic proportions; they may affect children and they have distinguishing features, e.g. rash. Table 13.2 shows the various types of infectious diseases, their incubation, quarantine and isolation periods and the relevant features of each.

TUBERCULOSIS

Although tuberculosis has shown a continuing decline in the UK, it still causes more deaths than any other notifiable disease. Children under 3 years of age are most susceptible, and lymphohaematogenous dissemination through the lungs often spreads to extrapulmonary sites, including the brain and meninges, eyes, bones and joints, lymph nodes, kidneys, intestines, larynx and skin. Increased susceptibility occurs again in adolescence, particularly in girls within 2 years of menarche.

Aetiology

The causative organism is the mycobacterium tuberculosis which is an acid-fast, non-motile rod. The organisms are sensitive to isoniazid and produce niacin and the enzyme catalase. Mycobacterium bovis now rarely causes tuberculosis in the UK. It is also sensitive to isoniazid, but does not produce niacin.

Spread of infection

Infants
Infants may acquire tuberculosis by:

1. Transplacental spread through the umbilical vein to the fetal liver,
2. Aspiration or ingestion of infected amniotic fluid,
3. Postnatal exposure to active tuberculosis in a close contact.

Children
Prolonged close contact with an active adult case usually leads to infection. The organism is inhaled through droplet infection, though the organism

Table 13.2 Infectious diseases

Disease	Incubation	Features	Quarantine	Isolation of infected children	Specific treatment
Chickenpox (varicella)	7–21 days	Macules at first on trunk later on face and extremities. Progress from macules to papules and vesicles. All three stages are present simultaneously	23 days	Until 1 week after the appearance of the rash	Calamine lotion, sedation
Diphtheria	1–6 days	Pharyngeal angina and toxaemia. Demonstration of presence of Klebs-Loeffler bacillus. Toxic neuritis	Until throat and nose swabs are negative	Until throat and nose swabs are negative on two consecutive occasions	Antitoxin — tracheostomy and respirator
Measles (morbilli)	7–14 days	Coryza, cough, conjunctivitis, photophobia, Koplick's spots. Maculo-papular rash on forehead, face, and spreading over trunk and limbs. Rash fades when the temperature subsides	16 days	Not less than 5 days from the date of the appearance of the rash	Rest; antibiotics for secondary infection
German measles (Rubella)	14–19 days	Fine pinkish macules on face, neck and spreading to trunk and limbs. Occipital lymph glands enlarged; fades in 24 hours	21 days	Until the rash disappears	No specific treatment
Scarlet fever	2–5 days	Diffuse, pinkish-red flush of the skin, with punctate 'gooseflesh' feel. Seen on face, neck, chest and abdomen. Whole body surface may be affected. Tongue whitish, then red and raw	—	During treatment (10 days) and until throat swabs are negative	Penicillin if severe
Poliomyelitis	5–21 days	Headache, sore throat, paralysis, stiff neck and back, weakness of various muscles	21–28 days	Minimum of 3 weeks	Rest; respirator (if required) (p. 395, 310)
Mumps	14–28 days	Pain chewing or swallowing, swelling of glands in the area in front of and below the ear	30 days	Not less than 2 weeks from the onset, provided that one clear week has elapsed since subsidence of the swelling	Rest, sedation
Whooping cough	7–14 days to catarrhal stage; a further 7–14 days to paroxysmal stage	Sneezing, lacrimation, coryza, troublesome cough at night which becomes paroxysmal producing a 'whoop'	21 days	Until the whoop has ceased for at least 2 weeks, may be longer	Sedation, ampicillin

Cont'd on page 244

Table 13.2 (*cont'd*)

Disease	Incubation	Features	Quarantine	Isolation of infected children	Specific treatment
Smallpox	10–17 days	Signs similar to influenza, appearance of pinkish lesions of macules 1–2 mm in dia. on the forehead temples, about the mouth spreading to the rest of the body. These increase in size, containing clear serum	About 18 days	Until all the scabs have fallen off and the lesions have healed	Symptomatic Broad-spectrum antibiotics against secondary infection
Enteric group	3–23 days	Gastroenteritis, blood and mucus in stools	23 days	Until stools are negative (3)	See p. 486
Infectious hepatitis	15–40 days	Severe headache, nausea vomiting, muscle pain, jaundice	42 days	7 days minimum	See p. 504

can survive in a dry state in dust. The bovine type is transmitted via unboiled or unpasteurised milk obtained from infected cows.

Pathogenesis
The primary complex in infancy and childhood consists of a small parenchymal lesion in any area of the lung with caseation of regional nodes and calcification. Post-primary tuberculosis in adolescents occurs in the apices of the lungs and is likely to cause chronic, progressive cavitary pulmonary disease with less tendency for haematogenous dissemination.

The primary lesions may heal or extend and undergo caseation. When an infection occurs a hypersensitive state develops. Hypersensitive syndromes include phlyctenular conjunctivitis (a brisk ocular inflammatory reaction to locally deposited tubercle bacilli), in which lacrimation and photophobia occur if ulceration is present; and erythema which consists of tender, mauve nodules on the front of the shins and sometimes on the exterior aspects of the forearm, disappearing in about 2 weeks.

Clinical features

New-born infant
The clinical signs of the new-born infant with tuberculosis are non-specific, but multiple organ involvement is usually present. The infant may look ill, with fever, lethargy, respiratory distress and failure to thrive.

Children
Pulmonary involvement is indicated by a brassy, non-productive cough or in young children, atelectasis distal to bronchial compression.

Meningitis may be suspected if there is vomiting, headache, lethargy, irritability, cranial nerve palsy, convulsions and coma.

Investigations
1. Skin tests, e.g. Mantoux or Heaf test.
   Mantoux test interpretation:
   Negative — no induration.
   Doubtful — 5 mm or less.
   Positive — 15 mm or more induration.

   Heaf test interpretation:
   Negative — no induration or erythema.
   Positive
   Grade I   — easily palpable papules around at least four puncture points.
   Grade II — coalescence of indurated papules to form a ring of induration.
   Grade III — 5 to 10 mm weal of induration.
   Grade IV — greater than 10 mm and a blister or central haemorrhage.
2. X-ray of chest.
3. Gastric washings on 3 consecutive days.
4. Lumbar puncture.
5. Examination of urine.

Prevention

1. Pregnant women with active tuberculosis can be treated with a combination of isoniazid and ethambutol. There is no evidence that these drugs are teratogenic to the human fetus. Rifampin (also known as Rifampicin) can also be given. However, streptomycin is potentially ototoxic to the developing fetus and should not be given unless rifampin is contra-indicated.
2. If the infant is asymptomatic, he should be separated from the mother until she is under effective treatment and her sputum is negative. Frequent skin testing of the baby is necessary and he can be given isoniazid. On the other hand the infant can be given BCG (Bacille Calmette-Guerin) vaccine within the first week of life.
3. Source contact should be identified, isolated and treated.
4. Good housing, good nutrition and good social circumstances.
5. X-rays of employees (i.e. nursing, medical and other staff) working with children.
6. Screening of schoolchildren.

Principles of treatment and nursing management
Treatment depends on the age of the child, duration of infection and general condition.

1. Hospitalisation is not necessary in all cases. Treatment can be given as an outpatient. However, if the child is ill and has signs of meningitis, then hospitalisation will be necessary.
2. When associated with bronchopneumonia, emphysema and collapse of segment, the treatment and nursing care is related to these conditions plus chemotherapy specific to tuberculosis.
3. Medication: isoniazid 10 to 20 mg/kg/d Para-amino-salicylic acid (PAS) 300 mg/kg/d or ethambutol 20 mg/kg/d.
4. Medication for tuberculous meningitis: streptomycin 20 to 30 mg/kg/d in addition to INAS and PAS. Rifampin has higher bactericidal activity but it is toxic to the liver. Corticosteroids may be used for suppressing inflammatory reactions in meningeal, pleural and pericardial tuberculosis.

5. Bed-rest is only indicated while the child feels ill.
6. Isolation of children is only necessary for children with draining lesions or renal disease, and those with chronic pulmonary tuberculosis. Most children are non-infectious and can attend school while being treated.
7. Normal nutrition for the age of the child.

Hospital-associated infection

An understanding of the importance of bacteriology in nursing is essential in order to recognise the dangers which are inherent in any activity within the hospital. The nurse has the greatest contact with the child and therefore has the greatest opportunity to infect the child, either directly or indirectly. By the same token she has also the greatest opportunity to prevent infection, where possible.

SOURCES AND PATHS OF INFECTION
Infections occurring within the hospital present special problems. Surveys have shown that about from 5 to 10 per cent of patients coming into hospital acquire some kind of infection. The infection occurring in hospital can originate from patients, staff, and visitors. The paths may be termed self-infection (endogenous), cross-infection, and infection from the environment (exogenous).

Self-infection finds its source in the patient's skin, nose, throat, mouth, intestine and infected lesions. In turn he may be a source of *cross-infection*. This may occur because of contact with nurses, doctors, visitors' hands and clothes, inadequately sterilised instruments, bedclothes and bedpans, food and some disinfectants.

Airborne transfer is another important pattern and is an example of exogenous or *environmental infection*. It can occur from the minute skin scales which are continuously shed and often carry staphylococci; from droplets of the nose and mouth containing organisms from respiratory infection; and from wound dressings containing *Staph. aureus* and nebulisers with Gram-negative bacilli. Dust from the ward itself, as well as from streets and buildings, can also transfer micro-organisms.

There are several factors which should be discussed in relation to the occurrence and effects of hospital infection.

The micro-organisms involved

Many of the factors have already been discussed in relation to the general concept of infection. There are, however, certain pathogenic organisms which are particularly associated with hospital infection. They are usually resistant to many antibiotics and flourish under conditions in which most disease-producing organisms cannot multiply. One example is aeruginosa (pyocyanea) a Gram-negative bacteria occurring in soil and water. This organism is found naturally in the alimentary tract and on the skin and occurs in suppurative conditions, urinary infections and burns.

Haemolytic streptococci are also a major problem since their effects are so serious: they are likely to cause complete failure of skin grafts if they gain access to full thickness burns.

Outbreaks of infection can occur as a result of agents of specific infectious diseases, food poisoning and errors in asepsis or sterile supply of infusion fluids or drops.

The patient

Children are particularly prone to infection, and the younger the child the greater the danger. Other factors, most of which are true for adults as well as children, are:

1. Poor general resistance either because of ill health or, in infants, because antibodies have not yet formed or are imperfectly developed.
2. Poor local resistance due to poor blood supply to tissues.
3. Surgical and nursing intervention which also allows access of bacteria to tissues which are normally protected.

Staff too are subject to infection from virulent organisms. It can occur through contamination with infected blood and exudates of patients with, for example, serum hepatitis.

The hospital environment

A wide variety of micro-organisms is likely to be found in hospital where many people, some with infections, are concentrated. Many organisms are antibiotic-resistant because the use of antibiotics has led to the suppression of sensitive bacteria.

Each area within a hospital has its own infection hazard. In the operating theatre, for example, there is the danger of wound infection since the wound is exposed for a considerable time to potential sources of infection. In the wards wound dressings, particularly those with drains, present a risk. *Neonatal wards* have a special hazard due to frequent handling of infants and the potential contamination of feeds, suction and resuscitation equipment due also to frequent handling.

The treatment of the patient

The results of infection are influenced by treatment. Correct surgical, medical and nursing procedures, including chemotherapy, can have a successful outcome, but treatment by immunosuppressive drugs or steroids can have an adverse effect.

Prevention of hospital infection

It will be seen from the above sources and paths of infection that prevention requires an understanding of the processes involved. The aim is to protect the patients against infection in hospital by means of a system of methods, including surgical asepsis and hospital hygiene, which recognises that *all* members of staff should understand the underlying principles of control of infection.

It has been suggested that some training programme should be instituted for all those involved in the work of the hospital, with refresher courses to bring the staff up to date with existing knowledge. Discussions can also be held where problems related to control of infection can be solved. The Working Party on Control of Hospital Infection (Control of Hospital Infection, 1975) further recommends the setting up of a Control of Infection Committee and the appointment of a Control of Infection Officer.

Full and up-to-date records should be kept and basic information about patients and staff should be recorded. There should also be routine monitoring of environment and equipment, involving the checking of air-flow in a ventilated area and the disinfection and sterilisation of equipment.

Application of the principles of aseptic technique and hygiene in the procedures carried out by all those involved in patient care is the essential parameter from which to start. Several important areas are considered here.

Ward lay-out

Spread of infection is most likely to occur in a large open ward. Where possible, smaller units with from four to six beds or individual rooms are more satisfactory. In a children's hospital or ward, single rooms or cubicles are ideal for infants or where reverse barrier nursing is required.

In all wards there should be adequate hand-washing facilities. Covered pails or containers should be available, particularly where there are infants, so that used or contaminated linen can be disposed of quickly. Linen disposal points should also be placed in areas where there is minimum contact with other rooms or equipment. Contaminated linen should be disposed of in closed bags in a central disposal area at the earliest possible opportunity.

Toilet arrangements

Intestinal infection is common in children and therefore extra care is necessary to achieve a high standard of cleanliness. Potties, bedpans and urinals should be disposable and the carrier made from materials which can be disinfected safely. Toilet seats should be washed frequently with a phenolic or hypochlorite solution.

Cotton napkins should be treated as contaminated and sealed in plastic or special bags, according to the policy of the hospital.

Hands

The hands of nurses, doctors, physiotherapists and others who handle patients are considered the most important vehicles of cross-infection. Hand washing should therefore be carried out conscientiously on arrival for duty, before and after aseptic procedures, and when attending to infants. Special hand-washing methods are necessary before attending patients in protective isolation, e.g. laminar flow (Fig. 13.4), and after attending a patient in barrier or source isolation. Any procedure such as bedmaking, toilet round, back treatment, temperature recording etc. should be followed by hand-washing. Most bacteria can be removed adequately by a thorough wash with soap and water but for more thorough hand-washing a liquid detergent preparation such as Hibiscrub (chlorhexidine) or Sterzas (hexachlorophane) can be used.

It should be recognised that soap containers may be a source of contamination. The containers should therefore be of a design which makes cleaning possible. Liquid dispensers must be regularly cleaned, maintained and filled.

Aseptic techniques

The term asepsis means 'free from sepsis' or 'exclusion of micro-organisms', and an aseptic technique is a method which aims at preventing micro-organisms from contaminating a wound or other susceptible site. This involves careful preparation of the equipment used in the procedure and the use of sterile materials supplied by a central sterile supply department (CSSD), where that service exists, or equipment effectively sterilised at local ward level. The technique of the procedures will vary from hospital to hospital, but the principles should be understood and obeyed within the limits of the environment. The technique should be simple and readily modified to any given situation. Any procedure which involves penetration of the skin, exposure of wounds or instrumentation should be carried out with sterile materials.

Masks

Masks are worn to protect the patient against organisms from the respiratory tract of the attendant. Most of these bacteria are dispersed on sneezing, talking or coughing although these microbes are normally not harmful to wounds. Experimental studies have shown that masks contribute little to the protection against infection of patients in wards and are therefore not worn routinely for all aseptic ward procedures. They are also not worn when attending pre-term or ill infants (although this may vary from hospital to hospital), except where the attendant is suffering from some upper respiratory infection. Whenever possible, such a person should not handle these babies.

Masks are generally worn during the dressing of

burns or of extensive open wounds, or as protection to the wearer while nursing infectious patients. Masks are of two types: (1) deflectors which should be impervious barriers preventing droplets from the wearer's mouth and nose from entering aseptic areas; (2) filter masks which gives some protection to the wearer against airborne bacteria.

Masks should be discarded after having been worn for an hour. In operating theatres, this is not practical and they should therefore be discarded at the end of a procedure. Masks should not be handled while worn and, when removed, should only be held by the tapes and disposed of immediately.

Protective clothing for staff

Many hospitals have dispensed with nurse's aprons, and for procedures such as dressings, toiletry, infant feeding and barrier nrusing, gowns are worn. The cotton gown is permeable to bacteria, and disposable plastic aprons have been recommended and are used widely. These can be disinfected with 70 per cent alcohol or swabbed with a solution of 0.5 per cent aqueous chlorhexidine. If gowns are worn a gowning technique such as the one illustrated in Figure 13.3 is useful to follow. This ensures that the two sides of the gown are not interchanged and that the outer side of the gown is not touched.

Protective clothing for parents

There is evidence that frequent and prolonged visiting by parents of their own children does not increase the infection rates. Some protection should, however, be provided for parents. This may be in the form of cotton gowns or plastic aprons. Parents will also need to be instructed in the policies regarding prevention of infection in hospital, particularly if they take an active part in the nursing of their child.

Baby baths

Where bath suites are not available, each baby

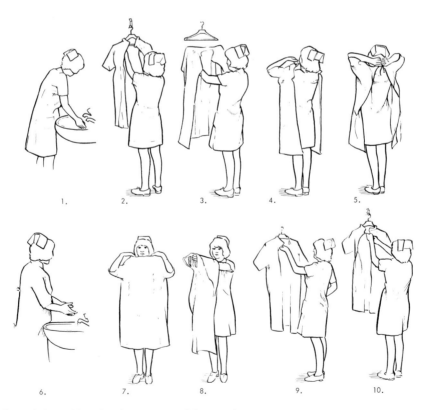

Fig. 13.3 Gowning technique. (Note that the outer part of the gown is not touched.)

should have his own bath and stand. These baths should be thoroughly washed after use with soap and hot water and dried. Traces of fluid should be removed and the bath inverted. On dismissal the bath should be disinfected before being issued to the next baby.

Linen containers

Covered linen containers should be available for each infant. Linen removed from the cot or the infant should be placed immediately into the respective containers. Some hospitals use two containers of different colours — one for used linen, the other for 'fouled' or contaminated linen. On completion of the procedure, these are taken, covered, to the disposal area. The pails should then be washed with soap and hot water or a disinfectant may be used, particularly where intestinal infections are present.

Preparation of infant feeds and milk kitchens

Milk is an excellent medium for growth of most pathogenic or potentially pathogenic organisms and contamination of feeds is a particular danger in a paediatric unit. Many organisms have been isolated from feeds, for example, salmonella, *E. coli*, β-haemolytic streptococci and many others.

Contamination of a feed can be due to poor hygiene, as well as faulty disinfection of bottles, teats, dispensing and mixing equipment. Water may be contaminated prior to use.

The initial contamination may be low but if stored at room temperature for a sufficient time, then organisms will grow and multiply. Preparation of feeds should therefore follow the same aseptic technique principles as those employed for other procedures discussed previously. These involve washing the hands, wearing a mask and gown and handling equipment which has been rendered sterile by immersion in hypochlorite. Bottles and teats should be cleaned thoroughly and all milk deposits must be removed. This is effectively done with a bottle brush. In large units, the brush is attached to a tap, the force of water and revolving brush cleaning the inside of the bottle. The teat can be treated with salt; this removes the milky layer from the inside of the teat. It is then rinsed and a jet of water is passed through the hole to remove any particle.

The equipment should then be completely immersed, for the recommended time and with air bubbles removed, in hypochlorite (125 parts chlorine per million).

Autoclaving of bottles and teats is a more reliable method. It is also possible to obtain commercially supplied pre-sterilised feeds. These bottles can be stored in a clean store room and at ward level. Before feeding the infant it is necessary to determine that the vacuum has not been broken (instructions are issued by the manufacturers). Each baby has his own teat which will fit any of these bottles. The teat is discarded every 3 to 4 days and a new pre-sterilised one issued; it is stored in hypochlorite between each feeding session.

Infant feeding routine

To ensure that the infant is not infected during feeding, it is necessary to plan a routine suited to the environment and the equipment available. The simpler the routine, the easier it will be to follow. Hand washing is an essential factor in preventing infection so that it is difficult to emphasise how often this should be done. Each situation must be assessed but the main principles should be observed, i.e. decontamination should follow any procedure in which the hands may become contaminated. With frequent washing, hands can become sore and chapped hands should be prevented. Paper towels make chapping more likely so that, whenever possible, hand cream should be applied.

The following routine has been found simple and presents few problems:

1. The pre-sterilised feed is taken to the baby's locker.
2. The nurse washes and dries her hands, puts on a gown and changes the infant's napkin. The soiled napkin is left in a closed container. The hands are washed and dried again.
3. The teat is put on the bottle and covered. The infant is fed. His napkin is changed again, if necessary, and the hands are washed and dried before removing the gown.
4. The teat is removed and cleaned and placed in Milton solution. The bottle is removed to a disposal point or if a conventional feeding

bottle is used, it is rinsed and placed in the bottle rack.

5. The soiled napkin and linen are disposed of, the containers are washed and replaced. Hands are washed and dried again, completing the routine.

Isolation of patients

The spread of infection can be controlled by isolating the patient. Two methods are used:

1. Barrier nursing or isolating the infected patient to prevent the transfer of his infection to others.
2. Reverse barrier nursing which aims at protecting a patient who is at special risk from infection.

In both methods single rooms can be used, although reverse barrier nursing can take place in plastic enclosures (laminar flow) in the open ward.

Barrier nursing

Where possible, barrier nursing should take place in a single room or cubicle. It should have a wash closet, wash-hand basin and shower, i.e. it should be self-contained. If no single rooms are available, an area near a wash-hand basin should be reserved. The bed is screened and essential equipment placed within this self-contained area. This is not a satisfactory method, particularly where infection is transferred by air, but may be used if no alternative method is available.

The following equipment will be required: pedal bins; plastic bags; individual thermometer (usually available); gowns or plastic aprons. Gowns should be changed daily or whenever soiled.

Gloves may be required for handling infected sites or contaminated materials.

Masks may be required for protection of members of staff. Equipment such as sphygmomanometer, stethoscope, bedpan carrier, etc. should be kept in the area until it is possible for terminal disinfection when the child is discharged.

Crockery and *cutlery*. Disposable items are useful, but if not available, the items should be placed in a plastic bag and washed separately. Food left-overs should be placed in polythene bags and discarded with ward waste.

Exudate. Precautions against infected exudate

such as pus and sputum are essential. This can be achieved by placing the contaminated material in sealed paper or plastic bags. 'Non-touch' technique should be used, i.e. wearing disposable gloves or using forceps.

Disposal of linen and personal clothing. Any clean linen or clothing which has been in the isolated area should be considered contaminated and should not be used for other patients. Contaminated or fouled clothing should be transferred to the hospital laundry in sealed impermeable bags. The laundry has a routine for linen contaminated by specific organisms.

Reverse barrier nursing (Fig. 13.4)

This form of isolation is used for children suffering from diseases in which there is increased susceptibility to infection. They require protection from the hospital environment. The amount of protection required varies with the type of patient. For example, children suffering from leukaemia who are treated with immunosuppressive drugs,

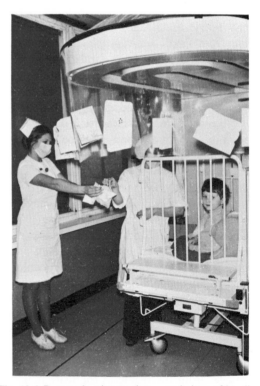

Fig. 13.4 Reverse barrier nursing — technique of handing equipment to a member of staff or parent under the laminar flow.

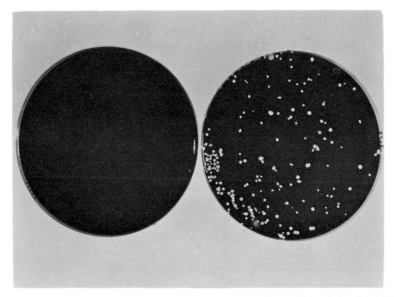

Fig. 13.5 Agar plates showing plates without bacteria (on the left) and with a colony of bacteria (on the right).

require maximum protection, including sterile food, toys and sometimes sterile linen.

Isolation area. This may be an area within the ward, where the child is isolated under a laminar flow, or in a single room.

Equipment. The child will require all his own equipment as described for barrier nursing. The difference lies in the fact that any equipment entering the isolated area is either treated chemically or by gamma rays. This includes toys, books, food and cutlery. The child's medicine glasses and plastic spoons are kept in a solution of Milton (hypochlorite). Clean linen from the laundry is usually considered satisfactory. Tins of food and

Table 13.3 Disinfectants which can be used for objects and for patients and staff

Purpose	Disinfectant	Strength
Floors, routine cleaning	Agnagel	1 in 80
Beds, lockers, cots, incubators, table tops	Savlon	1 in 100
Tents, canopies	Savlon	1 in 100
Dressing trolleys	Savlon	1 in 100
	Milton (before use)	1 in 80
Bedpan holders	Savlon	1 in 100
Combs	Soap and water, if necessary	
	Chlorhexidine	0.5% in 70% alcohol
Clinical thermometers	Chlorhexidine	0.5% in 70% alcohol
Suction and Dia-pump jars	Chlorhexidine	0.5% in water
Eating and drinking utensils (non-metal)	Milton	1 in 80
Hands	Hibiscrub	
	pHiso-Med	
	Hexachlorophane	2% bar soap
Skin preparation	Mediswab	70% alcohol
	Betadine antiseptic	
Umbilical cord	Methylated spirit	70%
	Mediswab	
Wounds	Chlorhexidine	0.5% Sterile
	Cetrimide	0.5%
	Aqueous solution — single use containers	

tubs of butter are immersed for 15 minutes before opening.

Staff and visitors. Any member of staff or visitor suffering from an infection should be excluded. All members of staff and visitors should wear a cap and mask. Hands and forearms should be washed up to the elbows and dried carefully. Gowns are worn and gloves should be worn by all who carry out procedures which involve puncturing the skin.

Monitoring of bacterial activity is essential. The air is tested for bacterial count indicating the efficiency of the ventilating system. Swabs are taken from the various areas of the child, e.g. nose, throat, skin, rectum, hair, etc. and micro-organisms identified and their sensitivity to anti-biotics obtained. Figure 13.5 shows a cultured Agar plate obtained from an air sample.

Cleaning and disinfection of equipment. Each hospital will have its own policy regarding the method and the substances to be used to disinfect equipment. Table 13.3 shows the type of substances which can be used and have been found to be satisfactory.

Chapter 14
Medical genetics

Genetics is the branch of biology concerned with heredity. It may be defined as the study of the way in which genes operate and the way in which they are transmitted from parents to offspring, while medical genetics is the study of the possible genetic factors influencing the occurrence of a pathological condition. Many cases of mental retardation, dwarfism and multiple congenital anomalies are associated with specific chromosomal defects. Many of the metabolic disorders are hereditary, and even in the case of some drug reactions the problem lies not only with the drug but also with the individual who has inherited an enzymatic defect that prevents normal detoxification.

General aspects of human genetics

The central structure of any living cell is its complement of *genes*, located on the *chromosomes* within the cell nucleus. The chromosomes derive their name because they take up certain basic stains very readily. They consist of protein and deoxyribonucleic acid (DNA). This chemical consists of long molecules coiled in a double helix and the strands of the helix are chains of sugars and phosphates. The two helices in a DNA strand are joined together by cross-bridges made by pairs of organic nitrogenous bases (purines and pyrimidines) joined to the sugar molecules. The organic nitrogenous bases are called nucleotides.

The principal bases in the DNA molecule are adenine (A), cytosine (C), thymine (T), and guanine (G) which are paired as: thymine and adenine, or adenine and thymine; cytosine and guanine, or guanine and cytosine. It is thought that the sequence of these bases is the important factor in heredity and that a gene may consist of a particular sequence of up to 1000 base pairs in a DNA molecule.

The genes, the basic units of heredity, are molecules of DNA. The capacity to replicate itself constitutes the basis of hereditary transmission. DNA also provides the *genetic code*, which determines the development and metabolism of cells by controlling the synthesis of ribonucleic acid (RNA). The sequential order of the components that make up RNA determines the amino-acid composition of proteins, which in turn determines the functions of proteins and thereby the functions of cells.

Many thousands of genes are carried by the chromosomes. In man, each cell normally has 46 chromosomes arranged in 23 pairs. One pair, the sex chromosomes, determines the sex of the individual. The female has two X chromosomes in every cell nucleus; the male has one X and one Y. The male sex chromosomes are said to be heterologous (of two kinds) and the female sex chromosomes are said to be homologous, i.e. each member of a pair has the same configuration and genetic material as the other member of the pair. Both the X and Y chromosomes have a genetic as well as a sex-determining aspect but it is now known that the genetic information is more extensive on the X chromosome than on the Y chromosome. The remaining 22 pairs of chromosomes, the *autosomes*, are homologous, since both members of a pair are usually identical in size, shape and genetic loci.

Recombination of chromosome occurs during *crossing over* (Fig. 14.1). This process takes place during meiosis, when reduction division occurs ensuring that the offspring has the same number of chromosomes as the parents. This reassortment does not provide new genes but the variation already existing in the parent is placed in new combination as his spermatozoa and ovum are formed. Fertilisation normally involves the rela-

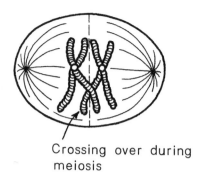

Crossing over during meiosis

Fig. 14.1 Crossing over during meiosis.

tively random union of two parental cells, each containing 23 chromosomes (haploid number) that carry new, unique combinations of old genes.

The exact location of a gene on a chromosome is its *locus* (Fig. 14.2). Each chromosome has thousands of loci arranged in a definite manner and the number and arrangement of genes on homologous chromosomes are identical. Genes that occupy homologous loci are *alleles*, or partner genes. Each individual has therefore two of each kind of gene, one on each pair of chromosomes.

Genes usually remain stable from generation to generation but it is possible for them to undergo a change or *mutation* and thereby transmit a new or altered pair. This change will then be transmitted to future generations. Mutations can occur spontaneously or may be induced by such environmental factors as radiation, viral infection or drugs.

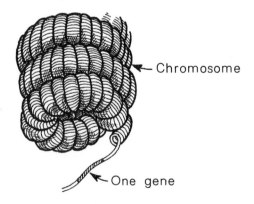

← Chromosome

← One gene

Fig. 14.2 Gene locus on chromosome.

Modes of inheritance

Through the process of reproduction, offspring are produced which, in multicellular organisms, follow a definite pattern of development. Although this developmental sequence of events is quite similar for closely related organisms, it is very specific for members of an individual species and consequently all members of a given species resemble one another. Yet the offspring within a species, and even from the same parents, are always different.

The numerous features by which we recognise an organism constitute its *phenotype*. There are many aspects to phenotypic characteristics which emphasise the similarities and differences of the organisms.

Numerous phenotypic traits, such as colour of eyes, appear to be transmitted from one generation to the next. However, offspring do not inherit phenotypes from their parents; rather they inherit the ability to produce these phenotypes. This ability resides in the *genotype*, and it is the material of the genotype that is transmitted from one generation to the next. The genotype is composed of numerous subunits, the *genes*, the material of which is able to reproduce itself exactly. Only rarely does this reproduction lead to a gene with properties different from that of the original. Therefore, there is continuity of the genotype from one generation to the next.

The expression of the phenotype is attributable not only to the genotype but to environmental conditions as well. These environmental conditions, however, do not affect the genotype. For example, tanning of the skin occurs after exposure to ultraviolet radiation; the effect, however, is transient, for once the opportunity for exposure to ultraviolet light is removed, the skin becomes light again. Environmental alterations of the phenotype do not reflect alterations in the genotype, but rather the response of the organism to its environment. However, the ability of an organism to respond to its environment is determined to a large extent by its genotype.

Genetic variation: mutation

The origin of inborn variation lies largely in variation at the loci, so that many pairs of loci contain different genes or *alleles*. The origin of these differences lies in *mutation* which can be defined as an event that gives rise to a heritable alteration in the genotype. Mutations are divided into two major classes; those involving a change in the structure or number of chromosomes and those involving a single gene. Under most mitotic and meiotic conditions newly-formed chromosomes and their genes are very exact copies of the originals. On occasion, however, imperfect self-reproduction of chromosomal DNA molecules may occur to produce the potential for new traits.

Mutation in any cell of the body except the germ cell is called somatic mutation. An example of this is observable in blue-eyed people. Blue colour in the eyes of a person is attributable generally to a lack of pigment; possibly a single chromosome locus is involved. The genes that produce this trait are *recessive* to those that generate pigment. If b represents the gene (allele) for blue eyes and B an allele coding for brown eyes, then the person with blue eyes would be represented by bb. If DNA changes were to occur in an egg or sperm (germ cell) there would be a probability that a newly-mutated gene would be passed on to the next generation. It is at least theoretically possible that two bb (blue-eyed) parents could produce Bb (brown-eyed) children through germ cell mutation.

Another example of single gene inheritance is the clinical disorder of syndactyly (webbed fingers or toes). The gene for syndactyly is represented by D and the gene for normal is d. Each parent is represented by two genes, each of which they received from their fathers and mothers. In this example, their genetic constitution has been desig-

nated Dd. The male parent (Dd) will be able to produce sperms that are either D or d. The female parent will be able to produce ova that are either D or d. Therefore the possible offspring are DD, Dd, or dd. Both parents have syndactyly and three of the four offspring may also have syndactyly (Fig. 14.3). Because they have the same physical characteristic, i.e. syndactyly, they are said to have the same phenotype, but their genetic composition or genotype is different (they may be either Dd or DD).

Since syndactyly is present if D is one gene of a pair of genes (Dd) as well as both genes (DD) it is a *dominant* trait. Normal digital spaces (d) are present only if d is on both genes (dd) and is a recessive trait.

Dominance is attributable to the presence of an allele whose action results in the production of a given phenotype, while the action of the recessive allele may be missing or in some way altered or masked.

If an individual's genetic constitution for syndactyly contains similar genes (DD, dd), the person is a *homozygote*; if it contains dissimilar genes (Dd), the person is a *heterozygote*. Besides dominant and recessive inheritance, there is an intermediate or co-dominant inheritance. In co-dominance, the two characteristics are expressed in the heterozygote. An example of this is in haemoglobinopathies, such as sickle cell anaemia. The S homozygote (SS) has sickle cell anaemia, the S heterozygote (AS) has sickle cell trait, with characteristics of haemoglobins A and S; the person without S is normal.

Inheritance is either *autosomal or sex-linked, dominant or recessive.*

Autosomal dominant inheritance has three criteria:

1. Every affected person has an affected parent.
2. Every affected person who marries a normal person has a one in two chance of having each offspring affected.
3. Every normal child of an affected person will have normal offspring.

Examples of disorders with autosomal dominant inheritance are: retinoblastoma, renal glycosuria, sickle cell trait, thalassaemia minor and major, haemophilia D and muscular dystrophy.

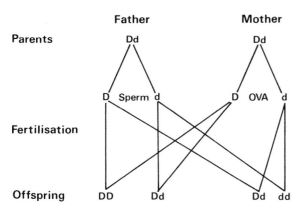

Fig. 14.3 Inheritance of syndactyly.

Autosomal recessive inheritance displays the following characteristics:

1. The vast majority of affected persons have parents who are normal in all outward appearance.
2. In affected families, each child has a one in two chance of having a genetic defect.
3. When an affected person and a normal person marry, their offspring will be normal in most cases.
4. If their offspring is affected, the 'normal' parent is a heterozygote.
5. When two affected persons marry, all their children will be affected.
6. The rarer the defect, the more likely it is that there is consanguinity in the family tree.

Where *sex-linked inheritance* is concerned one of the significant features lies in the direct correlation between transmission of a given chromosome, the X chromosome, and the transmission of specific hereditary traits.

With *X-linked recessive inheritance* there are two main characteristics:

1. The defect is carried by women and exhibited by men.
2. Affected men can pass the disease only through their daughters.

An example is haemophilia A. The female with her two X chromosomes must have the gene for haemophilia present in each X chromosome to this recessive disease. Since the frequency of this gene in the population is low, the chances of two affected X chromosomes occurring together, although possible, are highly unlikely. Therefore, haemophilia is very rare in females. Males, with their XY chromosome composition, require the haemophilia gene present only on one chromosome, i.e. the X chromosome, to have it expressed clinically. There is no homologous locus on the Y chromosome to neutralise the effect of the haemophiliac gene.

As far as X-linked dominant inheritance is concerned, no fully dominant X-linked gene has been discovered in humans with the exception of vitamin D-resistant rickets.

Cytogenetics

Cytogenetics is the study of the chromosomal structure of the cells. Because of the constancy of chromosome number and morphology (structure) it is possible to classify chromosomes. Each chromosome has basic characteristics in relation to:

1. The total length.
2. The position of the centromere.
3. The length of the arms.
4. The presence or absence of satellites.
5. The banding pattern.

Chromosomes can be observed by culturing lymphocytes in the presence of a stimulant and then allowing the dividing cells to accumulate in cell division, or mitosis, by adding a substance which blocks their completion. The chromosomes which are about to separate to form the nuclei of the daughter cells are then seen as double structures, called chromatids. They are connected at their centromeres, a constriction, which divides the chromosome into two arm lengths. The centromere may vary in its position.

The chromosomes are then photographed and each is cut out and placed in a ranking position according to size, shape and staining characteristics. In this way the characteristic karyotype is obtained (Figs. 14.4 and 14.5).

The chromosomes may deviate from the normal pattern either by being too few or too many, i.e. numerical abnormalities, or where the individual chromosomes may be abnormal, i.e. structural abnormalities. In some cases where, for example,

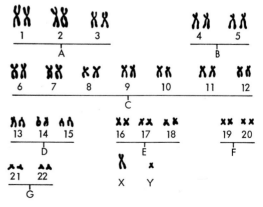

Fig. 14.4 Karyotype of a normal male.

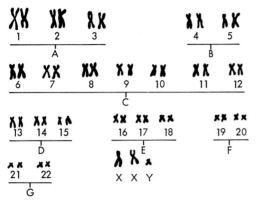

Fig. 14.5 Karyotype of a person with Klinefelter's syndrome (47, XXY).

two chromosomes fuse together, structural abnormalities may lead to numerical abnormalities.

Abnormalities of structures

1. *Non-dysjunction.* This is failure of a chromatid pair to separate in a dividing cell. If it occurs in either the first or second divisions of meiosis, it will result in gametes with abnormal chromosomal patterns. If it occurs in mitosis, *mosaic* patterns occur, i.e. one area of an organism will have one genetic pattern and another area of the same organism will have another genetic pattern. Patients with a mosaic constitution present an incomplete and variable clinical picture with features of each of the genetic syndromes represented in the mosaic.
2. *Translocation.* In simple translocation, there is

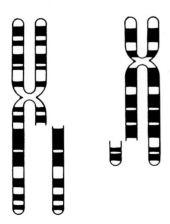

Fig. 14.6 Chromosomal translocation showing banding and separation of lower parts.

an exchange of chromosomal material between two non-homologous chromosomes (Fig. 14.6).

3. *Deletion.* In deletion, there is loss of chromosomal material due to breakage of chromatid during cell division.
4. *Duplication.* If breakage occurs in a chromatid during cell division, the broken part may realign itself so that many loci are duplicated on one chromosome and are absent from the other member of the pair of chromosomes.
5. *Inversion.* This occurs if, after fracture of a chromatid, the fragment reattaches itself to the same chromosome in a different order.

Abnormalities of chromosomal number

1. *Monosomy.* Chromosomal number is 45. Monosomy is due to the absence of one of a pair of chromosomes in the diploid cell. *Example*: monosomy 21–22 and the fetus is stillborn.
2. *Trisomy.* Chromosomal number is 47. Trisomy is caused by non-dysjunction of a chromosome pair during the first meiotic division, with the result that three chromosomes are present instead of the usual two. *Example*: trisomy 13, 18 and 21. Trisomy 13 and 18 are less common than trisomy 21, the latter being associated with Down's syndrome.
3. *Polysomy.* Chromosomal number is 48 or more. This occurs when one chromosome is represented four or more times. An example is XXXXY.
4. *Complex anenploidy.* In this situation two or more chromosomes have an abnormal variation in number; the structures of these chromosomes are normal. Examples are trisomy 21 and XXX in the same individual.

Heredity in health and disease

It has been known for a long time that the difference between health and disease is sometimes due to heredity. A percentage of infants born are more or less seriously incapacitated by genetic defects, while many pregnancies resulting in abortions or stillbirths may be due to genetic conditions.

Diseases due to simple recessive genes are generally more difficult to study genetically because the affected children are born to parents, neither of whom is affected. These include diseases such as juvenile amaurotic idiocy, a serious neurological disorder that is fatal early in life. Both parents may be heterozygous and carry one dose of the defective gene; although they themselves enjoy good health one in four of their children on average may suffer from the disease.

In some cases the dichotomy of hereditary versus environmental defect or disease cannot always be sustained and it is a fact that each of us will respond differently to exposure to diverse environments imposed by food, bacteria, parents and social conditions. There are also more subtle genetic differences such as blood groups or HLA type (human leucocyte antigen system) which may influence susceptibility to disease. However, it is difficult to consider that there are specific genes predisposing to disease. There are, however, a number of disorders which can be linked directly to the genetic make-up of the individual, for example, neoplastic disorders, mental disease and inborn errors of metabolism. The latter disorders will be discussed more fully in a subsequent section of this chapter.

GENETIC COUNSELLING

With the greatly advanced techniques of detecting genetic disorders by amniocentesis and biochemical identification of heterozygotes, the clinician will now be able to transmit that information to the people concerned. The purpose of genetic counselling is that the parents can decide whether or not to have more children. Genetic counselling also extends to other members of the family. This involves not only informing and instructing high-risk relatives but also reassuring low-risk relatives.

To provide such a service the consultant requires the following specific information:

1. An accurate diagnosis, since closely related disorders, especially biochemical defects, may have a markedly different prognosis and mode of inheritance.
2. A detailed family history with an accurate pedigree showing the affected and non-affected members.
3. A knowledge of the behaviour of the disorder from the literature.

With this information at hand, the risk of recurrence can be estimated.

Situations where fairly precise information can be given include those which show a clear-cut Mendelian inheritance, and even this may necessitate the study of many pedigrees. When it is found, the risks to subsequent offspring are too high to be acceptable to most people.

This is based on Mendel's first law which states 'that every trait in an organism is determined by a single pair of hereditary units or genes'.

For example
1. In Huntington's chorea (a disorder controlled by an autosomal dominant gene) the chance of any given offspring having the disease if one parent is affected is one in two and the risk is similar for subsequent siblings.
2. In fibrocystic disease, phenylketonuria (controlled by an autosomal recessive gene), one in four siblings on average will be affected in a family where the disease is occurring.
3. If the disease is due to an X-linked recessive gene, as in haemophilia, then an affected male married to a normal woman will have *all* carrier daughters but all sons will be unaffected. Of the daughters of a carrier female, half will be normal and half carriers, and of her sons half will be affected and half normal. If, however, there is no family history of such a disease, it is very important not to give the rather bad prognosis for relatives until the possibility of a mutation has been considered. If a mutation has occurred in the patient, then none of his sisters would be carriers.

There are situations where the risk cannot be predicted by a general theory. These conditions include:

1. Congenital dislocation of the hip where several factors have to be considered. Two of these are genetic; one affecting the development of the acetabulum and the other producing an increased laxity of all joints (a dominant trait). There is also an environmental component, namely the intra-uterine posture.
2. Hypertrophic pyloric stenosis which is believed to be a multifactorial inheritance. It is

commoner in boys than in girls, but when a girl has the condition she has more affected relatives than has a boy with the condition. The female baby is apparently normally more resistant than the male baby to the condition and, when she does develop it, this is because she has a very high concentration of predisposing genes.

3. Abnormalities of the central nervous system, i.e. anencephaly, spina bifida and hydrocephalus, may also be multifactorial or the environment may be partly responsible as well.

Another aspect of genetic advice is the detection of carriers in recessive conditions. As far as autosomes are concerned there are two which are of importance, fibrocystic disease and thalassaemia. In cystic fibrosis of the pancreas (frequency about one in 2000 live births) skin fibroblast cultures show cytoplasmic staining abnormality (metachromasia) not only in the affected children but also in their parents who will be found to be heterozygotes. Thalassaemia has a high frequency in Northern Italy and Thailand. Patients with two doses of the gene usually die young from gross anaemia but those who are heterozygotes may be mildly affected or not at all. It is important to detect the carriers by screening procedures. This is done by estimating the fragility of the red blood cells which are unusually resistant to haemolysis by hypotonic saline solutions. Normal red blood cells burst easily when in contact with hypotonic saline solution. The same applies to the more common X-linked conditions, e.g. haemophilia, where the sister of an affected man must be advised that she may be a carrier. In general, the assessments are made by biochemical methods.

In amniocentesis the genetic constitution of an unborn baby can be examined. The amnion is a fluid-filled sac in which the embryo develops, and by means of a hollow needle a little fluid can be removed. The cells in it are fetal and they can be sexed by the Barr body (a darkly-staining body under the nuclear membrane of mammalian somatic cells, present in normal females but absent in normal males), or grown and examined for chromosomal or biochemical abnormalities. The knowledge obtained could be useful in helping parents to decide whether to ask for a pregnancy to be terminated. There is therefore an important aspect of preventive medicine in medical genetics.

GENETIC ENGINEERING

Genetic engineering is the term used to describe the introduction of human choice and design criteria into the contruction and combination of genes. The term however, should mean the artificial interchange of hereditary material between species.

Transfer of genetic information from higher organisms into bacteria is now a possibility. It involves implantation of human genes into bacteria by recombinant DNA, in an effort to obtain new knowledge of genetic mechanisms at the molecular level and also to achieve such benefits as abundant and inexpensive supplies of human insulin, interferons and other proteins.

Essentially there are three types of vectors used in recombinant DNA technology (genetic engineering): the plasmids, phages and cosmids. All replicate within the host bacterial cell. Plasmids occur naturally in bacteria to which they confer resistance to various substances including antibiotics. They are stably inherited in an extrachromosomal state, and consist of a circular duplex of DNA.

After the foreign DNA has been incorporated into the plasmid, the plasmid is introduced into the host bacterial cell by exposing the latter to calcium salts which make the cell membrane permeable to the plasmid (Fig. 14.7).

The next step is to grow the host vector in culture to produce clones, i.e. where all the cells are derived from a single genetic constitution. Finally, a selection is made of those clones which contain the relevant DNA fragment. A number of techniques have been developed to detect the insertion of specific sequences.

There are a number of applications of recombinant DNA technology. For example, gene structure/mapping, population genetics in relation to disease and population structure, control of genetic disease, biosynthesis, e.g. insulin, growth hormone and interferon, and treatment of genetic disease by the insertion of a cloned normal gene.

With regard to insulin production, it is normally

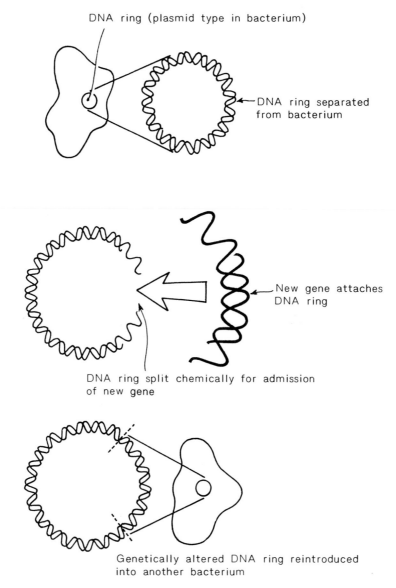

DNA ring (plasmid type in bacterium)

DNA ring separated from bacterium

New gene attaches DNA ring

DNA ring split chemically for admission of new gene

Genetically altered DNA ring reintroduced into another bacterium

Fig. 14.7 Diagrammatic representation of genetic engineering.

obtained from pig pancreas which has to be carefully purified before it can be injected into patients, and even then there is the possibility of producing sensitivity reactions. When using recombinant DNA technology, micro-organisms can be used to synthesise human insulin. It is not necessary to copy the gene for insulin to do this. From the known amino-acid composition of its two polypeptide chains, the sequence of codons is chosen and in this way an 'artificial' gene is made

which carries the necessary information for synthesising insulin. The chemically constructed gene is then inserted, with appropriate devices to ensure efficient transcription and translation into a plasmid, and cloned in *E. coli*. In this way it is possible to make milligram quantities of insulin per litre of bacterial culture. The 'artificial' gene may not be identical with the natural gene because of excess in the genetic code and it also does not take account of intervening sequences which are not transcribed but may be important in controlling gene action.

Some attempts have been made at gene therapy, but there are problems associated with it. It would only be effective in certain unifactorial disorders where only one gene is involved, and there are still technical problems to overcome. It must also be recognised that there are elements of hazard and much work requires to be done not only to ensure effectiveness but also to allay the fears of the general public.

Treatment of genetic disease is also a possibility though achieving a cure in the sense of replacing a mutant gene by a normal gene is as yet not possible. When a disorder is due to an enzyme block then the defective enzyme or protein might be replaced or its substrate restricted or the deficient product can be replaced. However, many enzymes have not been isolated or synthesised and even if they were given by injection they might not be effective because many perform their catalytic function within the cell. There is the possibility that the defective enzyme can be replaced by the transplantation of tissue possessing normal enzyme activity. Bone marrow transplant may also prove useful in certain inborn errors of metabolism.

Chapter 15
Inborn errors of metabolism

In general, only rare diseases are inherited in a simple manner while in common diseases there is usually no simple pattern of inheritance.

Metabolic processes proceed in an orderly sequence. Each step is controlled by a specific enzyme and each enzymic step is controlled by a single gene. Deficiency or absence of a particular enzyme will affect the metabolic pathway, i.e. block the metabolic process of that particular product and produce effects on body functions which can have serious consequences.

Nearly 200 human diseases can be classified as 'inborn errors of metabolism'. Disorders can be due to faulty metabolism of amino-acids, protein, carbohydrate, fats (lipids), water and electrolytes. Only some of the more common disorders will be discussed with examples for each of the substances mentioned.

Disturbances in amino-acid metabolism
At least 35 disturbances of amino-acid metabolism have been described in man. Some of these involve the whole body, others affect transport involving the surface membranes in the kidney tubules or the lining of the intestine.

DISORDERS OF PHENYLALANINE AND TYROSINE
The normal pathway for the degradation of the amino-acids phenylalanine and tyrosine occurs in a series of separate steps. Absence of a specific enzyme will prevent the conversion of phenylalanine to tyrosine, and lead to the condition of *phenylketonuria*. Further along the chain reaction, an absence of p-hydroxyphenypyruvic acid oxidase causes tyrosinaemia, or an absence of the enzyme homogentisic oxidase casuses alkaptonuria. As another pathway of metabolism, tyrosine is also converted to 3.4-dihydroxyphenalaline (DOPA),

and eventually to melanin by the action of the enzyme tyrosinase. The absence of this enzyme is responsible for the hereditary defect *albinism*.

Phenylketonuria
Phenylketonuria is transmitted by an autosomal recessive gene. In an affected family there is a chance of one in four of future children being affected. The incidence is at least one in 20 000 births.

Clinically, the classic picture is frequently represented by fair-haired, blue-eyed children with fair skins, eczema and mental retardation. Some may have convulsions.

Since screening of new-born infants is widespread, the presenting problem is hyperphenylalaninaemia in healthy new-born babies. However, hyperphenylalaninaemia is no longer synonymous with phenylketonuria since other causes have now been established.

Investigations

1. Urine test for the presence of phenylpyruvic acid (p. 566).
2. Guthrie test. This test is carried out in the first 10 days of life (when milk feeds are started the phenylalanine level rises) (p. 266).
3. Checking serum phenylalanine levels. If the infant is clinically suspect, a repeat test is done one month later. This will permit discovery of the infant with phenylketonuria who was not diagnosed in the newborn period. It is also important to recognise that affected infants who are totally breast-fed may not demonstrate phenylketonuria for many months.

Principles of treatment and nursing management

1. Dietary means (p. 263). The aim of treatment

is to reduce the serum level of phenylalanine to normal. Foods are given which are almost phenylalanine-free, giving just enough to support adequate growth without causing mental impairment. The diet is a very restrictive one with foods such as bread, meat, fish, dairy products, nuts and legumes being withheld. Preparations such as Minafen and Cymogran can be given. It is generally agreed that the diet should be maintained for 3 to 6 years, but some believe it should be maintained for life.

The diet will not reverse or improve existing mental retardation but, if it started before the age of 2 months, the child has a chance of attaining normal intelligence.
2. Basic nursing care.
3. Genetic counselling (p. 258).

If the mother has classic phenylketonuria, she can bear a normal infant, but there is an increased risk of bearing a child with non-phenylketonuric mental retardation, microcephaly and congenital heart disease. Dietary therapy during pregnancy has been shown to be ineffective in preventing the fetal effects of phenylketonuria. It is suggested that the treatment should start before conception.

DISORDERS OF CARBOHYDRATE METABOLISM
The principal disorders in this area involve, amongst others, galactosaemia, pentosuria, fructosuria, the glycogen-storage diseases and red blood cell enzyme defects.

Galactosaemia
This disorder is transmitted as an autosomal recessive inheritance. The basic defect is an inability to convert galactose to glucose due to the deficiency of either or both transferase and galactokinase.

Galactokinase deficiency is rarer and the condition is mild but cataracts are present. In transferase deficiency, there is greater toxicity with failure to thrive, vomiting, liver disease, cataracts and mental retardation.

Clinical features
After milk feeding has started, the infant develops vomiting and refuses feeds. This is followed by diarrhoea, loss of weight and dehydration. Cataracts are common. If untreated, he becomes mentally retarded and develops ascites, due to hepatic involvement.

Investigations
1. Urine tests for galactose and protein, which may be due to renal tubular damage.
2. Erythrocyte test for galactose. The condition can be confirmed by demonstration of enzyme deficiency in the peripheral red cells.
3. Galactose tolerance test. This is always abnormal in galactosaemia.

Principles of treatment and nursing management
1. Correction of fluid and electrolyte imbalance. If an infusion is required then the principles of care of the child with an infusion apply (p. 448).
2. Milk substitutes, such as low-lactose food, Nutramigen and soya bean milks, are given. As the child gets older, his diet will become more varied and he will probably be able to tolerate some galactose in his diet. Provided the treatment is started early, the child should develop normally.
3. Routine basic nursing care.
4. Daily urine testing.
5. Monitoring of blood glucose.
6. Genetic counselling. Since the heterozygotes can be identified by blood studies and the affected fetus identified by amniotic fluid or fetal blood analysis, a maternal diet free of galactose can be maintained during the pregnancy.

Glycogen storage disease
Glycogen storage diseases now constitute a number of separate entities, all of which are clinically and biochemically identifiable. Each has deficient activity of specific enzymes involved in the synthesis and degradation of glycogen causing an accumulation of abnormal glycogen in any or all of the tissues of the liver, heart, skeletal muscle, kidney and brain. When it involves the liver and kidney it is called *von Gierke's* disease. When the heart and voluntary muscles are involved, it is called *Pompe's* disease.

The inheritance is probably autosomal recessive (with the exception of type 8, which is X-linked recessive).

Clinical features
Clinical features vary with each type. In von Gierke's disease the new-born infant may present with hepatomegaly, respiratory distress, ketoacidosis and hypoglycaemic convulsions. As the child grows older, and in less severe cases, there will also be steatorrhoea, poorly developed musculature and delayed linear growth. Until about 6 years of age, bleeding and acute infections are the major clinical problems. The cause of bleeding is defective platelet adhesion. Accumulation of fatty cells (xanthema) and osteoporosis from a negative calcium balance of chronic acidosis with pronounced skin features such as prominent venous patterns are features of this condition. Linear growth and motor development are delayed but intelligence may be unimpaired.

Investigations

1. Urinalysis, e.g. acetone is found in the urine.
2. Blood analysis, e.g. low blood sugar level, hyperlipaemia and increased blood glycogen level.
3. Liver biopsy for testing of material for glucose-6-phosphatase. An open liver biopsy is usually preferred to ensure proper haemostasis.

Principles of treatment and nursing management
Nursing management will depend on the age and general condition of the child. The aim is to maintain plasma glucose levels by:

1. Dietary means (p. 218). Frequent feeding at 3- or 4-hourly intervals with glucose. It may be necessary to use intra-gastric infusion via a naso-gastric tube or a gastrostomy may be fashioned to provide overnight feeding. Protein content should be normal, with a low fat and adequate calorie intake.
2. Monitoring of blood glucose levels to determine the specific requirement of each child.
3. Nursing management of a child with:
   a. A naso-gastric tube (p. 512)
   b. A gastrostomy (p. 514).

4. Routine nursing care.
5. Genetic counselling. Since it is transmitted as an autosomal recessive inheritance, parents will require genetic counselling (p. 258).
6. Parental support is also very important and the parents should be encouraged to take part in nursing their child whenever possible.

Pompe's disease (type 2 glycogen storage disease)
In Pompe's disease the symptoms appear early in infancy. It is due to deficiency of the enzyme α-1.4 glucosidase (acid maltase). At autopsy there is massive accumulation of normal structured glycogen in liver, muscle, heart, tongue and nervous system.

Clinical features
The disease occurs in three different forms, one of which is the adult form.

1. Infantile form. The infant appears to be normal at birth but after about one month there is muscle weakness and poor feeding with progressive dyspnoea. He will develop macroglossia, an increased heart and heart failure. He is unable to swallow saliva; hypostatic pneumonia occurs and the child dies early in childhood.
2. Where the onset is in late infancy or early childhood the above clinical features apply with death at less than 20 years of age.

Investigations

1. Blood analysis. Normal levels of blood sugar, lipids, ketones, and uric acid are found.
2. Glucagon and epinephrine test. Responses are normal.
3. Liver and muscle biopsy. Cytoplasmic glycogen is found to be normal but on electromicroscopy marked lysosomal accumulation of glycogen is found.

Principles of treatment and nursing management
There is no effective treatment. Dietary regimens are unsuccessful since the usual pathway of glycogen metabolism is normal.

Nursing care must be based on the general condition of the child. For example:

1. Dyspnoea can be relieved by positioning and possible oxygen administration.
2. Feeding problems can be handled by giving small, frequent feeds or by giving these by intra-gastric infusion (p. 512).
3. Suction will be necessary since the child has difficulty in dealing with salivary secretions.
4. Care of pressure areas. There is muscle weakness and therefore limited mobility; handling should be gentle and general cleanliness is important.
5. Support for parents. This is a distressing condition and the parents will require full support. Every opportunity should be given to allow them to participate in nursing the child.
6. Genetic counselling (p. 258).

DISORDERS OF LIPID METABOLISM

Most of the disorders of lipid metabolism involve storage of phospholipids or glycolipids and these are associated with neurological involvement.

Serum lipids and lipoproteins are fairly constant throughout life, with the exception of the newborn period and early infancy when they are somewhat lower. The lipids include cholesterol (a basic substance from which the body synthesises the sex hormones and bile acids) and lipoprotein. All lipids are transported in serum as macromolecular complexes with proteins.

Lipid storage disease

Disorders of the serum lipoproteins are generally classified according to the major lipoprotein species involved. There may be excesses or deficiency and they may be due to a primary genetically determinent defect or to a secondary manifestation of another disease state. In some diseases there appears to be a definite ethnic factor, for example, Tay-Sachs' and Nieman-Pick's diseases which are more common in Jewish children. Both conditions lead to disorders of the central nervous system.

Clinical features in Niemann-Pick's disease

Manifestations occur early in infancy and consist primarily of liver and spleen enlargement and central nervous system involvement, with convulsions and mental retardation. They may also be diffuse pulmonary infiltration, cutaneous lesions, gastro-intestinal bleeding, thrombocytopaenia and anaemia.

Clinical features in Tay-Sachs' disease

The disease is clinically apparent by the age of 5 to 6 months. The enzyme hexosaminide A is absent, resulting in an accumulation of ganglioside in the ganglion cells. The destruction of the ganglion cells is accompanied by glial proliferation and myelin degeneration. This leads to psychomotor retardation, hypotonia, dementia and blindness.

Investigations

1. Blood analysis.
2. Liver and marrow biopsies. These will show foam cells.
3. Demonstration of sphingomyelinase deficiency in white blood cells and cultured skin fibroblasts.

Principles of treatment and nursing management

In both cases treatment is supportive:

1. General routine nursing care.
2. Management of pressure areas and prevention of breakdown of skin. Gentle handling of children.
3. Positioning the child in the most comfortable position and supporting his head.
4. Suction of bronchial secretions as required (p. 120).
5. Medication for concurrent infection and relief of convulsions.
6. Nursing management during a convulsive episode (p. 307).
7. Providing adequate nutrition. It may be necessary to give feeds by naso-gastric route (p. 512).
8. Support for parents. Encourage them to participate in the nursing care of the child.
9. Genetic counselling. Both diseases are transmitted as autosomal recessive inheritance and genetic counselling is essential.

Biochemical investigations

There are many biochemical investigations required to aid diagnosis and to determine efficiency of treatment. When frequent blood samples are required an indweling venous cannula is preferred to repeated venous punctures.

Guthrie's test

The Guthrie test is performed to detect cases of phenylketonuria in very early infancy. It is carried out by the sixth day of life when feeding is established, and the serum level of phenylalanine increases to detectable levels.

The Guthrie inhibition assay test is used. A strain of phenylalanine-dependent *Bacillus subtilis* is cultured in a medium on which is placed a filter paper disc impregnated with several drops of capillary blood, together with other discs containing varying amounts of phenylalanine (controls). The zone of growth around the disc containing the blood sample is proportional to the phenylalanine content.

More exact tests must be used to confirm the condition. These include fluorimetric methods or ion exchange column chromatography.

Requirements

1. Mediswabs.
2. Heel stab needle.
3. Guthrie's test card.
4. Elastoplast dressing.

Method

The skin is cleaned with alcohol (Mediswab) and allowed to dry. The heel is stabbed and a drop of blood is placed on each of the four rings in the special test card. Each circle must be completely filled with blood. Press the infant's heel against the centre of the filter paper until the circle is filled. The punctured area is cleaned and covered with Elastoplast dressing to stop bleeding. The test card is then completed in pencil and sent to the biochemistry department.

Screening test for galactosaemia

A reliable screening test for galactosaemia which may be used depends on the fluorescence formed when there is a breakdown of galactose. The test is performed on 0.025 ml of heparinised blood.

Diagnostic test for galactosaemia

For this test, 1 ml of heparinised blood is required.

Glucose tolerance test

This test measures the child's ability to stabilise his blood sugar level after taking some glucose. Intake of glucose raises the blood sugar level and insulin lowers it. The child should be having a diet containing adequate carbohydrate for at least three days before the test is performed. After a 12-hour fast for a child (4-hour fast for an infant), capillary blood is obtained for sugar determination. The child is given oral glucose (1.75 g/kg) and specimens of blood are taken at 30, 90 and 150 minutes.

Determination of fasting glucose and insulin

The child is fasted overnight and a specimen of blood is obtained at 8 a.m. to test for glucose and insulin. This is repeated on two subsequent days. Several urine specimens are tested for ketones. This may indicate the occurrence of ketotic hypoglycaemia.

Leucine sensitivity test

This test is performed when the history suggests that hypoglycaemia follows protein loading. A fasting venous blood specimen is taken for glucose and insulin determination. This is followed by L-leucine (0.15 g/kg) given orally. Specimens of blood are taken at 15, 30, 45, 60, 90 and 120 minutes after L-leucine has been given. Hydrocortisone and glucose should be available to combat the effect of L-leucine.

Glucagon test

Glucagon has a hyperglycaemic action. It mobilises glucose and raises the blood glucose level. As a test it is used to investigate both glycogen storage disease and insulinoma.

The child fasts for about 10 hours; younger children for as long as possible. Capillary blood is taken at 20 minutes and again immediately before the glucagon is injected. A dose of glucagon 1 mg is injected intravenously and the child is observed for signs of shock, nausea and vomiting.

Blood samples are taken at 20, 40, 60, 90 and 120 minutes after the injection. Failure of rise in blood glucose level is consistent with most forms of glycogen storage disease.

Tests for disaccharidase deficiency

Lactase deficiency is the most common primary disaccharidase deficiency. A diagnosis of disaccharidase deficiency may be suspected if acidic stools (pH < 6) are passed. It is further substantiated by a flat oral tolerance test when the affected sugar is ingested.

1. *Test of faeces.* Universal indicator paper is moistened with water and laid on a microscope slide. A small amount of faeces is then rubbed on to the paper.
2. *Lactose tolerance test* for disaccharide absorption. The child is fasted overnight and a specimen of blood is taken in the morning for fasting blood sugar estimation.

   The child is given a drink of lactose, 2 g/kg of body weight, dissolved in a glass of water. Further blood samples are taken at 30 minute intervals for 2 hours.

   Normally there is a rise in the blood sugar level. If there is no rise in the blood sugar level, the test is repeated using a mixture of glucose and galactose, 1 g/kg of body weight each.
3. *Sucrose tolerance test.* The procedure is the same as for the lactose tolerance test, except that sucrose 2 g/kg of body weight is used. If a repeat test has to be done a mixture of glucose and fructose (1 g/kg of body weight each) is used.

Sweat test (thermal)

In this procedure the aim is to encourage the excretion of sweat, so that the contents of the sweat may be analysed. It is an important aid to diagnosis in the condition of fibrocystic disease of the pancreas, where the concentration of sodium chloride in sweat is increased.

There are various methods of performing this test and mention will be made of two which are generally used: (1) production of sweat is stimulated by the application of general heat and (2) sweat glands in a limited area are stimulated by the use of chemicals. The first method is largely superseded by the second one which avoids the discomfort and danger inherent in severe general sweating.

Requirements

1. Dissecting forceps.
2. Dressing pack.
3. Skin cleansing lotions and methylated ether.
4. Square piece of plastic sheet, slightly larger than the swab.
5. 2.5 cm adhesive strapping, scissors.
6. Jar with lid containing a weighed swab (obtained from the biochemistry department).
7. Plastic bag.
8. Electric blanket or additional blankets and covered hot water bottles.
9. Bathing equipment and change of clothing.

Preparation and care of the child

It is important to remember that excessive sweating will lead to loss of water and sodium chloride, so that the child may become dehydrated, a condition which leads to respiratory distress and cyanosis. It is therefore necessary to prepare drinks containing salt, for example, orange juice in half-strength normal saline, or for infants quarter- or half-strength normal saline. This can be given during and after the test. While the test is in progress constant supervision is necessary. The room must be warm and the bed prepared by placing well-covered hot water bottles in it, or by using a well-protected electric blanket. The child is undressed and placed inside the plastic bag, enclosing the whole body except the head.

Before closing the bag the area between the two scapulae is washed with distilled water and any skin oils and inorganic salts are removed with methylated ether. A swab which has been previously weighed and is completely dry is placed on the cleaned area with a pair of forceps (fingers must not be used as the nurse's fingers contain inorganic salts which will be transferred to the swab, thus invalidating the findings). The swab is then covered with a piece of plastic or polythene slightly bigger than the swab and it is held in position by adhesive tape. The bag is closed at the neck and the child is covered with blankets.

Sweating should be profuse and beads of sweat on the forehead and neck will indicate when to remove the child from the sweat bag. During this time the child must be watched carefully for any signs of respiratory distress, cyanosis or dehydration. Whenever any of these signs appear, the doctor must be notified and the test abandoned. Oxygen should be administered and saline drinks given. When sweating is profuse, the swab is removed with a pair of forceps, placed into the jar provided, and sent to the biochemistry department for analysis. Meanwhile the child is given a drink and a bath is prepared and given. Cooling of the child must be avoided, therefore bathing and dressing should take place in a warm room and the clothing should be warmed.

Instead of using the plastic bag, blankets only may be used. The child is wrapped in the blankets overnight and the test is discontinued in the morning. The care of the child is the same as in the method described above.

Sweat test by iontophoresis

This method causes much less distress to the child; no special preparation is required and no special restrictions need to be placed on the child immediately before or after the test. The older child should be given an explanation to allay his fears and to gain his confidence.

Sweating is stimulated by means of a pad moistened with pilocarpine solution (e.g. pilocarpine 0.45 per cent in distilled water). The ionised drug is transported to the sweat glands under the influence of an electric field (a mild electric current is passed through the drug for about 5 minutes, using an iontophoresis apparatus).

Requirements

1. Sweat test box, containing battery, two leads and two electrodes.
2. Dressing pack, swabs.
3. Bowl and two gallipots.
4. White lint or several layers of gauze (to cover the electrodes).
5. Weighed filter paper in a container (to absorb the sweat).
6. Adhesive tape and waterproof tape.
7. Dissecting forceps.
8. 10 cm square of polythene.
9. Scissors.
10. Solution of pilocarpine nitrate 0.45 per cent in distilled water to stimulate sweating.
11. Magnesium sulphate 10 per cent (for the conduction of the current).
12. Methylated ether and deionised or distilled water.

Preparation of the equipment

1. Two pads, each of five thicknesses of lint, are made of slightly larger size than the electrode plates.
2. Polythene is cut to about 15 cm, large enough to cover the filter paper completely with about 2.5 cm overlap, or sufficiently large to cover the area between the scapula.
3. Strips of waterproof adhesive are prepared, to seal off completely the edges of the waterproof sheet. These are applied after the filter paper and polythene sheet are in position on the skin.

Method

Areas of the skin on which the electrodes are to be placed are cleaned to remove old sebaceous excretions and sweat. Ether is used, followed by distilled or deionised water and the areas are then dried.

One pad of lint is moistened with magnesium sulphate solution and placed on the child's thigh. The electrode plate is placed on top and, using waterproof adhesive, the assembly is strapped to the thigh sufficiently firmly to make good contact. This electrode is connected to the negative lead. The magnesium sulphate solution provides the electrolyte necessary for the conduction of the electric current.

The second pad is moistened with the pilocarpine solution and placed on a suitable area of the thorax where the filter paper can be applied flat, e.g. the area between the scapulae. The electrode plate and strapping is applied as before and the connection is made to the positive lead.

Great care must be taken to ensure that no part of the electrode plate or any bare lead touches the skin or a burn may be produced when the current is passed.

When both leads are securely in position, the doctor adjusts the current gradually to 4 to 5 milliamps and leaves it at this level for 5 minutes.

The child may feel a slight tingling sensation.

The electrodes and pads are then removed. A reddened area will be seen under the pilocarpine electrode. The area and some distance around is washed with distilled or deionised water to remove the pilocarpine and sweat already on the skin. The area is then dried completely, making sure that no threads or paper fluff remain which might adhere to the filter paper.

The filter paper is removed from the container with clean forceps and applied to the reddened area. The waterproof sheet is placed on top and is sealed off with waterproof adhesive to given an airtight seal. A cross of adhesive in the middle will help to hold the paper in better contact with the skin. The filter paper is left in position for 30 to 60 minutes, and it is then carefully removed with clean and dry forceps. Great care must be taken to ensure that the filter paper is intact and no part is broken off. It is placed at once in the container which must be closed and sent to the biochemistry department for analysis as soon as possible. The skin areas used are then cleaned and dried carefully and any adhesive removed. (Normal sodium levels are < 30 mmol/l [< 30 mEq/l] in fibrocystic disease the sodium level is increased, usually above 60 mmol/l [60 mEq/l]).

Precautions when performing the test

The dangers of burning have already been mentioned and great care must be taken to prevent this. Contamination with sodium must be avoided as this would invalidate the result. Soap and detergents much be excluded from any part of the test and any material used in the test must be kept clear of any surface which might be contaminated with sodium salts. The filter paper must be lifted and manipulated with forceps to prevent contamination from the operator's fingers and only distilled or deionised water must be used for cleaning the skin.

Evaporation of sweat must be avoided by ensuring an airtight seal between the skin and the waterproof covering, by rapid transfer of the damp paper to the bottle, and by airtight closure of the bottle.

Since the complete bottle and filter paper have been weighed no changes should be made on the outside of the bottle or container. A code or number is usually on the container and this code should be used for identification on the request form. Care must also be taken to avoid damage which might alter the weight of the container/bottle.

Chapter 16
Disorders of the endocrine system

The endocrine or ductless glands secrete substances directly into the bloodstream. These secretions are called hormones and they are transported by the blood to distant sites where they exert specific effects on cells.

The endocrine glands include the following: hypothalamus and pituitary gland; thyroid; parathyroid; pancreas; testis and ovary. Each of them have been studied experimentally and although the precise mode of action of their secretions is not fully known, certain effects of their decreased or increased activity have been recognised. An endocrine gland may be absent, infected or invaded by abnormal cells which will result in signs and symptoms of disease.

One of the major functions of the endocrine system is to keep the internal environment constant. This is achieved through a mechanism of negative feedback. For example the glucose level is controlled by two hormones secreted by the islet cells of the pancreas. Insulin secretion is promoted by a rise in blood glucose and when the level has fallen sufficiently, insulin secretion ceases. The other hormone glucagon is stimulated by a fall in blood glucose and its secretion stops when the glucose level rises to a certain level. In these examples the control over hormone secretion is exerted directly by the blood concentration of the islet cells of the pancreas.

The other mechanism involves a sequence of events which includes the hypothalamus. This gland secretes a specific releasing factor which passes via the adenohypophyseal vessels to the anterior pituitary gland which it stimulates to release the appropriate hormone. This circulates via the blood to the target gland which in turn is stimulated to produce its specific hormone. The importance of the hypothalamus has recently been recognised and it is now considered to be the controller of endocrine function. However, there is a very close interrelationship between the hypothalamus and the pituitary gland.

The position and relationship of these two glands to other structures such as the optic chiasma means that any lesions of the hypothalamus and pituitary may present with signs such as eye involvement.

Hypothalamus
The hypothalamus contains nuclei from which non-medullated nerve fibres arise. One group of nuclei has neuro-endocrine activity which controls the secretory activity of the anterior and posterior pituitary gland. Lesions of the hypothalamus lead to endocrine and autonomic disturbances.

Pituitary gland
The pituitary gland consists of the anterior (glandular) and posterior (neural) parts. Seven hormones which are secreted by the anterior pituitary gland have been identified. Three have metabolic activity: growth hormone, thyrotrophic hormone and adeno-corticotrophic hormone; three are gonadotrophic hormones: follicular stimulating hormone, luteinising hormone and lactogenic hormone; a seventh hormone is the melanocyte stimulating hormone.

The posterior pituitary gland stores and secretes oxytocin and vasopressin (anti-diuretic hormone — ADH).

Diseases of the hypothalamus

Diabetes insipidus
This condition is due to abnormality of the hypothalamo-neurohypophyseal system. It may be idiopathic (no cause found) or due to primary

tumours, encephalitis (causing destruction of the neurosecretory neurones), or hereditary factors, acquired as a dominant or sex-linked recessive disease. The condition is characterised by an inability to concentrate urine, polyuria and polydipsia (excessive thirst).

Clinical features

In early childhood, the onset of the idiopathic type is sudden. In other cases, where it is due to trauma, it may be abrupt or delayed following infections. Polyuria and polydipsia are the outstanding features. The urine is of low specific gravity and the amount passed is between 4 to 20 litres daily. Dehydration is *not* a feature since the child drinks large amounts of fluid. However, if fluids are restricted, severe dehydration, headache, vomiting, abdominal pain, restlessness and confusion will result. Sleep is disturbed by polyuria and thirst, contributing to restlessness.

The child's excessive thirst leads him to drink anything he can find — water from pools, even his own urine.

Investigations

1. Fluid intake and output measurements.
2. Testing urinary specific gravity; a specific gravity of less than 1.005 is evidence of the condition.
3. Pitressin test. This is a valuable test since it distinguishes between diabetes insipidus and pitressin-resistant renal diabetes insipidus. Five pressor units of vasopressin are given intravenously which, in diabetes insipidus, will induce a marked reduction in urine volume with increased specific gravity. The effects last for 1 hour.
4. Intravenous saline test. A 2.5 per cent sodium chloride solution is infused at 0.25 ml/kg wt/min. In the absence of ADH no change occurs in concentration (specific gravity) nor is the volume reduced.

Principles of treatment and nursing management

1. Treatment of underlying cause.
2. Pitressin tannate in oil, 5 units given intramuscularly. Dose varies with each child.

3. Pitressin snuff or Lypressin (nasal spray). N.B.: repeated use causes rhinitis (p. 372).
4. Drugs which suppress sodium resorption in the distal tubule, e.g. chlorothiazide. This leads to decreased urinary output.
5. Routine nursing care:
   a. During investigation include relevant observation; fluid charts, behaviour.
   b. Nutritional needs.
   c. Care of napkin area.
   d. Nose care when receiving 'snuff' treatment.

Other conditions involving the hypothalamus include: neoplastic processes, inherited autosomal recessive conditions, e.g. lack of subcutaneous fat, and accelerated growth or lesions of the hypothalamus which produce cerebral gigantism. The latter may be associated with cerebral injuries resulting from varying degrees of asphyxia occurring during pregnancy or during delivery of the child.

Precocious puberty

In this condition, secondary sexual characteristics appear before the age of 10 in boys and 8 to 9 years in girls. This includes appearance of pubic, axillary and facial hair, enlargement of external genitalia and deepening voice in boys, while in girls it includes menstruation, developing breast tissue and hair growth in pubis and axilla. It may be due to tumours of the posterior hypothalamus.

There is no known treatment but parents will require guidance and sympathy. In boys it may produce perverted behaviour which is generally met with understanding by the authorities.

Disorders of the anterior pituitary gland (adenohypophysis)

It is generally accepted that the essential lesion is in the hypothalamus and that the pituitary secretion is affected as a result of that lesion. The effects are therefore (1) oversecretion or (2) undersecretion of one or more trophic hormones.

There may, however, be lesions such as eosinophil adenomas of the anterior pituitary which cause gigantism or acromegaly, while compression of the anterior pituitary by chromophobe adenoma prevents secretion and gives rise to hypopituitarism.

INCREASED ACTIVITY

The following features can be recognised:

1. Increased growth, e.g. arms and legs, hands and feet enlarge if it occurs before epiphyseal fusion.
2. Acromegaly, i.e. assymetrical growth.
3. There may also be signs of thyrotoxicosis, hyperglycaemia and glycosuria.

Linear growth acceleration is due to increased levels of growth hormone in the circulation.

Principles of treatment and nursing management

1. Treatment depends on the presenting signs and symptoms, e.g. visual disturbances indicate removal of tumours by operative means or irradiation to arrest the tumour and halt the progress of the disease.
2. Cryosurgery. In this treatment a small canula is passed via the nose and a small volume of liquid nitrogen is introduced into the pituitary fossa. As it evaporates freezing takes place; temperatures of −25°C to −190°C can be obtained. At these temperatures crystals form in the gland, cell membranes are disrupted and the enzymes are destroyed.
3. Replacement of deficient pituitary hormone as a result of the treatment.
4. Routine nursing care plus:
   a. Careful observation during cryosurgery, e.g. transient diabetes insipidus may occur.
   b. Care of the child during radiotherapy (p. 106).
   c. Drugs to combat radiation effect.
5. Support for parents.

DECREASED SECRETORY ACTIVITY

Growth hormone deficiency

The child usually has a normal birth-weight and length, but during the first year of life there are already indications of retarded growth (Fig. 16.1). If the child is left untreated, the final height will probably be in the region of 140 to 145 cm.

Ossification is retarded and the closure of the anterior fontanelle is delayed up to a few years. The voice is high pitched. Hypoglycaemia is troublesome and children tend to waken at night, demanding food. This is due to thyroid and

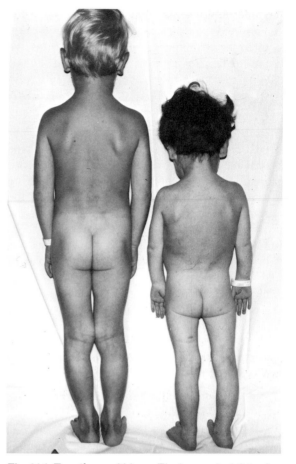

Fig. 16.1 Two 4½-year-old boys. The boy on the left is of normal height, the boy on the right is of small stature due to growth hormone deficiency.

adrenal deficiency which produces reduced tissue metabolism with a low blood sugar level (hypoglycaemia). There is also poor response to insulin.

Puberty is delayed and the genitalia remain small.

Investigation

1. Determination of fasting levels of growth hormone.
2. Determination of response to insulin (hypoglycaemia stimulates growth hormone secretion). The patient is fasted overnight or for 4 hours, if an infant:
   a. Fasting venous sample is taken.
   b. Intravenous insulin is given (0.1 units soluble insulin/kg/body wt).

c. Samples of venous blood are obtained at 30, 60, 90 and 120 minutes.

d. Glucose solution must be available to counteract the effect of insulin.

Principles of treatment and nursing management

1. Intramuscular injection of human growth hormone is continued for two years. This treatment is also effective where there is abnormality in the growth hormone structure. The defect seems to be inherited as an autosomal characteristic.
2. Routine nursing care.
3. Support and guidance for parents.

Corticotrophin deficiency

Clinical features

The features presented are those of adrenal insufficiency mainly of glucocorticoids and androgens (p. 278). The former produce anorexia, general weakness, frequent attacks of hypoglycaemia and hypotension. (Glucocorticoids are important for glucose formation and metabolism.) Androgen deficiency leads to incomplete puberty, that is scant secondary hair (pubic and axillary).

Investigations

1. Measurement of plasma cortisol level.
2. Measurements of serum electrolytes (low serum electrolytes are a positive finding).
3. Insulin unresponsiveness test (increases hypoglycaemia).

Principles of treatment and nursing management

1. During frank episodes glucocorticoid replacement is given.
2. Anabolic hormones (derivaties of androgens which promote protein storage and to some extent growth, are given). These also improve vigour, appetite and sexual development. Oestrogens should be used in girls.
3. Correction of hypoglycaemic attacks.
4. Routine nursing care.
5. Support for parents and child. This involves clear explanations regarding the cause and course of the disease, and during an episode, understanding of their anxiety.

Gonadotrophin deficiency

Clinical features

Secondary sex characteristics are poorly developed. In the male, the voice is high pitched; the testes are small. In females, menstruation may be slight or absent.

Principles of treatment

1. a. *Males.* Intramuscular injection of gonadotrophin and androgen. This should result in testicular enlargement.
   b. *Females.* Oestrogen therapy will lead to regular menstruation.
2. Support for parents and child. The treatment may be given as an outpatient. Since both parents and child will show a level of anxiety, the condition must be explained fully. Treatment is usually continued into adulthood. In the male, fertility may not be achieved and in the female, cyclical oestrogen administration is required throughout the reproductive period.

The thyroid gland

The thyroid gland lies at the sides of larynx and upper part of the trachea. Two hormones are manufactured in this gland, thyroxine and tri-iodothyroxine which consists of iodine and tyrosine.

The function of the thyroid hormones is to regulate the rate of metabolism in body tissues by increasing the energy available for cellular function, and heat production by the body. Deficient secretion of these hormones is termed hypothyroidism and increased secretion is hyperthyroidism.

Investigations

1. Blood levels of thyroxine and tri-iodothyroxine provide a direct indication of thyroid activity.
2. Determiniation of skeletal maturation, i.e. radiography to determine bone age.
3. In children over 2 years of age, serum cholesterol estimation is of value. (Cholesterol is raised if the child is suffering from hypothyroidism).
4. Radio-iodine tests. Thyroid hormones are rich in iodine and therefore iodine is a convenient

indicator of thyroid activity. Lowered uptake is found in hypothyroidism and raised in hyperthyroidism. Radioactive iodine is given either orally or i.v.

5. Thyroid scintiphotography is used in conjunction with the radio-iodine uptake test. Radioactive iodine is given orally and a scan camera picks up the impulses which are converted into photographic images.

6. There are other tests which can be carried out to aid diagnosis, e.g. biopsy and assessment of abnormal thyro-protein.

HYPOTHYROIDISM (CRETINISM)

The causes of hypothyroidism vary slightly with different age groups, but the clinical features are fairly similar. It is therefore convenient to look at the different causes in the two distinct age groups (1) neonatal period and (2) infancy and childhood.

1. NEONATAL PERIOD

Congenital thyroid hypoplasia

There is only a small amount of thyroid tissue and the severity of the hypothyroidism at birth depends on the extent of thyroid failure. It may function adequately for the neonate but will not be adequate for the 2-or 3-year-old. Despite the thyrotrophic hormone activity, the thyroid is generally not palpable.

Clinical features

Grunting respiration is an early manifestation and is due to partial obstruction of the airways by the large tongue. The cry is hoarse and throaty; the skin is wrinkled and dry, and the hairline is low; the hair itself is coarse, lustreless and straight. The fingers are short and frequently there is an umbilical hernia.

There is difficulty due to the large tongue, the lack of energy and drowsiness. A low body temperature and bradycardia (low pulse rate) are characteristic. Intestinal mobility is decreased, leading to infrequent bowel movements (Fig. 16.2).

Principles of treatment and nursing management

1. Drug administration. L-thyroxine sodium is given orally. The dose is small initially, about 0.0125 to 0.025 mg daily. Too large a dose

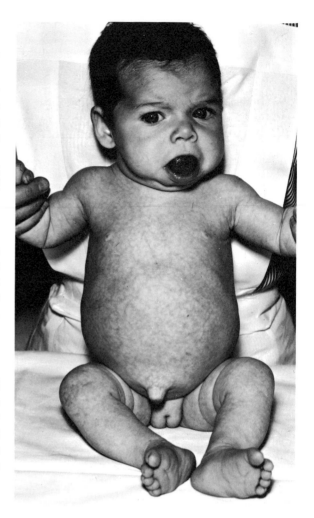

Fig. 16.2 Cretin. Note coarse features, large tongue and umbilical hernia.

would lead to sudden increased metabolic activity, to which the myocardium cannot respond. Treatment is life-long and the dose is gradually increased to meet the infant's needs.

2. The infant will be difficult to feed until the drug is effective; spoon feeding or naso-gastric feeding may be necessary to ensure adequate nutrition.

3. Careful observations:
   a. Pulse rate and rhythm.
   b. Level of alertness.
   c. Bowel movements (loose stools might indicate too high a dosage).

4. Routine nursing care.
5. Support for parents. This includes counselling and guidance because of the child's need to continue treatment throughout life. Frequent follow-up of progress, assessment and decisions regarding education for the child. The earlier the treatment is started, the less intellectual impairment is likely. However, the mental ability of the child depends on the degree of deficiency or inadequacy of the thyroid at the critical period in the development of the central nervous system and on the adequacy of the treatment.

Hypothyroidism due to inborn errors of thyroxine biosynthesis

This may be due to a defect related to an intra-thyroidal enzyme. There may be *thyroid enlargement* due to increased thyrotrophic hormone activity. Treatment and nursing management are along the lines described previously.

Maternal ingestion of 'iodide' substances

The mother has probably ingested iodide from drugs containing iodide, e.g. cough mixtures. Excess iodide causes defect in the binding of iodine to tyrosine. Iodide freely crosses the placental barrier causing thyroid swelling. If the swelling is large, it may cause obstruction of the upper air passages.

Treatment is along the lines outlined above. However, in these cases it may be necessary to carry out a tracheostomy or thyroidectomy to relieve respiratory obstruction. If there is no obstruction to breathing, then the drug can be withdrawn after several months provided the thyroid gland functions normally.

2. INFANCY AND CHILDHOOD

Hypothyroidism, in this group, can also be due to inborn errors of thyroxine biosynthesis. This can involve impaired uptake of iodine or defective enzymes. The treatment is life-long and is also based on L-thyroxine sodium which is increased in dosage with age.

Thyroidectomy may be required if the enlarged thyroid compresses the trachea or, if there is modular hyperplasia, there is a high risk of malignancy.

Chronic lymphocytic thyroiditis (Hashimoto's disease)

The gland shows a characteristic response to the antibodies, the cells becoming hyperplastic and failing to function. Girls are more commonly affected than boys. The thyroid is swollen and the child complains of discomfort. Disturbance of thyroid function is indicated initially by features of hyperthyroidism, such as sweating and agitation, but as the condition progresses, signs of hypothyroidism become evident.

The diagnosis is confirmed by tests for thyroid antibodies — tanned red cell agglutination, complement fixation and the immunofluorescent tests. They detect the presence of circulating antibodies to thyroglobulin, the thyroid epithelial cell microsomes.

Treatment aims at correcting the hypothyroidism with L-thyroxine sodium which is continued throughout life.

HYPERTHYROIDISM

Hyperthyroidism occurs when there is an excessive amount of circulating active thyroid hormone. It is most commonly seen as a result of increased production of thyroxine by the gland.

Neonatal hyperthyroidism

This is found in the infant whose mother is thyrotoxic. The maternal hormone has crossed the placenta and the new-born exhibits typical features of hyperthyroidism.

Clinical features

A persistently high fetal heart rate which persists after birth (190 to 220 beats per minute). The infant is very restless with warm, flushed skin and rapid breathing. Thyroid swelling and exophthalmos (bulging eyes) are obvious. In some cases the onset is delayed for a few days after birth and then progresses rapidly.

Principles of treatment and nursing management

1. Drugs: oral potassium iodide is given first and if the condition is not controlled, carbimazole 2.5 mg is added.
2. Observations:
   a. Heart rate.

b. Behaviour of infant, e.g. agitation.

c. Bowel movements.

3. Routine nursing care.

Hyperthyroidism in infancy and childhood

Hyperthyroidism tends to occur in increasing numbers with age. The greater incidence is between the ages of 11 and 15 years. The cause in this age group is now believed to be due to long-acting thyroid stimulator (**LATS**) a thyroid auto-antibody.

Clinical features

The onset is insidious. There is a sudden spurt of growth, tachycardia, nervousness, frequent rapid mood changes, insomnia, loss of weight and behaviour changes. As the condition becomes established there is intolerance to heat, palpitation, diarrhoea and further loss in weight.

The child looks flushed, has a staring 'glassy-eyed' appearance and varying degrees of exophthalmus. A fine tremor in the fingers can be detected when they are outstretched. The sleeping pulse is raised.

Principles of treatment and nursing management

1. This aims at reducing the child's excitability:
   a. Bed-rest.
   b. Drugs, e.g. phenobarbitone (30 mg twice daily).
   c. Drug to reduce the tachycardia.
   d. Carbimazole (10 mg 3 × daily).
   e. If hypothyroidism develops L-thyroxine sodium is added.
2. Operative treatment — thyroidectomy:
   a. Pre-operative treatment with above mentioned drugs, plus the addition of Lugol's iodine solution to reduce the vascularity of the gland.
   b. High carbohydrate diet to fortify the child against the operation.
   c. Partial thyroidectomy.
   d. Post-operative care:
      (i) Routine.
      (ii) Treatment for thyroid crisis, e.g. infusion of glucose/saline; sedation and sodium iodide.
      (iii) Observations for hypo- and hyper-thyroidism, laryngeal paralysis and hypoparathyroidism. Hypoparathyroidism may occur when parathyroid tissue has been removed during the thyroidectomy.
3. Routine nursing care.
4. Careful supervision and follow-up. Hypothyroidism frequently follows surgery when the remaining tissue is inadequate in meeting the metabolic needs of the body.

Disorders of the parathyroid glands

The parathyroid glands are ovoid bodies embedded in the thyroid gland. Parathormone is the hormone produced in the parathyroid glands. Its actions are as follows: (1) to maintain the concentraion of calcium in the extracellular fluid; (2) to cause a breakdown of bone substance by osteoclast formation; (3) to promote the renal tubular excretion of inorganic phosphate. It has a secondary action to stimulate absorption of calcium from both the intestine and renal tubule.

Investigations

1. Estimation of levels of serum calcium and phosphate.
2. Estimation of urinary excretion of calcium, phosphate and osteoclastic action (hydroxyproline).

As with other endocrine glands, the parathyroid glands may be the primary seat of disease, as in developmental anomalies or where there is over or underproduction of parathormone.

HYPOPARATHYROIDISM

This state can occur in both infancy and childhood. In infancy the causes are as follows: neonatal tetany, sex-linked hypoparathyroidism (sex-linked recessive inheritance) and congenital absence of the parathyroid glands.

Neonatal tetany

Clinical features

Tetanic convulsions begin between the third and 10th day of life. The convulsions are due to reduction in calcium concentration which causes an increase in the excitability of muscles and nerves. Tetany is characterised by spasms of the small muscles of the hands and feet and also spasms of the muscles which pull the vocal cords together (laryngeal stridor). Carpo-pedal spasms are not readily seen at this stage but there is a tendency to apnoeic attacks.

Principles of treatment and nursing management

1. Administration of calcium chloride given orally.
   This is usually effective within 48 hours.
2. In the acute stage, calcium gluconate 10 per cent solution is given intravenously.
3. Correction of hypoglycaemia if present.
4. Relief of convulsions with anticonvulsant (p. 307).
5. Administration of oxygen if apnoeic attacks are severe.
6. Routine nursing care.

Hypoparathyroidism in childhood
In childhood two types of hypoparathyroidism are recognised: (1) idiopathic and (2) pseudohypoparathyroidism. The cause in the former is unknown but an auto-immune reaction is suggested; the later (pseudo-hypoparathyroidism) is due to an unresponsiveness of the renal tubule to parathormone.

Idiopathic hypoparathyroidism

Clinical features
Onset is sudden with convulsions and tetany. Some children may be small but most are of normal height. Intelligence is normal at the time of onset but due to progressive intracranial calcification this may be impaired. There is a tendency to cataract.

Principles of treatment and nursing management

1. Vitamin D is given to raise the serum calcium level and maintain it. This is given orally and controls the convulsions and tetany.
2. Routine nursing care plus:
   a. Observation of general behaviour (mood changes).
   b. Observation of convulsions and tetany.

In *pseudo-hypoparathyroidism* the symptoms appear about 8 years of age. Convulsions and tetany are frequently seen. Dwarfism, moon-face and mental retardation are an important feature. Skeletal changes are also typical. Vitamin D_2 (calciferol) is given, but there is a possibility of vitamin D overdose. This is reflected by polyuria and the urine has a low specific gravity; there is constipation and anorexia. This is reversible when vitamin D is temporarily stopped. Phosphate absorption should also be restricted.

HYPERPARATHYROIDISM
This can be caused by adenoma and hyperplasia of the parathyroid glands.

Clinical features
Muscle weakness, lethargy, vomiting, anorexia, constipation, polyuria and polydipsia are characteristic features. Joints may be painful and swollen. The effects are due to hypercalcaemia.

Principles of treatment and nursing management

1. Removal of tumour (parathyroidectomy):
   a. Pre-operative care: i.v. infusion.
   b. Routine preparation (p. 128).
2. Correction of post-operative tetany, i.e. calcium and vitamin D is given.
3. Correction of dehydration by intravenous infusion.
4. Routine nursing care.
5. Support for parents.

The adrenal cortex

The adrenal cortex secretes three groups of hormones.

1. *Mineralocorticoids.* These influence the rate of sodium and potassium transported across cell membranes. *Aldosterone* is the hormone which acts predominantly on the distal tubules to cause sodium re-absorption and potassium excretion. Decreased activity of aldosterone causes severe sodium loss and potassium retention; this leads to hyponatraemia. Increased activity leads to sodium retention, resulting in polydipsia and hypertension.

2. *Glucocorticoids*. Their action is primarily on carbohydrate and protein metabolism. The main glucocorticoid is *cortisol* (hydrocortisone). Glucocorticoids promote the conversion of protein into glucose and increase glycogen deposition in the liver. In excess these hormones can cause hyperglycaemia. They have also an important function to increase the body's resistance to stress, e.g. infection, trauma.

3. *Androgens* (sex hormones). These are important in fetal development of the genital organs.

Investigations

The following are biochemical assessments of adrenal function:

1. Water excretion test. This is based on the inability of the kidneys to excrete a water load if there is serious adrenal insufficiency.
   a. It involves drinking large volumes of water after the bladder has been emptied. The fluid is taken within 20 to 40 minutes.
   b. Careful charting of hourly urinary output; urine is collected for 4 hours. The amount of urine passed varies with time. Normally 50 per cent of the urine is passed in the first 2 hours. If less is passed in that time or 50 per cent is passed in 4 hours then the test is negative.
   c. Cortisone acetate is given orally and water is given to drink 4 hours after; urine collection is started again as above. An increase in the percentage of urine passed would indicate a positive result and the greater the increase, the more indicative it is of adrenal insufficiency.
2. Urine test for chlorides. (See test for chlorides, p. 563.) One drop of 20 per cent potassium chromate sol. to 10 drops of urine. Add silver nitrate 2.9 per cent drop by drop (counting). Shake the tube after each addition until a yellow to brown colour develops. The number of drops of silver nitrate used gives the concentration of chloride in the urine as grams/litre.
3. Adrenal stimulation and suppression test (estimation of plasma levels).
   a. Corticotrophin stimulates production of cortisol.
   b. Dexamethasone suppresses cortisol levels.

DISORDERS OF ADRENAL CORTICAL FUNCTION

These include those which are due to insufficiency and those which are due to overactivity. In children, acute adrenocortical deficiency is more common than chronic insufficiency or excess hormone production. The disorders may be due to: (1) inborn errors of steroid biosynthesis when there is deficiency of the enzymes involved in the pathways of biosynthesis; (2) congenital defect of adrenal tissue, or damage to adrenal tissue (haemorrhage) or (3) interrelated disorders, e.g. renal tubular insensitivity to mineralocorticoids.

Inborn errors of steroid biosynthesis

This is a familial disorder transmitted as an autosomal recessive. Defective steroidogenesis results in adrenocortical hyperplasia where there is excessive production of androgens. This leads to abnormalities of external genitalia. The internal reproductive structures develop normally.

Clinical features

Since more than one steroid is involved there will be symptoms related to overactivity of androgens and underactivity of hormones such as aldosterone and cortisol, for example: (a) the testes remain undescended, small penis, clitoral enlargement, fused labia and single urogenital tube (androgen excess); (b) evidence of water and salt loss (aldosterone deficiency), i.e. failure to feed, hypotonia, vomiting and diarrhoea; (c) lack of cortisol leads to listlessness, anorexia, failure to thrive and hypertension.

Principles of treatment and nursing management

1. Correction of salt and water loss.
   a. Milk feeds are reconstituted with half-strength physiological saline. This prevents dehydration.
   b. If vomiting is present — intravenous replacement of both fluid and electrolytes.
   c. During fever, fruit juices reconstituted with normal saline are given.
2. Replacement therapy.
   a. Mineralocorticoid (if defect is 18 oxidase).
   b. Glucocorticosteroids. Cortisone acetate or cortisol is given. The drug is given

throughout the 24-hourly period, i.e. six times daily (adrenal activity is greatest during the night and it may be necessary to give a double dose at 10 p.m.).

c. Recognition of increased requirements during adrenal crisis and infection, i.e. increased dose of glucocorticoid.

3. If vomiting is present, drug administration is by intramuscular route.
4. Surgical correction.
    a. Pre-operative preparation:
        (i) Routine (p. 128).
        (ii) Specific, i.e. intravenous infusion of dextrose 5 per cent in half-strength physiological saline and intramuscular corticosteroid.
    b. Operation. Surgery of the perineum. The operative measures depend on abnormalities found during exploratory operation.
    c. Post-operative care:
        (i) Routine care (p. 131).
        (ii) Observation of symptoms indicating adrenal crises.
        (iii) Drug administration.
        (iv) Prevention of infection.
        (v) Continuation of intravenous infusion and gradual introduction of oral feeding regime.
5. Routine nursing care.
6. Support for parents. This includes: understanding of problems and genetic counselling by the specialist is essential; encouragement to take part in the nursing of their child; preparation of home; care and education of parents in the reappearance of the syndrome; frequent follow-up visits and close liaison between hospital, family doctor and home.

INFANCY AND CHILDHOOD

Adrenocortical insufficiency

It may be due to toxic destruction of the gland with associated deficiency of the salt and water-controlling fraction (Addison's disease), or to bilateral adrenal haemorrhage as a result of meningococcal septicaemia (Waterhouse-Friderichsen syndrome). The latter is found as an acute condition, the former as a chronic form.

Clinical features

1. Addison's disease. Anorexia, weakness, vomiting and diarrhoea leading to dehydration. Hypoglycaemia, convulsions and coma are also common features.
2. Waterhouse-Friderichsen's syndrome. Fever, nausea, vomiting and diarrhoea leading to dehydration. This may be followed by circulatory collapse, hypothermia, confusion and coma. Extensive purpura may also be present.

Principles of treatment and nursing management

A. Acute form

1. Treatment of infection by appropriate antibiotics, e.g. penicillin.
2. Replacement therapy. Intramuscular or intravenous hydrocortisone and intravenous aldosterone.
3. Relief of hypotension.
4. Intravenous infusion of plasma or blood.
5. Correction of fluid and electrolyte loss.

B. Chronic form

1. Intramuscular injection of deoxycorticosterone and cortisone acetate.
2. Intravenous infusion of glucose/saline.
3. Correction of hypoglycaemia.

C. Both forms

1. Routine nursing care plus: routine blood pressure measurements; care of the child with intravenous therapy; observations of signs of hypoglycaemia; daily weighing; fluid charts.
2. Protection from infection.
3. Support for parents. Recognition of their anxiety, particularly during a crisis; co-operation between hospital and community, close follow-up; explanation of long-term care of the child and need to keep in contact with hospital.

Adrenocortical overactivity

Adrenocortical overactivity in children is usually due to a secreting tumour in the adrenal cortex. The type of tumour can be identified by the hormones secreted and found in plasma and urine. The tumours may therefore give rise to (1) Cushing's syndrome, producing precocious puberty, large body with short limbs, moon-face, mood changes such as, euphoria, anxiety, depression, restlessness and apathy. Cushing's syndrome can also occur due to administration of corticosteroids or corticotrophin. In that case it is reversible on withdrawal of the drugs. Withdrawal must be gradual, since sudden withdrawal results in adrenal crisis. (2) Aldosteronism (rare in children). This is presented as polyuria, polydipsia, muscular weakness, cramp, headaches, hypertension, papilloedema and retinal haemorrhages. Due to loss of hydrogen ions there is alkalosis resulting in tetany and paraesthesia. Surgical removal is the only satisfactory form of treatment. (3) Increased androgens leading to masculinisation or feminisation. The former effects mainly females, the latter mainly males, though both sexes can be affected by either.

Principles of treatment and nursing management

1. Surgical removal, if the condition is due to tumours.
2. Routine pre-operative care (p. 128).
3. Specific pre-operative preparation:
   a. If there are features of Cushing's syndrome, corticosteroids must be given.
   b. If aldosteronism is present the serum potassium level is raised with spironolactone, 25 mg four times daily (a steroid which resembles aldosterone).
4. Post-operative management:
   a. Routine care (p. 131).
   b. May require steroid therapy.
   c. Measurement of blood pressure and central venous pressure.
   d. Accurate recording of fluid intake and output.
5. Routine nursing care.
6. Support for parents. Recognition of their anxiety, particularly during post-operative period.

Steroid therapy

Steroid hormones are normally secreted by the adrenal cortex. Their function has been discussed on page 277. Synthetic steroids are used for a variety of conditions, some of which have been discussed in relation to disorders affecting the adrenal cortex, i.e. as replacement therapy. There are, however, other clinical indications for systemic treatment with corticosteroids. These include the following:

1. In the treatment of leukaemia to suppress production of lymphocytes and shrinkage of lymphoid tissue.
2. In tissue transplantation to suppress the rejection phenomenon.
3. As an anti-inflammatory drug where disorders present with inflammatory signs and symptoms, for example nephrotic syndrome, thrombocytopaenic purpura and ulcerative colitis.

The choice of steroid depends on the disease and the effect it has. It is important that the nurse should be aware of the adverse effects of corticosteroid therapy, particularly if relatively high doses are required for anti-inflammatory activity.

1. Mineralocorticoid
a. Sodium and water retention; weight gain, oedema, raised blood pressure.
b. Potassium depletion; weakness, tiredness, alkalosis.
Observations: daily weighing, examination for oedema, measurements of blood pressure, fluid charts.

2. Glucocorticoid
a. The normal inflammatory responses to infection are reduced or masked. A latent tuberculosis foci may be reactivated.
   Nursing action: prevention of infection (isolation in hospital (p. 250).
b. *Osteoporosis* (steroids cause increased output of calcium and phosphorus). This interferes with skeletal growth. Steroids are gradually reduced and may be withheld for 48 hours to allow growth to take place.
   Nursing action: regular weight measurement. Protection against injury (fractures occur readily). Diet should contain calcium and protein.
c. Steroids produce insulin resistance and precipitate glyconeogenesis resulting in diabetes mellitus.

Nursing action: daily urine tests for evidence of glucose.

d. Steroids produce changed behaviour patterns such as increased excitability (affect the central nervous system).

Nursing action: observation of convulsions. Observation of behaviour, recognition of any deviation from the usual pattern. Keep the child calm, i.e. exciting situations should be avoided.

e. Moon-face, weight gain.

Nursing action: dietary control (low salt, high protein).

Diabetes mellitus

The syndrome of hyperglycaemia and glycosuria occurs whenever there is an absolute or relative insulin deficiency. Insulin is a protein hormone produced by the beta cells of the pancreatic islets. The rate of insulin release from the pancreas is determined chiefly by the blood glucose concentration. A rise in blood glucose concentration causes increased insulin secretion from these cells, whose membranes are freely permeable to glucose; a fall in blood glucose concentration causes decreased secretion.

The actions of insulin are many but the chief one appears to be its blood sugar-lowering effect. This it achieves by acting on cell membranes, promoting the transfer of glucose across the cell membrane and facilitating glucose phosphorylation within the cell. When insulin is absent or lacking, glucose remains in the circulation, resulting in hyperglycaemia. A raised blood glucose concentration means that the renal threshold is exceeded so that glucose appears in the urine (glycosuria). Excessive amounts of glucose in the fluid in the collecting ducts lead to an osmotic diuresis with an increased frequency of micturition. The loss of water and electrolytes which accompanies the frequency of micturition, causes thirst. If the fluid intake is insufficient, dehydration occurs. There is both intracellular and extracellular water loss as well as loss of cell potassium.

Because glucose cannot enter cells adequately, other sources of energy are metabolised to a greater extent, for example, protein and fat. Fat is the main source to be metabolised (protein tends to be spared), but there is failure to oxidise the circulating fatty acids; not all fats are broken down to CO_2 and H_2O; the molecules combine to form ketone bodies leading to ketoacidosis. The clinical features of diabetes mellitus are therefore related to the hyperglycaemia and ketoacidosis.

The manifestations of ketoacidosis include weakness, nausea, vomiting, abdominal pain and ultimately loss of consciousness (diabetic coma). Ketone bodies are excreted in the breath (giving it a characteristic odour of acetone) and also in the urine.

TYPES OF DIABETES

In children the most frequent type is where insulin production is inadequate. This can also be seen in neonates and some pubertal and post-pubertal cases of cystic fibrosis. Genetic factors are also believed to play a part and there may be destruction of beta cells due to immunological reactions and virus infections.

Juvenile diabetes mellitus

Clinical features

Glycosuria is usually the earliest sign which may be detected during routine urine tests. Polyuria and polydipsia may be present and bed-wetting in a child who has previously been dry at night is suspect. There may be weight loss, listlessness and muscular weakness.

When ketoacidosis is present, the features become more pronounced — anorexia, vomiting, abdominal pain, dehydration with sunken eyes, dry mouth and hypotension. The breathing rate is rapid and sighing; coma follows if treatment is not instituted immediately.

Investigations

1. Testing of urine — catheterisation may be necessary.
2. Blood sugar estimation. Normal blood sugar level is between 2.5 to 5.3 mmol/l (45 to 95 mg/dl); it is lower in the new-born period. In diabetes mellitus it may be above 11.1 mmol/l (200 mg/dl). A fasting level of 6.7 mmol/l (120 mg/dl) is diagnostic.
3. Blood pH, PCO_2 and bicarbonate are reduced.

Principles of treatment and nursing management

Stabilisation of diabetic state by:

1. Minimal biochemical disturbance:
   a. Subcutaneous injection of soluble insulin. This should at first precede each main meal and the dosage adjusted to maintain the urinary sugar at no more than 0.5 to 1 per cent and the fasting blood sugar between 80 and 120 mg/100 ml (4.4 to 6.7 mmol/l). This is changed to a single daily injection of insulin zinc suspension and crystalline (equal quantities). The combined dose approximates to ¾ of the total of soluble insulin given previously.
   b. Diet: apportioning of daily calories, for example:

   Carbohydrate 40 to 45 per cent.
   Protein 15 to 20 per cent.
   Fat 35 to 40 per cent.

   The carbohydrate intake is regulated throughout the day. It is convenient to calculate the amount of 10 g portions, with a total daily intake of 80 to 160 g, depending upon the age. The caloric intake is about 1000 kcal (4 MJ)/d at 1 year, increasing by about 100 kcal (0.4 MJ)/d for each year of age until puberty. Final stabilisation is only possible when the child is at home and normal activity is achieved.

2. Pre-coma and coma state:
   a. Weigh the child.
   b. Intravenous infusion of physiological saline (180 ml/kg body weight per day).
   c. Intravenous infusion of insulin. Once the infusion of saline has been established, insulin is given. An initial loading dose of 0.1 unit/kg of body weight of Actrapid or soluble insulin is given. This is followed by a constant insulin infusion of 0.1 unit/kg of weight/h. A syringe pump may be used. The rate of fall of blood glucose should not be too rapid because of the danger of cerebral oedema, which may follow a rapid reduction in blood osmolality.

   Soluble insulin can also be given intramuscularly when the dose is 0.05 unit/kg/body weight. Since it is given hourly it has the disadvantage in that the child is traumatised by repeated injections.

   d. Blood sugar level estimation after about 2 hours following the initial injection of insulin.
   e. Test urine for sugar and acetone (p. 564).
   f. Accurate fluid input and output chart.
   g. Hourly pulse measurement.
   h. Hourly blood pressure readings.
   i. Gastric aspiration if vomiting or if the stomach is distended.
   j. Observation of signs of infection and hypoglycaemia, and need to watch for signs of sudden change of level of consciousness, irritability, sweating and convulsions.
   k. Oxygen should be administered to all semi-comatosed or comatosed children unless their PO_2 is greater than 10 kPa (75 mmHg).

Dietary measures

1. When the child recovers from the acidotic state and is able to feed orally, he is given 180 to 210 ml milk with 5 g sugar. This is offered five times during the first 24 hours and, if this is tolerated, a controlled diet as described above is commenced.

2. Instruction of parents and child in dietary regulation, urine testing, blood sugar estimation and insulin administration is essential.
   a. The dietician will be responsible for teaching the parents and child how to control the diet. A diet sheet will be provided so that suitable alternatives can be chosen for a meal. Initially weighing may be advisable, but this soon becomes unnecessary as the family gain in experience.
   b. Urine testing. The parents and child are taught how to test urine for sugar and acetone. They will be issued with a test card and instructed to keep an accurate record. Clinitest tablets (sugar) and Acetest tablets or Ketostix are satisfactory.

   For assessing urinary sugar (g/100 ml):

Urine glucose (g/100 ml)	Blood glucose (mmol/l)	(mg/100 ml)
5	>20	>360
2–3	16–20	290–360
1	13–16	235–290
0.5	10–13	180–235
0–trace	<10	<180

The bladder should be emptied 30 minutes, prior to testing of urine, as this gives a truer indication of the blood glucose level at the time of testing.

c. Blood glucose monitoring. The parents and child are taught how to measure the blood glucose level by using a hypocount (Fig. 16.3) and are instructed to keep an accurate record. Both urine and blood sugar levels can be used as a means of determining the dose of insulin to be given on a sliding scale. For example, for a urine glucose level of 5 g/100 ml, 0.5 units/kg of body weight Actrapid can be given subcutaneously. The medical officer will prescribe a suitable regime.

Administration of insulin. The parents and child should be taught how to give the injection. It must be emphasised that this should be done regularly and throughout life. As the child grows older he will require increased amounts.

The parents and child should be competent in the following before returning home.

1. The site of injection — (upper outer aspect of thigh, abdomen, upper arm).
2. Method of administration.
3. Cleanliness of syringe and needle.
4. Prevention of infection — skin cleanliness, washing of hands.
5. Calculation of dose.
6. Availability of insulin.
7. Recognition of hypoglycaemia signs, i.e. irrita- bility, inability to concentrate, sweating, trem- bling, hunger pangs, faintness, headache, confusion and convulsions.
8. Knowledge of how to deal with hypoglycaemic state:
   a. Oral glucose, lump of sugar.
   b. Test urine.
   c. Give glucagon 1 mg i.m. if in coma.
   d. Seek medical assistance.
9. Carry identification card or disc stating that the child is suffering from diabetes mellitus.

Psychological aspect of diabetes in children
The nature of the illness presents many problems for parents and child. Because of the child's need for repeated injections and particularly in the initial stages, the parents tend to be over-indulgent and over-protective. Children quickly learn to use the situation and play on the anxieties of their parents. Difficulties can arise with respect to food intake and injections. Advice to parents should include guidance on the need for firmness tempered with understanding for the child's own difficulties and anxieties. The child must learn from the onset of the disease that he must obey certain rules regarding food and that he must accept the injections at the time stated. Although activity need not be restricted, it is important to recognise that there are greater energy require- ments during activity.

As the child grows older, he will realise the nature of his illness and that it is life-long. This can be traumatic and, particularly during puberty, lead to depression and feelings of inadequacy. For the child and young adolescent, holiday time can also present problems, and it may be wise to allow him to take part in group holidays for diabetic children. Here he can meet others with similar problems and learn to live within a community where his needs are recognised, but where he is not singled out as being special or different. Parents too will require understanding and help to cope with stressful situations. They should be encouraged to meet other parents with similar problems and to join the association formed for this purpose. The medical social worker will be able to give the address of the local group.

Schooling should not present any problems, but the school authorities must be aware of the child's

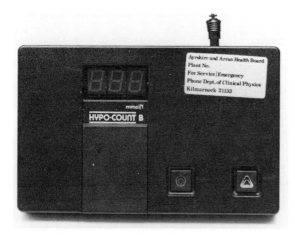

Fig. 16.3 Blood glucose monitor (Hypocount).

condition and be given clear instruction should help be required. This involves discussion of presenting signs of hypoglycaemia and how to handle the situation.

Hypoglycaemia

Hypoglycaemia means a blood glucose concentration below 40 mg/100 ml (2.2 mmol/l). Hypoglycaemia is a serious state, and the more so the younger the child.

Brain cells are least capable of survival if deprived of glucose (p. 296). Hypoglycaemia may occur in association with many diseases, for example in the neonate whose mother is a diabetic and who has been subjected to hyperglycaemia *in utero*; or as a complication of cold injury. (During the period of chilling the body stores of glycogen are adequate, but on warming an increased demand for glycogen occurs. The glycogen stores are diminished and the reserves cannot meet the demands on warming; see page 99.)

Choice of insulin

The choice of insulin will depend on the level of control desired or necessary, the age of the child and the duration of his diabetes. Insulins which are available at the present time are considered according to their length of availability in the body, i.e. whether short-acting, medium or long-acting.

Short-acting insulins

These insulins are mainly used in the treatment of diabetic ketoacidosis. It is, however, possible to give short-acting insulin in controlled cases. For example, the young active child may do well on one or two injections of soluble insulin and still maintain sugar-free urine. Each child will therefore require individual assessment based on his age, level of activity and evidence of pancreatic endocrine activity.

Insulins	Action begins (hours)	Action lasts (hours)	Peak of action (hours)
Insulin injection BP	1	8	3–6
Novo insulin	1	8	3–6
Actrapid MC	½	7	2½–5

Medium-acting insulins

These afford adequate 24-hour cover to certain children, e.g. young children with relatively mild and stable diabetes.

Insulins	Action begins (hours)	Action lasts (hours)	Peak of action (hours)
Insulin zinc suspension (semilente)	1½	15	5–9
Semitard	1½	15	5–9
Rapitard	1	22	4–12
Isophane (NPH)	2	24	4–12
Monotard	2	22	6–14

Long-acting insulins

Some of these can be used as a depot insulin in children of school age. Its action may not be sufficient to cover rises in blood sugar after meals, while it may lead to hypoglycaemia between midnight and breakfast.

Insulins	Action begins (hours)	Action lasts (hours)	Peak of action (hours)
Lente (IZS)	2	24	6–14
Ultralente	4	36	7–30
Protamine zinc	4	30	10–26

Mixing insulins

Two types of insulin may be given in one injection and to prevent contamination in the vial by traces of long-acting insulin on quick-acting insulin, the following methods are recommended (Craig, 1977).

Method 1. A volume of air, equivalent to the amount of insulin to be removed, is injected into both vials, while they are in the upright position. This is first done into the vial of the longer-action insulin. The needle is withdrawn and inserted into the second vial (shorter-acting) into which air equivalent to the amount of insulin is injected. The vial is then shaken and the insulin drawn off. The longer-acting vial is then shaken and insulin is also drawn off.

Method 2. Each vial is pierced by needles which act as air vents. A third needle is attached to the syringe and the required amount of insulin is withdrawn from each vial.

Leucine sensitivity

Leucine is an amino-acid and in susceptible children is known to provoke hypoglycaemia. Leucine is found in foods such as wheat, oats, rice, maize, eggs and cow's milk. The danger of leucine-induced hypoglycaemia lies in the risk of physical and mental retardation if it is not recognised and treated early.

Treatment aims at reducing leucine intake, by giving a low protein and high carbohydrate diet.

Part 5
Childhood disorders and their management

Chapter 17
Disorders of the nervous system

The nervous system is made up of three intimately connected parts; the central nervous system, the peripheral nervous system and the autonomic nervous system. The central nervous system consists of the brain and the spinal cord. The peripheral nervous system consists of the cranial nerves which arise from and travel to the brain stem and the spinal nerves which travel to and from the spinal cord. The autonomic nervous system is a part of the peripheral nervous system, but has its own particular anatomical features and special functions.

The peripheral nerves are made up of two kinds of fibres: (1) motor fibres, which are concerned with initiating movement of muscles, and (2) sensory fibres, which carry various sensations inwards to the central nervous system. Many nerves carry both motor and sensory fibres. These nerves branch repeatedly, carrying their fibres to every part and to all organs of the body.

The brain

The brain is a complex organ which is dominated by the cerebrum (Fig. 17.1). This is a twin structure, i.e. it is bilaterally symmetrical and consists of two parts called hemispheres, each a mirror image of the other. The nerves from one side of the body connect to one half of the cerebrum. The left half of the cerebrum is concerned with the right side of the body, and the right half of the cerebrum is concerned with the left side of the body. There are, however, some brain functions which are not mirrored, for example, control of speech is confined to one hemisphere.

The two hemispheres are separated in their upper parts by the median longitudinal fissure. This separation is not complete since at the base of the fissure, in the centre, a block of fibres called the corpus callosum connects the two halves of the

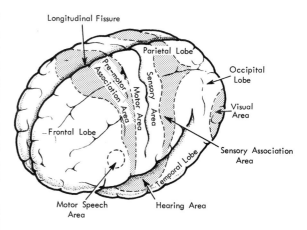

Fig. 17.1 The cerebrum of the brain, showing lobes and regions where specific functions have been identified.

cerebrum. These fibres are the means of communication between the two sides of the body.

A further structural variation is the division between 'grey' and 'white' matter. The 'grey' matter lies largely on the surface of the brain; the 'white' matter lies below, in the interior. The grey matter is known as the cortex and is 3 to 4 mm thick. It is wrinkled and fissured and envelops the entire surface.

There are recognised landmarks in the brain which have been artificially divided into lobes and regions. The occipital lobe is at the rear; the temporal lobes are at the sides; the frontal lobe is at the front behind the forehead and the parietal lobes are posterior to the frontal lobe. These divisions correspond very closely to regions which have particular functions in the control of bodily activity and in the processing of sensory information. In general terms, the cortex of the *parietal* lobes cortex contains those areas which are responsible for the co-ordination and control of sensory

289

input and motor output. The *frontal* and *temporal* lobes have much more diffuse and less understood functions relating to speech, learning, memory, intelligence and performance. The *occipital lobe* contains receiving centres for vision. There are also association areas of the cortex. These are concerned with treatment and analysis of sensory input and motor output. The association areas are found adjacent to the specific receiving zones.

Deep in the substance of the cerebral hemispheres are masses of grey matter. These constitute lower motor and sensory centres, and include lentiform and caudate nuclei (i.e. lower motor centres) concerned with modifying and co-ordinating *voluntary* muscle movement. Haemorrhage into this area results in jerky uncoordinated movements. Uncontrolled tremors of the hands follow degeneration of this tissue.

Thalamus (Fig. 17.2)

The thalamus consists of a large grouping of sensory relay and association nuclei transmitting sensations of pain, cutaneous and other sensory information to higher cortical centres. In the thalamus, white matter (which is widespread in the interior of the cerebral hemispheres) is found as a distinct feature. Examples are the corpus callosum and the internal capsule. The latter is a

narrow passage through which nerve fibres must pass. Damage to the areas leads to loss of sensation and paralysis on the opposite side of the body.

Hypothalamus (Fig. 17.2)

The term 'hypothalamus' refers to the grouping of small nuclei that are generally at the anterior portion of the cerebrum at the junction of the midbrain and thalamus.

This is an important structure and has a close link with the pituitary gland, which is actually innervated by neurons from the hypothalamus. This interrelationship has been found to be of crucial importance in the nervous regulation of endocrine gland functions. Minute nuclei which make up the hypothalamus are involved in eating, sexual behaviour, drinking, sleeping, temperature regulation and emotional behaviour. It is the major central brain structure concerned with the functions of the autonomic nervous system, particularly with its sympathetic division.

Meninges (Fig. 17.2)

These cover the brain and have a protective function. There are three membranes:

1. *Dura mater*. This is the tough outer membrane and has two layers. It lines the skull and by

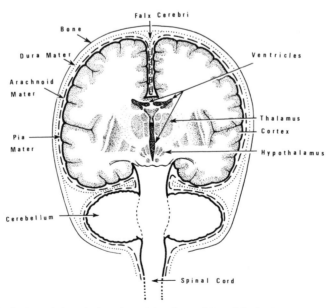

Fig. 17.2 The meninges of the brain and the spinal cord, nuclei and ventricles of the brain.

extending downwards through the foramen magnum also lines the vertebral canal. Between the layers lie the great venous sinuses.

2. *Arachnoid mater.* This is a thin fibrous tissue which loosely covers the brain and spinal cord. The space between the dura mater and arachnoid mater is the subdural space.

3. *Pia mater.* This is the innermost lining which is closely applied to all the folds and furrows. Between the arachnoid mater and pia mater is the subarachnoid space which contains cerebrospinal fluid.

The spinal cord is covered and protected by these meninges. The dura and arachnoid mater extend further down the vertebral canal than the spinal cord, thus forming a sac in the lumbar region from which cerebrospinal fluid can be withdrawn.

Ventricles and cerebrospinal fluid

Deep in each cerebral hemisphere is a cavity called the *lateral ventricle*. These two ventricles are connected by openings to a centrally place slit-like cavity, the third ventricle. A narrow channel (aqueduct of Sylvius) runs from the posterior part of the *third ventricle* through the midbrain below the cerebellum and widens to form the *fourth ventricle*. From this, a small channel continues down the spinal cord and its central canal.

Cerebrospinal fluid is formed in the choroid plexuses which are found as tufts of vascular tissue in the ventricles. Formation of cerebrospinal fluid is constant and under normal conditions circulates freely along the following path: from the fourth ventricle some of it flows into the central canal; some of it flows into the subarachnoid space, where it is reabsorbed by the arachnoid villi which project from the arachnoid mater into the venous sinuses. At various points, it collects to form pools of which the biggest is the cisterna magna, lying behind the medulla and above the foramen magnum. The normal flow of CSF is shown in Figure 17.7 (p. 300).

Composition of cerebrospinal fluid

It is a clear colourless fluid with a specific gravity of 1.005 to 1.008. Small amounts of protein (0.2 to 0.4 g/l), immunoglobulin (0.07 g/l) and sugar (2.5 to 4.8 mmol/l) are present as well as chlorides (0.72 to 0.75 g/l) and some urea. In diseases such as meningitis and encephalitis, the amount of protein is increased and sugar is increased in diabetes mellitus, but decreased in infection. The cerebrospinal fluid volume is as follows:

Infants: 40 to 60 ml
Young children: 60 to 100 ml
Older children: 80 to 120 ml
Adults: 130 to 150 ml

Fluid pressure

The normal pressure of the cerebrospinal fluid depends on a balance between its rate of secretion and its rate of absorption. The value in an adult in the lateral recumbent position varies between 100 and 120 mm H_2O. In the sitting position the

Table 17.1 Contents of spinal fluid

Contents	Values (normal)	Increased	Decreased
Protein	0.2–0.4 g/l	Meningitis Poliomyelitis	
IgG	0–0.07 g/l		
Sugar	2.5–4.8 mmol/l	Diabetes mellitus Uraemia	Bacterial meningitis
Cell count	0–5 mononuclear cells/mm^3	Encephalitis Bacterial meningitis Poliomyelitis Encephalitis	
Chloride	100–130 mmol/l	Uraemia	Meningitis

pressure can be 200 mm H_2O higher. The values in children vary with age and are as follows:

New-born: 50 to 80 mm H_2O
Infants: 40 to 150 mm H_2O
Older children: 70 to 200 mm H_2O

A rise in venous pressure which follows coughing or crying interferes with absorption and so raises the cerebrospinal fluid pressure. Compression of the internal jugular vein has a similar effect (Queckenstedt's sign).

Functions of cerebrospinal fluid

1. It serves as a fluid buffer, i.e. it forms a protective cushion for brain tissue.
2. It acts as a reservoir to regulate the contents of the cranium; if the volume of the brain or the volume of the blood increases, e.g. in cerebral tumour and overhydration, then the cerebrospinal fluid drains away; if the brain shrinks, more fluid is retained.
3. It is believed to serve as a medium for nutrient exchanges in the nervous system, and waste products from nerve cells are excreted into the cerebrospinal fluid.

Obstruction to the outflow of cerebrospinal fluid leads to hydrocephalus. It may be either internal when the excess fluid is in the ventricular system; or external when the excess fluid is in the subarachnoid space.

Brain stem

The brain stem links the spinal cord to the cerebrum. It is divided into three parts:

1. *Midbrain.* This contains nerve cells (nuclei) which receive certain specialised impulses from the eye and from the ear. It serves as a centre for both visual and auditory reflexes. The midbrain merges anteriorly into the *thalamus* and *hypothalamus*.
2. *Pons.* This contains the neurones of the sensory nuclei of the cranial nerves V, VI and VII. The white matter includes nerve fibres leading to the thalamus and links higher cerebral centres with the medulla and spinal cord.
3. *Medulla oblongata.* The group of neurones found in the medulla oblongata form the nuclei

of the cranial nerves VIII, IX, X, XI, and XII. In addition, several vital autonomic nuclei concerned with respiration, cardiac activity and gastro-intestinal function, are located in the medulla.

Cerebellum

The cerebellum lies above and behind the brain stem, and is also joined to it. It is separated from the cerebral hemispheres by a tough, tent-shaped sheet of meninges (tentorium). The cerebellum is similar to the cerebrum in that it has many fine convolutions of its surface grey matter. Deep in its substance are additional groups of neurones. The cerebellum contains centres which are concerned with balance, maintenance of posture and with the fine control of movement. It is linked to other parts of the brain and spinal cord by important nerve tracts.

Lesions of the cerebellum

Lesion of one side of the cerebellum will cause ataxia (unsteadiness) down the same side of the body, together with loss of tone, reduction of reflexes and a tendency to stagger to that side when walking. This is because the fibres from the cerebellum either remain on that side or, if they cross the midline, cross back again after a short distance.

Spinal cord

The spinal cord is continuous with the medulla oblongata and lies within the vertebral canal. Running through its centre is the spinal canal containing cerebrospinal fluid and connecting with the ventricles of the brain. Thirty-one pairs of nerves originate from the cord and are named according to their related anatomical sections — cervical, thoracic, lumbar, sacral. Each of these sections or segments receive sensory nerve roots and give off motor nerve roots on either side. These roots join to become peripheral nerves, which pass out between the vertebrae.

The spinal cord runs along the vertebral canal from the foramen magnum to the first lumbar vertebra. Below the first lumbar vertebra, many of the peripheral nerves pass in a downward direction to their exit foraminae in the lumbosacral region.

These resemble a horse's tail and so are called the cauda equina.

The spinal cord has two specific functions:

1. It acts as a centre for reflexes which are muscular and autonomic responses to body stimuli, e.g. stretch reflex (knee jerk), flexion reflex (removing the limb from painful stimuli).
2. It provides channels down the spinal cord (descending tracts) for nerve fibres from the cerebral cortex and other brain structures to the motor neurones. It also provides channels, which convey the bodily sensations up the spinal cord to the brain (ascending tracts).

The spinal cord differs structurally from the cerebrum in that the grey matter, containing nerve cell bodies, is found mainly in the central portion, and the white matter consisting of tracts of fibres, is situated in the areas surrounding the grey matter.

Lesions of the spinal cord
Complete destruction of the cord at any point produces paralysis (loss of power) and loss of sensation of all those parts of the body which are supplied by nerves leaving or entering the cord *below the level* of the lesion. A lesion in the neck, for example, paralyses the arms, legs and respiratory muscles. It is possible to determine the exact level of the lesion by determining the point where loss of sensation changes to normal sensation.

Partial cord damage produces different effects. For example, damage to one lateral half of the cord will affect:

1. One pyramidal tract, producing paralysis *on that* side below the lesion.
2. One side of the posterior columns, causing loss of position sense *on that* side below the lesion.
3. One spinothalamic tract, causing loss of pain and temperature sensation below the lesion, but the sensory loss will be on the other side of the body.

The spinal cord is only a part of the nervous system which, throughout the length of the body, forms the junction of the nerve paths arriving from and leaving for all regions with which the nerve fibres communicate.

The reflex
The simplest complete reaction of the system is a reflex one. There are many reflexes which are extremely complex, being a combination of a number of simpler reflexes.

A reflex is a reaction initiated by a stimulus to some nerve, which transmits the impulse to other nerves by connections within the central nervous system. Reflex action is an *involuntary* one caused by the stimulation of an afferent (sensory, ingoing) nerve ending or receptor. The nerves which are involved in transmission of the impulse and its reflection from the central organ, are known as a 'reflex arc'.

Receptors
These are special cells which are adapted to specific stimulation, e.g. touch, cold, pain, heat; others, called *proprioceptors*, are lying within muscles, joints, ligaments, fascia, etc. The reactions which are induced in these structures are followed by reflex reactions initiated from proprioceptors.

Reflex activity will be affected when there are lesions of the motor system. For example, lesions of the upper motor neurones show exaggerated tendon reflexes, while in lesions of the lower motor neurones tendon reflexes are absent (Fig. 17.3).

Structure of nervous tissue
The structural unit is the nerve cell with its own cell body, dendrites (ingoing fibres) and axon (outgoing) processes. The cell and its fibres constitute the neurone. There is no direct cytoplasmic continuity with other nerve cells, but neurones are linked in the nervous system at a synapse.

A *synapse* (Fig. 17.4) is a junction of neurones by which nerve impulses are transmitted within the nervous system. It is usually formed between the axon of one neurone and the cell body or dendrite of another. The two structures do not form an actual connection but rather a close approximation to one another. The nerve fibres end in small swellings which almost touch the cell body or dendrite of another neurone. There is always a gap between them.

The importance of the synapse is that all activity of the brain and all behaviour of organisms depend

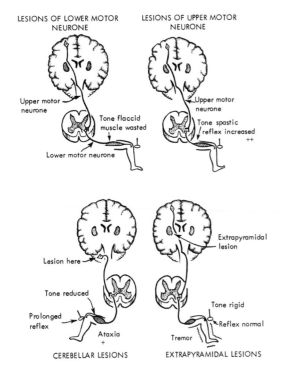

Fig. 17.3 Lesions of the motor system.

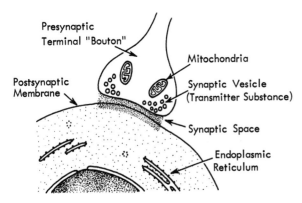

Fig. 17.4 Synapse.

on the interconnections and synaptic interactions between neurones. There are different types of synapse which, according to Eccles (1964), mediate postsynaptic excitation and postsynaptic inhibition. It is also suggested that presynaptic processes occur (inhibition and excitation).

The mechanism of synaptic activity is initiated by the arrival of axonal signals or impulses. These trigger off a chemical mechanism. The release of particular chemical substances which diffuse across the gap between the pre- and postsynaptic membrane interact at the postsynaptic side with specific receptors. This triggers off a sequence of postsynaptic events which result in the firing of the postsynaptic neurone.

The chemicals are known collectively as transmitter substances (excitatory and inhibitory). Substances which are known to play a part include acetylcholine, noradrenalin, serotonin and dopamine. To stop the activity of the transmitter at the postsynaptic site, the postsynaptic cell has a mechanism for destroying the transmitter almost as soon as it arrives. This is the action of enzymes which break down the transmitter molecules into inactive substances; for example, in the case of acetylcholine the enzyme is cholinesterase.

Certain drugs are known to interfere with transmitter substances — curare blocks the effects of acetylcholine at the neuromuscular junction. A similar blockage causes myasthenia gravis, the clinical features of which are skeletal muscle fatigue and weakness which rapidly become worse when the muscle is used, especially towards the end of the day. Nerve activity can be restored by the administration of a substance like physostigmine which inhibits the action of the enzyme. This prolongs the effect of acetylcholine which, if it persists, will lead to excessive activity at the neuromuscular junction.

A defect of neurohumoral transmission which affects children is the Riley-Day syndrome (familial dysautonomia). This is inherited as a recessive trait and has been found predominantly in Jewish children.

Nerve fibres

The axon, when it leaves the central nervous system, acquires a covering of fatty insulating material called myelin.

The myelin coat is incomplete and is interrupted at intervals along the course by nodes (nodes of Ranvier). Very small diameter fibres have no myelin sheath. Current flows in and out only at these nodes. Conduction of an impulse is more rapid in myelinated than in non-myelinated fibres. All the postganglionic fibres of the autonomic nervous system are non-myelinated and these are numerous in the central nervous system.

Nerve impulse

The function of the nerve fibre is to conduct the nerve impulse. The nerve impulse is usually generated in the nerve cell and travels along the axon. It is a physio-chemical change, e.g. oxygen consumption, carbon dioxide and heat output; energy substances are metabolised and various biochemical substances are formed. These activities occur not only in nerve cells but also in all other types of cells. However, the neurone is a specilised cell designed to conduct impulses and this involves a number of unique physico-chemical phenomena. The active nerve cell generates voltages which can be measured. These are centred on the cell membrane which allows the passage of potassium ions but not sodium ions. This means that there is a high concentration of potassium *inside*, and a low concentration of potassium *outside* the cell. This is reversed with respect to sodium, which is high outside and low inside the cell. In the resting state, the cell membrane is polarised.

Stimulation of a nerve causes loss of potassium and sodium enters the cell. These ionic movements provide an immediate source of energy for the conduction of impulses. However, this increased permeability to sodium ceases after 0.001 second but potassium moves out more freely. Once the action potential develops, current flows in where it occurs and flows out again at a more distant region (non-myelinated fibre). If stimulation occurs immediately after an action potential, the fibre will not respond. This brief period (about 1 millisecond) is called the absolute refractory period. The speed of an impulse depends on the size of the axon, the presence or absence of myelin, temperature, etc.

Damage to nerves

Peripheral nerves can be injured and injuries can be of varying severity, for example:

1. Pressure on the nerve, interfering with blood supply and oxygen, affects its function.
2. Damage to the axon may lead to death of the axon. If the endoneurial tubes are not broken, then regeneration of the nerve fibre can take place.

Repair begins about 20 days after nerve section and is complete in about 80 days. Cell repair may occur even if the axon does not regenerate.

Afferent neurones

If there is damage to the central axons of the posterior roots (e.g. due to syphilis), the ganglion cells show very slight changes. The synaptic terminals in the spinal cord swell after 24 hours, begin to disintegrate in 3 days, and disappear within 6 days. This will interfere with synaptic transmission of impulses.

Central nervous system

Most of the affected cells atrophy completely. The atrophy is more intense when fibres are cut close to their parent cells.

Regeneration of nerves

During degeneration, regeneration of the nerve fibre begins and the daily rate of growth is 0.25 mm in the junctional area of scab tissue, and 3 to 4 mm in the peripheral stump. Each structure of the fibre gradually regenerates and completion of the medullary sheath occurs within one year. Connections are established, though many fibres do so with new kinds of endings, for example a touch fibre connecting with a temperature receptor.

There may also be functional imperfections. Skin sensitivity is reduced and areas of anaesthesia may be present if skin receptors fail to establish central connections.

Pathway for voluntary motor impulses

The pathway for impulses, which control the movements of the skeletal muscles, consists of an upper and lower link. These two links are known as the *upper* and *lower* motor neurones. They are connected in the spinal cord. The upper motor neurones are those from the cerebral cortex to the spinal cord. The lower motor neurones are from the spinal cord to the periphery. Injury or lesions of the *upper motor neurones* lead to:

1. Slight wasting of muscles.
2. Weakness of muscle.
3. Spasticity, i.e. increased tone.
4. Exaggerated tendon reflex.

Injury or lesions of the *lower motor neurones* lead to:

1. Marked wasting of muscle.
2. Marked muscle weakness.

3. Flaccid tone.
4. Absent tendon reflex (Fig. 17.3).

In addition, lesions of other systems which influence motor activity also cause abnormality of function of the areas supplied by these systems, such as cerebellar lesions leading to decreased muscle tone, intention tremor and marked ataxia. The *sensory* system too will be affected if damage occurs in any part of the system. Damage to sensory fibres causes loss of sensation over the area from which the particular fibres have come, for example, loss of pain sensation (analgesia) and loss of light touch (anaesthesia).

Neurological disorders

Damage to any part of the brain will produce brain malfunctions. Tumour of the brain creates considerable pressure on other cells either killing them or distorting their activity. Small scars in the midst of healthy tissue may act as the focus for epileptic attacks; massive electrical discharges start at the focus and radiate until a large part of the brain is involved. Genetic disorders, in which particular enzymes or hormones fail to be produced, interfere with brain development, for example phenylketonuria, Down's syndrome (mongolism). There are also a variety of viral or bacterial diseases in which irreversible central or peripheral nervous system damage may result, for example meningitis or poliomyelitis.

Brain damage due to hypoxia

Cerebral hypoxia is defined as an inadequate supply of oxygen to the brain. This can be caused by acute cardio-respiratory failure, hypoglycaemia, anaesthetic drugs and prolonged convulsions.

Nerve cells in the brain are the cells in the body most sensitive to lack of oxygen. Unlike many other cells, these cells must have oxygen available to them at all times if they are to function normally. If nerve cells are deprived of oxygen for more than a few minutes, they die and once they are destroyed, they cannot regenerate. The supply of oxygen to the brain depends on the cerebral blood flow and the oxygen content of the blood. The cerebral blood flow depends on the cerebral perfusion pressure, which is the difference between arterial blood pressure and intracranial pressure. There is an intrinsic mechanism available known as *autoregulation* which ensures that the cerebral blood flow remains within normal limits. When the blood pressure falls, the arterioles of the brain dilate so that cerebral blood flow can remain fairly constant. Conversely, when the blood pressure increases, the arterioles constrict so that cerebral blood flow does not increase.

Psychological physiology

This section looks at the behavioural aspect of brain activity as distinct from the motor and sensory activity. The human brain is able to respond to stimuli other than internal and external environment. These concern many non-specific behavioural phenomena such as 'alertness', 'attention', 'arousal', 'sleep', etc. There are specific areas which are believed to serve general functions of inhibition, excitation and integration of brain activity. One of these areas is the ascending reticular activating system which is located in the brain stem; another is the diencephalon which contains the hypothalamus, thalamus, pituitary gland, optic tracts, etc. Impulses spread from the brain stem to the cerebral cortex which keeps the brain in a state of activity. It has been found that different regions are associated with specific functions, e.g. waking and deep sleep.

There are regions of the cortex called 'association areas'. These are concerned with relating cortical activity to behavioural variables like habituation, attention and learning. It is also interesting to look at the neurophysiological function of discrimination, i.e. the ability to select the various types of sensory information.

The neuronal basis of learning is also considered by many to be in the nature of physical-chemical changes. Learning, according to psychologists, can be defined as a semi-permanent change in behaviour and from the point of view of a physiologist it represents a change in neural substance. Biochemical studies relating to acetycholine and ribonucleic acid have been undertaken but no direct evidence is as yet available. However, it is accepted that changes in synaptic action during learning involve increased or decreased activity in excitatory and inhibitory neurones, with associated changes in RNA content.

Other areas of brain activity to be considered in

behavioural terms are intelligence, emotions and motivation, thinking and reasoning. The nature of these activities has not yet been defined, yet interference with any one of these has a profound effect on the behaviour of the individual. The causes of abnormal function of intelligence, for example, have been found to be related to enzyme deficiencies or genetic anomalies, but damage to brain cells due to infection or prolonged convulsions may also occur. Drugs too interfere with normal thought processes and emotions when they alter the neuronal environment.

The central nervous system is a highly complex one which is involved in every body function. Knowledge of its structure and function should therefore help in understanding the effect of damage to any part of this system on the behaviour of the individual and on the related function.

Defects of the nervous system

The fetal cerebrum appears as a recognisable structure at about 28 days' gestation, when the anterior end of the neural tube shows a globular expansion. Gradually differentiation into the various structures of the brain appears and differentiation of neuroblasts leads to formation of neurones and glial cells.

The brain of the full-term infant contains the full adult complement of neurones but its weight is only about one-third of that of the adult.

Abnormal influences occurring before the sixth month of gestation tend to affect development of the gross structure of the brain and to diminish the total neuronal number. Defects can occur due to pathological influences affecting myelination, i.e. retarding it. Loss of brain substance due to destructive lesions occurs in late fetal and early infancy periods. Among the many abnormalities are: (1) *microcephaly* where there is defect in the growth of the brain as a whole. The head is small in size, the frontal lobes are stunted and the cerebellum is often disproportionately large, and (2) *anencephaly* where there is an absence of the cerebral hemispheres. When it is replaced by a large fluid-filled cavity it is termed hydroencephaly. Head size may be normal or slightly enlarged and convulsions may occur. The diag-

nosis is confirmed by transillumination of the skull.

Disordered function of nervous tissue

From the discussion of the structure and function of the nervous system, it should be easier to understand abnormal function due to damage to any part of the system. The degree of impaired function depends on the damage done to he tissue. Nerve cells which are totally destroyed will not function and the effect of this can be readily recognised, for example, acute anterior poliomyelitis. Some nerve cells are partially damaged and can recover, others are extensively stimulated or 'irritated' into abnormal activity. Involvement of motor cells results in convulsions and, if sensory nerves are affected, there is pain and tingling.

THE NEONATE

Maldevelopment of the central nervous system is a common abnormality found in the neonatal period. The causes in most cases are unknown, though genetic factors are recognised as playing a part. Abnormalities of other systems may also be associated with maldevelopment of the central nervous system.

Spina bifida

In this condition the vertebral arches fail to fuse posteriorly. The functions of the vertebral column are to provide a rigid structure as part of the skeletal system and to give protection for the important communicating system of which the spinal cord is an integral part.

Instead of having a single spinous process projecting posteriorly, the arch on either side projects forming a bifid spine. It is always present in the lumbar, thoracic or cervical regions where meningocele or myelomeningocele defects are present (Fig. 17.5).

Meningocele

Meningocele is a protrusion of the convering of the spinal cord through the spina bifida and is visible as a bulge on the surface. The cystic swelling is covered by skin which may be very thin.

This abnormality may be corrected by surgery in certain cases. The operation consists of excision of the meningocele and closure of the dura mater.

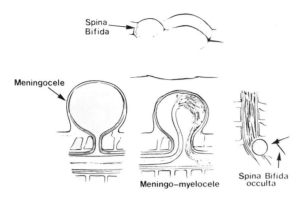

Fig. 17.5 Different types of spina bifida.

The skin is then closed over the defect. Hydrocephalus is a likely complication which may require drainage (p. 299).

Meningo-myelocele and myelocele

In these defects the spinal cord itself may enter the sac. The exposed nervous tissue will have suffered some intra-uterine damage. If the neural plate is left exposed after birth, further damage occurs as a result of infection and of drying of the nerves. The severity of neurological involvement depends on the extent of the malformation. This can range from paralysis of some muscles of the lower limbs, to gross deformity due to the paralysis of some groups of muscles and to overactivity of others.

The areas affected are the motor and sensory nerve supply to the lower limbs and the nerve supply to the bladder and rectum; normal sphincter tone is seldom present. In these lesions there is usually a leak of cerebrospinal fluid, even though the membranous sac is closed. The lower end of the spinal cord is imperfectly developed and the nerve roots, arising in the region of the exposed cord, may be deformed.

Principles of treatment and nursing management
1. Pre-operative care:
   a. Immediately following birth a sterile saline-soaked dressing covered with polythene should be applied, or the exposed lesion should be covered by a non-stick dressing, e.g. Telfa pads, to prevent the exposed nervous tissue becoming dry.
   b. Routine neonatal pre-operative care (p. 161)

with particular emphasis being placed on maintenance of body temperature which can quickly fall. In some centres the infant's trunk is placed in a plastic bag to help prevent the heat loss which can occur due to the wet surface of the lesion.
   c. A record of muscle activity in the lower limbs and anal sphincter will be made by the physiotherapist.
   d. Occipito-frontal head circumference is measured and charted.
   e. An X-ray of the spine will be ordered.
   f. A photograph of the lesion may be taken.
2. Operation. The exposed cord is enclosed in dural covering and the skin is sutured over the repaired dura. When the gap is large, a greater amount of skin has to be used to cover the defect. In these infants suction drains are inserted under the flaps.
3. Post-operative care:
   a. General neonatal post-operative care (p. 131).
   b. Oral feeding may be offered 4 hours after operation.
   c. If a wound suction drain is in place it should be checked hourly to ensure that no twisting or kinking of the tubing has occurred and that the negative pressure in the container is maintained. Fluid may stop draining approximately 2 or 3 days post-operatively, when the drain can be removed. The wound dressing will probably be left intact, with regular inspections, until the sutures are removed 10 to 12 days after operation.
   d. Due to lower limb paralysis, a full range of passive movements is performed daily. This helps to prevent fixed deformity of the joints and should be continued at home by the parents, after they have had a demonstration of the technique. If other congenital deformities are present, for example talipes equino-varus or dislocation of the hips, appropriate treatment is given.
   e. To prevent sores developing, some of these babies require more frequent repositioning than normal.
   f. Due to a defective nerve supply to the bladder, the infant may dribble urine continuously. Care must be taken that the

skin over the perineum and buttocks remains intact and regular nappy changing with careful cleaning and drying of the skin is essential.

A few of these infants have complete retention of urine and the surgeon may order gentle bladder expression to be carried out at regular intervals, probably 4-hourly.

Routine specimens should be examined for urinary infection to which these infants are prone and the appropriate antibiotic can then be prescribed.

A urinary ultrasound can be helpful in determining the presence of any anomalies.

g. Rectal prolapse may be an early problem due to pelvic floor muscle paralysis and strapping the buttocks should be attempted. If unsuccessful, a peri-anal suture may be required.

Some infants become constipated, therefore it is essential to record the type of faeces passed and also how often. It is unusual, however, for a neonate to be constipated severely enough to require medication.

h. Head circumference is measured and charted once or twice weekly. There is often an initial increase in the measurement following closure of the spinal defect and if this increase continues and hydrocephalus is developing the appropriate treatment will be given.

i. Support for parents. The infant is admitted to the neonatal unit soon after birth. The mother may or may not have held her baby but will be in a state of shock. It is vitally important that a great deal of time is given to the parents as this is a condition with many potential problems which some may find hard to understand or to accept. The full extent of the abnormality will be explained to the parents who should be given every opportunity to discuss their problems with the surgeon and senior nursing staff. It not only involves the immediate treatment but also subsequent treatments, nursing care of the infant, assessment regarding educational possibilities and any related problem.

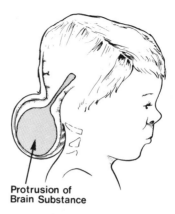

Protrusion of
Brain Substance

Fig. 17.6 Encephalocele.

Genetic counselling should be arranged as should any follow-up care; some parents find parent-group meetings and associations of benefit, and they should therefore be made aware of their existence.

Encephalocele (Fig. 17.6)

In this condition there is a defect in the occipital bone through which the meninges, containing brain tissue, protrude. These swellings may be very large, containing the cerebellum and the occipital lobe of the cerebrum. There may also be a massive quantity of cerebrospinal fluid in the swelling. Treatment consists of excision of the sac and salvaging as much of the brain tissue as possible, and then closing the defect. Nursing care is similar to that described for meningo-myelocele.

Hydrocephalus (Fig. 17.7)

Hydrocephalus in the neonatal period is almost always congenital in origin and may be associated with meningo-myelocele. In older infants and children it can follow meningitis, but in some cases there is no history of infection, nor is there any obvious anatomical abnormality.

Hydrocephalus is an abnormal enlargement of the cerebral ventricles caused by an increased pressure gradient between the intraventricular fluid and the brain.

Causes

Hydrocephalus existing alone without a spina bifida may be due to:

1. Stenosis and forking of aqueduct.

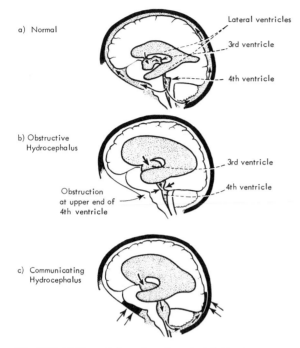

Fig. 17.7 (a) Normal flow of cerebrospinal fluid. (b) Obstructive hydrocephalus. (c) Communicating hydrocephalus.

2. Congenital obstruction or absence of the foramina of Monro, Magendie and Lushka (not common). Obstruction in the roof of the fourth ventricle leads to gradual development of hydrocephalus.

Types
Two anatomic types are distinguished:

1. Obstructive or non-communicating hydro cephalus where there is interference with the circulation of cerebrospinal fluid within the ventricular system itself and the fluid cannot reach the subarachnoid spaces, e.g. defect in the aqueduct or foramina of the fourth ventricle.
2. Communicating hydrocephalus, where the pathways inside the ventricular system are open and the ventricular fluid is able to move freely into the spinal subarachnoid space.

Clinical features
Where the degree of hydrocephalus is advanced, the head will be large and the fontanelles and

sutures wide. The forehead is bulging and there may be intraventricular haemorrhage due to birth trauma.

There is also the characteristic 'setting sun' sign of the eyeballs (Fig. 17.8). This is considered to be due to the expanding brain causing depression of the orbital roofs and downward displacement of the eyeballs. Cranial nerve paralyses are common, e.g. sixth nerve palsy, producing convergent squint as found in older infants.

Principles of treatment and nursing management

1. Special investigations, e.g. ventriculostomy and radiography.
2. Introduction of a drainage system (Fig. 17.8), e.g. Holter valve: medium and low pressure valves are available.

The valve consists of two reed check-valves made from silastic, which are housed in stainless steel tubes and which are connected to a reservoir of silastic. Each reed check-valve contains a slit that opens at a constant pressure and closes as soon as the pressure falls below 42 mm water (normal pressure valve).

The valve lies beneath the scalp behind the right ear and drains the right lateral cerebral ventricle into the superior vena cava. At the end of this catheter is a step-down filament

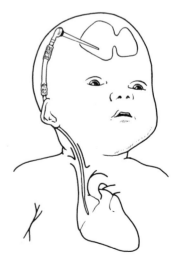

Fig. 17.8 Holter valve drainage system incorporating venticulostomy in a child with hydrocephalus (note also the 'setting sun' sign of the child's eyeballs).

which is directed into the right atrium of the heart. The valve and wound may become infected and to overcome this a ventriculostomy is performed and a reservoir is introduced. This allows repeated aspiration with a fine needle, of cerebrospinal fluid through the silastic cap. Through this cap, antibiotics, air and contrast media can also be injected directly into the ventricles.

3. Post-operative care: routine care (p. 131):
   a. Position of infant. The head of the infant should be raised to promote drainage. If drainage is excessive, the infant should be nursed flat or in the head-down position. Rapid drainage can be recognised by a grossly depressed anterior fontanelle, vomiting and, occasionally, shock. The infant should be positioned on the left side, as lying on the side of the valve should be avoided for the first week because of the danger of injury to the thin skin covering the valve.
   b. Feeding. If there is no vomiting, feeds can be started 6 hours after operation.
   c. Pumping of valve. This should not be done routinely but if it is necessary, then gentle milking is preferred to vigorous pumping.
   d. Open drainage. If there is an obstruction in the closed drainage system, cerebrospinal fluid may be drained into a water-sealed container, which should be changed at regular intervals. It may lead to loss of fluid and electrolytes, requiring adjustment to the milk formula.
4. An alternative treatment for infantile hydrocephalus is by drug therapy. The drug is isosorbide, a derivative of mannitol (osmotic diuretic). It is given orally in carefully controlled dosage and during its administration, biochemical studies are necessary to ensure that electrolyte balance is maintained. Biochemical complications such as hypernatraemia, acidosis and raised blood urea may occur. It had been found (Lorber, 1975) that infants with moderate hydrocephalus usually respond well, although some still require a shunt. Acetazolamide, which diminishes production of cerebrospinal fluid, has been found useful in mild, slowly progressive hydrocephalus, but it causes side-effects such as drowsiness and mental confusion.

INFANTS AND CHILDREN

Head injuries

Birth injury to the skull, leading to intracranial damage is a serious form of birth trauma. It may lead to extensive lacerations and gross cerebral damage which could be fatal.

Intracranial injuries may result in cerebral palsy, hydrocephalus and retardation in mental development. Head injuries in children are common and usually follow road accidents or falling.

Cerebral oedema may follow head injury. It is very dangerous and can result in intracranial hypertension. If it is due to vasogenic factors then fluid accumulates because of increased vascular permeability due to disruption of the endothelial cells or change in blood-brain barrier. The extent of the oedema depends on the systolic pressure, the duration and extent of the vascular injury and the opening of the blood-brain barrier.

The resulting damage and cerebral oedema may give rise to loss of consciousness, pallor and vomiting which may last from hours to several days.

Clinical features

The effects of head injury vary in severity with the cause of the injury and with the stage of skull development. There may be periods of unconsciousness, varying in time and depending on the severity and type of injury:

1. In severe injury or haemorrhage there is unconsciousness with pupillary changes, motor paralysis and changes in blood pressure, pulse and respiration rate.
2. Damage to the brain stem and the hypothalamus is followed by a rising temperature.
3. Convulsions (p. 305).

Principles of treatment and nursing management

1. Routine nursing care.
2. Observation of the state of consciousness (p. 302 and below).
3. Maintenance of clear airway.
4. Sedation (narcotics are not desirable since they depress brain activity).

5. Treatment of cerebral oedema. Control of intracranial pressure can be achieved by limiting fluid intake and by inducing diuresis. Mannitol or frusemide may be given. Accurate fluid intake and output records must be maintained. All vital functions must be monitored because of the danger of electrolyte imbalance. Urine should be tested for specific gravity and serum electrolyte levels should be monitored to identify any changes in electrolyte state.
6. Nutrition:
   a. If conscious — oral feeding.
   b. If unconscious — tube feeding.
7. Position of the unconscious child (p. 303).
8. Care of pressure areas (p. 94).
9. Neurosurgical treatment.
10. Support for parents. Recognition of their anxiety, particularly if the child is unconscious. Need to give information about the nature of the injury and the possible outcome. Advice about the level of activity permitted once the child returns home and to contact the general practitioner or the hospital if any complications are noticed.

Tumours

Tumours of the nervous system are said to be primary if they grow from the nervous tissue itself, or secondary if they are carried to the nervous system by the blood from a primary tumour elsewhere in the body (p. 116).

Tumours are not uncommon in infancy and childhood, and they tend to be gliomas which affect the supporting tissue of glia. The majority of tumours are: (1) *astrocytomas*, occurring in both cerebrum and cerebellum, the latter being more commonly affected; (2) *ependymomas*, arising from the lining of the ventricles, and (3) *medulloblastomas*, arising predominantly in the cerebellum.

General features of cerebral tumours

In infancy a tumour may not be evident because the open sutures delay the effect of intracranial pressure. Where the sutures have united and in the older child, the following symptoms are present:

1. There is increase in intracranial pressure because of the increase in mass within the skull.

2. Compression of the ventricles interfere with the flow of cerebrospinal fluid and there is increased pressure.
3. Destruction of brain tissue produces a *progressively* deteriorating function related to the area affected, e.g. weakness of muscles on the opposite side of the body. If the frontal lobe is affected, loss of memory and changes in personality occur.

Increased intracranial pressure produces the following signs and symptoms:

1. Headache, which is increased by coughing and stooping.
2. Vomiting, which usually occurs at the height of the headache.
3. Diplopia and blurring of vision.
4. Decreased pulse rate.
5. Dilation of the pupils and failure to react to light.
6. Papilloedema, i.e. swelling of the optic disc. This can be seen through an ophthalmoscope.
7. Increasing drowsiness progressing eventually to coma.
8. Convulsions.

Levels of consciousness

Before discussing the different levels of consciousness, it is necessary to define the term 'consciousness'. Consciousness is an awareness of the environment and of oneself. This depends on the brain and there are certain parts which are particularly concerned with this function.

These are the reticular system in the brain stem and the cerebral cortex. Depression of neuronal activity interferes with the functions of the nervous system, but all functions are not equally affected. From the higher cortical centres to the lower brain stem and spinal cord, different effects can be recognised which can be divided into three stages. However, these are arbitrary and are a continuum.

Stage 1: impaired mental ability. This occurs when the cerebral cortex responsible for higher intellectual functions is affected, e.g. inability to concentrate, forgetfulness, etc.

Stage 2: depression of consciousness. This stage is an important aspect of diagnosis and the observation and recording of the rising and falling levels of consciousness is an important nursing function:

1. Alertness. This indicates normal consciousness. The individual is able to respond in a normal and rational fashion.
2. Stage of automism. The individual is aware of his surroundings but may show abnormality of mood, i.e. he may be irritable or elated and may show defects of memory and judgement.
3. Confusion. The patient may be disorientated in time and space. He is unable to think and speak in a logical and coherent way.
4. Delirium. During this stage, he is restless and may be violent and is not capable of rational thought.
5. Stupor. In this stage, the patient becomes quiet and does not communicate. He is conscious but has a glazed look and appears not to understand when spoken to.
6. Semi-comatosed state. The patient passes into periods of unconsciousness and may be roused to a stuperous state.
7. Coma. The patient does not respond to the environment in any meaningful way; he does not speak, does not obey commands, does not open his eyes and cannot be roused.

Each stage merges into the other when the level of consciousness decreases or increases. The older child's response to spoken stimulus and the infant's and young child's spontaneous movement or crying in response to auditory or tactile stimuli, may indicate that his level of consciousness is satisfactory.

Stage 3: depression of reflex activity. Depression of reflex activity involves the neurones of the lower brain stem and of the spinal cord. Muscle tone gradually diminishes and is finally absent. Eye movements disappear and the eyeballs become fixed. The pupils gradually become fully dilated, do not constrict when stimulated by light and may be unequal in size. The corneal reflex is one of the last to disappear, that is the eye does not close when the cornea is touched with cotton wool.

CARE OF THE UNCONSCIOUS CHILD

Principles of nursing management

When the child fails to respond to any stimulus and cannot be roused, then he is said to be in a state of coma or unconsciousness. There are many causes of coma or unconsciousness and all involve some kind of insult to the brain. These include direct injury; pressure, due to bleeding, abscess or tumour; infection, such as meningitis, encephalitis; biochemical disturbances such as electrolyte imbalance; lack of oxygen; drugs and poisons. The period of unconsciousness can vary from a few minutes, as found in epilepsy, to a prolonged time, following extensive damage. However, the principles of care apply whatever the cause or duration of period of unconsciousness.

1. *Adequate ventilation*:
   a. Safe positioning of the child, usually semi-prone or prone (Fig. 17.9).
   b. Clear airway. Suction equipment must be available (p. 120).
   c. Resuscitation trolley (p. 118).
   d. Care of artificial airways, e.g. tracheostomy and endotracheal tube (p. 386).

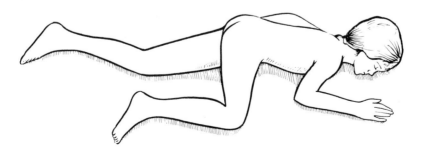

Fig. 17.9 Position of the unconscious child.

e. Oxygen administration (p. 382).
2. Prevention of inhalation of vomit by passing a naso-gastric tube and aspiration of gastric contents.
3. Replacement of fluids and electrolytes intravenously.
4. *Nutrition*:
   a. Initially there may be inadequate absorption and intravenous feeding may be instituted (p. 455).
   b. Naso-gastric feeding (p. 512).
5. *Administration of drugs*:
   a. Intravenously (p. 449).
   b. Intramuscularly (p. 175).
   c. Via naso-gastric tube.
6. *Monitoring of vital functions*:
   a. Levels of consciousness (p. 302).
   b. Temperature, pulse and respiration (pp. 102–104).
   c. Blood pressure measurement (p. 460).
7. Observations. These include colour, e.g. cyanosis, convulsions (p. 307), limb movement, abdominal distension, incontinence of urine and faeces (older child), measurement of head circumference.
8. *Routine nursing care*:
   a. Pressure area care (local relief of pressure) and general care by frequent change of position.
   b. General cleanliness.
   c. Hair care.
   d. Mouth care: this can be achieved by low oral suction to remove excess secretion and gentle brushing of teeth (p. 96).
   e. Eye care. Recognition of the danger of keeping the eyes partially open leading to exposure keratitis and corneal ulceration. It may be necessary to tape the eyes down or cover them with a pad of paraffin gauze.
   f. Elimination of waste matter:
      (i) *Urinary output* must be measured accurately and catheterisation may be necessary.
      (ii) *Faeces*: lack of bulk in diet may lead to constipation which can be corrected by inserting a suppository or giving an aperient, whilst a fluid diet may produce diarrhoea, causing damage to the skin surrounding the anus.

9. Understanding of special needs of the unconscious child and recognition that, though unconscious, thought processes and sense of hearing may remain intact. Communication should be maintained throughout and care taken not to make adverse comments which might distress the child (p. 112).
10. Support for parents. This is an extremely anxious time for the parents and every opportunity should be given to them to take part in some aspect of care. Daily progress reports should be given to them and every effort made to relieve their anxiety. This should include frequent interviews with the medical staff; senior nursing staff should be present to ensure consistency in information given to parents.

Pain

Pain is an unpleasant sensory experience quite distinct from other sensory states such as touch, warmth and cold. It is usually associated with tissue or cell damage and serves as a warning that such damage is taking place. Pain gives information about the condition of the body but not about the nature of the stimulus: Pain cannot be defined in words which are meaningful to someone who has not experienced it. It is a subjective sensation, though it may be accompanied by various physiological responses such as reflex withdrawal movements, changes in vasomotor tone, in blood pressure and in heart rate. Some responses limit the damage produced, e.g. an external stimulus may lead to appropriate action being taken (as in reflex withdrawal) or where the pain is well defined and recognised as in acute appendicitis, appropriate treatment can be given.

Not all pain serves as a protective early warning system. Exposure to X-rays does not cause pain until some time later when inflammatory changes develop and in cases of cancer, pain may only occur when the damage cannot be repaired.

Components of pain

Pain is not only a physical phenomenon but it has also a large psychological component. There is an important aspect of the significance of the pain which may not have the same effect on children — for example, knowledge of the consequence of a disease might affect the experience of pain just as it can block pain. While the adult identifies the pain with some specific disease, for example pain in the chest with heart disease, the child is frightened of the pain itself but does not identify it with a specific disease. Fear of the disease may increase the intensity of the pain. The desire to do something pleasurable may have the effect of decreasing pain. Pain sensitivity varies greatly with individuals. Some people appear to be insensitive to stimuli (even though their nerve apparatus is intact), others may be hypersensitive. The reaction of the individual to the pain of disease will depend on the cause of the pain, its location, its severity, his pain-sensitivity and his psychological make-up. Pain is whatever the patient says it is and where it is. What is important from the nurse's point of view, is the ability to assess the significance of the patient's description of his pain and to describe the pain in the terms used by the patient.

Quality of pain

The quality of pain varies according to the stimulus and the site of stimulation. Older children will be able to describe pain in terms such as 'pricking', 'burning', 'tearing', etc. The small or younger child will cry and the intensity of the pain will produce a different cry, for example a sharp pain may produce a piercing cry.

Assessment of pain

This involves careful observation of the child, e.g. response to pressure or movement, furrowed brow, facial contortion, gritted teeth, sound indicating pain and whether accompanied by pallor, sweating, tachycardia or vomiting.

Relief of pain

No child should be expected to suffer pain unnecessarily. Nurses do not prescribe drugs and it is therefore essential that the medical officer is notified as soon as possible if a child is in pain. In some cases pain-relieving drugs are prescribed in anticipation of pain and these should be given when the situation demands.

Convulsions — epilepsy

Nerve cells function by discharging electrical impulses and normal function is disturbed when neurones display abnormal electrical activity. This is characterised by involuntary muscular contractions and disturbances of consciousness.

Abnormal activity in cerebral neurones can cause motor or sensory disturbances as well as disturbances of consciousness. They may be localised to certain muscle groups or generalised throughout the body. They consist of vigorous involuntary muscle spasms which may be sustained (tonic) or intermittent (clonic). When generalised, such spasms are called 'convulsions'. Initially the contractions are tonic so that the body is contorted into a fixed position. Fatigue of neurones changes this pattern to clonic contractions leading to violent irregular involuntary movements.

When sensory areas of the brain are involved, sensory disturbances occur. These occur as prodromal signs and involve sense of smell, taste, sounds and sight. They are considered to be warning signs (aura) of a more severe attack to follow.

Causes

The term convulsions is generally used when spasms are not repeated over a prolonged period of time and where the cause can be identified.

Epilepsy is common in children and this term is referred to in children who are subject to recurring seizures or lapses of consciousness. The majority of convulsions are related to specific events. These include: birth injury, neonatal tetany, tetany of rickets, infection, tumours and injuries.

The most common cause of convulsions in the pre-school child is the high temperature in response to an acute infection. The mechanism is not clear, but it is known that temperatures above about 40°C cause damage to cells, especially in the brain. The rate of rise and height of the temperature appears to be more important than the infection, but pyrogens (p. 99) are also believed to affect the hypothalamic thermostat.

Convulsions may also occur in the following situations:

1. Lack of oxygen. A severe reduction of oxygen in the brain is a common cause, e.g. cardiac arrest, fall in blood pressure.

2. Reduction in PCO_2. Hyperventilation or over-breathing lowers the carbon dioxide pressure in the blood, resulting in convulsion.
3. Reduction in blood glucose concentration (hypoglycaemia). Glucose is used in brain cell metabolism; lack of glucose is as damaging to brain cells as lack of oxygen. This is a danger in pre-term babies and in children where an overdose of insulin has been given.
4. Water and electrolytes across the cell membrane is responsible for the excitability of neurones and therefore any disturbance of electrolytes may precipitate convulsions, e.g. water intoxication, low serum calcium below 8 mg/100 ml, low magnesium or hydrogen ion concentration.
5. Local lesions, e.g. tumour or infection.

Types of seizures

Various clinical types of epileptic seizures are recognised.

Grand mal or major fit. This may start abruptly with loss of consciousness or there may be a short warning or aura. The type of aura is important because it indicates where, in the brain, the abnormal discharge starts.

The sequence is as follows:

1. Aura.
2. Tonic phase, i.e. rigid contraction of all muscles. During this phase the tongue or cheek may be bitten. Muscular contraction prevents breathing and the child may become cyanosed and is unconscious.
3. Clonic phase. During this phase, jerky movements begin which may become violent. Injury may be caused by the violent movement and there is often incontinence of urine and faeces.
4. Coma. Muscles are completely relaxed. It may last for 10 minutes to several hours and is followed by a period of confusion during which the child may be restless.

Petit mal. These attacks consist of brief periods of loss of consciousness, but there are no generalised convulsions. Petit mal attacks may be frequent in childhood and tend to disappear at puberty. When they persist into adulthood, they tend to become more like grand mal.

Many attacks occur each day. Each attack consists of momentary loss of touch with the surroundings. The eyelids may flicker, the head may nod, he may drop what he is holding, he may repeat words and he then continues his previous activity as if there has been no interruption. This type of seizure is easily missed and often only a close observer is aware of the occurrence.

Infantile spasms. These have also been called 'salaam fits'. The onset is before the age of 12 months. Numerous attacks occur each day and consist of sudden transient jerks of the whole body, head and limbs. Most often the head and trunk flex suddenly forward while the hands rise up alongside the head. These spasms occur in children who have been brain damaged at birth.

Psychomotor seizures (temporal lobe epilepsy). These are relatively uncommon in childhood and cause sudden disturbance of behaviour. The child may show sudden fear, or other aura and the attack itself frequently consists of abnormal repetitive movements, for example jaw movements, eye fluttering or blinking, staring and clasping or fumbling with the hands. There may also be violent tantrums and dream-like states.

Status epilepticus. Epileptic attacks usually occur at well-spaced intervals, but sometimes one seizure passes into another in quick succession so that consciousness is not regained. The attacks may last for many hours. The temperature rises to high levels and unless the convulsions are stopped, the patient will become exhausted and die.

Electroencephalography (EEG)

Electroencephalography may assist in diagnosing epilepsy. It is a method of recording the electrical activity of the brain (Fig. 17.10). It is used as an aid to diagnosis in cases where there is a history of convulsions or to identify the cause of depression of the nervous system. Electrodes are placed at various points on the scalp and connected through a valve amplifier to an ink-writing oscillograph. Small potential changes can be recorded and these reflect electrical activity in the underlying brain. Recordings are usually made from the frontal, parietal, occipital and temporal regions.

The brain waves vary in frequency and amplitude and are classified in terms of their dominant frequency (Fig. 17.10).

Alpha waves. These are seen in most normal people when they are awake and in a state of

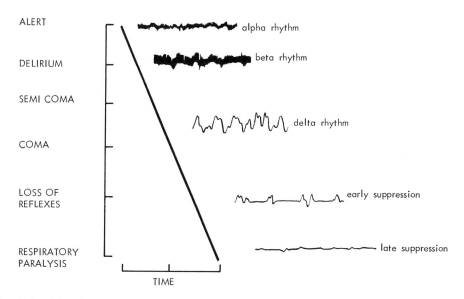

Fig. 17.10 Electrical activity of the brain during different levels of consciousness.

mental rest. *Beta waves*. These are frequently seen in children. *Delta waves*. These are seen in young children and in deep sleep.

The procedure is carried out in a quiet room. An explanation should be given to the older child, and reassurance can be given that it is not a painful process. He should be kept calm and relaxed, though sedation is not desirable as it alters the brain activity and therefore the pattern.

EEG examination can help if it is taken during an attack, as between attacks, the pattern may be quite normal. In an attack of grand mal, high frequency, large amplitude spikes are recorded all over the scalp. This indicates that the activity may involve the reticular activating system in the brain stem (p. 296) so that all parts of the cortex are stimulated and become active at the same time. In attacks of petit mal, the pattern is different, i.e. spike and dome pattern all over the brain. It may also show abnormal discharges arising from one point only, suggesting a lesion of the brain at that point.

Principles of treatment and nursing management

Emergency treatment

1. Protection of the child and correct positioning, e.g. lateral position (Fig. 17.9).
2. Clearing and maintaining the airway.
3. Administration of oxygen and pharyngeal suction.
4. Treatment of specific conditions, e.g. hypoglycaemia, hypocalcaemia, pyridoxine deficiency.
5. Control of seizures by parenteral anticonvulsant therapy, e.g. phenobarbitone, diazepam, or paraldehyde (0.15 ml/kg of body weight).
   Note: When intramuscular paraldehyde is given, it must always be taken from a sealed ampoule because paraldehyde in a bottle can undergo dangerous decomposition. Paraldehyde should not be administered from a disposable plastic syringe but a glass syringe should be used.

Elective treatment

1. Maintenance control of seizures, e.g. dipropylacetate (Epilim), phenytoin, etc.
2. Advice and guidance for parents:
   a. Care during seizures.
   b. Need to take drugs regularly as directed.
   c. Reassurance to parents by answering any questions regarding the education of the child and prospects and type of work.

Ketogenic diet. Fasting causes cessation of grand mal seizures in the majority of epileptic children, the effect usually appearing shortly after ketosis has appeared on the third day. A strongly ketogenic diet has a comparable anticonvulsive effect after ketosis has developed.

In fasting:

1. The body uses up fat stores from adipose tissue.
2. Fluid intake is restricted.
3. There is an increase in acid-forming salts.

The diet consists of medium chain triglycerides (MCT) given in the form of oil. The diet is based on the child's caloric requirements when 60 per cent of these calories are from MCT oil (MCT = 0.03 mJ/ml), the remaining 40 per cent being provided by normal dietary food. The child is gradually introduced to the MCT oil which is mixed with some food. The diet must be explained clearly to the parents and also to the child if he is old enough to understand.

Method. The child is fasted for 48 hours, when ketone bodies can be detected in the urine. He is then gradually introduced to the MCT oil, when 10 to 15 ml are given first. This is followed by daily increase of 15 ml until the maximum amount is reached.

The diet has its limitations because of the effect such a restricted diet has on the child; emotional disturbances are believed to be associated with the diet.

Breath-holding attacks

Breath-holding attacks are quite common in children between the ages of 6 months and 4 years. They usually occur when the child is crying as a result of injury, anger, frustration or fear and may be followed by pallor, cyanosis or temporary loss of consciousness. There may also be a few convulsive movements of the limbs which may be interpreted as epileptic seizures. The child may, therefore, be referred to the hospital for investigation, where an electroencephalography usually shows normal patterns.

An attack may last for a few seconds or longer and can be quite alarming to the onlooker. The child should be handled gently during the attack from which he generally recovers spontaneously. As this is a very frightening experience for both the onlooker and the child, calmness is essential and he should be comforted and reassured during and after the attack.

Infections of the nervous system

The nervous system can be infected by bacteria and viruses. The mode of entry can be via the respiratory system, circulatory system and the skin. Any part of the nervous system can be affected and the various stages of infection and inflammation can be recognised. The process may be acute as in poliomyelitis, subacute as in some forms of encephalitis and chronic as in neurosyphilis.

Meningitis

This is an infection of the meninges. Normally the blood-brain barrier is an effective protective mechanism, but when the invasion of micro-organisms is extensive this barrier breaks down. The areas involved are usually the pia and arachnoid mater, i.e. those nearest the brain tissue. Bacterial meningitis is one of the few infections which are related to levels of development, e.g. less than 2 months — *E. coli*, group B beta haemolytic streptococcus; 2 months to 6 years — *Haemophilus influenzae, Neisseria meningitidis*; children over 6 years — *Neisseria meningitidis, Streptococcus pneumoniae*.

Mode of entry

1. Trauma or surgical procedures.
2. Upper respiratory infection.
3. Lymphatics, e.g. mastoid, possibly sinuses.
4. Circulatory.

Once entry has been achieved into the meninges the organisms spread into the cerebrospinal fluid. Subdural effusions occur frequently. Extension of the infection into peripheral cranial nerves or compression of these nerves by increased intracranial pressure can produce deafness, blindness or paralysis of facial and other muscles of head and neck.

Three main types of meningitis are recognised:

1. Pyogenic, i.e. pus-forming bacteria. These include bacteria such as meningococci, pneumococci and influenza bacilli and staphylococci.
2. Viral. Caused by a number of different viruses, e.g. poliomyelitis virus.
3. Tuberculosis. Caused by the tubercle bacillus.

Clinical features

There are certain features which apply to all types of meningitis. Before any meningeal signs appear, there is a history of pyrexia a few days prior to the appearance of specific features. There may be a 'cold' and sore throat followed by headache which spreads backwards to produce pain in the neck and back. This is accompanied by vomiting and photophobia. The child becomes irritable and restless, producing a typical high-pitched meningeal cry. Petechiae are present in meningococcal meningitis.

On examination, Kernig's sign is positive. To test for this, the hip is first flexed and then an attempt is made to straighten the knee. If the sign is positive, movement is restricted and is accompanied by pain.

In infants, there may be neck retraction or the body may be arched (opisthotonus) due to neck spasm.

Pyogenic meningitis

This type of meningitis follows an upper respiratory infection or may follow pneumonia. Newborn infants may be infected by *E. coli* via the umbilical stump or via the alimentary tract. Staphylococcal meningitis may follow ingestion of infected milk if the mother suffers from breast abscess. Cerebrospinal fluid which contains leucocytes is turbid, its sugar content is reduced and Pandy's test is positive.

Principles of treatment and nursing management

1. Identification of organism, e.g. lumbar puncture, blood culture, throat swab and umbilical swab.
2. Chemotherapy/antibiotics — these may be given intramuscularly, intrathecally or intravenously (if infusion is given), e.g. chloramphenicol, penicillin, kanamycin and sulphonamides.
3. Observations, recording and relief of convulsions.
4. Nutrition:
    a. Oral, if conscious.
    b. Intra-gastric, if unconscious (p. 512).
5. Intravenous infusion if dehydration is present.
6. Routine nursing care.
7. Tepid sponging.
8. Support for parents.

Viral meningitis

The onset and features are similar to pyogenic meningitis. The cerebrospinal fluid is usually clear but contains lymphocytes; sugar and chloride are normal.

Principles of treatment and nursing management are as for pyogenic meningitis.

Drug therapy will be related to symptoms. Since no specific drug deals with viral infection, antibiotic therapy will only be of value if there is any additional bacterial infection.

Tuberculous meningitis

This type of meningitis occurs more gradually than the others. The child has become infected with mycotuberculosis elsewhere in the body, though he may present, for the first time, signs and symptoms of meningitis. It affects children of all ages but is more common between 1 and 5 years of age. The cerebrospinal fluid shows fewer cells, and both sugar and chlorides are very low.

Principles of treatment and nursing management are as previously described. However, the following drugs are specific for this infection: PAS — para-amino-salicylic acid, given orally; INAH — isonicotinic acid hydrazide, given orally; streptomycin, given intrathecally, intramuscularly or orally; rifamycin, which has higher bactericidal activity but is toxic to the liver.

Encephalitis

Inflammation of the brain is called encephalitis, and if the meninges are involved, it is called meningoencephalitis. The conditions are characterised by inflammatory and degenerative lesions of the brain and cord.

There are a variety of micro-organisms responsible and some are part of specific infectious diseases. Other causes have been attributed to vaccination. Diseases such as measles, German measles, chickenpox and smallpox have been followed by encephalitis as complications.

Other organisms which may produce encephalitis are the viruses of herpes simplex, herpes zoster, mumps, poliomyelitis, coxsackie and ECHO viruses.

Characteristic features

These consist of headache, vomiting, confusion,

delirium, coma and epileptic fits. Unless the meninges are also infected, there is relatively little neck stiffness.

The effects of encephalitis vary with the type of organism responsible. Some children show changes in personality with a tendency to epilepsy. There is also progressive mental deterioration which is more pronounced in subacute forms of encephalitis.

Principles of treatment and nursing management
Basically as for meningitis.

Poliomyelitis (acute anterior poliomyelitis)

This is an acute virus infection in which the clinical signs consist of increased temperature, headache, neck and back stiffness and sometimes flaccid paralysis of various muscle groups. The causative agent belongs to the enterovirus family. The virus enters the body by way of the oropharynx. It is present in the throat, blood and faeces 3 to 4 days after exposure. The characteristic lesions of poliomyelitis are found in the grey matter of the spinal cord, the medulla, the precentral gyrus of the cerebral cortex and the deep nuclei of the cerebellum. There may also be cardiac involvement (myocarditis).

Clinical features
These vary from minor to major illness. In the minor form there is headache, sore throat, a slight rise in temperature and vomiting sometimes occurs. In most cases the condition improves, but in some, symptoms recur and the major form appears. This is characterised by high temperature, severe headache, stiff neck and back, deep muscle pain, weakness of various muscles and loss of superficial and deep reflexes. The site of paralysis depends on the location and lesions in the spinal cord or medulla. In the bulbar form, the cranial nerve nuclei are involved with resulting paralysis of the pharyngeal, laryngeal, facial and other muscle groups innervated by the cranial nerves.

Difficulty in swallowing, nasal regurgitation and nasal voice are early signs of bulbar involvement. When respiratory muscles, diaphragm and intercostals are affected then respiratory failure follows. In this case a ventilator will be required to maintain life (p. 395).

Principles of treatment and nursing management

1. Routine nursing care.

Pre- or non-paralytic stage
2. This stage requires no specific treatment except relief for the headache. Rest is of the greatest importance, particularly during this stage, since physical exercise greatly increases the probability of paralysis.
3. Positioning of patient and supporting painful limbs. Bed appliance should be used to keep the weight of bedclothes off limbs. If the joints are painful and if muscles are in spasms then hot packs may give relief. Movement should be limited for a few days; this interferes with the care of pressure areas. However, when pain subsides full routine nursing care can be given.
4. Passive physiotherapy, e.g. moving each joint through its full range twice a day.

Paralytic stage
5. Treatment of respiratory paralysis. This may involve performing a tracheostomy and connecting the ventilator to the tacheostomy tube. The lungs are inflated by positive pressure (p. 395).
6. Occupational therapy, e.g. play and school work according to the child's age and general condition.
7. Rehabilitation of the severely paralysed child. This involves decision-making with respect to:
   a. Home care.
   b. Institutional care (See Handicapped child in the community p. 68).

Cerebral palsy

This term covers a number of conditions, which have various causes. The single most important cause is intracranial birth injury which may present as spastic paralysis. It may also be due to developmental defect, intra-uterine cerebral degeneration or in the postnatal state, following meningitis, encephalitis or trauma.

Clinical features
In the more severe cases, symptoms are evident from birth. The infant shows irritability and may vomit. Milder cases may not show motor de-

ficiency until the child fails to perform particular motor skills at certain periods of his development — he may not sit up at about 6 months or walk at about 1 year.

Three types of malfunction can be recognised and these depend on the area affected. However, a mixture of two or more malfunctions are often presented.

1. *Spasticity* (increased muscle tone). Spastic weakness is the more common manifestation. Both sides are affected and the legs more severely than the arms. A characteristic 'scissors gait' and exaggerated tendon reflexes, etc. are present. The more severe cases have marked spasticity of all extremities and may involve bulbar muscles leading to dysarthria (difficulty in articulation) and dysphagia (difficulty in swallowing).

2. *Ataxia* (unsteadiness). The lesion is in the cerebellum and is indicated by unsteadiness. The muscles are flaccid and muscle tone is decreased.

3. *Athetosis*. Here the basal ganglia are affected producing slow writhing movements, which are involuntary.

There are also varying degrees of mental retardation. Deformities may occur as the result of spasm or from the pull of stronger muscle groups.

Principles of treatment and nursing management
This will depend on the extent and type of involvement. The mild cases will probably manage reasonably well. Each child has to be assessed and decisions are made on these assessments. The moderately-affected group requires:

1. Physiotherapy.
2. Speech training.
3. Corrective orthopaedic measures.
4. Evaluation of physical and mental ability.
5. Educational programme.

Severely affected children. The care of these children requires skill and, if they are nursed at home, then effective supporting service must be available. Specific nursing measures aim at: (a) prevention of pressure sores; (b) maintaining a clear airway; (c) finding the most suitable way to feed the child and ensuring an adequate intake of food; (d) establishing a system of communication so that the child can make his needs, wishes and desires known, and (e) encouraging the child to make use of his abilities and helping him to develop to the full limits of his capabilities.

Breathing difficulties may be due to mucus and this can be aspirated when necessary. The child's position can be changed frequently and a position adopted which povides the greatest comfort and aids breathing.

Feeding difficulties may be due to difficulty in sucking and swallowing. Feeds or solids should be given slowly and in a form that the child can manage. As the child grows and develops he should be encouraged to feed himself, however, this will depend on his ability to control his hands adequately.

Orthopaedic correction may be required to aid development and to maintain good body mechanics. This may involve tendon lengthening or division, tendon transfer, arthrodesis (surgical fixation of a joint, e.g. wrist) and neurectomy, i.e. division of a nerve to relieve tightness of muscle.

Parents must be supported and helped to accept the child's disabilities. They should be guided in the care of the child until they feel secure in their ability to do so alone.

Procedures related to the nervous system

Neurological examination
A careful neurological examination is essential to localise any specific neurological condition. This involves examination of the following:

1. Behaviour and mental status — the child's ability to relate to others, his level of ability and activity, e.g. hyperactivity or hypoactivity:
    a. Attention span, e.g. does he move quickly from one activity to another?
    b. Speech development — expressive, e.g. talking and vocabulary or aphasic receptive, e.g. understanding.
    c. Ability to read — graded reading paragraphs.
    d. Ability to write, draw and copy, e.g. control of pencil and handedness should be noted.
    e. Testing of arithmetic — test for possible mental slowness.
2. Motor examination:
    a. Assessment of muscle strength — standing, walking, respiratory muscles.

b. Assessment of muscle tone.
c. Tests of fine motor co-ordination.
d. Involuntary movements.
e. Examination of reflexes, e.g. presence, absence, increase or decrease of reflexes.
3. Sensory examination:
a. Taste, smell, sight, hearing and touch.
b. Eye movements.

The equipment required should therefore serve the needs of the examiner, for example:

Toys suitable for all age groups (bricks of various shapes, size and colour), paper, pencil, crayons, books or special reading material.
Fine paper, bell (hearing test).
Tendon hammer to test reflexes.
Ophthalmoscope for examination of eyes.
Auriscope for examination of ears.
Measuring tape used to measure head circumference when a hydrocephalus is suspected, or limbs where shortening of one or more limbs is suspected.
Cotton wool.
Skin pencil.

Lumbar puncture

This procedure is carried out for the following purposes:

1. Diagnostic: to obtain cerebrospinal fluid for examination in cases of suspected meningitis.
2. To relieve cerebrospinal fluid pressure in hydrocephalus and meningitis.
3. To administer a drug, e.g. penicillin.
4. To administer spinal anaesthesia.
5. For X-ray examination of the ventricles.

Principles involved

The spinal cord ends at the level of the first lumbar vertebra but the meninges, i.e. dura mater, arachnoid, and pia mater, are prolonged below it. The space between the pia mater and arachnoid is known as the subarachnoid space, which contains cerebrospinal fluid.

Normal spinal fluid is a clear, colourless fluid. Table 17.1 shows the normal and abnormal values of its contents.

The total volume is 20 ml in a new-born infant, increasing with age until it reaches the total of 100 to 150 ml in adulthood. The initial pressure is 70 to 180 mm of spinal fluid.

In disease, the amount and type of fluid may be altered and can show the following: (a) *clear fluid, but a positive Pandy's test*. (Pandy's test is a qualitative test which indicates increase in protein. When phenol 1–15 is added to the clear cerebrospinal fluid, it becomes cloudy.); (b) *purulent fluid* indicating infection by organisms such as meningococcus, bacillus coli, etc.; (c) blood which may be found in subarachnoid haemorrhage. The pressure may be raised in hydrocephalus, tumour of the brain or where infection of the meninges is present. Measurement of pressure can be accurately recorded only in the older child.

Requirements

1. Sterile dressing pack; additional sterile hand towels and drapes.
2. Lumbar puncture needles of required size.
3. Glass manometer and a small piece of rubber tubing or three-way tap.
4. 2 ml syringes and hypodermic needles.5 and 10 ml syringes.
5. Test tubes and centrifuge tubes (sterile).

Additional equipment

6. Cleansing lotion (Betadine, methylated spirit).
7. Phenol 1–15.
8. Antibiotic or substance to be injected.
9. Local anaesthetic.
10. Air-strip dressing or wound sealing aerosol.

Preparation of the child

This is a frightening operation and some sedation is usually given prior to the procedure. A local anaesthesia may also be given in some cases. It is very important that the child is prevented from moving while the procedure is in progress and this can be achieved by placing the child on his side, the back level with the table edge (Fig. 17.11). The nurse's right arm is placed under the child's knees, grasping his arms. The nurse's left arm is placed round his neck bending his back. This increases the intervertebral space, but care must be taken not to flex the head excessively as it might lead to respiratory and circulatory difficulty. Alternatively, the child may be placed in the sitting position, supported by a nurse.

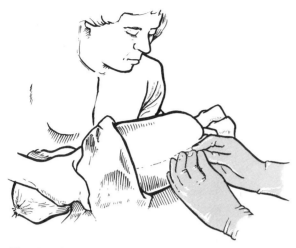

Fig. 17.11 Position of the child during a lumbar puncture.

Method. After cleaning the skin and anaesthetising the area, a spinal needle is introduced between the interspace until it enters the subarachnoid space. If the spinal fluid pressure is to be measured, the manometer is attached to the spinal puncture needle and the initial pressure reading is obtained by measuring the level of the fluid column after it comes to rest. Cerebrospinal fluid is then allowed to drop into the various test and centrifuge tubes for comparison, and laboratory examination.

After-care of the child
Once the needle is removed, pressure is applied to the puncture site or a dressing may be applied. Sometimes a wound-sealing aerosol is used. The child is dressed and gently returned to his bed, with one pillow under his head. If postpuncture headache is severe, the foot of the bed can be raised and glucose fluids given. Oxygen may also relieve the headache. If there is any pain in the neck, legs or back, it must be reported; it may be due to bleeding into the theca or to infection.

Cisternal puncture
In this procedure a needle is inserted into the cisterna magna. This is the largest of the subarachnoid cisternae or spaces. It lies in the angle between the cerebellum and the medulla and can be reached by passing a needle between the first cervical vertebra and the skull.

This procedure is more dangerous than the lumbar puncture and injury to the medulla may occur, therefore cisternal puncture is seldom used for routine examination of the cerebrospinal fluid, but where there is a block, i.e. some obstruction in the spinal canal, cisternal puncture is the method of choice. It is carried out for the same reasons as lumbar puncture and the requirements are the same. Special cisternal puncture needles may be used for the older child.

Preparation of the child
Pre-operative preparation is the same as for lumbar puncture, but the position of the child is different. The child either lies on his side, the shoulders in vertical line and the head slightly flexed, or he may be in the sitting position with the head slightly flexed. It may be necessary to shave the nape of the neck. During the procedure the child must be held firmly so that no movement takes place. The after-care is the same as for lumbar puncture.

Subdural puncture and ventricular puncture
This procedure is carried out to determine the presence of subdural haematoma and the presence of a hydrocephalus. If a haematoma is present, the cerebrospinal fluid will be grossly xanthochromic or bloodstained and will be more abundant. These procedures can only be carried out in infants where the sutures of the skull have not closed. In older children, when the anterior fontanelle and the sutures have closed, the procedure is carried out by a neuro-surgeon.

Requirements
As for lumbar puncture. A shorter and graduated needle may be used.

Preparation of the child
The scalp has to be shaved and the child restrained, lying on his back with the top of his head level with the edge of the table. The nurse holds the head, tilting it slightly forward. The needle is inserted into the extreme lateral corner of the anterior fontanelle. When fluid has been withdrawn, firm digital pressure is applied over the punctured areas and the child's head is raised. Pressure is maintained until no further leakage of cerebrospinal fluid occurs.

Air encephalography and ventriculography

This procedure is carried out to obtain an X-ray film of the cerebral ventricles. A lumbar puncture is made, cerebrospinal fluid is withdrawn, and air is injected. The X-ray (positive) will show lighter areas corresponding to the ventricles. The shape, size and position of the ventricles may give valuable information as to the position of tumours in the cranial cavity or, in an existing hydrocephalus, the degree of dilation of the ventricles.

Requirements

The same as for lumbar puncture with the following additions:

1. 100 ml measure for cerebrospinal fluid.
2. 20 ml syringe.
3. Extra pillows (if the procedure is carried out outwith the X-ray department).
4. Vomit bowl.
5. Resuscitation trolley (Ch. 6).

Preparation of the child

The child is prepared as for a general anaesthesia. Food and drink are withheld for 3 hours prior to the examination. He may be heavily sedated or a general anaesthesia is given.

Method

The child is positioned sitting upright well supported with pillows.

The head should be resting on the pillows ensuring a clear airway. A lumbar puncture is performed and the amount of fluid withdrawn is replaced by air. The amount varies with the age of the child. The whole procedure can be carried out in the X-ray department and throughout the procedure the child must be observed carefully for signs of shock or distress. Collapse may occur and is due to the change in intracranial pressure. The child should be laid flat immediately and oxygen administered.

On return to the ward, the child is nursed flat. Any restlessness and headache may be alleviated by raising the foot of the bed and administering oxygen. The oxygen assists in absorption of air which has been injected. The body temperature may fluctuate considerably following this procedure. Hyperpyrexia is not uncommon, nor is a sudden drop in body temperature leading to shock. Temperature, pulse and respiration should be measured 4-hourly for a 48-hourly period following this examination, and more frequently, if necessary.

Ventriculography

This procedure is similar to that of air encephalography except that the air is injected directly into the lateral ventricles.

Infants

Where the sutures of the skull have not yet closed, the procedure is the same as for a ventricular puncture (p. 313). The scalp may have to be shaved. The preparation and care of the child are the same as in air encephalography.

Older children

The child is prepared as for a general anaesthesia and the scalp is shaved. The procedure is carried out by a neuro-surgeon who performs bilateral burr holes in the skull on either side of the midline in the occipital region. A cannula is inserted into the burr hole and passed through the cerebral substance into the posterior horn of the lateral ventricle.

The post-operative care of the child includes observations for cerebral irritation, levels of consciousness and signs of infection.

Angiogram

This is an X-ray examination of the blood vessels of the head and neck. Contrast media is injected into the carotid or vertebral arteries and it is possible to demonstrate tumours, abscesses, intracranial haemorrhage and occluded arteries.

After-care

Discomfort may be experienced particularly at the injection site. The child should be kept warm and carefully observed for hypersensitivity, convulsions and hemiparesis.

Brain scan

It is possible to demonstrate pictorially discrete solid tumours in the brain. This is achieved by radionuclide scanning, after the intravenous injection of radioactive compound. The techniques are safe, non-invasive and have, as their basis, the concentration of special readionuclides or radioactive compounds in or around the tumour tissue. Most tumours, irrespective of histology, label positively and most scanners produce scans with dimensions equivalent to the anatomical scanned.

After-care
No special after-care is required, but any linen which may contain radioactive material must be dealt with according to the policy of the hospital (p. 106).

Computerised axial tomography (CAT)
Computerised axial tomography is a sophisticated scanning technique used for the diagnosis of many neurological disorders. It provides visualisation of the brain through a series of segmental pictures and is most accurate in determining lesions with significant differences in densities, such as intracranial haematomas, vascular tumours, brain abscesses, hydrocephalus and cystic lesions of the central nervous system. It can also be accurate in defining cerebral oedema, low-grade astrocytomas, and some congenital malformation of the central nervous system. A CAT scanning has limited effectiveness in the evaluation of subarachnoid haemorrhage, meningitis and changes in blood vessels.

The main problem with CAT scanning in children is movement artifacts. It is important that the child holds perfectly still and to ensure that, sedation is usually necessary for children under 4 years of age, and for the hyperactive or retarded child.

Echoencephalography
The transducer is applied directly to the skull and ultrasound can display the position of the midline of the brain and the walls of the lateral and third ventricles. Deviation of the brain midline to eiher side suggests the presence of an expanding intracranial lesion. Widening of the distance between the ventricular walls suggests internal hydrocephalus. It is a very useful technique for screening head injuries and, when using a grey scale, it can show delineation of the ventricular system and of intracranial pathology in infants under 1 year, before complete calcification of the skull.

This is a non-invasive examination and there is no special preparation or after-care required. The child can be reassured that it will not be painful and a simple explanation can be given of the technique if the child is old enough to understand.

Chapter 18
Psychopathological conditions

In Chapter 1 we dealt with the growth of the body and it was shown that this growth follows certain patterns. This chapter discusses behaviour and the relationships between physical and mental growth — in particular the conscious and subconscious processes: learning and perception, intelligence and personality.

Learning and perception

The two terms learning and perception are fundamental to the development of behaviour. In order to learn we must first be capable of perceiving. The patterns of stimulation reach the brain by way of the sense organs and are then transformed into perceptions. The consequences in the nervous system of the perceptions are what we know as learning.

The individual gains experience by the perceptive process and he continually uses this experience when faced with new stimuli. There are various learning processes through which the individual passes, for example elementary (reflex) with which the newborn infant is endowed, learning by trial and error and imitative learning. The mechanism by which learning is made possible requires motivation to direct activities towards a definite end. It is considered as the energy force and guiding process in satisfying physiological needs and drives and also the highest human ambitions.

Learning is the product of constant experiences. The infant must learn to talk, dress and feed himself. He has to learn social habits acceptable to the community and, as an adult, must learn how to perform certain tasks to fulfil the role/s he has assumed within the community. Learning is a conscious and unconscious process which produces some change in behaviour. It involves thinking, reasoning and remembering.

According to Piaget (1924), there are four principal stages in the development of thought. Each stage is related to different age groups, for example; pre-logical thought from the age of $1\frac{1}{2}$ to 2 to 4 years; intuitive thought between 4 and 8 years; concrete thought between 8 and 12 years and finally, the formal thinking of the adolescent.

Intelligence

It is difficult to define intelligence. Some define it as the ability to learn, others as the ability to adapt adequately to the environment, and others as the ability to reason.

Measurement of intelligence

Intelligence tests were first introduced by Binet and Simon in 1905 and now many different tests are available. The areas tested are usually performance, for example fitting shapes into appropriate spaces, and verbal ability. The former can be used for people whose verbal ability is inadequate, for example for those with poor vision and hearing or for children whose handicap seems more severe in verbal than in other areas. In the verbal ability tests the emphasis is on verbal comprehension, especially in vocabulary tests. Binet and Simon made two basic assumptions. First, intelligence is a composite of many abilities and second, that the nature of intelligence changes with age. This means that the tests should contain tasks which are encountered by almost anyone and that the items selected should be graded by age and level of difficulty.

Binet also introduced the concept of mental age

(MA). If a given child can solve the problems posed for a 9-year-old, that child is said to have a mental age of 9. Mental age is therefore independent of chronological age (CA or the actual age). Thus if a 6-year-old child can pass the test set for a 9-year-old, his mental development is greatly accelerated.

The mental age of any child is computed by finding his basal age (the age at which he successfully completes all items) and adding it to a number of age units, in months. This corresponds to the number of items passed at higher levels. For example, a child who passes *all items* up through age scale 7 has a basal age of 7. If he passes on *four* of the six of age scale 8, each of these passes are worth 2 mental age months; on scale 9 he passes *two* of the six and none on scale 10. His mental age would be 7 + 8 + 4, i.e. 7 years plus 12 months = 8 years. This type of test is called age scaling.

To determine if the child is above or below average, it is necessary to know both his mental and chronological age. This allows for immediate comparison and is called the intelligence quotient (IQ). The formula for the IQ is:

$$IQ = \frac{\text{Mental age}}{\text{Chronological age}} \times 100$$

For example, if a 6-year-old has a mental age of 8 his IQ would be

$$\frac{8}{6} \times 100 = \frac{800}{6} = 133.3$$

An IQ is therefore a measure which compares the intelligence of a child with that of other children of the same age. There are a number of tests available, for example the Stanford-Binet, the Wechsler Intelligence Scale for children and the Raven's Matrices. The Wechsler test can be used as a diagnostic instrument in classifying mental deficiency, for example:

	IQ
Mental defective	69 and below
Borderline mental defective	70 to 79
Dull normal	80 to 89
Average normal	90 to 109
Bright normal	110 to 119
Superior	120 to 129
Very superior	130 and above

Other tests are used in assessing educational retardation and concept learning. Some studies of concept formation can help to identify the effects of brain damage, for example testing memory and ability to think.

Personality

Personality is generally accepted as the relatively permanent emotional qualities underlying the person's behaviour, his drives and needs, attitudes and interests, his intellectual, motor and cognitive skills. However, personality changes throughout life from infancy to adulthood and is influenced by the complex interactions of biology and environment. Personality can therefore be considered as the sum total of all our physical and psychological characteristics. A number of theories have been propounded and these attempt to classify individuals in terms of their characteristics.

Freud is the founder of psycho-analysis and he introduced concepts such as the dynamics of personality of which the 'id', 'ego' and 'super ego' are components. He believed that personality develops and grows as a result of a variety of processes, stresses and experiences, such as maturation, deprivation, conflict and anxiety and that the individual passes through various stages of development. Every stage of development has opportunities for stress which might interfere with the process of personality development. He introduced the concept of 'aid techniques' where the individual identifies with others, i.e. he incorporates some qualities or behaviour of another person in order to be more acceptable or to avoid rejection. An important aid in the development of a stable personality is the defence mechanism of the ego, i.e. facilitates growth of personality by protecting the ego from stress. Each of the mechanisms (repression, denial, fixation, regression) is designed to avoid guilt and anxiety. Examples might be regression, where the child already has bladder control, but when under stress, starts wetting himself; of fixation, where there is arrest of personality growth at a particular stage, for example school-phobia, where the child appears to be afraid to be separated from his home and mother.

Carl Jung introduced the concepts of introvert and extrovert and the idea that the self consisted of thinking, feeling, sensing and intuition. More recent psychologists, like Carl Rogers, see two components of personality in the organism and the self. The individual constantly strives to develop and expand the self. He must learn to have respect for and faith in himself. This largely depends on his experiences and his ability to adapt to different situations; recognition and acceptance of variations in behaviour and awareness of his feelings, attitudes and impulses. As he matures, he will grow more tolerant, more flexible and more creative. Rogers' theory of the self plays an important part in psycho-therapy and can be applied to children in play therapy.

An extension of the concept of self is that of identity. As the child progresses from infancy to adulthood he passes through various states which follow a pattern; he creates a succession of potentialities for vital interaction with other people or groups of people. The infant's utter dependence and trust in others changes to independence and identification. With each developmental stage the child will go through some change which he either incorporates or rejects resulting in conflict.

The above theories fail to explain the great variety of personality types, but nevertheless, behaviour forms can be recognised in relation to (1) hormonal influences, (for example excess thyroid activity leads to increased activity (p. 273) while decreased thyroid activity leads to lethargy and dullness) and (2) physical characteristics which are recognised in behavioural terms, for example short and plump people are considered as unstable and tolerant.

Personality assessment

Personality measurement is believed to be important in understanding the individual child as a whole. The tests in use are (1) projective tests and (2) psychometric measurements.

Projective tests

This type of test includes the Rorschach and the Children's Apperception Test. The former is said to be applicable from 3 years upwards. The test itself consists of 10 symmetrical ink blots. Each blot is presented individually and the child is asked to describe what he sees. The observer records what the child says and at the same time notes other features of his behaviour, for example length of time it takes to respond, facial expression. The descriptions are scored on such dimensions as colour, involvement perceived, figures seen. Scoring is a problem and its use for testing or measuring children's personality is still doubtful.

The Children's Apperception Test (CAT) is also claimed to be useful with children between the ages of 3 and 10 and is used in child guidance clinics. It is supposed to measure oral conflicts, sibling rivalry, etc. The supplementary test measures such behaviour as fears in play, interpersonal problems in classrooms, etc. It consists of cards with ambiguous pictures and the child is asked to tell a story about it. The stories are recorded and scored. Like the Rorschach Test, its value as a personality assessment is doubtful, since the interpretation is highly subjective and cannot be quantified.

Psychometric techniques

Psychometric techniques are a more recent development and are based on measurements of traits and factors. The psychometric approach is complementary to other personality investigations. Professor H. J. Eysenck (Britain) and Professor R. B. Cattell (USA) are two exponents of these techniques.

1. Junior Eysenck Personality Inventory. H. J. Eysenck claims that there are just two fundamental trait dimensions of personality: normal–neurotic and introversion–extroversion. The normal–neurotic dimension refers to the general adjustment of a person to his circumstances and the stability of his behaviour over a period of time. The introversion–extroversion dimension reflects the degree to which an individual is generally outgoing and participative in his interactions with other people.

The test itself has implications for personality theory, education and therapy. It consists of 60 questions, 24 each for the scales of extroversion and neuroticism and 12 for the lie scale (to estimate the reliability-validity of the test). The information obtained so far shows that there is a relationship between neuroticism and performance and that the learning process differs in extroverts and introverts in certain respects.

2. Cattell's Children's Personality Questionnaire. Cattell et al have devised a questionnaire which measures a set of 14 distinct personality traits, for example, the individual answers questions which are two-dimensional (do you have many friends? or just a few good friends?). Each of the 14 characteristics can be measured and interpreted in terms of primary personality traits. A profile of the child's personality can be drawn and described. It is constructed in such a way that profiles so obtained, can be used to predict success or failures for certain occupations, and to diagnose accepted clinical abnormalities in personalities.

Abnormal behaviour (psychopathological states)

Psychopathological behaviour has been defined as behaviour that deviates from the norm. However, this definition also includes any behaviour which might be considered unusual, for example creative and eccentric. It is therefore necessary to clarify what is really meant by abnormal or deviant behaviour which is also pathological. Psychopathological behaviour can be defined as the inability to behave in a socially acceptable or appropriate way so that the consequences of that behaviour are disturbing for the individual and/or for society. This may be due to some organic defect (brain damage) or functional defect (lack of motivation, skill or knowledge). It is important to recognise that appropriate behaviour is a culturally determined act. What is acceptable in one community, may be considered abnormal in another.

In medicine, pathological behaviour is viewed as symptomatic of a disease (mental illness) and each pattern of behaviour can be placed into major diagnostic categories. These are neurosis, psychosomatic illness, personality disorder and psychosis. In children, it should also include aspects of normal development, stress reactions, brain syndromes and mental handicap.

Children's behaviour varies widely and it is often difficult to determine the borderline between normal and abnormal. The way a child responds to any given situation is also difficult to predict. However, if the behaviour pattern persists (for example thumb-sucking is normal in infants and toddlers but is not normal in older children) then treatment may be necessary.

Causes of psychiatric disorders in children
To determine any single cause is not possible, but one can look at various factors which might contribute to a particular situation. The following factors can therefore be considered:

1. Heredity.
2. Environment.

Heredity
Genetic endowment may determine the reaction of an individual to situations. It can also affect certain physical and mental states. Phenylketonuria, for example, is an inborn (genetic) condition which can affect mental or intellectual functions. It can also be assumed that a child's intellectual potential is limited by the kind of brain with which he is endowed, but whether he reaches that potential is not predetermined and depends on other factors, for example environment. In theory, it is also possible to explain vulnerability as a hereditary predisposition. However, this must also be looked at in terms of development (both perinatal and postnatal). There are critical periods when the fetus and the infant are vulnerable, for example, the central nervous system is sensitive to oxygen lack and drugs given during the first trimester of pregnancy may interfere with cell differentiation, causing abnormalities. Mental illness therefore may be ascribed to causes other than hereditary.

Environment
When one considers the total personality and the pattern which emerges, it is important to recognise the part environment plays. The term 'environment' is generally considered to consist of the external environment (i.e. the physical surroundings) and the internal environment (i.e. the physiological state) each of which may influence the child's own attitudes and behaviour and also perhaps the attitudes and behaviour of others towards him.

1. The child's environment is affected by any *genetically transmitted* (inherited) *disorder* (in particular any neurological disorder) he may have. If the child is handicapped in any way, he is exposed to greater than normal stress, not only in his relationship within the family but also within his peer group. It has been noted that the 'battered' child tends to be the child who is 'different' in some way, though this is not the only factor. The hyperkinetic child can create stress within the family, thereby influencing his parents' attitude to him and often increasing the stress for both.

2. *Psychological factors.* These are related to the experiences the child has in his daily life. The child who is subjected to disturbing events and experiences in his day-to-day life, will find it more difficult to cope with traumatic events. The child who has a close emotional bond with his parents (preferably both) should be able to overcome any sudden change in his daily routine. The birth of another child should not produce resentment in such a child, for example, but if the relationship is already tenuous, then it is more likely that behaviour difficulties will occur. The mother, in particular, carries much of the burden in ensuring that her child develops satisfactorily. Maternal deprivation has been shown to affect young children adversely, however, the long-term effects have not been shown to be significant (Bowlby, 1961). Parental inconsistency in attitudes or an ineffectual and absent father are also causes of emotional disturbances and later delinquency.

3. *Social factors.* There is a close relationship between emotional disturbances and social and cultural deprivation. Poverty by itself, is not necessarily a causative factor, but where there is also overcrowding, malnutrition and severe or chronic illness in parents, then the stress can be overwhelming, resulting in emotional disturbances.

Types of psychiatric conditions

Stress reactions

Children show stress under different conditions. For example, babies may cry easily and show disturbed sleeping and feeding patterns when they feel insecure or if tensions are present in the home. The older infant and the toddler show signs of anxiety if there is a change in their daily routine such as separation from parents. The schoolchild may show stress if the demands made of him are not realistic or, if he feels unable or unwilling to meet these demands. The stress reaction exhibited by individuals varies. It may present in a mild transient psychosomatic reaction form like abdominal pain. (A psychosomatic reaction is a reaction characterised by an active interplay between psychological and physical factors.)

Children have special ways of coping with stress. They use 'play' as a means of coming to terms with a frightening or difficult situation — a child who is afraid of going into hospital, for example, may 'play at hospital', thereby acting out a stressful situation and coming to terms with the problems. The child may also reject a loved one if he feels his trust has been betrayed. The child admitted to hospital will show his resentment in several ways such as withdrawal or direct aggressive behaviour. These reactions are not abnormal and are a form of defence mechanism. Defence mechanisms are processes for handling stress in every day life. Internal stress is dealt with by repression and denial, while displacement means the re-channelling of inner conflict to a substitute object. Play is a good example, where the stressful situation is substituted by a less personal level, and resolution of the stress can be achieved.

Neurosis

Neurosis is a generic term. It is a less severe form of behaviour disorder, which may be troublesome enough to require treatment. Many of the disturbances are a more extreme form of normal defence mechanism used in an attempt to resolve a persistent conflict. The presenting symptoms may therefore be similar to stress reactions but are of longer duration.

The main causes are to be found in day-to-day experiences and are probably due to misinterpretation (conscious or unconscious) of such experiences.

The underlying psychopathology is difficult to ascertain, but from infancy there are predominant modes of feelings relating to other people and events. If during the development of the child there is overwhelming stress or trauma at any particular stage, then emotional arrest may occur.

Anxiety is a common feature even in young children and is an appropriate reaction to some circumstances of stress and danger. When anxiety persists and causes distress to the child or those concerned with him, then it must be considered abnormal. Some of the anxiety can be coped with and does not require special treatment. When the anxiety is not related to external situations or when it occurs in situations which normally do not produce anxiety, then help will be required.

Expressions of anxiety

The child may feel and appear anxious. He would show physical signs such as frequency of micturition, nausea, vomiting, headaches and sleeplessness. Other behaviour forms include regression or aggression directed towards the object or cause of the anxiety.

Enuresis is usually considered an expression of anxiety. School refusal, with or without associated somatic symptoms, is also often an expression of anxiety which may interfere with learning and may therefore lead to educational underfunctioning. Where the child feels less able than his peers, it can also lead to aggressive behaviour both at home and at school.

Psychosomatic disorders are characterised by definite abnormalities of physiological function or organic structures. The disorders seem to affect those organs which are under the control of the autonomic nervous system such as skin (eczema), respiratory system (asthma), cerebrovascular system (headache, migraine), musculoskeletal systems (inability to move or write) and gastro-intestinal tract (nausea, vomiting, constipation, diarrhoea). Some stress situations can produce bodily manipulation, for example, hair-pulling.

Management

Careful assessment of the total situation is essential. Sometimes an anxiety-laden situation can be resolved if the parents are given an explanation and reassurance; while the child should be encouraged to talk to an uninvolved adult. Anxiety may be caused by excessive demands made on the child, or by parental depression. Relief of the child's difficulties may be achieved once the parent has been treated. Drugs play a small part in managing anxiety in children. Some children may be given tranquillisers for a short time and these are usually given where there is a crisis, such as examination of the child.

Group therapy is useful for some adolescents, and in the form of play, for younger children. Adolescents can also take part in psycho-drama.

PSYCHOSIS

Psychosis is a generic term. It applies where there is continuous bizarre and unpredictable behaviour. Two types can be identified in childhood:

1. Early infantile autism.
2. Childhood schizophrenia.

Early childhood autism

The word autism means withdrawal and loss of contact with reality or other people. This non-relatedness to other people may not be noticed during infancy but may already be present. A great deal of research into early childhood autism has been undertaken and there have been advances in the understanding of the condition. A useful definition has been proposed by Rutter (1970) that the diagnosis of autism should be restricted to cases in which there is: 'an onset before 30 months of age, of a disorder involving an autistic-type failure to develop interpersonal relationships, a delay in speech and language development and ritualistic and "compulsive" phenomena'.

There are certain features which can be recognised:

1. *Withdrawal.* Autistic children do not respond when spoken to and do not make contact with others. They do not appear to be deaf since they often can reproduce phrases and songs (which they must have heard). Eye-to-eye contact is lacking. The child is said to sit for long periods, preoccupied with his hands, gazing at objects. This preoccupation with objects continues and becomes more striking as he becomes older, when there is apparent fascination with shiny surfaces and mechanical objects. There are also sudden mood changes and temper tantrums.
2. Failure to respond to tactile and painful stimuli is also a feature.

3. Speech is often affected. The child is generally able to speak at about the usual age, but he loses this facility by the age of 2 years. There is also a tendency in some children to repeat a phrase or word exactly (echolalia).
4. Intellectual retardation is often found in these children when first examined, but there is a tendency for improvement when the child begins to emerge from his withdrawal.
5. Ritualistic and compulsive behaviour is a feature of autism, the child insisting on a particular routine in his daily life, resisting any change. The same applies to objects to which he becomes extremely attached and from which he cannot be parted.
6. Unusual postures and movements are also often present. These include hand flapping and fingers flicking near the eyes. Facial grimaces, jumping and walking on tip-toe are also seen.

The cause of autism has not been determined, though various theories have been put forward. These include the assumption that (a) the environment, particularly parental attitudes, and personalities exert a fundamental influence on the child. This is based on the observations in the social interaction between a parent and an autistic child. It is, however, important to consider how very difficult it is for anyone to interact normally with such a child and this therefore cannot really be considered a cause for the condition. (b) it may be due to organic brain disease. (This is explained by the presence of cerebral dysfunction, for example disorders of communication and sensory disorders. It is also not uncommon for these children to develop epileptic fits); and (c) autism may be genetically determined.

The features also vary with the age of the child. In *babyhood* there may be failure to cuddle or come for comfort; he may not respond appropriately to being picked up and may lie limp and unresponsive. Lack of eye contact may give the impression of distance or non-recognition. The older baby may show little curiosity or interest in his environment. Play tends to be unimaginative. Pre-verbal communication such as babble is abnormal; sleep may be disturbed and there may be prolonged screaming.

In *childhood and adolescence* the autistic child may show an abnormal response to sounds; he may be terrified of some and fascinated by others. Speech may be impaired and some children may be mute all their lives. Those who develop speech may show abnormalities such as echolalia and telegrammatic constructions. As they grow up speech tends to remain pedantic with abnormalities in intonation and timing.

There may also be abnormalities in visual perception and the autistic child may appear to concentrate more on the periphery, or on parts and details of a picture or environment, than on the whole. They may be fascinated by texture and may make extensive use of their sense of smell, taste and touch when exploring their environment.

Autistic children also tend to show from an early age exaggerated and stereotypic movements which are of absorbing interest to them. These include: rocking and turning, hand flapping and finger posturing. Many of these activities appear to have ritualistic functions and are intensified under conditions of excitement or stress. Some autistic children may be abnormally restless, destructive or have excessive temper tantrums.

In adolescence, sexual behaviour may be inappropriate and without inhibition. Some autistic adolescents may make exploratory sexual contact with complete strangers.

Principles of treatment and management
There is unfortunately no medical or psychological treatment which is known to be effective. Parents need help in coping with their child. Serious behaviour problems such as noisiness, restlessness, or self-injury may be partially alleviated with drugs such as chlorpromazine or thioridazine. Sleeplessness may respond to sedatives such as chloral hydrate, and convulsions will have to be controlled with anticonvulsants. Hyperkinesis is a problem, and where it is sustained and severe, an additive-free diet (p. 221) may be tried.

Training and education are of great importance and various methods are advocated — for example, use of operant conditioning, where positive reinforcement (rewards) and negative reinforcement (punishment) are used. The general aim is to use the most suitable method for that child to help him to overcome his handicap, to develop social skills and encourage practical skills. Patience is an essential attribute since progress is generally extremely slow.

Whatever the approach adopted, it is important to involve all those who are directly involved in the care of the child. This includes parents, nurses or other residential staff. For parents it is of vital importance that they feel that they are contributing to their child's treatment. It is also important that parents are aware of self-help groups such as the Scottish Society for Autistic children and the National Society for Autistic Children where they can get support, and are made aware of the range of services available for autistic children.

Childhood schizophrenia

This is a psychotic state which begins early in childhood. The onset is more insidious. The child behaves in a peculiar manner until the more obvious signs appear. These include hallucinations, delusions, blocking of thought, blunting of the emotions and frequent mood changes.

Management

The child or adolescent is often very disturbed by his symptoms and he often reacts with anxiety or depression. Drugs like the phenothiazines are effective in relieving the symptoms.

Hyperkinetic syndromes

Hyperkinesis or overactivity is a term which is commonly used in children who exhibit restless and fidgety behaviour. It should however be reserved for those children where there is a chronic, sustained, excessive level of motor activity relative to the age of the child. It occurs mainly in boys and is accompanied by distractibility and short span of attention, impulsivity, excitability and explosive outbursts of such as temper tantrums and low frustration tolerance. Their behaviour tends to be aggressive and anti-social and there may also be learning problems and emotional lability.

The behaviour pattern is often apparent from an early age and mothers may describe their babies as unusually active, alert and requiring little sleep. The cause of this condition is not clear. Some believe that it is associated with brain damage. Whilst some hyperkinetic children may suffer from brain damage, many do not, and likewise most brain-damaged children do not present with the hyperkinetic syndrome. Hyperkinetic behaviour is common in mentally retarded patients, particularly those with epilepsy and with more severe degrees of retardation.

Treatment and management

It is important that there is a consistent handling policy and to involve all those directly in contact with the child in a common approach. Space is important since it is difficult to manage such a child in a confined and crowded environment. The parents may have to be provided with a suitable house e.g. ground floor with an attached garden.

Drugs such as major tranquillisers of the phenothiazine and butyrophenone groups are probably the mainstay of treatment. These drugs may be palliative. Other drugs such as imipramine (antidepressant) and lithium carbonate have also been used.

Some success has been achieved by using operant conditioning techniques. Behaviour modification in the form of a token reinforcement programme produced good results from relatively short courses of treatment. It has also been suggested that food additives can exacerbate hyperkinesis and therefore additive-free diets have been developed and used and in some cases found to be effective (p. 221).

School refusal

Many children are absent from school due to illness, but there are others who are absent without any acceptable reason. Some are kept at home by their parents to help a house-bound parent. Absence from school is also known as 'truancy' when the child does not attend without the knowledge or consent of his parents and school authority. These children leave home in the morning, some go to school to register, but others make no attempt to go to school. They roam the streets or return home and many show anti-social behaviour. There is another group of children who, for some reason or other, seem unable to make themselves go to school and sometimes openly refuse to do so. There are signs of anxiety when the time comes to go to school and although they set out for school, some never arrive there but return home in panic. Sometimes there are other signs such as loss of appetite, abdominal pain, vomiting, syncope, headache, diarrhoea and other physical signs associated with psychosomatic states. Most of these symptoms disappear at the weekend and during school holidays. The onset may be sudden in younger children who tend to cling to their mothers and refuse to leave them to go to school. The cause of the fear of going to school is often difficult to elicit. It may be because he feels that he cannot meet the demands made by the school, even though he has no difficulty with his school work. Any situation, either at home or at school, could produce this response, e.g. illness of one parent, humiliation at school or a poor relationship with teacher or other children.

Older children. The onset is more gradual. There may have been periods of reluctance to attend school or outright refusal. There is gradual withdrawal from group activities and a tendency to prefer staying at home. Depression often accompanies this behaviour and there may also be changes in personality.

Management

The management depends on identifying the true situation. If it is truancy then the cause should be investigated. However, these children are dealt with by the educational system or in persistant cases through the courts, particularly if it is associated with anti-social behaviour.

The true case of school refusal must be distinguished from all other types first and the management will be geared to the underlying psychological factors. Each case should be carefully studied and any complaints about the school should be listened to and, where possible and appropriate, the necessary action should be taken, for example allocation to school or class. Although initially the child may be kept away from school, the aim should be to return him to school as soon as possible. Liaison between clinic/hospital and school is important so that the treatment given will have a chance of success.

Tensions and anxiety in the family can be contained either by the general practitioner or the clinic. Drugs such as diazepam or chlordiazepoxide can be useful in reducing anxiety in the child to allow him to go to school. In some cases, the child will have to be referred to the child psychiatric service and inpatient care may be necessary.

The handicapped child and his needs

The birth of a handicapped child is a traumatic event for parents. Throughout pregnancy, both parents have had anxious thoughts about the type of child they will have. The first questions that are always asked are whether the baby is a boy or girl, and if the baby is 'normal' or 'all right'.

The 'normal' child has to reach maturation with a minimum of function, but he is able to respond in a generalised way to communicate his primitive needs, i.e. states of comfort and discomfort. He gradually moves from the highly dependent state to one of greater independence so that by the age of 5 years, he is able to join the larger school community.

The handicapped child has not only to overcome or learn to live with his handicap, he also has to overcome the barrier or rejection. The impact on the parents is such that there is numbness, grief, disgust and a feeling of helplessness. Such feelings interfere with the way the mother, in particular, perceives the initial cues from her baby and her response to them. There is a need to support the parents and to discuss with them all the different aspects of the handicap and its implications for the child and parents.

The blind child can smile early in infancy but as he grows he smiles less frequently and the response is due to touch rather than sight. Sensory stimulation is limited. He has to wait to be touched by objects and people because he cannot reach out and locate objects. He tends to find pleasures in rocking, twisting, thumb-sucking rather than through manipulation. He is often left in one area, for example a play-pen, and has little social contact with other people.

The child who is over-protected also becomes overdependent and retains much of the infantile behaviour. He also has difficulty in adapting to any stress or crises during development.

Each handicap produces its limitations when forming early relationships. For example, the blind child can only hear an angry tone of voice and there is no relief by seeing a smile afterwards, although a change of voice should give some relief. The deaf child will have difficulty in communicating and will feel insecure in a world of silence. He does not readily tolerate frustration resulting in periods of anger, rage and tantrums. Such outbursts, provoked by nearly all crises, may produce violent behaviour that is directed against the child himself.

Some severely handicapped children withdraw and create their own little world.

Management

Where possible, the child should remain with his parents and the child without parents would be better in a foster home. Facilities should be made available in the community to help the family at all levels.

Forms of psychiatric treatment

Behaviour therapy or behaviour shaping. This technique is based on the principles of learning theory. The aim is to let the child unlearn and relearn, using the method of rewards or nonrewards. A child may be rewarded when he makes a good or desirable response; no reward is given if the desired response is not forthcoming.

Psycho-therapy. This is based on interviews. The aim is to find the cause or to treat the child. The child is encouraged to speak and to express his feelings. At a superficial level the therapist listens and directs any difficulties the child may have into more positive channels. Parents too are involved. They are interviewed together with the child and also on their own.

Play therapy. This is a good method for children. They often find it difficult to express their fears and anxieties in words but can express them through play. The child is allowed free undirected play while the therapist observes. Where necessary he helps him to verbalise his feelings and emotions, so that the child can learn to deal with his problems in a rational adaptive way.

Group therapy. This is more suitable for older children and adolescents. The aim is learning to relate to others in the group, sharing their problems and learning not only from the therapist but also from other members of the group. Group method varies from a very directive approach from the therapist, to near non-directive approach. It is hoped that the child may gain insight into his own and other people's behaviour.

Chapter 19
Mental retardation

Mental retardation can be defined as a limitation of intelligence sufficient to interfere with normal adaptation to the environment. It is manifested by abnormal development and is associated with difficulties in learning and social adaption.

It perceives the state as a condition of arrested or incomplete development which is especially characterised by subnormality of intelligence.

Classification used to be based on intelligence only, but today it includes concepts of 'social competence or adaptive behaviour'. The following classification is a useful one since it indicates different aspects of development, social competence and behavioural variations which will influence the individual's ability to adapt to the environment.

Level I: Where there is some motor and speech development, but he is incapable of self-maintenance. He needs complete care and supervision.

Level II: The individual can contribute partially to self-support under complete supervision. He is capable of developing self-protection, and able to achieve skills to a minimum useful level in a controlled environment.

Level III: He is capable of self-maintenance in unskilled or semi-skilled occupations. He requires supervision and guidance when under mild social or economic stress.

Level IV: He is capable of social and vocational adequacy with proper education and training. He frequently requires supervision and guidance when under serious social or economic stress.

Causes of mental retardation

In many cases the cause of mental retardation is unknown. In others, the cause has been identified. The causes are said to occur in the prenatal, perinatal and postnatal periods.

Prenatal period
Mental retardation occurs due to genetic chromosome abnormalities, hereditary disorders or infectious diseases. Retardation before birth may also be due to anoxia, metabolic disorders and trauma.

Chromosomal abnormalities (p. 253)
These comprise the largest number of known genetic causes and the most common are the trisomies, which involve an additional chromosome, viz. 47 instead of the normal 46. For example, G-trisomy, when chromosome 21 is trisomic, trisomy 17–18 (E syndrome), trisomy 13–15 (D syndrome). Partial or complete deletion of the short arms of chromosome 5 is also known as 'Cri du chat' syndrome. Abnormalities in sex chromosomes, such as Klinefelter's syndrome (XXY), Turner's syndrome and various mosaics, may also be associated with mental retardation.

Hereditary causes
The defect is transmitted via genes (p. 254). Most of these are sex-linked recessive defects, e.g. Lowe's syndrome (oculocerebrorenal syndrome) and Hunter's syndrome. Metabolic disorders, such as phenylketonuria (p. 262), galactosaemia (p. 263), Tay-Sachs disease, etc. are also due to autosomal recessive disorders.

Infections
Infections due to rubella virus and cytomegalovirus have also been identified as a cause of mental

retardation. These viruses can pass the placental barrier and interfere with normal development of fetal tissue.

Perinatal period

Perinatal complications such as breech presentation, bleeding, high forceps delivery and asphyxia neonatorum may increase the risk of mental retardation due to brain tissue damage. Malnutrition *in utero* and toxins may also cause mental retardation.

Postnatal period

Postnatal infection by viruses and bacteria, poisoning by substances such as lead and severe head injuries may all be causes of mental retardation. Malnutrition may have a major effect on brain development and mental retardation can result where famine and hunger are commonplace.

The pathology of mental handicap

There are a number of syndromes which contain normal intelligence, mild handicap and also severe mental handicap. Down's syndrome is an example. A small proportion function in the mild retarded range. It is known that mosaicism permits degrees of gradation from superior intelligence to the least able for Down's syndrome in the range of profound mental handicap. A number of mildly handicapped persons include other chromosomal abnormalities, e.g. Klinefelter's and Turner's syndromes. Such errors may lead to cerebral dysfunction which in turn gives rise to other symptoms of intellectual deficit.

There is little evidence that mildly mentally handicapped people have structural abnormality of the brain, but in some cases neurological abnormality may be present. Some children with structural abnormality of the brain function normally, while others have behaviour disorders of the most varied kind; still others have epilepsy, and the most common clinical effect of brain damage is intellectual retardation. However, the great majority of severely mentally handicapped have demonstrable abnormalities of the brain.

Brain function in the mentally handicapped shows variation. For example, there is slowed reaction time to both visual and auditory, simple and complex stimulus-response situations, which is characteristic of many mentally handicapped;

the electroencephalogram is often abnormal and there is psychological dysfunction, such as poor arousal, deficient short-term memory and poor attention span.

Down's syndrome (Fig. 19.1)

Down's syndrome is the most common specific type of mental retardation occurring in about one in 600 live births. The cause is a chromosomal defect and is often linked to older mothers where non-dysjunction is more likely to occur. However, recent studies have shown that the father may be the carrier of the extra chromosome. Chromosome 21 (Denver system) is especially liable to this error although it can also involve D 13–15 (15) where an additional member (trisomy) will be seen. Another type is mosaicism when faulty chromosomal distribution occurs in the developing embryo after fertilisation.

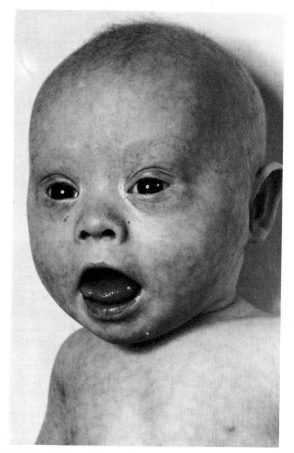

Fig. 19.1 Infant with Down's syndrome.

Clinical features

The clinical features of Down's syndrome are usually easily recognised by the characteristic facial features which resemble those of the Mongol people. The term Down's syndrome is preferred to mongolism, since the latter implies a relationship between the condition and the Mongolian people.

These children present with nystagmus, squint, speckling or mottling of the iris, epicanthic folds or fold, transverse palmar creases or crease; often there is an associated congenital abnormality such as congenital heart disease, congenital dislocation of the hip; there is a tendency to leukaemia.

The infant tends to be placid, rarely cries and there is muscular hypotonicity. Microcephaly, brachycephaly and a flattened occiput are characteristic. The mouth is often held open because of a large protruding tongue which may also be fissured. The hands are short and broad and hyperextension is possible. The little finger is curved in and the middle phalanx is poorly developed. Dermatoglyphs are peculiar — a single or 'simian' transverse crease is found across the palm. There are fewer whorls and loops open to the radial side but there are more ulnar loops than in normal subjects.

They tend to be cheerful, happy, friendly and fond of music, but like normal children they can exhibit a range of personality attributes. In adolescence, sexual development is usually delayed or incomplete. Males have small genitalia and may be infertile. Females menstruate at the average age and a few Down's syndrome women have reproduced; about half of their offspring have had the syndrome.

Mental development

The range of mental handicap varies from only mildly retarded to more severely retarded. Those children whose syndrome is due to mosaicism tend to have a higher IQ than those found in children with trisomy 21. They are markedly deficient in the development of language and it is often difficult to understand the speech of these people. However, they are quite good at rote learning and mimicry.

Although Down's syndrome is the most described and best known of the conditions associated with mental retardation, there are many conditions which produce a characteristic physical appearance usually associated with mental retardation, for example, facial asymmetry, microcephaly, dwarfism with characteristic facies (De Lange syndrome).

Investigations

1. *Neuroradiology* may reveal abnormalities in the structure of the skull, e.g. intracranial calcification or raised intracranial pressure.
2. *Echoencephalography* may show tumours and haematomata.
3. *Brain biopsy* is only useful in a small number of mentally retarded children. It is also not readily acceptable to parents who see the removal of even a small piece of brain tissue as adding damage to the already inadequate brain.
4. *Biochemical studies* determine the level of various metabolic substances which are known to affect brain tissue if they are present in abnormally large or small amounts, e.g. hypoglycaemia in pre-term new-born infants, accumulation of glycogen in muscle and neurones, fatty deposits in the brain and high phenylalanine levels.

Treatment and management of the mentally retarded child

When the condition is due to inherited disorders of metabolism, then the relevant dietary management can either prevent damage to the brain tissue or limit the damage. Conditions which have a specific cause, e.g. cretinism, are treated with the relevant drugs; other which have no specific cause, e.g. Riley-Day syndrome, may have some of the symptoms relieved by suitable drugs which, however, have no effect on the damaged brain tissue.

Once mental retardation is established, there is little evidence that improvement can be achieved by either drugs or any other forms of treatment. The aim, therefore, is to utilise the existing social and educational services so that the child can develop to the limit of his potential.

At the present time the care of the mentally retarded child is either custodial (i.e. hospital) or community, e.g. the child's own home. The choice of environment will largely depend on the degree of retardation and the presence of other abnormalities.

When a mentally retarded child is admitted to a sick children's hospital or ward in a general hospital, it is important to recognise that the child has different needs and that nursing requires a different approach. The child's lack of, or limited reasoning ability makes it imperative that explanations are kept simple and that the words and sentences used are related to the age and degree of retardation. Fear and anxiety have to be allayed positively, primarily by giving physical support rather than by reasoning, e.g. holding and comforting the child. However, it should also be understood that because of the physical strength of some of these children, particularly older ones, it is wise to have help when performing procedures such as dressings, administering oral or parenteral drugs.

The nursing function can therefore be clearly defined where abnormalities or other conditions exist, which require specialist nursing, e.g. naso-gastric feeding, suction, etc. but the social and educational aspects are not, strictly speaking, within the nursing function, though nurses must be aware of the needs of such children and provide a suitable environment.

The education of the mentally retarded child requires teachers who have been specially trained and the local Education Authority has a duty to provide education suitable for this category of child whether in custodial or community care.

Pre-school training

Little children need to explore within safe limits and, even for the normal child, this can be difficult to achieve. For the mentally retarded child, limited understanding and reasoning means that a higher level of supervision is necessary and unless the environment is safe, exploration may have to be limited. Toilet training will also take longer and greater patience will be required. Learning is by imitation as in the normal child but, at a comparable age, the mentally retarded child has less ability to control and foresee the consequences of his action or behaviour. Toys should be of good quality and should serve a number of functions including development of motor skill and control, which he can learn in the home environment, provided he receives the requisite time and patience from his parents and family.

Special schools and day-care centres

The functions of these establishments are to teach the educable child some of the normal school subjects, e.g. reading and writing, and to teach him simple skills. The aim is to allow each child to work and learn at his own pace and thus to achieve his potential.

Community responsibility

Mentally retarded people have to be protected just as the community has to be protected. Children of low ability tend to fall prey to undesirable influences and a number of them are involved in a variety of crimes. Clinics or centres should be available where these children can receive support and training so that those who are able can play a limited but useful part. This includes vocational training, guidance centres for employment and later employment suitable for them.

It should be recognised that any type of abnormality, but particularly one affecting the intellect, creates stresses and strains within the home. The fact that the mother in particular is often isolated because of the unacceptable behaviour of the child, means that there is often tension within the home. There is a need to provide relief of some kind, e.g. during the holidays, the child might be taken into care so that the mother and probably the rest of the family too, can recuperate. Feelings of guilt also produce conflict in the parents, and it can often be found that where a mentally retarded child is one of a number of children in the family, then he will often receive more attention than the other, normal children.

The parents will therefore require a great deal of guidance and support which they often get from other in a similar situation. However, it is also necessary that the support comes from professionals like the general practitioner, clinical psychologist, teachers and geneticists who should explain the condition and the likelihood of producing a similar abnormality in future children.

Chapter 20
Disorders of the visual system

Most disorders of the eyes are due to functional or physical abnormalities of some part of the eye or its attachments. In order to understand abnormal function, it is therefore necessary to have some understanding of the normal structure and function of the eye.

The infant's visual system

At birth the human eye is about half the size and weight of that of the mature adult. Anatomically it is the same, but the relation of the parts to each other is different from that of adults and not all parts develop at the same rate. For example the cornea is much closer to its final stage of development than is the iris. The retina is fairly well developed in the new-born, but the macula is only partially formed. The optic tract is only partially myelinated at birth and this reduces the conductivity of the nerve fibres and electrical activity is dispersed to surrounding tissue. Myelination of the optic tract is essential for effective vision.

Ocular control also is different in infants. At birth the eye operates like a fixed focus camera and no accommodation of the lens occurs for targets presented at different distances. The distance of around 20 cm appears to be the ideal focal distance. This state persists for the first few weeks of life.

General description

The anterior segment of the eye, the *cornea*, is transparent and permits rays of light to pass through to the interior of the eye. The remainder of the eye is opaque. The wall of the eyeball contains three layers:

1. External supporting layer (sclera) consists of dense connective tissue which is white, except for the covering of the anterior portion of the eye (cornea), which is transparent.

2. Middle layer (choroid) contains blood vessels and is bluish in colour. Anteriorly it forms the ciliary body. This circular structure gives rise to ciliary processes which extend inwards and continue forwards to form the *iris* of the eye. The iris surrounds an aperture called the pupil, which can alter its diameter by a change of tone of the smooth muscle in the iris. The pupil contracts when the eye is exposed to bright light and dilates in dim light.

3. Retinal layer. This consists of two parts, an outer pigmented layer which lines the whole of the inner surface of the choroid and an inner *nervous* layer which contains the photo-receptors (rods and cones).

The retina consists of several layers of which the light-sensitive receptors are outermost. It also contains three layers of neurones from inwards outwards, ganglion cells, bipolar cells and light-sensitive rods and cones. The light travels through the ganglion cells and bipolar cells before finally reaching the rods and cones.

The cones are adapted to daylight and colour vision and enables us to see objects in clear outline and detail. One area, the fovea centralis, contains only cones and it is here that the image of small objects falls when the eye is used in discriminate vision. In all other areas both rods and cones are found. The entrance of the optic nerve (optic disc) is insensitive to light and constitutes the 'blind spot'.

The rods contain rhodopsin or visual purple, which is bleached by light. They are concerned with dark adaptation, which is the ability to see in dim light.

The lens. The crystalline lens, which is attached to the ciliary body by means of the suspensory ligament, is a biconvex structure enclosed in a highly plastic capsule.

The ability of the eye to focus on objects at varying distances (known as accommodation) is due to a mechanism which allows changes of curvature of the anterior surface of the lens. This is due to the action of the ciliary muscles (Fig. 20.2B).

Contraction of the ciliary muscles increases the curvature of lens. This brings near objects into focus. When looking at distant objects, the ciliary muscle relaxes, the suspensory ligament is pulled towards the edge of the choroid and the lens becomes less convex.

The space between the cornea and the anterior lens surface is called the anterior chamber and the narrow circular space between the iris, lens and the ciliary body, is called the posterior chamber. Both chambers contain *aqueous humour*, a thin watery fluid containing crystalloids in concentrations similar to that of plasma. The fluid is formed by dialysis of crystalloid fluid from the capillaries of the ciliary process. It passes from the posterior chamber into the anterior chamber. From the spaces of Fontana the fluid passes across the endothelium lining the canal of Schlemm which drains the fluid into the ocular veins.

The vitreous body is a transparent gel which occupies the intra-ocular space between the lens and the internal layer of the retina. Its function is to maintain intra-ocular pressure.

The ocular muscular apparatus (Fig. 20.1)

Apart from the intrinsic muscles which are concerned with accommodation, there are extrinsic or external muscles which are responsible for eyeball movement.

The movements of the eyeballs are brought about by six voluntary muscles to each eye, arranged in three opposing pairs and controlled by three cranial nerves III, IV and VI. These muscles and their functions are as follows:

Superior rectus — turns the front of the eyeball *upwards*.

Inferior rectus — turns the front of the eyeball *downwards*.

External and internal recti — turns the eye outwards and inwards respectively.

Superior oblique muscle — turns the eyeball obliquely outwards and downwards.

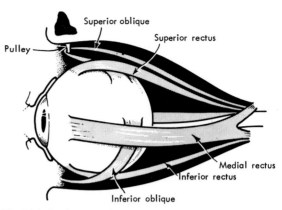

Fig. 20.1 Ocular muscular apparatus — causes of squint.

Inferior oblique muscle — turns the eyeball upwards and outwards.

Partial paralysis or overaction of any of these muscles will result in the formation of two images (diplopia). It also gives rise to strabismus (squint).

Eyebrows are arched encumbrances of skin lying on the orbits containing short hair. They have a protective function.

Eyelids are two thin movable folds. The upper eyelids are more movable than the lower ones. Their function is to protect the eye; frequent blinking keeps the eyes moist and free from dust.

Eyelashes are attached to the free edges of the eyelids. Short, thick, curved hairs are arranged in double or triple rows. Ciliary glands are found close to the free margin of each lid which open near the attachments of the eyelashes. Infection of the follicle leads to stye formation and the glands may become infected.

Conjunctiva. The conjunctiva consists of transparent mucous membrane which lines the inner surface of the eyelids and is reflected over the front part of the sclera and cornea. Inflammation of the conjunctiva may occur.

Lacrimal apparatus. This consists of (1) the lacrimal gland and (2) the lacrimal canal, sac and nasolacrimal duct which conveys the fluid into the nasal cavity.

The lacrimal gland produces tear fluid which keeps the conjunctivae moist.

Functions of the eyes

All the transparent structures of the eye play a part in forming images of external objects on the retina.

The ability to bend rays of light (refraction) depends on the structure through which they pass, i.e. cornea, aqueous and vitreous humour and the lens. The lens also changes its curvature so that it accommodates to objects at varying distances. Rays of light ordinarily travel in straight lines. A convex lens bends the light rays so that they meet at a point of focus behind the lens. Accommodation depends also on pupillary constriction which shuts off the more peripheral parts of the lens. Accommodation can be paralysed by atropine and homatropine. Loss of accommodation (presbyopia) can occur due to sclerosis of the lens substance.

The eye of the newborn baby is different from the adult eye. For the first 2 months the eyes show rough movements in response to stimuli. The cornea occupies a larger part of the outer coat of the eye; its curvature is greater. The eye is hypermetropic (long sight). The iris is incompletely

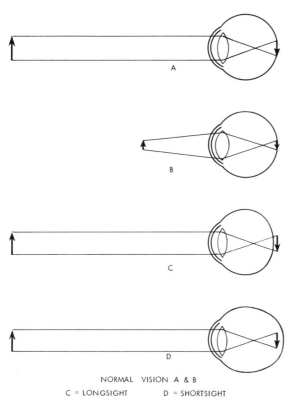

NORMAL VISION A & B
C = LONGSIGHT   D = SHORTSIGHT

Fig. 20.2 Diagram of normal, hypermetropic and myopic eye.

coloured, the sclera is thin and appears blue and the lens is relatively spherical.

Defects of vision

REFRACTIVE ERRORS

These arise when the parallel light rays are not brought to focus on the retina when the ciliary muscle is at rest.

Hypermetropia (long sightedness)

The image of a distant object comes to focus behind the retina as the axial length of the eyes is too short (Fig. 20.2C). It may also be due to insufficient curvature of the cornea and lens. Most infants are hypermetropic at birth and only gradually develop normal refraction. Abnormal hypermetropia may lead to convergent strabismus (squint). Hypermetropia can be corrected by a convex lens which increases the convergence of light rays incident upon the retina.

Myopia (short sightedness)

The image of the distant object comes to a focus in front of the retina (Fig. 20.2D). This may be due to increased curvature of cornea and lens, but is more commonly due to an abnormally large eye. Myopia is a developmental abnormality which progresses during the years of body growth. The danger of the increase in size results in stretching and patchy degeneration of the retina. Vision is poor and can be corrected by concave glasses which cause divergence of the incident rays.

Astigmatism

In this condition the refractive power is different in the different curvatures of the cornea. It may also affect the lens. The focus for horizontal rays differs from that for vertical rays.

Strabismus and amblyopia (squint)

In this condition, the visual axis of one eye is not directed at the object observed by the other eye (normal eye). This condition is found in approximately 2 per cent of all children. If the squinting eye is 'turned in', the squint is convergent; if 'turned out', the squint is divergent.

Causes

Any disability which makes it harder than usual for the child to learn to use his two eyes together may be cause. Normally, vision of nearby objects involves (1) increased convexity of the lens and the simultaneous constriction of the pupil, and (2) convergence of the visual axis, i.e. the direction of light rays focused on the macula. This accommodation/convergence reflex is gradually acquired in the early years of life.

The following situations produce a squint:

1. High degree of refractive error. This makes objects blurred. The child attempts to compensate for the error and also attempts to prevent squinting. When he is unable to achieve a clearer image, he tends to use one eye for fixing and suppresses vision in the other eye.
2. Extra-ocular muscle imbalance. There appears to be a fault in the muscles which move the eyes, resulting in an abnormal convergent or divergent resting position of the eyes.
3. Eye muscle paralysis. This leads to squinting and consequent double vision.
4. Stress. A latent squint may become obvious during some intercurrent illness.

Types of squint

1. Pseudo-squint. This is common in young children but generally disappears with facial development.
2. Latent squint. This is found where there is extra-ocular muscle imbalance.
3. Concomitant (non-paralytic squint). The angle of deviation remains unchanged whatever the direction of gaze. It may be either convergent or divergent, turned upwards or downwards. It may also be intermittent but is generally present at all times.
4. Incomitant (paralytic) squint. This is not so common and may be due to dysfunction of the VIth cranial nerve.

Principles of treatment and nursing management

1. Investigation. It is essential to confirm the presence of a doubtful squint.

   a. Tests. The cover test is useful and consists of covering each eye in turn while the child looks steadily at some object. Assessment of vision in both eyes is very important and testing for refractive errors is essential. Children of all ages are often not aware of poor vision and accept as normal their poor vision. Tests should be carried out in pre-school children and schoolchildren should have assessments at regular intervals. To examine young children, a cycloplegic drug is used. This paralyses accommodation which is the desired effect, although it also acts as a mydriatic (dilates pupil). Atropine 0.5 per cent may be used twice daily for two days prior to the examination, although there is a danger of toxicity if the atropine is absorbed through the lacrimal passages. Atropine ointment 0.25 per cent is considered safer than drops.

   b. Ophthalmoscopy. This instrument enables examination of the fundus. The infant is probably better lying on a couch or bed, while the older child can be examined while sitting. Both eyes should be open and he should be asked to fix his eyes on a distant object.

   c. Photography of the face; external eye, anterior segment, lens and fundus can be photographed.

   d. Radiological examination. This is useful in the early diagnosis of orbital lesion, e.g. optic nerve tumours.

   e. Testing visual acuity using test card (Fig. 20.3). The test card used for children from 3 to 6 years of age is the 'E' test card, and the Snellen alphabet card is used for children over the age of 6.

2. Spectacles to correct refractive error.
3. Surgical treatment may be necessary where correction cannot be achieved by other means. This involves shortening, lengthening or repositioning of the extra-ocular muscles.

   a. Pre-operative care. See page 128 for routine preparation — there is usually no specific preparation.

   b. Post-operative care. Routine (p. 131) — arms should be restrained to prevent rubbing of eyes. In some units, the eyes may be covered. In these cases, it is important to anticipate the child's anxiety. He will not

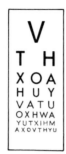

Snellen's Test Card (for older children who can read)

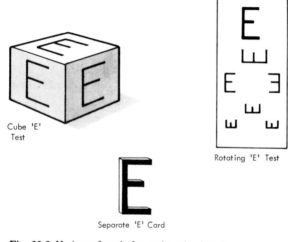

Cube 'E' Test

Rotating 'E' Test

Separate 'E' Card

Fig. 20.3 Variety of cards for testing visual acuity.

be able to see and sounds which are unfamiliar to him will make him anxious. When approaching the child, the nurse should speak to him so that he is aware of her presence, and before touching him explain what is going to happen. The child is usually allowed to go home on the third post-operative day.

RETINOBLASTOMA
This is the only malignant tumour that occurs in the eye in childhood and it develops within the first few years of life. Treatment consists of enucleation of the affected eye with the removal of as much of the optic nerve as possible but, if it is diagnosed early, radiotherapy is effective.

DISORDERS OF THE LENS

Cataract
This term is used to describe a lens which is partially or completely opaque. The lens can be seen as a white or grey area. The opacity is due to degeneration of lens proteins and, in some cases, calcification. Five types of cataract are recognised and four of these apply to children.

Developmental cataract. This is present at birth or develops within the first few years of life. Cataracts may be hereditary and may be transmitted as an autosomal dominant.

Secondary type is often associated with some coexisting ocular or systemic disease, e.g. rubella cataract, which may occur in an infant whose mother has had rubella during the first three months of pregnancy.

Galactosaemia cataract is an inborn error of metabolism (p. 263). It is reversible with treatment, but where a complete lens opacity develops, surgery is effective.

Diabetic cataract is rare in children. In the early stages the lens opacities are reversible with correction of the metabolic state, but when complete, surgery is effective.

Tetany cataract (due to reduction of calcium ion concentration). This is not reversible but can be arrested with systemic treatment.

Principles of treatment and nursing management
1. Except where cataract is reversible, the treatment is by surgery.
2. Pre-operative care:
   a. Conjunctival swab.
   b. If the child is old enough the operation should be explained to him. He should also be shown how to close his eyes gently.
   c. Eyelashes may be trimmed.
3. Post-operative care:
   a. Position: the child is propped up with his head supported on pillows.
   b. Restlessness and crying should be avoided and sedation may be necessary.
   c. Normal nutrition.
   d. Immobilisation of arms.
4. Dressing (if required).

Conjunctivitis

Inflammation of the conjunctiva is a common condition caused by various bacteria, often associated with the common cold. Other causes can be irritation from dust, smoke and intense light.

Clinical features

There is redness due to hyperaemia and increased lacrimation (watering) which is followed by a mucoid or mucopurulent discharge which may be scanty or profuse. Photophobia and smarting or itchiness are common symptoms.

Principles of treatment and nursing management

1. Swab for bacteriological investigation.
2. Bathing the eye and lids (p. 339).
3. Application of local antibiotics (p. 336).
4. Arm restraint for infants to prevent rubbing eyes.

Ophthalmia neonatorum

This is a purulent conjunctivitis which occurs in new-born infants. It is acquired from an infected birth canal during the birth of the infant. The main causal organism used to be the gonococcus and may still be in some cases, but other micro-organisms such as *staphylococcus, pneumococcus* or viruses are now generally responsible.

Clinical features

Both eyes are usually affected. If the causal organism is the gonococcus, the symptoms appear within 12 to 48 hours after birth, the discharge becoming copious and purulent. The condition may subside in two to three weeks, leading to conjunctival hypertrophy and chronic inflammation. Complications frequently follow, such as corneal ulceration leading to corneal scarring and interference with vision.

In non-gonorrheal cases, the symptoms are milder and recovery is more rapid.

Principles of treatment and nursing management

1. Prevention by antenatal examination, investigation and treatment of any vaginal discharge of the expectant mother.
2. At birth, the infant's eyes should be swabbed and antibiotic drops instilled.
3. Preventing the infant from handling eyes, i.e. immobilisation of arms.
4. Swabbing of eyes and instillation of antibiotic drops (pp. 339 and 336).
5. If gonococcal infection — barrier nursing.

Disposable gloves should be worn when carrying out eye care.

DISEASES OF THE LIDS

The lids are modified folds consisting of four layers: the skin, muscle, fibrous tissue and conjunctiva. Inflammation of the lids is called *blepharitis*. The ulcerative type is caused by bacterial infection, usually staphylococci, affecting the hair follicle and the meibomian glands. Other types include seborrhoeic and non-ulcerative blepharitis.

Clinical features

There is itching, burning and redness of lid margin, oedema of lids, falling out of lashes and conjunctival irritation.

Principles of treatment and nursing management

1. Local swabbing of lids.
2. Application of antibiotic or other chemotherapeutic substance (p. 338).
3. Prevention of rubbing eyes.

Chalazion or meibomian cyst

This is usually a chronic infection of the meibomian gland in the tarsal plate where the duct is blocked and the secretions of the duct are retained. The gland swells slowly until it becomes obvious, distorting the lid.

Clinical features

Symptoms may be absent until a round mass is felt. With larger swellings, there is conjunctival irritation. The swelling may burst or may require incision to clear the contents.

Principles of treatment and nursing management

This may include surgery as indicated above. Post-operative care includes application of ointment and general care of the eyes.

Hordeolum externum (stye)
This is an acute infection involving the follicle of an eyelash. It is usually caused by staphlylococcus.

Clinical features
There is localised swelling at the lid margin which is painful. The pain is due to increased pressure in the region.

Treatment
Application of ointment (antibiotic) (p. 338).

Examination of and nursing procedures relating to the eyes

EXAMINATION OF THE EYES
Examination of the eyes is a routine admission procedure carried out by medical staff and, if requested, by the ophthalmologist, for special diagnosis, e.g. cataract, refractive errors. The doctor uses an ophthalmoscope which consists of a light reflected by a mirror with a central hole. The light rays are reflected on to the patient's eye and then back to the person examining the eye. It also contains a circular disc of lenses which vary from the resting mark 'C' (clear glass) to $+1$ to $+12$ and back from -12 to -1 to suit the eyesight requirements of the individual operator. The ophthalmoscope is used to examine the retina. With it the doctor should be able to detect papilloedema (due to swelling of the optic nerve) and disease of the retina such as retinal detachment or haemorrhage.

To examine an infant or young child, it is usually necessary to dilate the pupil. Atropine 0.5 to 1 per cent or ointment 1 to 2 per cent can be used; the action starting in 15 minutes and the effect lasting 10 to 12 days. Alternatively, hyoscine — scopolamine 0.25 to 0.5 per cent may be used; its action is quicker than that of atropine and its effect lasts 2 days.

The actions of atropine and hyoscine are as follows. The pupil dilates (mydriasis) due to blockage of cholinergic tone on the sphincter pupillae. The ciliary muscle of the lens is also paralysed producing impairment of accommodation, the lens being fixed for far vision.

Preparation and position of the child
The examination should take place in a part of the ward which can be darkened. Whenever possible, the nurse should explain clearly to the child the steps of the procedure and warn him of the effect of the drug on his vision. He must be told that he may see double, or that his vision may become blurred for a while. He should also be told that the examination is painless and that his co-operation is necessary.

Older children, where the condition permits, can be examined sitting on a chair, while infants will be examined lying on a flat surface. The nurse should hold the infant's head to restrict movement and be prepared to evert the eyelids at the doctor's direction.

Instillation of drops
Drops are instilled for many reasons, some of these being:

1. To enlarge the pupils in order to facilitate examination of the eyes and in traumatic affections of the cornea, iris and ciliary body.
2. To contract the pupils; this is usually used to counteract the effects of the mydriatic.
3. To counteract infection. Antibiotics such as chloramphenicol, or chemotherapeutic agents such as albucid may be used.
4. To induce local anaesthesia, where a foreign body is to be removed from the cornea.
5. To lubricate — bland oily drops such as cod liver oil or castor oil are used in the treatment of burns or abrasions.

Requirements

1. Eye drops; these come in single dose packs or in bottles with a dropper.
2. Cotton wool balls or paper tissues.

Method
When the procedure is to be carried out on a young child or infant, two nurses should be available. It must be carried out quickly, as no child will remain still for long while a drop shimmers at the end of a dropper.

The child or infant should be lying flat, but an older child may be in the sitting position. Holding the dropper ready, the nurse rests one hand on the child's forehead, keeping the dropper at a sufficient distance for safety in the event of a sudden jerk. With the other hand, she simultaneously draws the child's lower lid gently downwards and attracts his gaze upwards (Fig. 20.4). One or two drops are instilled into the lower recess of the conjunctiva and any excess which may trickle down the cheek is mopped up immediately.

Test for visual acuity

Visual acuity is assessed by comparing the child's acuity with an arbitary standard of normality. Each eye is tested separately, while the other eye is covered. For children who cannot read, finger tests or the 'E' test are used, and for those who can read the Snellen's test is used.

The child stands 6 metres from the test card and he is asked to read from the top line. Each size of letter is designated a number which is the distance in metres at which the average normal person can read the type. For example, if he can read size 6 letters at 6 metres, his vision is described as 6/6, i.e. average normal; if size 4 his vision is 6/4, i.e. better than average. If he cannot read letters smaller than 12 at 6 metres his vision is 6/12. A person is regarded as blind if his vision is below a certain value, e.g. less than 3/60 — that is, he cannot identify at 3 metres when an average person can identify at 60 metres.

Slit-lamp microscopy

This procedure enables the conjunctiva, cornea, anterior chamber, iris, posterior chamber and lens to be examined in greater detail. The structures are viewed through a binocular microscope while

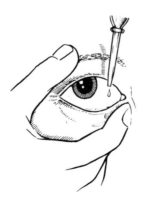

Fig. 20.4 Instillation of eye drops.

illuminated by a narrow beam of intense light which can be moved gradually across the eye.

Correcting lenses

Refractive errors are corrected by suitable lenses. The unit of measurement of the refractive power of the lens is the dioptre (D). This is calculated as; the refractive power of a convex lens being equal to 1 metre divided by its focal length. Therefore, a spherical lens has a refractive power of dioptre when it is capable of converging parallel light rays to a focal point 1 metre beyond the lens. If it bends the light rays twice as much, it is said to have a strength of +2 dioptres. Two types of lenses are used:

1. Convex, which corrects the vision on a hypermetropic (short eye). This is denoted by the sign +. The range is +0.25 D to +20.00 D. The rays are brought to focus in front instead of behind the retina.
2. Concave lens. This lens corrects the vision in a myope, where the eye is longer and the focus in front of the retina. It is denoted by the sign −, and the range is −0.25 D to −20.00 D, but −20.00 to −30.00 is not uncommon.

Eversion of lids (Fig. 20.5)

The lids require to be retracted in order to carry out certain treatments.

1. *Lower lid.* The lid is drawn down and the child is asked to look up. The infant or toddler can be encouraged to look up by using a toy, placed or held in a strategic position to attract and hold his attention.
2. *Upper lid.* This is more difficult. The nurse holds the upper lid with a swab and gently everts it upwards. Where applicable, the child should be asked to look down.

Taking a conjunctival swab for culture

This procedure is necessary to determine the causal organism and to institute drug treatment. This is a simple procedure and should not cause any pain. Nevertheless, it can be frightening. To swab the eye of an infant or young child, two nurses should be available. The equipment required is a sterile culture swab, e.g. throat swab and Agar slope in tube.

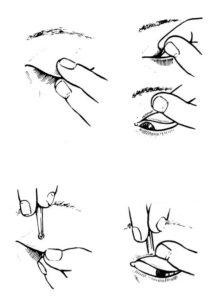

Fig. 20.5 Eversion of eyelid by hand and by glass rod.

Method

An explanation should be given to the older child. He is asked to look up and keep his eyes open. The infant and toddler's eye should be opened by the operating nurse while the assistant restrains the child. The lower conjunctiva is swabbed gently, care being taken not to touch the skin of the eyelids or the eyelashes. A representative sample of the exudate should be obtained and sent to the bacteriology department.

Cutting eyelashes

Before intra-ocular operations are performed it may be necessary to trim the eyelashes. It is a simple procedure but may frighten the child. If it is to be carried out, it is essential to reassure the child and prevent him from moving his head.

Method

A pair of blunt-ended, well-sharpened scissors should be used. The blades should be smeared with a layer of soft paraffin. This prevents the fine lashes from falling on to the conjunctiva, causing irritation. The lashes adhere to the paraffin. The older child should be asked to keep his eyes closed and not to screw them up. The nurse can apply a little traction to the upper lid. This will separate the two rows of lashes without opening the eyes.

They should then be trimmed separately, as close to the level of the skin as possible.

Occlusion

This means covering an eye. It is generally the good eye which is occluded by fixing an adhesive or Elastoplast patch on the face and forehead. It may also be fixed on a spectacle lens, if worn.

The reason for this procedure should be explained to the child, if old enough. He should be told that he has to use the uncovered eye to improve vision in that eye. The parents should also have a full explanation of the reasons and the desired effect. They should also be shown how to replace the patch. As part of the treatment, the child may be attending the orthoptic department. The orthoptist tests the visual acuity and supervises the occlusion. This also involves tests for binocular vision. The instrument, an amblyoscope, presents a picture to each eye in the line of the visual axis, this allows the angle of the squint to be measured and measures the ability of the child to use both eyes. The pictures are, for example, a parrot and a cage. If there is any binocular vision, the bird will be seen in the cage, even only momentarily.

Regular assessment of binocular vision will be made, using different pictures.

Application of ointment

Reasons for application:

1. Where infection of the eyelids is present.
2. In conjunctivitis, to prevent the eyelids from sticking together and to allow the escape of discharge.
3. Where corneal ulcers are present or to prevent their formation.
4. To dilate the pupils.

The following substances may be used: Albucid 2.5 per cent, chloramphenicol, penicillin, hydrocortisone and atropine.

Requirements

1. Dental rolls.
2. Wool balls.
3. Gallipot.
4. Eye lotion for cleansing purposes.

5. Ointment in nozzled tube.
6. Disposal bag.

Method

The child is placed in a comfortable position and, provided he is old enough to understand, the procedure is explained to him. The eye is bathed, if required, from the inner to the outer aspects of the eye. The dental rolls are used for bathing the canthus and the wool balls for the eyelids. Both are used once only. The ointment is then applied to the lower fornix.

An ointment is sometimes applied externally to the eyelids. In such a case, the ointment is gently worked into the roots of the lashes, or smeared along the lid margins with a sterile swab.

Irrigation of the eyes (Fig. 20.6)

This is a gentle method of washing away fragments of mucus, foreign material and clumps of dead cells from the conjunctiva. To avoid irritation of the conjunctiva, the lotion should be of the same concentration as lacrimal secretions, e.g. normal or half-strength normal saline.

Requirements

1. Jug of lotion at a temperature of 37.2°C.
2. Lotion thermometer.
3. Undine or eyebath.
4. Wool balls.
5. Container for returned fluid.
6. Water-repellent towel.
7. Disposal bag.

Method

Older children may use an eyebath, but the undine provides a more thorough irrigation. The procedure should be explained and the child reassured that it is not painful, in fact, he may find it soothing and quite pleasant. The water-repellent sheet/towel is placed round the child's shoulders. The undine is filled with the solution. The container is held at the side of the face just below the eye to be treated. It is advisable to try the lotion on the child's cheek first to accustom him to the sensation. The flow is then directed from the inner canthus to the outer. This is in an endeavour to prevent the spread of infection to the lacrymal duct. The child should be encouraged to

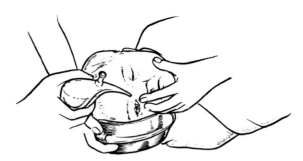
Fig. 20.6 Irrigation of the eye.

move his eyes freely. Finally, in the older child, the upper eyelid is everted and irrigated, but in an infant, it is easier to pick up the upper eyelid and pull it gently away from the globe and then irrigate. During the procedure, it is advisable to rest the hand holding the undine on the child's forehead and to hold the point of the undine at a safe distance, in the event of a sudden jerk (Fig. 20.6).

When the irrigation is completed, the eyes are wiped gently, using each cotton wool ball once only.

Removal, care and replacement of artificial eye

An artificial eye is usually made of plastic and it is shaped to fit the socket. The scleral and iris colour should match the natural eye. Since it is a foreign body it may act as an irritant to the conjunctival sac, it is therefore important that the eye is kept clean. To keep it clean it should be removed every day. Removal, care and replacement of an artificial eye will be carried out by the parents, but as the child grows older, he should be taught to carry out the necessary procedures. Both parents and child will require a great deal of encouragement from the nursing staff until they feel able to take over this function.

Removal of an artificial eye

The following requirements should be available:

1. Glass rod.
2. Packet of wool balls.
3. Solution of sodium chloride 0.9 per cent.
4. Container for the solution.
5. Drops or ointments as prescribed.

For irrigation of the socket

1. Undine.
2. Container for return fluid.
3. Water-repellent sheet for protection of the child.

Method

The nurse washes and dries her hands. The artificial eye is removed by lifting the lower edge of the eye over the lower lid and easing it out of the eyesocket, using a glass rod.

Care of the artificial eye

The eye is kept clean by washing it daily in lukewarm water. If soapy solutions are used, the eye should be rinsed in cold water. When it is not used, it should be wrapped in cotton wool to prevent scratches and for night storage it should be kept in clean cold water. Should it become scratched and lose its lustre, it should be returned to the eye clinic where it will be repolished. The surface of the eye eventually becomes rough and irritating, when it may be necessary to replace it with a new one.

Replacement of an artificial eye

In the early post-operative period, the socket is irrigated before the eye is replaced. When the socket is found to be clean and the prescribed drops or ointment have been applied, the eye is moistened and gently replaced. Care should be taken to ensure that the eye is put in correctly.

Removal, care and replacement of contact lenses (hard lenses)

Young children can be fitted with contact lenses. These are designed to be worn during the day and removed before going to sleep. Contact lenses resemble thin shells which fit in front of the eye under the lids. They are made of soft plastic material which can be easily damaged. They are also very expensive and the child must learn how to care for them and not to mislay or lose them. When contact lenses are obtained, the wearer is issued with a special box and instructions on how to care for them.

Removal of contact lenses

The following equipment should be available:

1. Rubber suction cup (or tube) (if necessary).
2. Special box containing normal saline.

Method

A rubber suction cup of the required size may be used. The child is either sitting or lying with the head resting back. Two nurses should be available. The operating nurse washes and dries her hands. The child is asked to look down and the upper lid is raised. The suction end is moistened, squeezed free of air and is then applied to the surface of the lens. The lens is then lifted downwards and out over the lower lid.

Care of the hard lens

The lens is washed gently and carefully in a small bowl of cold water, dried on a soft tissue and either returned to the box or replaced on the eye. It should never be washed in too hot water or placed in a chemical solution and, when replacing a lens, it should be put into the correctly labelled compartment, i.e. right or left.

Care of the soft lens

The lenses are washed and kept clean. They are placed in a special container, each lens fitting into its space. The compartments are marked 'left' and 'right'. The container is filled with normal saline, which must be prepared freshly each day. For most types the container and the lenses are placed in a pan of water which is boiled for about 10 minutes (a few types do not require boiling). Lubrication of lenses is not necessary since they are kept in saline.

Replacement of the lens (hard and soft lenses)

Each lens slips easily into the respective eye, fitting snugly below the upper and lower lids.

Extraction of the soft lens

Two methods may be used:

1. By applying gentle pressure on the eyelids the lens is squeezed out.
2. The lens is eased out by raising the lower edge of the lens and lifting it out.

Chapter 21
Disorders of the auditory system

Hearing, like many somatic senses, is a mechano-receptive event. The ear responds to mechanical vibrations of the sound waves in the air which are then converted to electrical impulses. The ear can be affected by disease which can lead to disturbance of hearing and which presents many problems for the infant, child and adult.

Applied anatomy and physiology (Fig. 21.1)
For convenience the ear can be divided into three areas: the outer, the middle and the inner.

Outer ear
This includes the *auricle*, and the *external auditory meatus*.

The auricle is composed of cartilage and is closely adherent to the skin. Sound waves are funnelled by the auricle into the external auditory meatus, which is about 2.5 cm long. The outer third is cartilage which contains hairs and ceruminous glands, and the inner two-thirds lie in the temporal bone. The skin of the inner part is very thin, adherent and sensitive. At the medial end of the meatus is a depression in which wax, debris or foreign bodies may lodge. At birth there is no osseous external meatus but this develops with the growth of the tympanic bone.

Middle ear
This includes the tympanic membrane and the ossicles — malleus, incus and stapes. The tympanic membrane lies at the end of the external auditory meatus. It forms the lateral wall of the middle ear which is really a small air-filled cavity in the temporal bone. In the neonate the tympanic membrane is almost horizontal and thicker than in the older child.

The three small ossicles transmit and amplify the movements of the membrane to the inner ear.

Functions of the ossicles. The malleus is attached to the tympanic membrane and its free head articulates with the incus. The incus articulates

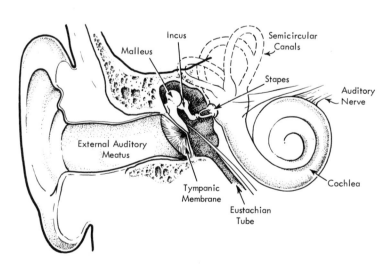

Fig. 21.1 The principal structures of the ear.

341

with the stapes and the footplate of the stapes fits against the oval window. The fluid of the inner ear is in contact with that part of the stapes. Ligament attaches the stapes to the oval windows; it is lax enough to allow movement of the stapes.

As the tympanic membrane vibrates in response to sound waves hitting its outer surface, its movements are transmitted by the ossicles to the fluid of the inner ear. The three ossicles form a lever system which diminishes the amplitude of the sound waves and increases their force on the inner ear.

Also in the middle ear is the opening of the Eustachian tube and the attachment of the tensor tympanic muscle which maintains the correct tension of the tympanic membrane (Figs. 21.2 and 21.3).

The Eustachian tube is about 3.5 cm in length in the adult but only 1.7 to 2.2 cm in the infant. It is more horizontal and wider in infants and this causes milk or vomit to enter the middle ear. Repeated nasal infection also causes blockage of the Eustachian tube, interfering with the mechanics of hearing. It is normally filled with air and the pressure is the same on both sides of the tympanic membrane.

On the posterior wall of the middle ear is the doorway to the mastoid air cells. These are hollow spaces in the mastoid process of the tympanic bone which lies just behind the ear. Infection can be transmitted via the doorway (aditus) from the middle ear to the mastoid air cells (Fig. 21.4).

The bony roof of the middle ear cavity is thin and the temporal lobe of the brain rests on its upper surface. An infection of this region could therefore result in meningitis or cerebral abscess.

The medial wall has two openings (windows). (1) The oval window opens into the internal ear and is covered by the stapes, and slightly below it and actually in the internal ear is (2) the round window which is covered by membrane. The facial nerve passes through the middle ear from the internal auditory meatus. It is relatively unprotected in children under 2.

Inner ear
This includes the cochlea and the vestibular apparatus (semicircular canals and otolith organs).

The cochlea. The cochlea is a system of coiled tubes around a central bony pillar. At the lower end are the oval and round windows. The lumen is divided into compartments. In the middle compartment lies the basilar membrane which separates the scala tympani (lower compartment) from the scala media (middle compartment). The specialised organ of Corti is situated on the basilar membrane. The compartments are filled with fluid; the upper and lower ones with perilymph and the middle one with endolymph (a fluid similar to that of intracellular fluid). The organ of

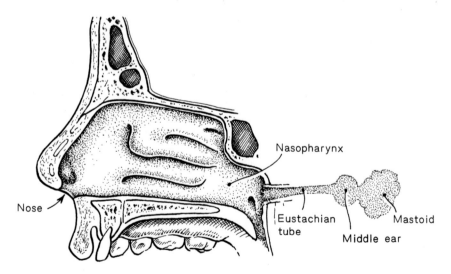

Fig. 21.2 Relation of Eustachian tube to nasopharynx, middle ear and mastoid.

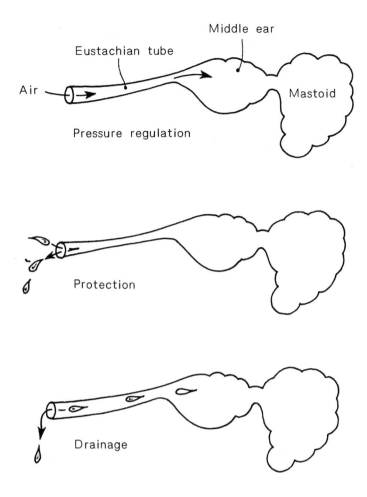

Fig. 21.3 Physiological functions of the Eustachian tube in relation to the middle ear.

Corti is the receptor organ for sound and consists of a complicated arrangement of rods and hair cells. They are innervated by nerve fibres of the cochlea division of the eighth nerve.

Mechanism of hearing. Sound consists of vibrations in the air. These vibrations vary in frequency from 20 cycles per second for the deep notes and up to 10 000 to 20 000 cycles per second (Hz) for the very high notes. The ear is less sensitive for low frequencies. Hearing is most acute at about 1000 cps (Hz).

The loudness of sound is measured in decibels. The decibel scale is a logarithmic scale where an increase of 10 decibels means an increase of 10 times in sound power. The following table indicates the intensity of the various sounds:

0 dB	Threshold of hearing. This is the lowest level; auditory acuity being greatest in the region of 1000 to 4000 cps/Hz.
40 dB	Talking in whisper.
80 dB	Traffic noise.
120 dB	Pneumatic drill.
140 dB	Jet plane at take-off.

Sounds over 120 dB produce pain in addition to sound.

Mode of action (Fig. 21.5). The external ear collects the sound waves and transmits them to the

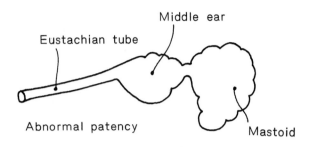

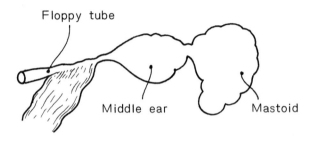

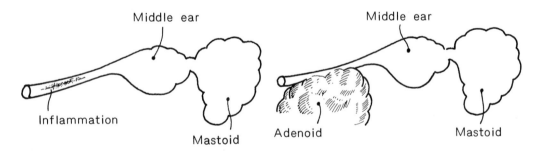

Fig. 21.4 Disorders of the Eustachian tube.

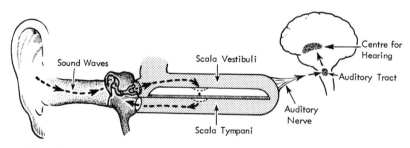

Fig. 21.5 The transmission of sound waves.

ear drum. The three small ossicles act as levers and transmit the sound to the oval window. As the oval window is pushed in by the action of the stapes, the fluid moves, causing bulging of the round window. The movement of fluid stimulates the organ of Corti. The fluid (endolymph) in the cochlea allows the large but weak vibrations of the air to be changed into smaller but more powerful vibrations in the fluid. The vibrations in the fluid are converted from mechanical into electrical energy, i.e. nerve impulses. This is due to stimulation of the localised nerve cells producing nerve impulses which are transmitted in the auditory nerve to the cochlear nuclei. Further connections along the auditory pathway are made until the fibres pass via the posterior limit of the internal capsule to the auditory cortex where interpretation of sound takes place.

Low frequency sounds cause the whole of the basilar membrane to vibrate; high frequency sounds cause only the base of the basilar membrane close to the oval window to vibrate.

Vestibular apparatus. This is the other part of the inner ear. It is not part of the hearing mechanism. It consists of two parts, the otolith organs and the semicircular canals. The otolith organs are the saccule and utricle which consist of modified hair cells. Embedded in the hair cells are chalk particles known as otoliths. The chalk particles are heavy enough to be pulled on by gravity. The saccule is connected to the middle compartment of the cochlea. This means that the hearing and balance parts of the inner ear are closely connected.

There are three semicircular canals, each lying in a different plane in space. They all open into the utricle which is joined to the saccule.

When the head is rotated, messages are sent to the brain from these sense organs into the semicircular canals, and the sense organs in the utricle and saccule provide information about the position of the head when it is not moving.

The control of balance is co-ordinated by the brain at an unconscious level. This control depends on accurate messages sent to the brain about our position in space which are derived from three separate sources:

1. The eyes.
2. The sense receptors in limb muscles and joints.
3. The organs in the labyrinths of the inner ear.

Conflicting information from any one source could lead to imbalance, just as damage to the labyrinth or its nerve connection with the brain would interfere with balance and may cause vertigo.

Disorders affecting the ear

Impacted wax
This is not a disease. Cerumen is normally secreted by the ceruminous glands. Some children appear to have a greater accumulation of wax which may become impacted. Cerumen is golden brown in colour and has a soft consistency when secreted, but if it lodges in the meatus it loses water by evaporation. It thus becomes harder and darker in colour. It can cause deafness and sometimes irritation of the meatal skin.

Principles of treatment and nursing management
1. Soft wax can be removed by a wool-tipped probe.
2. Syringing of ear (p. 352).

Furunculosis (boils)
This is a swelling at the outer end of the meatus spreading to soft tissues around the auricle, involving regional glands. It is relatively common because the soft tissues of the child's meatus swell easily. Pain can be severe and is aggravated by chewing. Hearing may also be affected.

Principles of treatment and nursing management

1. Antibiotics.
2. Local heat.
3. Routine nursing care.

Acute suppurative otitis media (in infants)
This is an infection of the lining of the middle ear. It not only involves the middle ear but also the 'middle ear cleft'. The mucous membrane of the Eustachian tube, the middle ear and the mastoid antrum and air cells are continuous and any infection at the nasopharyngeal end of this system may spread to all these areas.

Infants are particularly prone to infection of the middle ear and mastoid. This is due to several factors:

1. The infant's Eustachian tube is short, wide and horizontal and infected material passes readily from the nose into the tube. This is made easier by the fact that the infant lies passively on either side allowing both Eustachian tubes to become involved.
2. The infant's middle ear contains embryonic mesodermal tissue which is gradually absorbed during the first 6 to 8 weeks of life. It forms a ready medium for pathogenic organisms.
3. The lymphoid tissue of the nasopharynx and pharynx is still developing and therefore active. It is prone to infection. Associated with this is the poorly developed immunity in the infant.

Clinical features
Pain is indicated by persistent crying and head-rolling. Pyrexia is usually present and there may be food refusal. If other infections, e.g. gastroenteritis, are present, there may be vomiting and diarrhoea. Discharge is a late feature and might be due to the relative thickness of the tympanic membrane or to the ease with which the secretions can escape along the Eustachian tube. However, discharge indicates perforation which may become chronic.

The causative organisms are the staphylococcus, pneumococcus and *H. influenzae*.

Principles of treatment and nursing management

1. Antibiotics. This might be the choice if the infection is severe.
2. *Myringotomy*. An incision is made through the ear drum.
3. Dry mopping of the ear (p. 352).
4. Introduction of a grommet. This keeps the incision open to allow air into the middle ear until the Eustachian tube regains its normal function.
5. Routine nursing care.

Acute suppurative otitis media in children
The infection occurs frequently in young children aged 2 or 3 years. The infection arises in the nasopharynx and repeated upper respiratory infec-tion, enlarged adenoids and recurrent attacks of acute tonsillitis, rhinitis or sinusitis, all contribute to the infection into the Eustachian tube in children.

The organisms responsible are the same as in infants but *B. coli* and *B. Proteus* have also been isolated.

Clinical features
Pain is the first complaint. The child may waken crying or screaming. He will put his hand to the affected ear. Discharge may appear either running out of the ear or may be quite thick. There is an increase in temperature and pulse rate.

Principles of treatment and nursing management

1. Antibiotics if indicated, either oral or intra-muscular.
2. Local treatment, i.e. dry mopping (p. 352).
3. Routine nursing care.

Perforated tympanic membrane
The tympanic membrane may be injured by the penetration of a sharp object, a blow on the ear, or by unskilled attempts at removing a foreign body or infection. If the drum is injured, a sharp pain and a loud noise are experienced at the time of the injury. The pain is of short duration, but some degree of deafness and tinnitus (ringing in the ear) may follow.

Principles of treatment and nursing management

1. Initially, little active treatment is given. A sterile dressing may be inserted and no water is allowed to enter the ear.
2. Antibiotics may be given prophylactically.
3. Nursing care aims at promoting healing of the damaged tissue. This involves local treatment of tympanic membrane, relief of pain and routine nursing care.

Acute mastoiditis
Acute mastoiditis is the result of extension of infection through the posterior wall of the middle ear involving the mastoid air cells.

Clinical features
There is severe pain and swelling behind the ear

and discharge from the ear. Temperature is highly elevated and the pulse rate is increased. There may also be increasing deafness.

Principles of treatment and nursing management

1. Antibiotics. The appropriate antibiotic is given depending on the sensitivity of the predominant organism. Crystalline penicillin is given until the sensitivity reports are received.
2. Pre-operative management:
    a. Routine (p. 128).
    b. The hair of the affected side is shaved.
3. Drainage of mastoid cavity. This may last about three weeks.
4. Cortical mastoidectomy (Schwartze operation). This is reserved for cases with intracranial complications, such as sinus thrombosis, or those where no improvement has taken place in spite of adequate treatment. In this operation, the cortex of the mastoid is cleared. Debris, pus and granulations are removed, with the formation of one large cavity. The object of this operation is to drain the mastoid antrum and cells, but to leave untouched the tympanic membrane, ossicles, etc. It should leave the child's hearing unimpaired.
5. Post-operative nursing care: wound care, relief of pain, nutrition and routine nursing care (p. 131).

Deafness in infancy and childhood

Deafness means loss of hearing and some degree of deafness is fairly common in children. Audiometry tests of schoolchildren indicate that about 9 per cent of the school population have some degree of hearing loss. Most have a slight defect but there are some with serious loss of hearing and those who are classified as deaf mutes.

The function of hearing, the development of an understanding of the meaning of sounds, the discrimination of the sound of speech and the development of speech, are interdependent. Speech is an imitative process dependent on hearing, but if the infant is congenitally deaf he will not be able to speak unless special instruction is given.

Normally, as the infant grows he imitates noises and eventually produces meaningful sounds leading to words. Hearing develops in the newborn baby as the embryonic tissue and fluid are absorbed from the middle ear. The young infant responds to loud sounds by blinking, extension of arms and starting to cry, but he does not appear to respond if the sound is quiet. As he grows, he responds by turning his head towards the sound, and by 3 months he will attempt to imitate certain sounds. Talking in the form of babbling, cooing and responding to the sound of his name, can be demonstrated by 6 months of age. By the end of the first year of life the young child is able to show evidence of understanding of speech and of using speech by manipulating sounds into some form of language.

Hearing impairmant is one of the most handicapping of conditions. Severe hearing loss prevents or seriously interferes with the acquisition of language and speech so essential for social competence. A less severe loss is less debilitating but can nevertheless present many problems for the young child.

Causes (Fig. 21.6)

Hearing loss can be congenital or acquired. In the latter case children have already heard and acquired language and speech, and this will influence their education and training.

Genetic. It is considered that almost half of all cases of deafness are of genetic origin. There appears to be a high rate of deafness in children of parents who are blood relations. This indicates that many cases of genetic deafness are recessive in type, although a small percentage may be transmitted by sex-linked genes which may be either recessive or dominant. The chances of producing deaf children depends on the type of genetic transmission.

The majority of children with congenital deafness do not show other defects, but there is a significant group of children whose deafness is part of other abnormalities, for example, Hurler's syndrome (gargoylism) and osteogenesis imperfecta.

Embryopathic causes. It has been recognised that virus infection during the first trimester of pregnancy, particularly rubella virus, is responsible for damage to the organ of Corti. Drugs too are known to interfere with embryonic development if taken during the critical period of pregnancy.

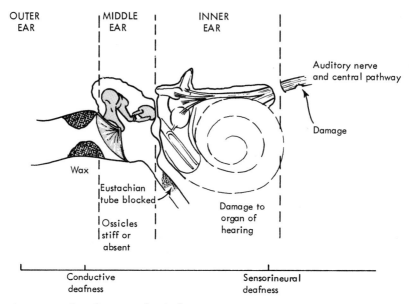

Fig. 21.6 Diagrammatic representation of areas causing deafness.

Perinatal causes. Lack of oxygen immediately prior to birth and also immediately after birth can cause a high frequency loss due to damage in the cochlear nuclei. Neonatal jaundice causes a specific type of high frequency loss which is also due to damage in the cochlear nuclei.

Acquired deafness. Total deafness may follow infection such as labyrinthitis or meningitis (particularly tuberculous meningitis). Middle ear disorders of any type may cause hearing loss of varying degree. Injury as a result of fracture of the temporal bone may also lead to deafness.

The hazards of ototoxic drugs and noise exposure are recognised as causes of deafness, for example, streptomycin used in the treatment of tuberculosis.

Detection and screening for deafness

The parents are generally the first people to recognise the infant's or child's inability to hear. However, where deafness develops gradually it is difficult (1) to recognise it as it occurs and (2) to accept that the child has a hearing defect.

The majority of hearing defects are detected during routine pre-school and school medical examination. Detection and screening is normally the responsibility of child and health medical offi-

cers and health visitors. For audiometry tests an audiology technician or a specially trained screener is usually employed to test schoolchildren. In all cases a careful case history is an important aspect of detection and decision regarding treatment. The methods used for screening depend on the age of the child. Figure 21.7 shows an example of a normal audiogram.

Infant and very young child. Distraction methods are used to perform screening tests on babies and young children (6 to 15 months). Operators work in pairs, one to observe the child who is sitting on the mother's lap and the other to make the various sounds. The tester stands behind the mother and out of the child's field of vision. She moves slowly and quietly from side to side to the required distance. The sounds are made on a level with and slightly behind the child's head. The observer sits in front of the child.

The following sounds are used:

1. Speaking in a conversational voice.
2. Whispering voice.
3. Using the 's' sound, as in 'bus'.
4. High-pitched rattle.
5. Tinkling sound, e.g. cup and spoon.
6. Rustle of cellophane.
7. The sound of a bell.

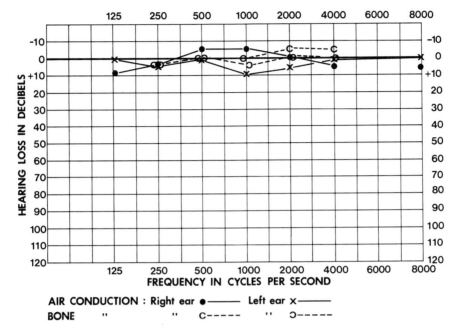

Fig. 21.7 Normal audiogram.

The sounds should not be too loud; quiet sounds of 35 dB are considered acceptable for testing purposes. Response to loud sound would fail to detect a partially hearing child. It has been found that young children respond better to interesting sounds and for this reason a high-tone rattle is used. If the baby is tired, irritable, wet or hungry, he may not respond to sounds, while signs of recognition of sound can be seen on the changes of expression on the baby's face, even if he does not turn towards the sound. The observer's task is to record these changes.

Toddlers. This age group can be quite difficult. The toddler tends to be very active and a combination of baby tests and speech tests can be used. Responses in this age group should be obtained to a soft voice at a distance of 3 metres.

Pre-school and up to 7 years of age. More complex speech test can be used. This depends on his development. For example, the 2- to 3-year-old can be asked to point to varying number of toys, parts of the body, etc. The tester moves slowly away to a distance of 3 to 6 metres. Each ear is tested separately.

School screening. Audiometry is performed on older schoolchildren. The audiometer is an elec-tronic instrument capable of generating pure tones ranging from 125 cps (Hz) to about 12 000 cps (Hz). A tone is chosen by manipulating a control. This tone is fed into the child's ear by means of a headphone. The volume control is adjusted until the child signals that he can hear the note emitted. The volume and frequency are then recorded. The threshold of hearing for each of the test frequencies is charted in the form of an audiogram. Hearing loss is expressed in decibels (dB), which are logarithmic units of relative intensity (p. 343).

Children are tested for five frequencies: 250 cps (Hz), 500 cps (Hz), 1000 cps (Hz), 2000 cps (Hz) and 4000 cps (Hz) at 25 dB made at regular intervals.

Types

There are two main varieties of deafness — conductive and perceptive. In *conductive* deafness there is some obstruction, defect or lesion of the external meatus, tympanic membrane, middle ear cavity or ossicles that interferes with the passage of sound waves through these to the oval window. The causes of conductive deafness include wax or debris; blockage of the Eustachian tube caused by effusion of thick and tenacious mucus; this is followed by absorption of air from the middle ear space so that the drum is pushed into the middle ear and cannot move freely. Perforation of the membrane is also a cause of conductive deafness. Bone-conducted sounds may persist longer and air-conducted sounds are less well perceived.

Perceptive deafness is nerve deafness (sensori-neural) caused by damage to any part of the ear central to the oval window. The structures involved are the cochlea, the auditory nerve and the cochlear nuclei in the brain stem. In nerve deafness both air-conducted and bone-conducted sounds are less well perceived.

Figures 21.8 and 21.9 show audiograms of individuals with conductive and perceptive deafness, respectively.

Management

The treatment of deafness depends on the type and the cause of deafness. In conditions where deafness can be treated the appropriate measures should prove effective. These include:

1. Removal of any obstruction of the Eustachian tube, i.e. myringotomy and suction of thick mucus.

2. Removal of adenoids. This allows the Eustachian tube to function normally. Complete removal of adenoids is not easy and recurrence of lymphoid tissue occurs frequently.

3. Treatment of nose, i.e. chronic rhinitis, sinusitis should be treated in the usual way.

Hearing aids. For older children clinical audiometry indicates the degree of deafness and also the frequency range. Hearing aids can be designed therefore, to overcome some of the acoustic problems of the individual child.

It is extremely important that the child should learn to speak. The ideal system is by hearing sounds and imitating them. This means that a hearing aid should be provided as soon as deafness is suspected. The hearing aid by itself is not enough, the child must receive auditory training, i.e. he has to be exposed to speech in a carefully planned way.

The hearing aid should have an automatic volume control. This is important because children live in an atmosphere of sudden noise. The aid will assist the deaf child to use his residual hearing to discriminate between different sounds, to acquire language, understand and eventually learn to speak. The aid must be checked daily to

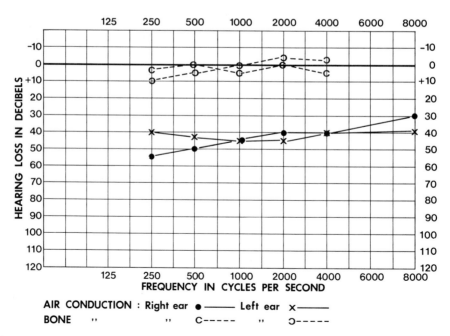

Fig. 21.8 Conductive deafness.

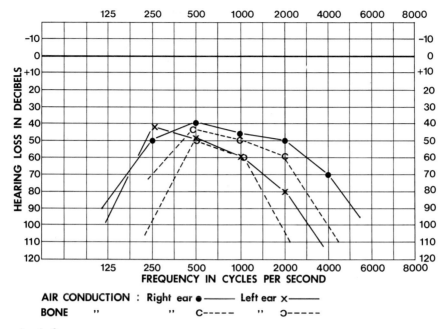

Fig. 21.9 Perceptive deafness.

ensure that it is working properly. Batteries must be replaced and parents should be taught how to detect and correct simple faults. The hearing aid must not be covered by clothing, as this will distort and prevent the flow of sound. It should be worn at chest height and not under the arm or on the hips. Ear moulds must be a good fit as it would otherwise develop whistling, causing discomfort and irritation. It is also important that the child feels confident in using and handling the aid and he should be encouraged to care for the equipment as soon as he is able or old enough.

Education of the deaf child

Once the diagnosis of deafness is made, a careful assessment of the child's and family's needs must be considered. This involves co-operation between the otologist who will decide on the degree of deafness and offer the appropriate amplification. The paediatrician and psychologist also have a role in assessing the child so that school placement can be decided upon.

The teacher of the deaf, together with the parents, will introduce a system of training suitable for each child. Acceptance on the part of the parent is a most important aspect of the

educational programme and school placement depends on the degree of deafness. The deaf child may be placed in a hearing school, a partially hearing unit or a school for the deaf.

The development and use of spoken language is extremely important. Parents, nurses and others caring for these children should have some idea how to speak to these children. When talking to a deaf child the following points should be considered:

1. Lip-reading should be taught. The child should be able to see the face of the speaker clearly.
2. Simple sentences should be used rather than single words. This helps to make language meaningful and it is important to specify clearly what he is to do by using words indicating specifics, e.g. put the book on the table.
3. Language should be used rather than gestures. Body language has a place but it is more important that the child should learn to watch the speaker's face and learn to interpret lip movements; however, exaggerated lip patterns should be avoided.
4. Patience is essential and shouting should be avoided.

5. To gain a child's attention it is better to move into the child's field of vision rather than to touch him. This means that he should be approached from either the side or the front but *not* from behind.

It is essential that the family learns to accept the handicapped child totally. To do so, the parents as well as older children, need the support of the community in which they live. Parents should be encouraged to express their fears and hopes, and contact with others in similar circumstances can be a comfort. The National Deaf Children's Society exists which provides help by relieving parental stress, giving advice and providing financial help for holidays.

Procedures relating to the ear

Examination of the ear is carried out by the medical officer, but nurses are responsible for carrying out certain procedures and assist in others. The following procedures will be considered:

1. Examination of the ear.
2. Swabbing of an ear.
3. Syringing of ears.
4. Insufflation of the ear.
5. Installation of ear drops.

Examination of the ear
The following equipment will be required:

1. Aural specula.
2. Cotton wool holder.
3. Cotton wool.
4. Head light or head mirror.
5. Light or an auroscope and container.
6. Salvage and disposal bag.

Method
Whenever possible, the nurse must give an explanation to the child. He should be held in a comfortable position and with the smaller child, the arms will require to be restrained. Older children are usually co-operative and do not require to be held. Infants and younger children may either be sitting or lying down, with the ear to be examined, uppermost or directed towards the examiner. The child should be prevented from moving his head during the examination.

Swabbing of an ear (mopping)
Swabbing may be carried out twice daily or as often as necessary. It is the method of choice for cleaning an ear when infection is present. The external auditory canal should be cleaned only as far is it can be seen and it is therefore necessary to have a good light available. A speculum should be used and the hand holding the speculum should rest against the child's head so that the speculum will move with any sudden movement of the child thus avoiding injury.

Requirements

1. Aural specula and cotton wool holder.
2. Cotton wool balls.
3. Light.
4. Receptacle for used instruments.
5. Disposal bag.

Method
The procedure should be explained to the child if he is old enough to understand. He is held in a comfortable position and with the smaller child, the arms will require to be restrained by another nurse. A wisp of cotton wool is attached to the cotton wool holder. It should be firmly attached to prevent it coming off the applicator whilst cleaning the ear, and sufficient cotton wool must be left at the tip to prevent the applicator touching the tympanic membrane.

The pinna of the ear is pulled backward in the younger child (0–2 yrs) and backward and upward in the older child, and the external canal cleaned.

Syringing of ears (Fig. 21.10)

Reason
This is an effective way of cleaning an ear and is useful in removing exudate from the canal. It facilitates removal of cerumen or foreign bodies and can be used as a means of applying heat to the tissues of the canal. If it used for the removal of cerumen, this can be softened by instilling warm olive oil 20 minutes before syringing. There are other substances available, such as Cerumol and

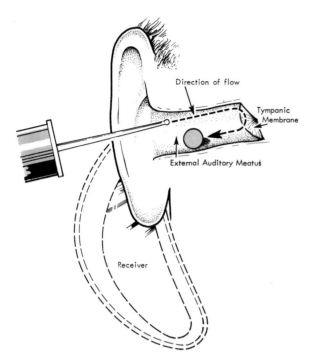

Fig. 21.10 Syringing of the ear, showing the direction of the flow of fluid.

Cerummex which are also useful in softening hard wax (cerumen).

Requirements

1. Aural syringe and speculum; aural angled forceps.
2. Cotton wool balls and holder.
3. Jug containing the solution at a temperature of 35.5 to 36.6°C.; e.g. sodium bicarbonate 4 per cent or normal saline.
4. Lotion thermometer.
5. Waterproof sheet.
6. Container for returned fluid.
7. Container for used instruments.
8. Disposal bag.

Method and care of the child

The procedure should be explained to the older child and he should be asked to report any discomfort or nausea. The child is held or placed in a comfortable position and a repellent sheet is placed around his shoulders.

The lotion is tested with a lotion thermometer.

The pinna of the ear is pulled upwards and backwards (if an older child) and backwards and downwards if a younger child. The tip of the syringe is placed at the entry to the canal and the fluid is directed gently to the roof of the canal. It may be necessary to repeat the irrigation until the wax has been cleared. Observations should be made for any signs of pain or dizziness and should these occur the operation is discontinued and the fact reported. When wax or pus has been cleared, the ear is mopped dry with cotton wool.

If both ears require syringing, the containers are marked to indicate each ear. The returned fluid is kept for inspection and the result recorded on the Kardex. It is also desirable to use separate nozzles for each ear and for added protection, rubber tips can be fitted to the metal nozzle.

The child should be left dry and comfortable on completion of the procedure.

Insufflation of the ear

Reason

This treatment is carried out when infection of the external canal is present. The drug, which is in powder form, is sprayed into the canal by means of an insufflator.

Requirements

1. Insufflator.
2. Drug to be given.
3. Cotton wool balls and cotton wool holder.
4. Receptacle for used instruments.
5. Disposal bag.

Method

The ear is cleaned with dry cotton wool. The insufflator is filled with the powder to be used and directed into the canal. The bulb is squeezed gently but firmly; too feeble a 'puff' may be useless.

Instillation of ear drops

Reasons

Drops may be instilled to soften wax, for the relief of pain or to kill insects. Substances which may be used include: alcohol 70 to 90 per cent to kill insects; Cerumol to soften wax, and antibiotics such as chloramphenicol.

Requirements

1. Individual, single dose dropper pack or drug contained in a bottle.
2. Dropper and angled aural forceps.
3. Container for used instruments.
4. Disposal bag.

Method

Whenever possible the nurse should explain to the child what is going to be done. He should be lying down with the affected ear uppermost. The substance may be slightly warmed; this can be achieved by warming the bottle or dropper in the hand. The required number of drops are then gently inserted into the canal. The child should remain in that position for a short time until the drops are absorbed.

Objective audiometry (electrocochleography)

This is a method of measuring auditory function, by determining the hearing threshold and making a differential diagnosis between sensory and neural lesions. Children are examined under general anaesthesia which does not affect the results.

Technique

A thin needle electrode is placed through the tympanic membrane to rest on the promontory of the cochlea. An external sound stimulus, usually in the form of clicks, produces action potentials from the eighth nerve and cochlear microphonics. Most of the information comes from the base of the cochlea which is associated with higher frequencies and a distinctive pattern emerges when sufficient stimuli are provided.

Chapter 22
Disorders of the throat

Structure and function of the pharynx
(Fig. 22.1)

The pharynx is the space behind the nose and the mouth which extends downwards to the upper end of the oesophagus. Its structure is complicated because it serves as a passage for both air and food.

The nasal part (nasopharynx) lies above the soft palate and the Eustachian tube opens into this part. The oral part is in the upper section behind the mouth and the laryngeal part lies behind, communicating with the larynx. The lining of the nasal part consists of mucous membrane whose surface epithelium is of the ciliated columnar variety. The rest of the pharynx consists of stratified squamous epithelium. The *adenoids* are situated in the nasopharynx and the *tonsils* are found in the oropharynx, at the back of the mouth, one on either side.

The anatomy of the pharynx and the nasopharynx in the infant and child differs slightly from that in the adult. For example, the retropharyngeal lymph glands are present in infancy but atrophy shortly after the first year of life. The growth of the tonsils varies. At birth they are small but enlarge rapidly in the first few months of life. There appears to be a decrease in rate of growth until about 2 years of age when the growth tends to be rapid. It is believed that this increase in growth is due to the developing immunity which the child needs to combat the growing contact with different organisms. The same applies to the adenoids, though these are not so readily observed.

The tongue of the infant fills its mouth and is in contact with both hard and soft palates. This is necessary for sucking. Infants are nasal breathers and this presents problems if there is obstruction to the nose, such as a bilateral atresia of the opening of the nasopharynx. During nasal breathing the pharynx is normally shut off from the mouth by the opposition of the tongue and the palate. Later the tongue moves away from its close opposition to the palate, and closure of the posterior part of the mouth depends on muscle tone.

Deglutition is initiated in the mouth and is under voluntary control. Difficulties may occur during the transition from semi-solid to solid food. Deglutition starts by the tongue pressing the food against the hard palate which is then squeezed backwards into the pharynx. The tongue forms a steep slope and food is directed into the oesophagus. Food is prevented from entering the nasopharynx by a forward movement of the posterior pharyngeal wall to meet the soft palate.

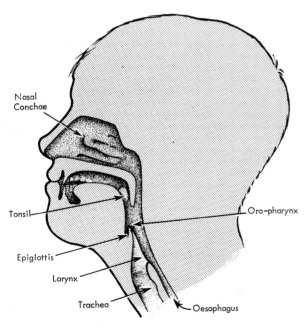

Nasal Conchae

Tonsil

Oro-pharynx

Epiglottis

Larynx

Trachea

Oesophagus

Fig. 22.1 The naso-/oropharynx and larynx.

At the same time there is closure of the naso-pharynx by the action of various muscles. The superior constrictor muscle becomes particularly active where a cleft palate exists. Food is prevented from entering the larynx by the soft palate, which can shut off the nose from the mouth and by the sphincter at the laryngeal inlet, which can separate the larynx from the pharynx. As far as speech is concerned, clarity of enunciation depends on the ability of the nasopharynx to be closed completely.

Functions of the pharynx
The pharynx fulfils four main functions:

1. It allows air to pass between the nose and the larynx.
2. It provides a passage to the mucus of the nose and saliva of the mouth.
3. It initiates the mechanism of deglutition.
4. It assists in speech.

The tonsils. Tonsillar tissue is lymphoid tissue, but differs from the lymph glands in that it has no afferent lymphaticus. From the standpoint of its structure, the most important function is the production of lymphocytes and their action against bacterial toxins. The fact that the growth of the tonsils is most active in early childhood indicates that the function of the tonsils is related to the production of immunity at a time when the child is in greatest need of immunity.

The adenoids. Like the tonsils, these are composed of lymphoid tissue. They are situated in the nasopharynx. Their function is the same as that of the tonsils.

There is another collection of lymphoid tissue found at the back of the tongue (lingual tonsil). The three groups of tissue make up a continuous ring (Waldeyer's ring) encircling the nasopharynx and pharynx. All food and air must pass through this ring.

Abnormalities, injuries and infections of the pharynx
There are a number of congenital abnormalities which may be found, though most are not common. These include amongst others, abnormalities of the tonsils, e.g. absence of tonsil (rare), bifid uvula and insufficiency of the soft palate and cleft palate (Chapter 26). Atresia of the choanae is the most common congenital abnormality of the nasopharynx (Chapter 23).

Injuries of the pharynx can occur when an object is accidentally pushed backwards and lacerates the palate. Scalds of the pharynx can have serious consequences such as oedema. Gross oedema of the arrytenoids and ary-epiglottic folds may require tracheostomy to relieve the respiratory difficulties (p. 386). Foreign bodies in the form of small objects, e.g. nail, fish bone, hair grip, etc. may lodge in the body of the tonsil. Examination and removal may be carried out under anaesthesia. Larger objects may be lodged in the hypopharynx leading to obstruction of the larynx. To remove these objects, the child should be turned upside down and slapped on the back in an effort to dislodge the object. The Heimlich manoeuvre may be performed which uses an upper abdominal thrust to create sufficient diaphragmatic pressure in the static lung air below the foreign body to expel the obstruction. This manoeuvre, however, is not recommended for infants and young children because of the risk of injury to the abdominal organs. If the obstruction persists, the foreign body can be removed by bronchoscopy or as a life-saving measure a tracheostomy may be performed.

Throat infections

The throat may be infected by many different types of pathogenic organisms and viruses.

Acute tonsillitis
This is a common complaint in childhood but is less frequently met with in children under 3 years of age. It is infectious and spreads rapidly by droplet infection. The incubation period is 2 to 4 days. The organism usually responsible is the haemolytic streptococcus, particularly the B (beta) haemolytic streptococcus, but organisms such as staphylococcus and pneumococcus may also be responsible.

Acute tonsillitis is usually described as falling into three categories, depending on the degree of the inflammatory process: (1) catarrhal; (2) follicular and (3) parenchymatous. In catarrhal tonsillitis there are inflammatory changes in the mucous membrane covering the tonsils. In follicular tonsillitis, the crypts become involved, the cells lining them swell and they disintegrate with a necrotic ulceration of parts of the epithelial lining. These ulcers fill with yellow exudate. In parenchymatous tonsillitis the infection spreads beyond the crypts resulting in congestion and swelling of the whole organ.

Clinical features

The onset may be rapid, the child feeling shivery, with pain in the throat (though the young child does not indicate when his throat is sore). He has difficulty in swallowing and his speech is thick. The temperature is high, rising to 39.4°C or higher and in young children it may be accompanied by convulsions. The cervical glands are enlarged and tender.

Tonsillitis may be present with other conditions and differentiation of the cause is important. Examples are: (1) diphtheria: this is slower in onset and toxaemia is greater. On examination, there is a membrane on the tonsils. The causative organism is the Klebs-Loeffler bacillus, which is identified by bacterial examination of a throat swab. (2) Glandular fever: the onset is similar to acute tonsillitis but there is a greater amount of pain and greater glandular involvement. Diagnosis is made by examination of the blood which will show a typical mononucleosis. (3) Scarlet fever: this is identified if the tonsillitis is accompanied by a rash and the typical raw red appearance of the tongue. Another distinctive feature is the presence of albumin in the urine.

Principles of treatment and nursing management

1. Isolation of the causative organism precedes the treatment although, if severe enough, antibiotic therapy is started before the result of the throat swab is obtained (p. 361).
2. Fluids only during the acute stage.
3. Relief of pain and restlessness.
4. Tepid sponging may be indicated if the rectal temperature rises above 39.4°C (p. 92).
5. Anticonvulsant drug is given if convulsions are present.
6. Routine nursing care.

Chronic tonsillitis

Chronic tonsillitis is the result of repeated attacks of acute tonsillitis. The tonsils are unable to resolve completely from an acute attack; the crypts retain purulent material and the regional glands remain enlarged. Finally, the tonsils show permanent enlargement and a spongy appearance. Fibrous tissue forms, preventing release of infected material.

Clinical features

The child tends to be pale and lethargic. He is easily tired, his appetite is affected and he may also complain of abdominal pain. He has frequent attacks of tonsillitis and his speech is nasal and thick.

Treatment is by tonsillectomy.

Peritonsillar abscess (quinsy)

Infection may spread beyond the tonsils so that pus collects in the space between the tonsil and its bed, but it is not common in children under 10 years of age. The throat is very painful and saliva may dribble from the mouth, because swallowing is so painful. Cervical glands are enlarged and the soft palate is very swollen.

Principles of treatment and nursing management

1. The treatment is the same as for tonsillitis but also involves incision of the abscess.
2. Pre-operative care: routine (p. 128).
3. Post-operative care: routine and special care of drainage of the incised abscess. The child is kept on his side and suction may be used. Gargles can be given to him if he is able to use these.
4. Antibiotics are given.
5. Routine nursing care.

Acute retropharyngeal abscess

This condition affects infants under 1 year old. It is due to an inflammation of the retropharyngeal lymph glands which suppurate. The abscess is limited to one side of the midline, bulging forward into the infant's oropharynx.

The onset is acute, following an upper respiratory infection. There will be pain and the infant will refuse feeds. Temperature is raised, pulse rate is increased and there is a high degree of toxaemia. Breathing difficulties may occur if the swelling extends towards the larynx.

Principles of treatment and nursing management

1. Treatment consists of incision and drainage performed without general anaesthesia.
2. Pre-operative care (p. 128).
3. Post-operative care: to ensure that the exudate is allowed to drain, thus preventing pus being inhaled.
4. Antibiotics are given.
5. Routine nursing care.

Hypertrophy of the nasopharyngeal tonsil (adenoids)

The adenoids are lymphoid tissue which enlarge during the first few years of life, particularly if there have been repeated infections of the upper respiratory tract. Adenoids may be present at birth and may cause difficulty in feeding. This is due to the need of the infant to stop feeding in order to breathe. (Babies are nasal breathers.) There may also be nasal discharge and a tendency to otitis media. Pre-school children and older children present a typical picture of mouth breathing, nasal catarrh, otitis media and deafness. Speech is also affected with the voice assuming a characteristic toneless quality.

Treatment is by surgical removal and, where mouth breathing has become habit, breathing exercises will be useful.

Tonsillectomy and adenoidectomy

This used to be a common operation, but in recent years the need for surgery has been questioned. Tonsils and adenoids used to be removed as part of the treatment of conditions such as nephritis and rheumatic fever, diseases associated with the haemolytic streptococcus. Enlargement of tonsils is no longer considered to be a reason for removal since it is argued that this is an important immunological function of these tissues.

However, there are situations when tonsils and adenoids are considered to interfere with the health of the child, and no longer serve a protective function. The decision to remove these tissues depends not on their size but on their appearance, e.g. presence of a band of congestion and of purulent material. Removal may also be necessary when they are considered to be the cause of conditions such as acute nephritis, otitis media and deafness.

Contra-indications for this operation have also to be considered. For example, it should never be performed if the child is suffering from haemophilia, leukaemia or during an epidemic of poliomyelitis. The latter is based on evidence (Medical Research Council, 1955) which showed that 59 per cent of those who had tonsillectomy developed symptoms of poliomyelitis within three weeks of the operation.

The timing of the operation is also important. In general, it should not be performed if any infective process is active.

Pre-operative care

The child has been examined as an outpatient and will generally be admitted as a 'cold case', i.e. from a waiting list. The parents will be advised that the child should be free from upper respiratory infections when presenting him for operation. Any other condition, e.g. diabetes mellitus, will be dealt with in conjunction with the physician responsible for the child's stabilisation.

For admission procedure, see page 76.

Immediate pre-operative care

This follows the general pattern of pre-operative care as described in Chapter 7. Sedation and premedication is prescribed. However, there are some differences in pre-operative care which might be considered. Generally a number of children of varying ages will be operated on, most of them being reasonably well. Many units return the children to the same ward and those waiting for the operation see them returning. It is important that they should be kept calm and comforted and, as far as possible, should not see the other children. A nurse who knows the children, or the play leader, has an important role to play here. There is no need to keep the child in bed and therefore a suitable waiting area could be a playroom.

Technique of the operation

General anaesthesia is always given prior to the operation. The child is placed on his back with the head slightly lowered and the neck extended. The mouth is held open with a gag, e.g. Davis-Boyle gag, and the tongue is pushed out of the way. Suction must be available to prevent inhalation of blood. The adenoids may be removed first, using an adenoid curette. The tonsils are removed by dissection or the guillotine. Whichever method is used, it is important to remove the tonsils completely. Bleeding is controlled by inserting a pack of gauze into the post-nasal space, which must be removed after the operation. Continued bleeding can be dealt with by ligating the vessels on the tonsil bed.

Post-operative nursing care

The principles of post-operative nursing care aim to promote healing and to prevent any complications.

On return from theatre, the child is already conscious but sleepy. He should be placed in the lateral position as this allows secretions to drain. However, since the cough reflex is present, there is not the same danger of secretions entering the larynx. Constant supervision is essential. This means regular recording of pulse rate, rhythm and volume. A rising rate would suggest the possibility of bleeding. Restlessness is always a problem in the post-operative period. The child will be uncomfortable, may cry and feel frightened. He should be comforted and if excessively restless, sedation may be prescribed. Sweating, pallor and excessive swallowing are also indications of bleeding. He should be encouraged to swallow and sips of water may be given. The oftener he swallows the more confident he will become. Once the child is able to drink he can be offered light food, e.g. ice cream and jelly are readily acceptable. After the first 12 hours he can eat bread and drink milk. Hard foods should be avoided.

The sloughs which form in the tonsil bed gradually dry up and harden. Separation of sloughs occurs 7 to 10 days after the operation. The child can be allowed out of bed on the second day after operation and if no complications are present he can go home.

Preparation for home

Full instructions should be given to the parents regarding eating and activity. Full activity should be achieved about a week after operation and any complications arising, e.g. rise in temperature or haemorrhage, must be reported to the general practitioner as soon as possible. In the event of haemorrhage, the parents should be told to contact the hospital immediately. If the child is old enough, gargles or mouthwashes can be used or drinks of water can be given after a meal. This ensures that the mouth is kept clean and healing can take place under the best possible conditions.

Complications

Haemorrhage is the most frequent complication. It may be either reactionary or secondary occurring from the tonsillar bed or from the nasopharynx.

Reactionary haemorrhage. This occurs within the first 24 hours after operation and usually within the first 4 hours. It can be recognised by the following signs and symptoms:

1. A slight oozing of blood from the mouth is usually seen during the first half hour in either method, when the vessels are not ligated — should this increase plus an increase in pulse rate, then it indicates that bleeding is excessive.
2. It will be noted that the child makes frequent swallowing movements in his sleep. This precedes vomiting of fresh blood.

Should any of the above be noted, the surgeon should be notified. Meanwhile, the foot of the bed is raised lowering the patient's head and placing him in the lateral position. If the child is restless and apprehensive, a sedative may be given. Blood loss should be replaced as soon as possible and is usually carried out before the bleeding point is treated.

The following measures can be employed. If the bleeding point is from the adenoid bed, ice packs can be placed on the bridge of the nose. To stop bleeding it will probably be necessary to do so by ligating the vessel, which is done under general anaesthetic. This can be dangerous because the child may have swallowed a great amount of blood and vomiting may occur with the possibility of inhalation of stomach contents.

Secondary haemorrhage. This occurs between the fifth and 10th post-operative days. It is more liable to occur if sepsis is present. The treatment is the same as for reactionary haemorrhage, however, it may be more difficult to ligate the bleeding point since the mass of friable tissue is more difficult to ligate.

Bleeding of the adenoid bed presents a more serious problem, because blood may trickle into the stomach over a considerable period and bleeding may not be recognised until the child has a large vomit.

Principles of treatment and nursing management

1. Treatment consists initially of sitting the child up.
2. If this is not adequate in controlling the haemorrhage, a pack is inserted under general anaesthesia. The post-nasal pack consists of a gauze swab of appropriate size rolled up and tied at its middle with ribbon gauze. The ends of the ribbon gauze are held in the nasopharynx and by a pair of crocodile forceps passed through the nose. One end of each ribbon is brought out of each nostril. The two ends are tied tightly after the main pack has been placed into the nasopharynx. A nasal pack is then introduced. The pack is removed in 12 hours. The nasal pack is removed first, the ribbon gauze is cut near the knot and the nasopharyngeal pack is then removed via the mouth. Another method which may be used is by introducing a small balloon catheter into the nasopharynx through the nose. The balloon is inflated to maintain pressure on the bleeding point.
3. It may be necessary to replace the blood loss.
4. Careful observations of vital functions will be necessary at frequent intervals. It is also necessary to ensure that the nasal pack does not slip out of place as this could obstruct the child's airway. Other complications such as carbon dioxide retention and hypoxia could occur, because a posterior nasal pack may depress the soft palate, causing airway resistance.
5. Following the removal of the nasal pack the child should be told not to blow his nose for at least 48 hours.

After-care at home

Any period of hospitalisation may have an effect on the child. There are, no doubt, variations in the extent and type of disturbance since each child reacts differently. The younger the child, the more traumatic the experience will be. Parents will need guidance as to the care of the child in the post-tonsillectomy/adenoidectomy period, i.e. amount of rest, type of food to eat, recognition of complications and what action to take.

Most children settle down fairly easily to normal home routine, but some anxiety can be expected. This will show itself particularly at night-time. He may not wish to sleep alone or he may be frightened to go to sleep. This situation requires a great deal of patience and understanding. The way the parents handle it will depend on the ideas they hold and the relationship they have with the child. In simple terms, if the child is frightened of sleeping alone, then he should not be left alone. Once he is able to overcome this anxiety he will revert to the previously established routine.

Nursing procedures related to the treatment of the throat

Examination of the throat

Examination of the child's throat is part of the routine examination of the child and is generally carried out by the medical officer. The nurse's responsibility lies in assisting the doctor by holding the child and preparing him for the examination.

Requirements

1. Head light or head mirror and lamp.
2. Tray containing:
   a. Tongue depresser.
   b. Post-nasal mirror.
   c. Laryngeal mirrors, curved and straight.
   d. Fine dissecting forceps.
   e. Dental rolls.
   f. Throat swabs.
3. Box of paper tissues.
4. Receptacle for disposables.
5. Receptacle for used instruments.

Preparation of the child

The small child should be sitting on the nurse's knee, facing the doctor, with his head tilted back and supported. The child's legs may be held between the nurse's knees, while the nurse supports his arms with one hand. Although this is not a painful procedure, children tend to be frightened. It is therefore essential to reassure and calm the child both before and during the examination.

Taking a throat swab

A throat swab is taken routinely or as a diagnostic test to determine the presence of micro-organisms and their sensitivity to drugs.

Requirements

1. Tongue depresser (a good light source).
2. Sterile throat swab.
3. Disposal bag.

Preparation of the child and method
The procedure should be explained to the child if he is old enough to understand. Two nurses will be required, one to hold and reassure the child, the other to swab the throat. The child may be either lying or sitting in the position described above.

The cotton wool holder is removed from the tube and the most representative exudate or area is swabbed. It is important to avoid contact with any other part, e.g. mouth and teeth. The cotton wool holder is then replaced in the tube, which is labelled and sent to the bacteriological department.

Gargles

These are excellent for cleansing and soothing purposes, but can only be given effectively to children of 7 years of age and upwards. The solution should be warm. The following lotions can be used:
sodium bicarbonate (one rounded teaspoonful to 300 ml of water), hypertonic saline (one teaspoonful to 300 ml of water) and glycothymoline 1:8.

Chapter 23
Disorders of the respiratory system

Disorders of the respiratory system present many problems from birth throughout childhood. They involve problems with inspiration, expiration, and gaseous exchanges at alveolar level, mechanical hindrance to lung movements and mechanical/nervous interference to pulmonary ventilation. A brief discussion of the structures involved in respiration and their function should help the reader to understand disease processes and their effect on function.

The respiratory system can be divided into upper and lower tracts. The upper respiratory tract consists of the nose, nasopharynx, sinuses and larynx, and the lower respiratory tract consist of the trachea, bronchi, bronchioles and alveoli (Figs. 23.1 and 23.2). Normally, the upper respiratory tract is discussed in conjunction with the ear, nose and throat, but since it is part of the air passage system, it has been included in this chapter.

The upper respiratory tract

The nose
The interior of the nose is divided into right and left halves by the nasal septum. Each half is incompletely divided into four regions containing the nasal passages which run backwards, leading into the nasopharynx. The area just within the nostrils is lined by skin containing coarse hair. The rest of the interior is lined by mucous membrane.

The function of the nose is to carry air to and from the lungs and to warm it as it is inspired. The hair inside the nostrils and the cilia covering the mucous membrane serve to remove dust and other impurities from the air.

When infection occurs, the main local effects are irritation of the mucous cells causing production

of excess mucus, swelling of the mucous membrane due to local oedema and congestion with blood (Fig. 23.1). The nasal passages tend to become blocked by the mucosal swelling and excessive secretions. Initially when viral infection occurs, the discharge is clear, but when there is a secondary invasion by bacteria, the discharge becomes yellowish or greenish due to the presence of pus (dead neutrophils and granulocytes).

Sinuses
The paranasal sinuses provide a system of air spaces situated within various bones in the face. They are lined with secretory mucosa and obtain their nerve and blood supply from the nose. Infection of the epithelial lining of the sinuses may spread from the nose leading to engorgement of the blood vessels, increased secretion of mucus and oedema. This is called *sinusitis*. Accumulation of secretions causes discomfort and pain which is relieved by drainage. This may occur spontaneously or surgical intervention may be necessary. Spontaneous drainage tends to be into the bronchi leading to *bronchitis*.

Larynx
The larynx is situated in front of the pharynx and above the commencement of the trachea. It consists mainly of the thyroid and cricoid cartilage, and seven other cartilages which are joined together by membrane. A cartilaginous structure overhangs the entrance to the larynx. This is the epiglottis which guards the glottis during swallowing, preventing food from entering the larynx and trachea. Inflammation of the epiglottis can result in obstruction to the airway.

The interior of the larynx contains two folds of mucous membrane which stretch across the cavity of the larynx from the middle of the thyroid

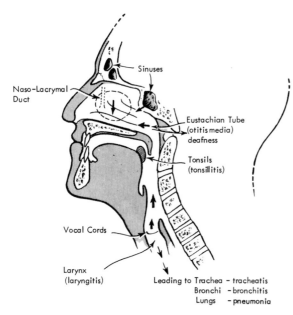

Fig. 23.1 Spread of common cold infection.

cartilage to the arytenoid cartilage. These are the vocal cords or folds. During ordinary breathing the vocal cords lie at some distance from the midline and respired air passes freely between them without setting them into vibration. During deep forcible inspiration they are even more abducted, while during speaking or singing they are adducted. These changes are effected by minute muscles. In children, the vocal cords are shorter than in adults.

The larynx serves the functions of respiration and phonation but at the same time it takes part in deglutition, during which it may close in order to prevent food entering the lower respiratory tract. It also closes during regurgitation of food preventing food aspiration. These reflex closures depend on neuromuscular co-ordination which may not be fully operative in infants, leading to spasms.

Conditions which may effect the larynx fall under three headings:

1. Congenital abnormalities, such as:
   Atresia of the larynx.
   Laryngeal web.
   Laryngeal cyst.
   Laryngomalacia (congenital laryngeal stridor).

2. Injuries — foreign bodies.
3. Infections — laryngitis, oedema of the larynx.

The lower respiratory tract

The structures which comprise this part of the respiratory tract are the trachea, bronchi, and bronchioles and the lungs (Fig. 23.2).

The first three, trachea, bronchi and bronchioles, are tubes which convey the air into and out of the lungs. The trachea commences at the lower border of the larynx and passes behind the sternum into the thorax. It is a wide, flexible membranous tube, stiffened by regularly spaced incomplete rings of cartilage. The tube is lined by mucous membrane, the surface epithelium being ciliated columnar in character. Soon after entering the thorax the trachea divides into right and left bronchus. Each bronchus divides into several branches which plunge into the substance of a lung. Within the substance of the lung the bronchi divide into innumerable branches of progressively diminishing calibres until the branches are of very narrow diameter, when they are called bronchioles. These tubes are lined by mucous membrane surmounted by ciliated columnal epithelium,

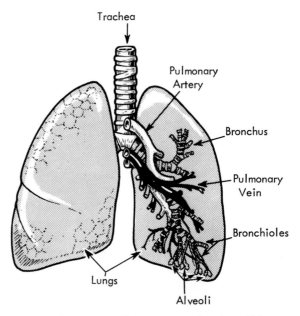

Fig. 23.2 The lower respiratory tract: trachea, bronchial 'tree' and lungs.

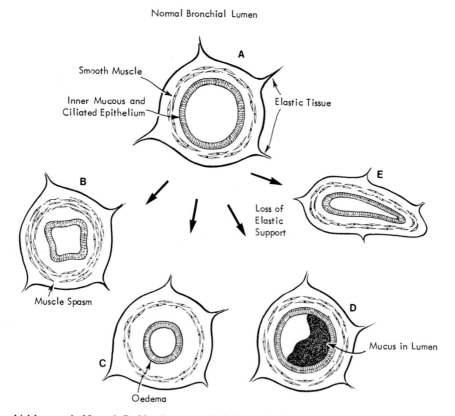

Fig. 23.3 Bronchial lumen. A, Normal. B, Muscle spasm. C, Oedema. D, Mucus in lumen. E, Loss of elastic tissue.

continuous with the lining of the trachea. Smooth muscle is found longitudinally in the larger bronchi and trachea. In the smaller bronchi and bronchioles it is confined to the posterior wall. The whole extent of the bronchial tree is richly supplied with elastic fibres which, together with all the other tissues mentioned, can be changed by disease, and so affect the normal functions (Fig. 23.3).

Lungs

Anatomically, the fundamental unit of lung structure is considered to be the secondary lobule. Many hundreds of these go to make up each lung. Each lobule is a lung in miniature with a bronchial tree and a circulation of its own. Each respiratory bronchiole terminates in an alveolus. The alveoli consist of large flat thin epithelial cells and it is here that the exchange of gases between the air and blood takes place.

The apices of the lungs reach just above the clavicle and the bases rest on the diaphragm. Both lungs are divided into lobes, the right into three, the left into two. Nutrition is brought to the lung tissues by the blood via the bronchial arteries; blood returns from the lung tissue via the bronchial veins.

The lungs have also a pulmonary circulation which is concerned with transporting deoxygenated and oxygenated blood. The lungs are supplied with deoxygenated blood by the pulmonary arteries coming from the right ventricle. The arteries divide and subdivide into progressively smaller branches, penetrating every part of the lungs till at last they form capillary networks which surround and lie on the walls of the alveoli. The walls of both the alveoli and the capillaries are extremely thin and it is here that the respiratory gases are interchanged. The oxygenated blood is returned to the left atrium by the four pulmonary veins.

Pleura

Each lung is enclosed in a double sac, one of which covers the surface of the lung (visceral pleura) and the other lines the inner surface of the thoracic wall and part of the diaphragm (parietal pleura). The two surfaces are smooth and moistened with serous fluid. The surface tension properties of this fluid keep the two surfaces together, so that the lung follows the movements of the chest wall. The pleural fluid also reduces friction during the breathing process.

Inflammation of this membrane is called pleurisy; accumulation of fluid is known as pleural effusion and leads to impairment of breathing. Other causes of restriction of ventilation, in addition to pleural effusion, are shown in Figure 23.4.

The function of the lungs is ventilation: to take in air containing oxygen and convey it to the blood and to eliminate air containing carbon dioxide received from the blood. The mechanism involves the rhythmic act of quiet breathing. It is an active inspiratory movement in which the diaphragm descends and the chest wall expands and is pulled outwards by contractions of the external intercostal muscles. Expiration is a passive process in quiet breathing. These activites are controlled by 'centres' in the brain stem which stimulate the motorneurones of the diaphragm and intercostal muscles (Fig. 23.5). Since the lungs are elastic, they follow the thoracic expansion passively and air is drawn into the depth of the lung. As the lung expands air flows through the open larynx until the pressure nears atmospheric. At the end of inspiration the external intercostal muscles and the diaphragm relax and the elastic recoil of the thoracic wall and the lungs causes passive expiration.

In quiet breathing, an adult breathes 6 to 7 litres of air per minute with a breathing rate of 12 to 14 per minute. The amount of air inspired or expired per breath (tidal air) is approximately 500 ml. At rest an adult uses about 250 ml of oxygen per minute and expires about 200 ml carbon dioxide per minute. In heavy exercise, the pulmonary ventilation volume may exceed 80 litres per minute and oxygen usage may rise above 3.5 litres per minute.

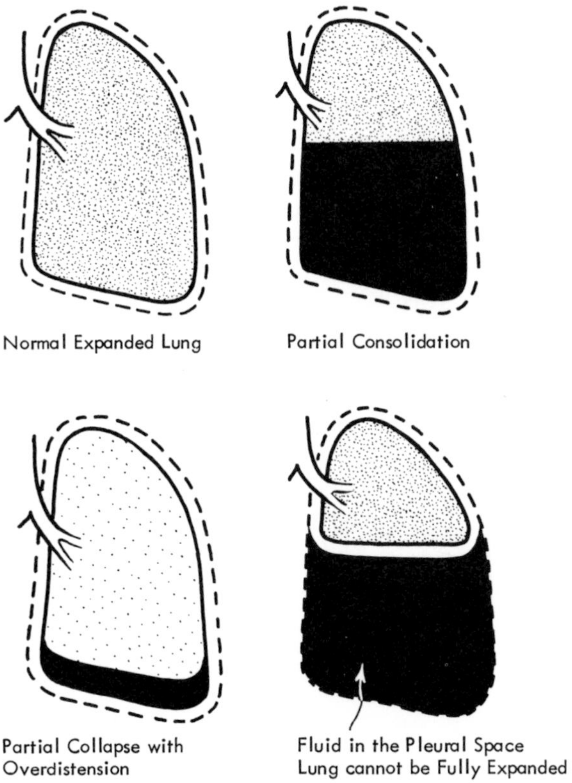

Normal Expanded Lung

Partial Consolidation

Partial Collapse with Overdistension

Fluid in the Pleural Space Lung cannot be Fully Expanded

Fig. 23.4 Restriction of ventilation of lung.

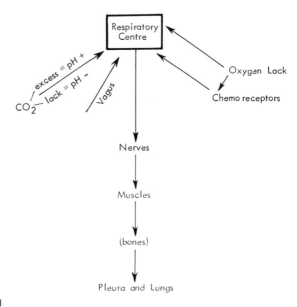

Respiratory Centre

CO_2 excess = pH +

lack = pH −

Vagus

Oxygen Lack

Chemo receptors

Nerves

Muscles

(bones)

Pleura and Lungs

Fig. 23.5 System responsible for lung expansion. Ventilatory failure can result from a failure of this system at any point.

The values in infants are different. They have a large surface area in relation to weight and a high metabolic rate. The airways have a greater relative diameter, and the anatomical dead space is proportionally larger. The ribs are almost horizontal at rest, and inspiration cannot raise them much more. Inspiration is mainly diaphragmatic and anything impeding this movement will cause respiratory embarrassment. These factors make breathing in infants less efficient than in the adult and an increase in alveolar ventilation is achieved by increasing breathing rate (18 to 40 per minute) which requires a high oxygen intake. The basal oxygen requirements at birth are 23 ml per minute. With increasing age the rate per minute falls and the basal oxygen requirement rises (Fig. 23.6).

Lung volumes

To determine volume changes a spirometer is used. The individual breathes into a mouthpiece and causes a bell to move up and down. A record can then be obtained of the volume of air an individual inhales, exhales, or leaves in the lungs. The volume changes of the spirometer bell are

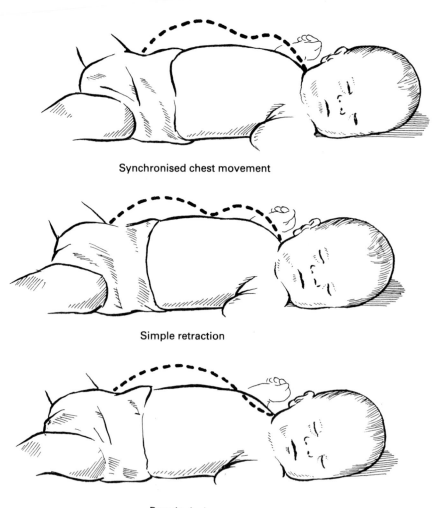

Synchronised chest movement

Simple retraction

Paradoxical

Fig. 23.6 Variety of chest movements during breathing.

equal to those of the lungs. It is also possible to establish lung volumes under differing conditions.

Tidal volume is the volume of air breathed in or out during quiet breathing (about 500 ml).

Inspiratory reserve volume is the maximal volume of air which can be inspired after completing normal quiet inspiration, i.e. inspired from the end inspiratory phase (2000 to 3200 ml).

Expiratory reserve volume is the maximal volume of air which can be expired after a normal tidal or quiet expiration (750 to 1000 ml).

Residual volume is the volume of gas which remains in the lungs after a maximal expiration (1200 ml).

Lung capacities

Vital capacity is the maximum volume of air which can be expelled from the lungs by forceful effort following a maximal inspiration. This depends on the size of the person and is usually of the order of 4.8 litres in men and 3.2 litres in women. It is increased in swimmers and divers and decreased in older people and in diseases of the respiratory apparatus, e.g. respiratory obstruction, pleural effusion and pulmonary fibrosis.

The vital capacity is also altered by posture, being greater when measured in the upright position owing to the decreased pulmonary blood volume in the standing subject. Another important measurement is the 'timed vital capacity'. Normally 80 per cent of the vital capacity should be expired in the first second. This is a more sensitive index of the severity of the obstructive diseases than that provided by the vital capacity itself, but it does not differentiate between the various causes of obstruction.

Respiratory function in children

Respiratory function varies with the age, size and build of the child. It is quite difficult to obtain values for young children (1 month to 5 years). For example, the dead space values in the new-born are 7 ml; at 5 years 50 ml; at 10 years 75 ml; and at 15 years 125 ml. The tidal volume in the new-born is 18 ml; at 5 years 200 ml; at 10 years 300 ml; and at 15 years 500 ml. The vital capacity is 90 ml in the new-born; 1200 to 1300 ml at 5 years; 1900 to 200 ml at 10 years; and 3300 to 3500 ml at 15 years.

Alveolar ventilation

Ventilation involves the gaseous exchange of oxygen and carbon dioxide by diffusion between the alveoli and the pulmonary capillary blood. This exchange depends primarily on the volume of alveolar ventilation and volume of blood flow through the pulmonary capillaries, which are in close contact with the ventilated alveoli. Each lung normally has the same ventilation/perfusion ratio, i.e. receiving 2 litres of ventilation and 2.5 litres of blood. Non-uniformity of this ratio leads to abnormalities of oxygenation of arterial blood. Examples of causes of uneven ventilation include asthma and pneumothorax, and non-uniform blood flow may occur in conditions such as emphysema and fibrosis, where there is a regional reduction in the blood flow.

In breathing, work has to be done in overcoming the elastic resistance. Both the lungs and the thoracic cage are elastic structures and this makes breathing possible (Fig. 23.7). *Compliance* is the term used to express the stretchiness of both

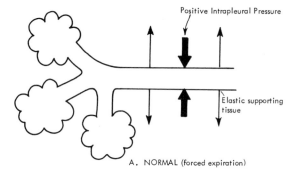

A. NORMAL (forced expiration)

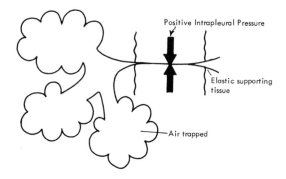

Fig. 23.7 Elastic supporting tissue, normal in (A), damaged in (B).

lungs and the chest wall, and is the measure of ease with which the lung and chest wall expand when the pressure inside them is increased. If the lungs of a patient expand less easily, their compliance is said to have decreased. Compliance of the lung can be measured on anaesthetised patients. Intrapleural pressue is estimated from oesophageal pressure, by using a small swallowed balloon. Oesophageal pressure is similar to pleural pressure, because both the oesophagus and the pleura are elastic sacs containing only a small quantitiy of fluid and both are contained in the thorax.

Increased compliance is associated with a flaccid paralysis of the muscles of the chest wall. It also occurs where an open pneumothorax is present. Decreased compliance increases the work of breathing and is found in diseases such as pulmonary fibrosis and congestive cardiac failure. Deficiency of surfactant also reduces compliance. Surfactant is a detergent-like substance present in the alveoli which reduces the surface tension of the alveolar fluid. The substance is believed to be liberated from the pneumonocytes lying adjacent to the alveolar lining membrane. Its action is to reduce the surface tension of the alveolar fluid, thereby enabling the alveoli to expand more readily during inspiration, thus increasing the compliance of the lung. The importance of these findings is that in atelectasis of the new-born, and in congestive atelectasis, there is a reduction in surfactant action leading to a failure of the lung to expand.

Transport of oxygen and carbon dioxide in the blood (Fig. 23.8)

Two important factors should be considered when discussing the transport of both oxygen and carbon dioxide. These are, tension and quantity. Briefly, tension is the driving force of a gas from one region to another. Oxygen passes from alveolar air into the pulmonary capillaries because the tension of the oxygen is higher in the alveolar air than in the blood. Transfer of oxygen in the tissues is due to higher tension in the blood than in the tissue.

Oxygen tension in the lungs is 100 mmHg and it leaves the lungs at that tension until it reaches the tissue capillaries. As it passes through the tissue capillaries, the oxygen tension falls steadily from 100 mmHg to 40 mmHg, which is the same as that of the surrounding tissue fluid. When the venous blood returns to the heart and back to the lungs its oxygen tension is 40 mmHg.

In the lungs it comes in contact with the oxygen of the alveolar air at a tension of 100 mmHg. The tension of oxygen in the lung capillaries then builds up gradually from 40 mmHg to 100 mmHg. The quantity of oxygen in the blood will depend on the amount of haemoglobin present and its property of combining with oxygen. One gram of haemoglobin has the ability to combine with 1.34 ml of oxygen. Each 100 ml of arterial blood passes to the tissues carrying about 0.3 ml of oxygen in solution and about 19 ml in combination with haemoglobin. When the oxyhaemoglobin is exposed to tissue oxygen at a tension of 40 mmHg, dissociation occurs and about 30 per cent of the

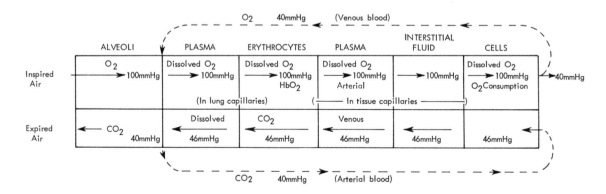

Fig. 23.8 Flow chart indicating the transport of oxygen and carbon dioxide in the blood.

oxygen present is liberated and diffuses out into the tissue fluid (i.e. 5 to 6 mm/100 ml).

This means that the venous blood leaves with an oxygen tension of 40 mmHg and an oxygen content of about 14 ml per 100 ml of blood.

Carbon dioxide transport in the body

Arterial blood reaches the tissues with a carbon dioxide tension of 40 mmHg, and a carbon cioxide content of 48 ml per 100 ml. Since the carbon dioxide tension of resting tissue is 46 mmHg, carbon dioxide diffuse rapidly into the blood and is formed into carbonic acid in the corpuscles. At the same time carbon dioxide combines with haemoglobin since it is in reduced form. It reaches the lungs at a carbon dioxide tension of 46 mmHg and diffuses through the alveolar tissues where the carbon dioxide tension is 40 mmHg.

The amount of carbon dioxide in the blood is greater than oxygen carried per 100 ml of blood. Only a small amount is lost through the lungs, i.e. 4 ml carbon dioxide per 100 ml. This indicates that carbon dioxide is not only a waste product but has important functions in maintaining blood pH and influencing the respiratory centre. Should the level of carbon dioxide in the blood be too high, the respiratory centre is stimulated and respiration is increased. Increased respiration washes out the increased carbon dioxide from the lungs, leading to a fall in carbon dioxide tension in arterial blood. A new equlibrium will then be set up with the carbon dioxide in the arterial blood at the correct level.

Blood reaction

In ordinary circumstances, the blood pH is 7.35 to 7.4. It is only in severe acidosis that the pH falls as low as 7 and only rarely that it rises to 7.7, even in severe alkalosis. This pH range of 7 to 7.7 is that compatible with life and corresponds to a change of hydrogen ion concentration from 100 to 20 ng (10^{-9} g)/l.

To maintain normal blood reaction, the body has a system which mops up hydrogen ions as they are formed. This is performed by the buffer anions. Two substances act as hydrogen acceptors, plasma proteins and haemoglobin, the latter being the more powerful one. The reaction involves carbon dioxide which is in a dissolved form when passing from tissue plasma, due to tension gradient (as in oxygen). It thus gains entry to the corpuscles where it is converted to carbonic acid (H_2CO_3). As more carbon dioxide combines with water to form carbonic acid a second reaction takes place which involves the release of hydrogen ions. Haemoglobin acts as the acceptor of hydrogen ions. Another function of haemoglobin is that of aiding carbon dioxide uptake and it does so more effectively when it is reduced, that is when it contains less oxygen.

As a result of the reaction, carbon dioxide is converted into bicarbonate ion. The change of concentration of bicarbonate ions is dependent upon the amount of carbon dioxide taken from the tissue or given off in the lungs. The body also reacts to a respiratory acidosis by increasing hydrogen ion secretion into the renal tubules, and by retention of bicarbonate ions by the kidneys.

Common respiratory problems

There are certain manifestations of respiratory disorder which are found in many diseases. These include *dyspnoea*, *hypoxia* and *hypercapnia*.

Dyspnoea is an unpleasant awareness of breathing, e.g. breathlessness.

Hypoxia implies lack of oxygen by the cells of the body. Four varieties have been classified:

1. Hypoxic = when the arterial oxygen tension (PO_2) is low due to respiratory failure, characterised by reduced arterial oxygen tension.
2. Anaemic = inadequate oxygen-carrying capacity of the blood.
3. Stagnant = due to poor circulation.
4. Histotoxic = inability of cells to use oxygen due to poisoning.

Hypercapnia denotes the presence of excess carbon dioxide in the blood. Effects on the body include peripheral vasodilatation, respiratory acidosis, stimulation of ventilation and cerebral depression.

Respiratory system at birth

Mature physiological responses are present in the respiratory system of the normal new-born.

However, the number of bronchioles and alveoli are not yet complete and increase throughout childhood until puberty. Anatomical differences of the airway and pulmonary vascular bed in various age groups result in variation in response to stimuli.

At birth the airway has little smooth muscle. By 4 to 5 months of age enough muscle is present to produce airway narrowing in response to irritative stimuli. By 12 months of age the quantity of smooth muscle is comparable to that of an adult.

Before the new-born takes his first breath of air, the terminal bronchioles and alveoli are not collapsed but are normally filled with fluid and glandular secretions. Some of the fluid is amniotic fluid but most of it is produced by the lining of bronchioles. Most of this fluid passes into amniotic fluid via the nose. The fluid in the alveoli is related to an active pulmonary vascular resistance present before birth. When air-breathing begins, the hormone bradykinin reduces the vascular resistance and the pulmonary flow increases. In order that the lung tissue (alveoli) can expand, the surface tension has to be reduced. This is achieved by the action of surfactant (a surface active agent). The first breath of life requires very high intra-thoracic pressures to expand the lungs with air. To keep enough air in the alveoli and prevent alveolar collapse, surfactant must be present to lower inspiratory pressure.

Pre-term infants lack surfactant and therefore much greater effort is required with each breath. Surfactant also serves to protect the alveolar cells from the direct exposure to oxygen, which is toxic.

Breathing difficulties in the new-born are related to both anatomical and functional differences. The following factors are involved:

1. New-borns are nasal breathers and total airway obstruction will occur unless the nasal passages are patent or an artificial airway is supplied.
2. Because the ribs of new-born babies are nearly horizontal the antero-posterior diameter of the thoracic cage imparts a limited amount of increase with inspiration. However, since the diaphragm is displaced upward by the relatively large liver, the result is inefficient chest wall function. In addition, ventilation is largely diaphragmatic.
3. The new-born larynx is situated nearer to the head than later in life so that the glottis is located at the level of the interspace between cervical vertebrae 3 and 4. The laryngeal reflexes are very active and the epiglottis longer.

Diseases of the respiratory tract

From the moment of an infant's birth, his life is dependent on the normal functioning of the respiratory tract. Like most bodily systems the respiratory tract may show lesions either congenital or acquired which will affect its function. This chapter considers some common disorders and principles of treatment. Related nursing care and procedures are presented for general, rather than specific conditions.

Respiratory failure
Respiratory failure denotes inadequate pulmonary function in delivering sufficient oxygen to meet the demands of the body and to eliminate carbon dioxide.

Respiratory failure is common in infants and children. In infancy it is because the chest wall is soft and compliant, the pleural pressure is at end-respiration zero and the alveolar diameter is small. The combination of these factors increases their tendency to develop atelectasis (p. 378). Once the alveoli collapse, they are more difficult to re-expand because the compliant chest wall prevents the generation of adequate pleural pressure to do so. This requires increased respiratory work, which the infant finds difficult to achieve and, therefore, many infants stop breathing (apnoea).

With growth, the chest wall stiffens, a negative end-expiratory pressure develops and the alveoli grow. By the time the infant is 1 year old, the number and size of his alveoli have increased nearly 500 per cent, i.e. six times from 20 million to 120 million. Despite this growth, the infant's airway resistance remains high, relative to his increased ventilatory needs. Small changes in airway diameter significantly alter his resistance to gas flow. Thus infection, aspiration of foreign material, and oedema all narrow his airway and increase resistance to breathing and therefore can cause respiratory failure in infants of this age.

Other causes of respiratory failure may be due to prematurity or hyaline membrane disease, congenital anomalies such as diaphragmatic hernia, congenital heart disease and abdominal wall defects. In older children, trauma and foreign body aspiration as well as chronic lung diseases such as cystic fibrosis and asthma can lead to respiratory failure.

Clinical features

Young infants. Irritability, poor activity and convulsions are commonly signs of respiratory failure. Wheezing in an infant may be diagnostic of asthma, and retractions of the sternum may indicate airway obstruction, while flaring of the alae nasi and the use of the accessory muscles indicate increased breathing work, as seen in restrictive lung disease (Fig. 23.9).

Older infants and children. Evidence of fatigue, restlessness, mental confusion and sweating are easily recognised. In addition, there will be flaring of the alae nasi and chest retractions with the use of accessory muscles.

Cyanosis can be a feature in all children. Cyanosis indicates oxygen desaturation and, to recognise it, it is necessary to examine the mucous membrane and nail beds. Since cyanosis may not adequately correlate with the arterial PaO_2, it is important to evaluate the blood gases of children suspected of having respiratory disease and of being cyanotic.

Management of respiratory failure

The management of respiratory failure depends on the presenting features. Type I respiratory failure (where there are abnormalities within the lung itself, e.g. partial obstruction or collapse of the alveoli resulting in hypoxaemia without carbon dioxide retention) is treated by the administration of humidified oxygen (p. 382). In type II respiratory failure, there is widespread hypoventilation of lung alveoli with a reduction in tidal volume and vital capacity. This can occur in head injury, drug ingestion, acute bronchiolitis or severe acute asthma, when the work of breathing is very high and leads to muscle fatigue when the ventilatory requirements cannot be met. Oxygen administration has to be carefully controlled. The Venturi oxygen mask or head tent, which delivers between 26 and 30 per cent oxygen concentration, is useful (p. 384). In very serious cases intubation will be necessary delivering 100 per cent oxygen (p. 393).

DISEASES AFFECTING THE UPPER RESPIRATORY TRACT

Nose

Congenital abnormalities of the nose do occur but are fortunately rare. Any osseous obstruction

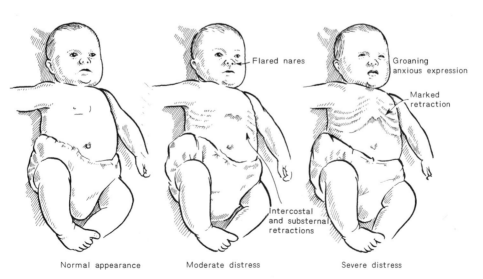

Normal appearance   Moderate distress   Severe distress

Flared nares

Groaning anxious expression

Marked retraction

Intercostal and substernal retractions

Fig. 23.9 Types of breathing movements.

would have to be dealt with as an emergency. An example is choanal atresia in infancy, which may be either complete bilateral, complete unilateral, incomplete bilateral or incomplete unilateral (atresia). Treatment is by operative means which aims at rupturing the membraneous atresia, or removal of the osseous atresia.

Nasal injuries may occur during labour, particularly during a difficult labour where the child's soft nasal framework may be damaged. The injury is present at birth and may be suspected when the nose is twisted to one side. Nasal breathing may be affected.

By far the most common disturbance of upper respiratory function is that produced by *infection and allergies*. All the regions of the upper respiratory tract may be involved. The most common infecting agent is a virus which is inhaled and the most likely areas are the nose and the throat. *Coryza* means simply a 'cold in the head' and *rhinitis* refers to inflammation in the nose. As with all infections, the effects can be local or general (systemic). Local effects are irritation of mucus cells producing excess mucus, swelling of the mucosa due to local oedema and stimulation of pain receptors, especially in the larynx, trachea and bronchi. The nasal passages tend to become blocked by mucosal swelling and excess secretions. Damage to mucosal cells encourages secondary invasion by bacteria, such as streptococci, pneumococci, staphylococci, etc.

Young children suffer frequently from these infections which tend to spread along the respiratory pathways into the sinuses causing *sinusitis*, downwards into the larynx leading to *laryngitis* and into the lower respiratory tract resulting in *bronchitis* and *pneumonia*.

Sputum

Sputum is excess mucus from the respiratory tract which cannot be removed by ciliary action. It accumulates and stimulates nerve endings in the mucous membrane, thereby initiating a cough reflex.

Sputum is formed in response to physical, chemical or infective irritation of the mucosa of the respiratory tract. The offending irritant is diluted and buffered by the mucus and expectorated. In addition, when the respiratory tract is inflamed, sputum contains the product of an inflammatory reaction. Young children cannot spit and so must swallow secretions from the respiratory tract. Their removal can be facilitated by getting the child to cough while the chest is inverted (postural drainage), since simple drainage is then easier than swallowing uphill.

Infants

Since the nasal passages are small, infection of nasal mucosa will further decrease the lumen and interfere with nasal breathing. Young infants mainly breathe through the nose and therefore any nasal obstruction will make sucking and breathing difficult and also interfere with sleep.

Children

The young child too is subject to nasal infection, but can cope with breathing by using his mouth. Nevertheless, difficulties with sleeping and irritability produce many nursing problems.

Many serious infections (including measles, diphtheria, meningitis and whooping cough) present upper respiratory symptoms at their onset and may be confused with coryza. Allergic conditions, such as hay fever, may also be confused with coryza, but differentiation is usually evident on the persistence of the allergic condition and specific diseases present their own signs.

Acute laryngitis

This is a relatively common infection in children affecting the larynx and it may also occur in the course of pertussis (whooping cough), bronchitis, etc. Symptoms and signs include hoarseness of voice and a harsh cough. There is usually a history of a 'cold' with the child wakening during the night with a harsh, barking cough and inspiratory stridor. Initially, there may be dyspnoea, if laryngeal oedema is present, and the temperature is often highly elevated.

Principles of treatment and nursing management

1. Humidified environment (Croupette) is effective (p. 381).
2. Drug therapy, antibiotic.
3. Sedation, if the child is restless.
4. Adequate fluid intake.
5. Routine nursing care.

If the cough is troublesome and the child is unable to feed, a naso-gastric tube can be passed.

Acute obstructive laryngitis (croup)

Croup is a term used to describe a condition which is characterised by a harsh cough, hoarseness and laboured breathing. Obstruction may be due to either spasm or to infection and infiltration of the larynx and adjacent structures. The obstruction may be partial or complete.

There are a number of conditions which resemble the above, but there are important differences. For example, *spasmodic laryngitis* occurs generally between the ages of 2 and 4 years. It comes on suddenly at night and follows a mild upper respiratory infection. The temperature is elevated. In (diphtheritic laryngitis the onset is more gradual and the cough is not barking but stenosis (narrowing) becoming increasingly severe. *Laryngospasm of tetany* is shorter lasting but may occur several times a day.

Principles of treatment and nursing management

1. Drugs are given in response to the causative organism. For example, broad spectrum antibiotics if secondary bacterial invasion is suspected, or in the case of diphtheritic laryngitis, diphtheria antitoxin is given.
2. Surgical intervention. This aims at relieving the obstruction by creating a tracheostomy (p. 386).
3. Nursing care:
   a. Positioning of the child so that he can breathe more easily (p. 109, 380).
   b. Humidity (p. 381).
   c. Oxygen administration to relieve anoxia (p. 382).
   d. Adequate hydration.
   e. Adequate nutrition.

THE LOWER RESPIRATORY TRACT

Laryngo-tracheal-bronchitis

This is an acute fulminating respiratory infection characterised by tracheitis, bronchitis, potential obstructive laryngitis, severe dyspnoea and a highly elevated temperature. It occurs mainly in infants and children. It generally follows a viral infection producing a 'cold'. The majority of cases are estimated to be due to myxoviruses. Super-imposed on the original infection is bacterial infection, in particular, haemolytic streptococcus, staphylococcus and Type BH influenzae.

The pathology is much the same as in previously described infections of the respiratory tract. Oedema is extensive with copious, thick mucus constantly being secreted which threatens to block the subglottic area of the larynx and bronchi. Involvement of smaller bronchioles often occurs as an extension of the disease.

Clinical features

This is a rapidly progressing illness with a high temperature, severe dyspnoea and toxaemia. Cough is very irritating but not productive. Initial hoarseness is followed by stridor (harsh sound) and later loss of sound (aphonia). The latter is partly due to dyspnoea. Respiratory movements show retraction of the supra- and infrasternal spaces. The child's facial expression is anxious and the initial flushed appearance changes to paleness as breathing become more difficult (Fig. 23.10).

Principles of treatment and nursing management

1. Oxygen with high humidity (p. 381–382).
2. Suction, to remove secretions (p. 386).
3. Antibiotic (broad spectrum).

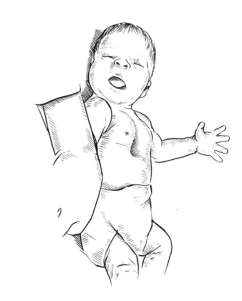

Fig. 23.10 Deep substernal retraction.

4. Sedation, if the child is restless. Recognition of the danger of carbon dioxide retention.
5. Observation of cardiac activity.
6. Routine nursing care.
7. Adequate fluid intake and naso-gastric feeding, if the child is too distressed to feed.

Bronchial asthma

This is a condition which is characterised by a paroxysm of dyspnoea of a wheezing type, which is due to the narrowing of the lumen of the smaller bronchi and bronchioles. It is often associated with other allergic conditions such as eczema. Two main causes are often cited: (1) external factors, which include pollen, dust, sometimes food, animals or drugs; and (2) internal (intrinsic) factors believed to be some infecting agent producing upper respiratory infection or affecting the lower respiratory tract. Whatever the cause, the clinical features are the same.

It may develop gradually during bronchitis or begin abruptly after exposure to an allergen. Attacks are paroxysmal with a feeling of tightness in the chest, dyspnoea, wheezing and may be accompanied by coughing and sputum. These attacks may last a short time or develop into status asthmaticus, lasting for some days. Termination of the attack is recognised by coughing which is moist and productive.

The child is extremely anxious, with laboured, wheezing breathing and profuse sweating. Expiration is prolonged. In the chronic state there are obvious chest contour changes.

The dyspnoea is caused by narrowing of the airways and is typically worse on expiration than on inspiration. This is because inspiration expands not only the lung alveoli but also all the airways. Inspiratory expansion of the airways aids inflow of air, but during expiration there is a rise in airway resistance due to the narrowed lumen, making expiration difficult, prolonged and wheezy (normally expiration is passive and inspiration is active).

Wheezing is associated with increased velocity of air flow due to the narrowed airways. This increased velocity leads to air turbulence and thereby can be felt as vibrations on the chest or heard as rhonchi (snoring sound) with a stethoscope.

Principles of treatment and nursing management
1. Mild attack:

   a. Give salbutamol or terbutaline in nebulised form 2- to 4-hourly. These can be given either via a face mask or a mouthpiece (Fig. 23.11). Salbutamol is given as 0.5 to 1.5 ml of 0.5 per cent ventilator solution which is made up to 2 ml with normal saline. Terbutaline is given in nebulised form 2- to 4-hourly in doses of 2 to 5 mg. Many children will respond completely and may be able to go home on oral therapy.

   b. Guidance to parents with regard to management of the child and, if a nebuliser is to be used, then full instructions on its use must be given.

2. Severe attack:

   a. Oxygen is required for any child who is cyanosed. The oxygen should be administered with caution since the child with respiratory difficulty may be dependent upon his low PO_2 to stimulate breathing.

   b. If the child does not respond to the nebulised salbutamol, aminophylline is given intravenously slowly over 15 to 20 minutes to avoid the dangers of cardiac dysrhythmias, nausea, vomiting and convulsions. Alternatively, intravenous salbutamol can be given.

   c. Careful monitoring of cardiac action.

   d. If the child is in status asthmaticus or if there is little or no improvement, steroid therapy may be given (Hydrocortisone intravenously, followed by prednisolone orally for 5 to 7 days.)

   e. It may be necessary to ventilate the child if the level of consciousness falls or if there is respiratory failure as is indicated by arterial $PCO_2 \geqslant 65$ mmHg (8.4 kPa).

   f. Intravenous fluids may be required to correct acid-base imbalance and to replace fluid lost from the respiratory tract and poor fluid intake. Overhydration should be avoided because it is believed to increase the risk of interstitial lung oedema.

   g. Physiotherapy should be given once the acute attack has abated.

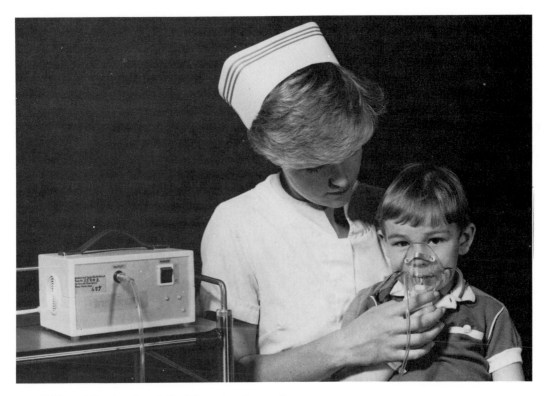

Fig. 23.11 Child receiving drug in nebulised form via a face mask.

Subsequent management

1. Meeting nutritional needs. Inititally a light diet should be given and once the child's condition improves this can be changed to a more normal diet for his age.
2. An adequate fluid intake should be maintained. Large amounts of oral fluids are not advisable during respiratory distress since gastric dilatation may limit diaphragmatic activity and thereby increase respiratory difficulty.
3. Medication should be given as prescribed. This may include an antibiotic in addition to bronchodilators either as inhalers or taken orally.
4. Physiotherapy should be continued. The child and his parents should be taught breathing exercises suitable for each child. Guidance should be given when exercises are most effective. For example, it may be possible to prevent asthma from developing by performing exercises at the first sign of an impending attack.
5. Support for the parents is important. The condition must be explained to them and they should be helped to understand the aims of the treatment. There is a danger that the child will be over-protected, and to avoid this the parents must be reassured and guided so that they can help him to become an independent person and live as full a life as possible. The importance of medication must be explained to them and they should know how to recognise specific symptoms and how to deal with episodes of asthma. Above all the child will need love and security as well as understanding of his difficulties. It is also important that they should provide a calm atmosphere during an attack.
6. The schoolchild will spend many hours at school. It is important that the school is informed of the child's condition and the treatment he is having, so that the teacher can create an environment which, if not free from anxiety, will at least be tolerable for the child.
7. Preventive measures may be indicated where the cause is suspected. Attacks may be precipi-

tated by infection, exercise, emotion or allergens and, if psychological problems are present, then help should be available. Frequent assessments should be made so that inadequate control can be recognised and the necessary action taken.

Bronchiolitis

This is an acute respiratory disorder of infants, occurring in epidemic form every two or three years during winter and early spring. A virus (respiratory syncytial virus) is the most common cause of this serious infection.

The features show an acutely ill infant with respiratory difficulties, particularly inspiratory, resulting in visible subcostal and intercostal recession (p. 371). Expiration is also difficult, with wheezing and grunting. Cough is very troublesome. The respiratory rate is rapid leading to insensible water loss from the lungs. Hypoxia is reflected by the restlessness of the infant and cyanosis may be present. Blood gases show a very low arterial PO_2 with a raised PCO_2 and a low blood pH.

Principles of treatment and nursing management

1. Oxygen with high humidity to combat anoxia and liquefy secretions.
2. Suction to remove pharyngeal secretions.
3. Adequate fluid intake.
4. Drugs: usually broad spectrum antibiotics.
5. Sedation to allay anxiety and restlessness; need to recognise danger of carbon dioxide retention.
6. Routine nursing care. (p. 109).
7. Support for parents. During the acute period the parents will require help to overcome their anxiety. When the child's condition improves, they can play a more active part in the nursing management.

Cystic fibrosis of the lungs

This is part of the inherited disorder affecting exocrine glands throughout the body. Secretions containing organic products, especially mucus, are concentrated or viscous in nature. These glands are also found in the lungs (see cystic fibrosis of the pancreas, p. 506). Small and large bronchi are filled with mucopurulent material and changes of chronic bronchitis, bronchiectasis and pulmonary fibrosis occur. This leads to obstruction of the airways. It resembles the condition of bronchiolitis in chronic form, resulting in generalised obstructive emphysema, i.e. loss of elastic supporting tissue which leads to collapse of the small airways, trapping air in the alveoli. The lungs cannot be emptied and the chest is constantly expanded, giving the appearance of a barrel. Infection occurs frequently and damage to the lung tissue leads to replacement by fibrous scar tissue.

Principles of treatment and nursing management

1. Drugs, i.e. broad spectrum antibiotics to combat infection.
2. Ultrasonic nebuliser (Figs. 23.12 and 23.13) with medication, to provide small amounts of medication in droplet form to penetrate the respiratory tract (p. 382).
3. Physiotherapy, including postural drainage (p. 377, Fig. 23.14).
4. Specific medication, e.g. pancreatic enzymes.

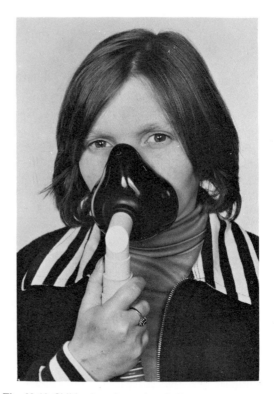

Fig. 23.12 Child using ultrasonic nebuliser.

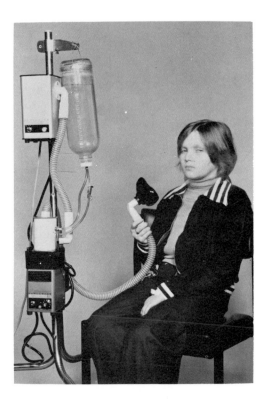

Fig. 23.13 Child with ultrasonic nebuliser, showing fine spray.

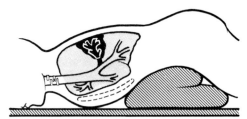

Postural Drainage Position. Lower lobe, dorsal bronchi

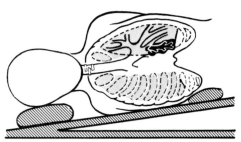

Postural Drainage Position. Lower lobe (left) lateral basal bronchi

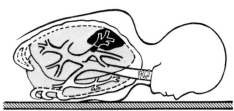

Postural Drainage Position. Upper lobe (right), sub-apical or dorsal bronchi.

Fig. 23.14 Postural drainage.

5. Routine nursing care and special emphasis on nutritional needs; the diet should be of high protein, high caloric value with a low fat intake (p. 507).
6. Specific nursing procedures:
   a. Humidity (p. 381).
   b. Oxygen in the acute periods (p. 382).
   c. Suction (p. 386).
7. Support for parents and home care. The child will require frequent hospitalisation and every effort should be made to help the parents to participate in the care of their child and learn to handle the equipment they may have to use at home. They should also be shown and be able to perform physiotherapeutic functions, and understand the dietary regime and medication. Regular medical follow-up care will be necessary and guidance given regarding routine immunisation and recognition of any complications. Play and school participation will depend on the severity of the illness.

Pneumonia

This is an acute infection of the alveolar spaces of the lung. It may involve an entire lobe (lobar pneumonia) or be more patchy (lobular). When it is restricted to alveoli adjoining the bronchi, it is termed broncho-pneumonia. Lobar pneumonia is more common in children over 2 years of age, while infants are more liable to suffer from broncho-pneumonia.

The causes of pneumonia are bacteria (such as pneumococcus, haemolytic streptococcus, staphylococcus) viruses and aspiration of material (non-infective).

Bacterial pneumonia

The organisms reach the lungs via the respiratory passages, finally lodging in the alveoli where they proliferate and set up inflammatory processes leading to consolidation. This refers to the presence in the alveoli of material which excludes the entry of air. The alveolar surface area available for gas diffusion is reduced, and the alveoli are filled with inflammatory oedema, bacteria and leucocytes.

Clinical features

Many cases of pneumonia are preceded by an upper respiratory infection. In infants and children, there may be convulsions at the onset of the condition. Temperature is highly elevated with rapid, shallow breathing and increased pulse rate. The cough is usually dry and very troublesome. There may also be gastro-intestinal disturbances. Cyanosis is often present and is closely related to the extent of pulmonary involvement. In the newborn baby, who appears to be susceptible to staphylococcal and *B. coli* infection, the effect and disturbance of function are often extremely serious.

Principles of treatment and nursing management

1. Drugs, usually antibiotics (broad spectrum).
2. Administration of oxygen and increased humidity. (pp. 381–382).
3. Physiotherapy.
4. Routine nursing care, which may also involve:
   a. Naso-gastric feeding until the infant is able to feed normally. (p. 109).
   b. Intravenous feeding if gastro-intestinal symptoms are prolonged.
   c. Fluid replacement, if the child is dehydrated.
5. Support for parents. The infant or young child is often very ill and this causes great distress to the parents. Where possible, they can help with some procedures and they should be kept informed about any treatment. As the condition improves they will be able to take a more active part in preparation for the child's return home.

Aspiration pneumonia

This form of pneumonia is due to foreign material which has entered the respiratory tract. In infants this presents a serious problem. Aspiration of amniotic fluid may be the causative agent in the new-born infant, while in the infant and young child, aspiration of oily substances, e.g. lubricant used for naso-gastric catheter, may be the cause.

Talcum powder, which consists mainly of magnesium silicate, has an irritant effect on the airways and may lead to conditions similar to acute bronchiolitis or broncho-pneumonia. Tear gas, used in riot control, can also affect children. In addition to acute irritation of the eyes and upper respiratory tract, exposure to these gases can result in pulmonary oedema and pneumonitis. Irritation caused by foreign material leads to oedema in the finer air passages and provides a suitable medium for bacterial growth.

The treatment aims at removing the irritant. For aspiration of bronchial contents, postural drainage (Fig. 23.14) may be attempted or intubation and bronchial toilet performed. Aspiration of talcum powder may require artificial ventilation using high ventilator pressure to overcome the high airway resistance. Other treatment is similar to that for bacterial pneumonia.

Atelectasis

The term denotes a shrunken and airless state of the lung, or part of the lung, which may be acute or chronic, complete or incomplete. It is a particularly serious problem in the new-born infant.

Failure of the lungs to expand adequately after birth depends on a number of factors, such as diminished nervous stimulus to breathing and crying, fetal hypoxia (due to oversedation or anaesthesia of the mother), prematurity, excessive amounts or tenacity of intrapulmonary secretions.

The pre-term infant is much more likely to be affected and the commonest cause of death in these infants is failure of gas exchange. The condition is also related to a deficiency of the surfactant material which lowers surface tension in the alveoli (p. 370). Surfactant activity is also reduced with increased body temperature. In fetal atelectasis, a mucus plug often obstructs the bronchus leading to the collapsed area. Atelectasis leads to hypoxia which induces pulmonary artery vasoconstriction. To overcome this, the blood is diverted through the foramen ovale and ductus arteriosus and there is a lowering of pulmonary blood flow. (For a description of fetal circulation, see p. 399).

Respiratory distress syndrome (hyaline membrane disease)

This condition is generally found in pre-term

babies within the first days of life. It is believed to be due to lack of surfactant (an enzyme which lowers the surface tension of the alveoli). This leads to dilated alveolar ducts and intense congestion. Hyaline membrane is found within the alveolar ducts and there may be intrapulmonary haemorrhage. This hyaline membrane appears to be mainly composed of fibrin derived from the pulmonary capillaries, and which also inactivates surfactant.

Clinical features

The infant presents with dyspnoea and a rapid breathing rate (over 50 per min). The Apgar score (Table 23.1) at birth is low. There is nasal flaring, retractions of the costal margins and lower sternum, grunting respirations and cyanosis. Symptoms are usually present immediately after birth but may be delayed for 2 to 4 hours. Oedema often becomes severe during the first 12 hours. Periods of apnoea occur with increasing frequency in babies whose condition is deteriorating.

Principles of treatment and nursing management

1. Prompt resuscitation with early endotracheal intubation (p. 393). This reduces the anoxia and acidaemia.
2. Oxygen administration for central cyanosis.
3. Minimal disturbance to reduce breathing difficulties. Feeding and crying have been shown to cause a fall in arterial PO_2 (p. 109).
4. A naso-gastric tube may be passed to aspirate gastric content, to prevent regurgitation and aspiration.
5. Intravenous feeding may be given or an intra-venous infusion set up to correct metabolic acidosis.
6. Adequate warmth and humidity. For each baby there is an ideal environmental temperature range; this ensures least use of energy and oxygen. The skin temperature should be maintained within the range of 36.2 to 36.8°C.
7. Antibiotics are usually given either as prophylaxis or because infection by B-streptococcus makes it difficult to differentiate between pneumonia and respiratory distress syndrome.

Pleurisy with effusion

This is a serous effusion into the pleural cavity. It is frequently due to tuberculosis in children, but it may also occur as a complication of pneumococcal pneumonia. The effects of the effusion depend on the size and the rate of accumulation of fluid. Large collections of fluid may greatly reduce the vital capacity by reducing pulmonary volume.

The onset is often insidious, with loss of weight. In the acute stage pain may be felt in the chest, hypochondrium and shoulder. There is a slight increase in temperature. Treatment consists of treating the cause and removing the fluid by aspiration (p. 389) (nursing care p. 109).

Pneumothorax

This denotes air in the pleural cavity. It may occur as a result of intratracheal intubation or as a result of injury to the chest. However, it is most frequently seen in staphylococcal pneumonia with bullous emphysema when it is termed spontaneous pneumothorax. Air enters from the lung. As pleural pressure is on average subatmospheric or

Table 23.1 The Apgar score chart is used to assess the new-born infant's condition 60 seconds after birth. The higher the score the better the infant's condition. A score of 10 indicates an infant in optimum condition. A score of 2 or less indicates an infant in a poor state (Chart was developed by Dr Virginia Apgar)

Sign	Score		
	0	1	2
Skin colour	Generalised cyanosis or pallor	Peripheral cyanosis	Good, pink
Muscle tone	Flaccid	Flexion movements of the limbs or trunk	Good muscle tone
Breathing	Absent	Gasping	Rhythmic or crying
Heart rate	Absent	Under 100/min	Over 100/min
Reflex response	Absent	Poor response	Brisk response

negative and air in the lungs is on average at atmospheric pressure, air is sucked into the pleural cavity. The rise in pleural pressure tends to cause the mediastinum to move towards the other side. Occasionally a large amount of air enters the pleural space when there is a valve-like situation at the point of entry; air therefore enters more easily than it can leave. The pressure of the air in the pleural cavity rapidly exceeds that of the atmosphere (tension pneumothorax) which causes severe pain, dyspnoea, cyanosis and circulatory collapse.

Treatment consists of removing the air by inserting a catheter into the pleural cavity and connecting it to tubing placed under water (underwater seal drainage, see p. 390, Fig. 23.21) (nursing care p. 392).

Nursing care and procedures related to respiratory tract diseases

Nursing care aims to complement medical and surgical treatment. The primary aim is to provide an environment which will ensure the successful outcome of the prescribed treatment. The following areas will be considered:

1. Position of the child.
2. Handling the child.
3. Specific procedures:
   a. Cleansing of nostrils.
   b. Maintaining humidity.
   c. Administration of oxygen.
   d. Oro/nasal pharyngeal suction.
   e. Tracheostomy.
   f. Chest aspiration.
   g. Underwater seal drainage.
   h. Bronchoscopy.
   i. Naso-tracheal intubation with positive pressure ventilation.

POSITION OF THE CHILD

Principles involved
These are to improve respiratory function by finding the best possible position for the infant/child and to ensure that the infant/child maintains that position. This is based on the observation that breathing is more efficient in the upright position. In the lying position, movements of the diaphragm are hindered by the abdominal contents. Therefore, if dyspnoea is marked, orthopnoea (upright position) is preferred. In severe dyspnoea the accessory muscles are used, in particular, the sternomastoids. In dyspnoea of pulmonary oedema due to left heart failure, sitting up tends to reduce venous return to the right atria and lungs and hence pulmonary capillary pressure falls, especially in the upper parts of the lungs.

Infant
It is quite difficult to find a suitable position for the infant and maintain it. If he is nursed in an incubator or Belfast cot, the mattress part or cot can be tilted so that the infant's chest is raised. Care should be taken to prevent the infant sliding down. This can be achieved by adjusting the angle of elevation. Nursing the infant in a larger cot would entail the use of pillows, with the infant resting against two or three pillows. It is important to ensure that the infant's chin is not resting on his chest, as this could impede breathing movement.

Young and older children
Older babies and toddlers, as well as children of pre-school and school age are easier to maintain in an upright position. Two or three pillows may be required and a bed-rest can be used to act as base. There is nevertheless a problem in preventing the toddler and older baby from sliding down and constant adjustment will have to be made.

HANDLING THE CHILD

Infant
This will depend on the severity of the condition. Handling should be gentle, particularly if breathing difficulties are also accompanied by pain. Nappy changes should be carried out with minimal movement of the infant, for example, turning the infant on his side rather than lifting the legs up to cleanse the infant and change the nappy. The method of holding the legs over the abdomen tends to increase respiratory distress. If

the infant is to be bottle-fed, then he should be lifted gently and sat on the nurse's knee. Constant observations are necessary and changes in breathing should be noted, either in relation to feeding or handling.

Children

Handling should be gentle, particularly if breathing difficulties are also accompanied by pain. Two nurses should carry out any nursing functions, one to hold the child, while the other, for example, makes the bed. Bigger children should be lifted up by two nurses, particularly if the respiratory distress is obvious and any movement or exertion might increase the distress.

SPECIFIC PROCEDURES

Clearing the nostrils

Upper respiratory infections involve primarily the nose. Excessive nasal secretions lead to breathing difficulties, particularly in the infant. The secretions also tend to harden, blocking the nostrils.

Infants

Infants cannot clear their own nostrils, except by means of sneezing. It is therefore the nurse's function to remove any debris. This can be achieved by using a fine roll of cotton wool and gently easing the matter out. Great care should be taken not to injure the mucous lining; damaged tissue encourages bacterial growth. If there is crusting, this should be softened first with a warmed solution of saline or sodium bicarbonate. However, it is important to recognise that there may be an element of danger if the debris is pushed further into the nostril as it may be inhaled.

Toddlers

The toddler is still too young to know how to blow his nose, though some make a good attempt at it. Two nurses may be required, one to hold and comfort the child, the other to carry out the procedure. During the acute stage, the nostrils tend to be sore and there is great resistance to any attempt at cleaning. Gentleness is essential and if the discharge is fluid, it can be mopped with cotton wool. If crust is present, it should be soft-

ened first before removing it. The method of removing debris is the same as as for infants.

Older children

Catarrh is also a problem leading to a condition known as sino-bronchitis. It is therefore important that nose-blowing should be taught and encouraged. As soon as nasal obstruction is obvious, it should be removed by blowing the nose. However, even older children may require help and the method could be much the same as that used for the toddler. Paper handkerchiefs should always be available and provision made for disposal as soon as possible. A disposal bag should be placed in a convenient place for the child to use.

Maintaining humidity

A moist atmosphere is provided by nebulisation of water, either into an incubator, into a plastic tent or through a machine like the Croupaire. Oxygen or air can be used as the vehicle.

Humidaire/Croupette (Fig. 23.15)

These are useful tents for younger children suffering from laryngo-tracheal-bronchitis. Nebulisation is the means by which water and medicated solutions are broken into small particles. These are small enough to be inhaled. To obtain very small particles, it is necessary to use an ultrasonic nebuliser which produces particles which are less than one micron (0.001 mm). Cooling can be achieved by placing ice in the compartment.

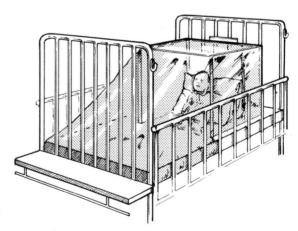

Fig. 23.15 A child with bronchitis in bed under a Croupette (tent).

Ultrasonic nebuliser

This is a useful form of inhalation for children suffering from cystic fibrosis with chronic respiratory difficulties. The function of the nebuliser is to provide advantages of high density, homogeneous ultrasonic aerosols in respiratory diseases especially where output volumes of not more than 3 ml of aerosol per minute are indicated.

Reasons and effect of humidity

Humidity is provided in cases where the bronchial secretions become thick due to evaporation of water from the lungs. Thick, tenacious secretions cannot be evacuated by ciliary action unless their viscosity is decreased. It does so by increasing the moisture in the lungs and at the same time reducing insensible water loss from the air passages and lungs. Another reason for providing humidity is to reduce the irritant effect of oxygen administration.

Preparation of the equipment

Clear instructions are usually given with the various tents and machines. The Croupette and Humidaire are commonly used for infants and toddlers while an oxygen tent is more suitable for the bigger child. Proper maintenance of the equipment is essential. This is particularly important regarding the Diapump which is used for suction. The glass jar should be filled with distilled water and care must be taken to ensure that sufficient amount of water is present to obtain the desired humidity. The glass jar should be checked for any cracks and screwed carefully into the fitting, otherwise vaporisation cannot occur. The filter too should be checked for patency and any blockage removed by passing a stream of water through it. The Diapump is fitted with two glass jars, one containing the filter, the other a cork ball which occludes the entrance to the mechanism when suction is used. The filter must be clean to be effective (see p. 118, Fig. 6.8).

If ice is placed in the compartment, a pail or basin should be placed under the outlet on the floor for the melted ice.

Preparation of the child

It is most important that the child should not be alarmed or frightened when first placed in the tent.

Fear will cause distress, and consequently increase breathing difficulty. If the child is old enough, an explanation should be given and the nurse should stay with him until he has settled down. The acutely ill child tends to settle down quicker than the less ill child; this may be due to the fact that he is very exhausted and finds relief in the tent. It is also a good idea to place a soft toy in the tent and ensure that the child can see out of the tent at all times. This will reduce his sense of isolation.

Care of the child

All nursing care can be carried out while the child is in the tent — changing his nappy, washing and feeding. However, it might be necessary to lift the infant out for feeding purposes. Misting of tent walls is a problem for the baby and child and therefore frequent wiping of walls should be carried out. This is important to allow observation of the child and to allow the child to see out. The high humidity moistens the child's clothes and bedclothes. A wet child will not only be uncomfortable but will lose heat more rapidly, which can be an additional problem. Sponging and drying the child should be done whenever necessary. Pressure areas too will require attention, since these children tend to remain in the same position unless moved at regular and frequent intervals.

As the child's condition improves, he should be allowed gradual reduction in humidity and the tent left open until he is able to breathe normally at room atmosphere.

Administration of oxygen

Administration of oxygen is necessary for the correction of anoxaemia (low arterial oxygen tensions) or anoxia (absence of adequate tissue oxygen). It can also be used as a diagnostic test for anoxaemia when changes in arterial blood-gas levels, oxygen saturation and the patient's colour are used to evaluate the response. The treatment should be controlled by blood-gas measurements to monitor the child's need for and response to therapy.

It is important to remember that although an important gas, oxygen can have toxic effects under certain conditions. For example, in chronic carbon dioxide retention, which may be found in advanced cystic fibrosis or cerebral trauma, there may be cessation of respiration; or it can cause constriction of retinal and cerebral vessels which may lead to irreversible brain damage and, in new-born pre-term infants, may lead to retrolental fibroplasia; or it can produce changes in pulmonary tissue leading to fibrosis and bronchiolar epithelial changes. The pulmonary effects appear to be dose-related, e.g. high concentrations for short periods or lower concentrations over long periods may have the same effect. It is suggested that oxygen should be given at the lowest concentration for as short a time as possible to achieve satisfactory arterial oxygen pressures.

Property and function of oxygen
Oxygen has the following properties:

1. It is colourless, tasteless, odourless and cannot be detected readily.
2. It is slightly soluble in water and can be passed through water when necessary for humidification with little loss of gas.
3. It supports combustion and is therefore extremely dangerous. Sparks from static electricity or mechanical equipment must be prevented. Smoking must never be allowed in the vicinity of the gas. Flammable solution such as alcohol or oils should also be avoided.

The *function of oxygen* in humans and animals is the oxidation of some of their foods to carbon dioxide. Oxidation is employed as a source of energy, i.e. oxygen is necessary for the process in which food is broken down to supply energy.

Indications for oxygen therapy
When oxygen deficiency occurs, the following signs can be observed:

1. Rapid, shallow breathing while the body is at rest.
2. Increased restlessness.
3. Dyspnoea.
4. Hypoxia or hypoxaemia.

In this chapter oxygen therapy is primarily concerned with disorders of the respiratory tract, but oxygen administration is often necessary due to disorders of the cardiovascular system, severe anaemia, carbon monoxide poisoning and cyanide poisoning.

Methods of administration
Several methods may be employed. The one of choice is dependent on the age of the child and is the one which will give an acceptable concentration of oxygen with the least disturbance to the child. Some means of humidification should be available. For the infant and the toddler, the croupette or Humidaire is effective, while the incubator is used for small, low-weight babies, new-born babies and pre-term babies. (The incubator is described in Chapter 10.)

The following will be considered:

1. Catheter.
2. Mask — funnel.
3. Tents.

1. *Catheter*
This method is used when a child cannot tolerate a mask and when it is undesirable to place the child in an oxygen tent, e.g. the child with extensive burns. It is not suitable for young children, but could be used for the 10- to 11-year-old.

It is a useful method in bronchitis where there is CO_2 retention. Since the catheter is inserted into the nostrils, is essential that these are clean and clear of any obstruction. A two-pronged plastic nasal catheter is inserted for $\frac{1}{4}$ to $\frac{1}{2}$ inch (0.6 to 1.25 cm) into each nostril. Before insertion, it should be connected to the oxygen supply and the flow commenced. Once inserted, it is fixed to the cheek using Micropore or similar adhesive strapping. The oxygen is turned on before insertion into the nostrils to prevent trauma due to sudden release of oxygen pressure, and the rate is adjusted to the prescribed level. A flow of 2 to 3 litres per minute produces a concentration of up to 35 per cent. Humidification is usually required but lubrication should not be used. It is also important to use pressure tubing to prevent kinking and the tubing should be checked regularly to ensure that the oxygen flow is not impeded. To obtain humidity, a nebulising attachment can be used.

If the child is co-operative and restful, there is generally no problem in nursing. The restless, disorientated child may require restraining though it would probably be better to use a more suitable method like a tent.

2. *Oronasal mask* (*Venturi mask*)

This is a quick and effective method. The masks are disposable (Fig. 23.16). They are suitable for young children over 4 years of age and infants. One to 4-year-olds do not tolerate masks over the face.

Method. The purpose of the treatment should be explained to the older child. A suitable size of mask is chosen. It is assembled and the oxygen is turned on at a slightly higher rate of flow than will be required. The mask is then applied to fit snugly over the child's face. Humidity is obtained by the moisture collected in the mask. The mask should be removed at hourly intervals to wash the child's face and cold cream can be applied to the areas where the mask rests on the face.

The Venturi mask provides a concentration of 24 to 28 per cent at a flow of 4 litres/min and a concentration of 35 per cent at a flow rate of 8 litres/min.

3. *Oxygen tents* (Fig. 23.17)

The concentration of oxygen within the tent will depend on the efficiency of the tent and the rate of flow of oxygen. The Mark V Refrigeration tent is one of choice for bigger children. The plastic tent must be tucked in enclosing the whole bed. This type of tent is more comfortable and most nursing procedures can be carried out through sleeves. An explanation should be given to the child as to why he is placed in such an environment and any fears should be allayed. Since the plastic canopy is clear, he can see the rest of the ward and the other children and will therefore not feel quite so isolated. He is also able to move about and read or draw while in the tent.

A high initial flow is necessary to provide the desired concentration, e.g. 10 to 12 litres/min for 20 minutes. Oxygen and air are circulated by a fan and a high ventilation rate can be used to wash out the CO_2. A small bottle containing distilled water

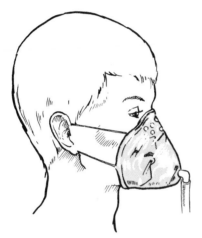

Fig. 23.16 Disposable oxygen mask.

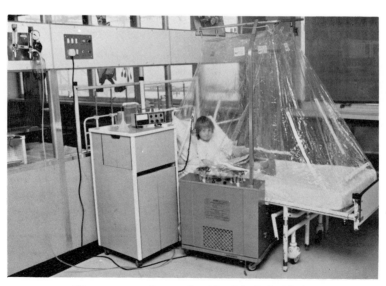

Fig. 23.17 Child in an oxygen tent. (Note oxygen analyser at the side of the bed with the sensor inside the tent.)

is situated at the side of the machine to add humidity to the tent. The following concentrations can be obtained:

8 litres/min = 50 to 57 per cent and CO_2 concentration from 0.8 to 1.1 per cent.

Humidaire/Croupette. These are two very similar tents useful for younger children suffering from laryngo-tracheal-bronchitis, where additional moisture is also provided (RH 100 per cent). The Croupette is the smaller of the two and more difficult to achieve complete leakproof enclosure, but is useful for small infants nursed in a cot. Assembly is easier for the Croupette than the Humidaire which requires two nurses to assemble. The Humidaire box should be placed at the foot of the bed to prevent injury to the child. It is also less frightening in that position. The following concentrations can be obtained:

2 litres/min = 39 to 43 per cent.
10 litres/min = 61 to 67 per cent.
20 litres/min = 70 to 80 per cent.

Cooling can be achieved by placing ice in the compartment and allowing drainage of water into a container at the foot of the bed or on the floor beneath the outlet.

Care of the child in a tent. These children are usually very ill and distressed. The small child cannot understand what is happening but he should be spoken to and reassured if apprehensive. There is generally no resistance to going into a tent and the relief can be observed by the facial expression and the gradual improvement in breathing. The temperature within the tent should be checked and maintained at 17.7 to 21.1°C (64 to 70°F).

All nursing care can be carried out through the sleeves or pockets, but it will be necessary to flush the tent after each procedure to ensure an adequate concentration of oxygen within it. As breathing becomes easier and the child's condition improves, he may be able to be weaned from tent care gradually. The infant can be lifted out for feeds, but a supply of oxygen should be available and may be given via a funnel placed over the child's face. Frequent changes of position are advisable and change of clothing and a sponge-down will keep the child comfortable.

To ensure that the oxygen level is maintained it is important to analyse the tent air at regular intervals. Tent oxygen analysis is carried out with *oxygen analysers*. Three types are in use today:

1. *Mira* Method — the instrument is placed on a flat surface, dial facing upwards. A sample of air is taken via the small polythene tube suspended into the centre part of the treatment chamber. The aspirator bulb is squeezed four

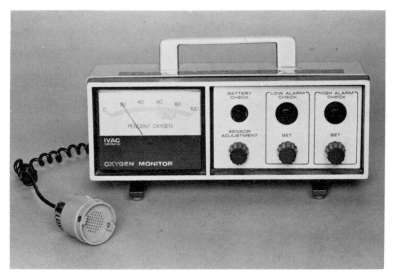

Fig. 23.18 Oxygen monitor.

to six times to obtain a sample of the air. The switch is pressed and held for 2 to 3 seconds. The point at which the pointer stops at the gauge is recorded.

2. *Photoelectric cell analyser.* The probe is inserted into the chamber, the switch compressed and readings taken.

3. *Paramagnetic oximeter.* This can be used for continuous oxygen analysis. The dials are pre-set to low and high levels and a bleep will be heard should the concentration of oxygen fall or rise to below or above those levels (Fig. 23.18).

The importance of oxygen analysis cannot be stressed too much. This is because of the danger of oxygen toxicity, particularly in the young infant. This could lead to injury of pulmonary epithelium and, in the pre-term baby, to retro-lental fibroplasia.

Oro/nasal pharyngeal suction

Suction of the oral and nasal pharynx may be required when secretions interfere with breathing. The sterile catheter is connected to the suction apparatus and the tip is inserted into the respective orifice. Care should be taken not to move the catheter round the orifice. It should be inserted and suction carried out during withdrawal. There is

danger of contamination from aspirated infected material and the low vacuum apparatus is considered less of a danger, but some form of filter is necessary or desirable. The bottles must be emptied with care, cleaned carefully and filled with Hibitane solution. A new sterile catheter is used for each suction session and the tubing is changed.

High vaccum suction should be used for thick or tenacious fluids. Low vacuum suction is less damaging to the mucosa of the mouth and respiratory tract. It is preferable for less viscid fluids and for large quantities of non-viscous material. The vacuum gauge should be checked to prevent applying excessive vacuum.

Testing the suction apparatus

If the joints are not airtight a vacuum cannot be obtained. It is therefore important to test the jars and tubing so that any fault can be determined and corrected. If there is no vacuum, the gauge will not show any reading.

Tracheostomy (Figs. 23.19 and 23.20)

A small transverse incision is normally made in the skin and the thyroid isthmus is divided. The incision in the trachea is made below the first tracheal ring (otherwise laryngeal stenosis may occur). If too low, the incision can disappear behind the

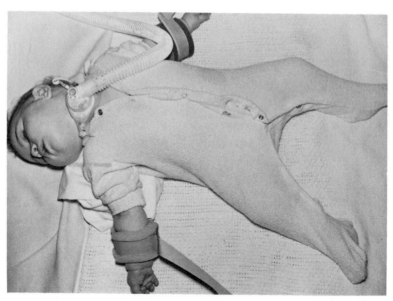

Fig. 23.19 Tracheostomy, showing administration of oxygen and humidity via the tracheostomy tube. (Note the position of the child's head and arm restraints.)

sternum when the neck is flexed. Different types of tracheal incisions are used — some cause difficulties when replacing the tube.

Types of tubes used

1. Plastic tubes (these are generally used now):
   a. With inflatable cuff but not in small sizes, as it decreases the possible lumen size. It can be used for older children and provides a seal.
   b. Plain, without cuff. 'Portex' has a narrow orifice; when inserting the connector for inflation of the lungs, it tends to decrease lumen further, causing resistance to gas flow.
   c. Great Ormond Street infant's pattern. This one has the advantage in that it can take the same size of connector for all tube sizes. The orifice at the flange is larger than the rest of the tube.
2. Silver tubes. Assorted sizes available with inner and outer tubes. These have been largely superseded by plastic tubes.

Reasons for tracheostomy

The operation of tracheostomy is performed for the relief of an airway obstruction, either partial or complete at or above the level of the subglottic area. There are a number of conditions which cause obstructions:

1. Laryngo-tracheo-bronchitis which is an inflammatory condition with oedema a prominent feature.
2. Inhaled foreign bodies.
3. Oedema due to inhaled steam.
4. The unconscious patient may need assistance in ventilation.
5. Cystic hygroma.

Recognition of need for tracheostomy

Respiratory emergencies can occur in any type of unit and nurses must be able to recognise the warning signs of obstructive respiratory events. This is heralded by any of the following:

1. Increasing breathing difficulties.
2. Increased breathing rate.
3. Change in breathing pattern.

4. Increased muscular effort — use of accessory muscles of respirations.
5. Sternal retraction. p. 371
6. Increasing tachycardia, cyanosis.
7. Increasing anxiety and restlessness.

Preparation of the child

The preparation depends on the circumstances and the conditions prevailing. If the child is old enough, and sufficiently capable of understanding, some explanation should be given, emphasising particularly the relief he will obtain from the treatment. If an anaesthetic is to be administered, preparation and pre-medication will be given as instructed. When the operation is carried out as an emergency, local anaesthesia is sometimes used. While the operation is in progress, preparation for the return of the child must be made. This includes the following:

1. Sterile equipment — spare tracheostomy tube, tracheal hook, sterile suction tubes, disposable gloves, swabs, saturated solution of sodium bicarbonate or normal saline, sterile water for clearing catheters.
2. Equipment for bronchoscopy.
3. Suction equipment.
4. Oxygen supply.
5. Humidity.
6. Oral hygiene tray.
7. Pad and pencil for the older child.

Care of the infant

Position. The infant has a short neck and the chin can easily obstruct the tracheostomy tube. The head should therefore be extended at all times (Fig. 23.19). A sponge-rubber wedge or small pillow under the neck and shoulders would be useful and the head of the bed or cot elevated. The position is not comfortable and requires constant adjustment.

Restraint. Small arm restrainers to prevent the child from pulling at the tube will be necessary.

Aspiration

Two nurses will be required for this procedure.

Technique. Strict aseptic technique should be used. This means that the catheter must not touch anything outside the tube and must be discarded

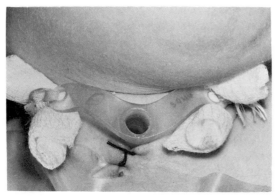

Fig. 23.20 Tracheostomy tube in position. Note the gauze pads to protect the skin.

if it does. Each unit will have its own policy, e.g. the use of sterile gloves or if hand-washing is adequate.

Catheter size. This should be half the diameter of the tracheostomy tube.

Method. The catheter is attached to the suction tubing and suction started. The catheter is pinched to prevent suction when entering the tube. It is passed down as far as the point of the tube and the trachea. Suction is applied only when the tube is being withdrawn. It should not be left in one position and should not move from side to side, Vacuum should be 25 cm (10 inches) Hg.

Duration of suction should not be longer than one breath. If excessive suction is used, it could lead to collapse of lung due to withdrawal of residual air. If the catheter has to be inserted three times successively, oxygen may be given via the tracheostomy tube. Suction should only be left on for 10 seconds because of the danger of hypoxia.

Signs of need for aspiration

1. Sounds of bubbling in the tube. The only exception to the rule is when frank pulmonary oedema is present — suction might increase the oedema. Increase in oedema may also occur in infants when a larger tube is used.
2. Signs of oxygen deficiency — restlessness, increased pulse rate, cyanosis as a late sign.
3. Routinely: aspiration should be performed every 10 minutes, hourly or as often as is necessary.

4. Bronchial toilet: a straight catheter will probably enter the right bronchus, it is therefore advisable to use an angled catheter which is first passed into one bronchus, then into the other.

Humidity

Since the nasal passages are bypassed, humidity is essential to prevent drying of mucus. Oxygen too must be passed through a humidifier, though this is not as effective. A nebuliser should be used. If crusting of secretions does occur water or normal saline 0.5 to 2.0 ml is gently instilled down the tracheostomy tube and left down for *5 seconds* before aspirating. Mucus solvent, i.e. acetylcysteine, may also be given in the liquid (see also p. 394).

Changing of tube

This is to be done only by trained staff. Extra tubes of assorted sizes must always be available and all must have tapes attached. It is advisable not to change the tube in the first 48 hours so that the track has a chance to become well formed. Early replacement can be difficult. When replacing a tube, the tape must be kept firmly tied around the neck. To prevent chafing, a pad may be placed beneath it. If it becomes loose, it must be reported immediately. If dressings are used, these are changed when required under aseptic technique.

Older child

The care of tracheostomy is basically the same regarding care of tube, aspiration, oxygen and humidity. The difference lies in the greater level of anxiety and the need to give constant reassurance and encouragement. In the initial stages, a nurse should be specially assigned to look after the child. Sedation may also be necessary in an effort to calm him.

Speech

The loss of speech can be very alarming to a child. For this reason it is essential that the reasons are carefully explained and reassurance should be given regarding return of voice. Children tend to adapt readily after the initial shock and provided the child is able to communicate his wishes and needs in some way, he will learn to accept his temporary state. A pencil and paper to jot down what he wants is essential (provided he can write). A small handbell near the child or other means of calling attention should be instituted. Speech is quickly restored once occlusion has taken place. Parents will experience an anxious time and their needs too must be catered for. It will be frightening for them to watch their child in such an ill state and the anxiety of the child trying to speak but unable to do so must increase their helplessness. However, there is a place for parents in caring for their child, particularly since they know the child intimately and can anticipate his needs. They will need a full explanation of the treatment and the aims of the procedures so that they can co-operate fully.

Removal of the tube

As the child's condition improves, he will get used to the tube and will show signs of apprehension when the time comes to remove it. This period requires patience and persuasion on the part of the nurse to prepare the child for the change and help him to overcome his fears. This procedure may take some days, when the tube will be occluded for an increasing period every day until it is finally removed. This allows the child to get used to breathing normally and to gain confidence in breathing without the tube. Alternatively the tube may be removed under anaesthesia. The wound is allowed to close itself. Careful observation is required and any signs of distress reported immediately.

Chest aspiration

Reasons

This procedure is carried out for diagnostic purposes to obtain a specimen of pus or serous fluid for examination, or as a therapeutic measure to relieve pressure within the pleural cavity caused by air (pneumothorax), blood (haemothorax), purulent fluid (pyothorax), or a combination of these conditions. Normal pressure in the pleural cavity is negative to atmospheric pressure and an increase in the pressure, decreases the lungs' ability to expand.

Technique

The aspiration is carried out by the medical officer, by inserting a needle attached to a syringe into the pleural space. The skin is cleansed and a local anaesthetic may be given. If it is done for diagnostic purposes, the needle is withdrawn after obtaining a specimen, and the puncture is sealed. Antibiotics may be introduced in some cases, when a special two-way syringe or a syringe with a two-way tap is used. This is to prevent air entering and to maintain a closed circuit.

Preparation of the child

If possible, an explanation should be given to the child. The form this takes depends on the age and the level of understanding of the child. It is vital that he keeps still and avoids coughing during the procedure. Sedation may be given, where this is considered necessary or desirable.

Position of the child

Infants. The infant is placed across a pillow, the affected side uppermost. The nurse raises the shoulder and arm of that side to increase the intercostal space. The infant must be held securely and prevented from moving. Constant observations must be maintained and the slightest change in colour and breathing reported. The resuscitation trolley and oxygen must be readily available.

Older children. The child is either placed in the same position as that described for the infant, or held in the sitting position. The position of choice should be ascertained beforehand, to minimise the amount of movement. If the child is to be treated in the sitting position, he should be resting his chest on pillows. The shoulders should be raised by the nurse to the hunched position. This will increase the intercostal space, thereby making the procedure easier. Observations of the child are the same for the infant.

After-care

After the procedure, the child is gently moved back into his bed/cot, maintaining the upright position, and he is made comfortable. The pulse, respiration and temperature should be measured and recorded and the child should not be left alone until the nurse is satisfied that there is no respiratory distress. Discomfort felt at the time of aspiration should be temporary and indeed there should be relief of breathing difficulty once the pressure has been relieved.

If a specimen has been obtained, this should be labelled clearly according to the policy of the hospital and sent to the appropriate department.

Lung puncture

In this procedure a transpleural needle is inserted into a diseased part of the lung in order to obtain secretions for culture or cytology, or both. Sputum is difficult to obtain in children and many of the diagnostic procedures, e.g. naso-pharyngeal and throat swabs, blood cultures and tracheal suction, are either unreliable or indeed traumatic. Lung puncture, although not without danger, has been found to be a reliable means of obtaining material for examination.

It is useful in a critically ill child in whom specific aetiology is of utmost and immediate importance so that the most suitable treatment can be instituted.

Preparation of the child

The procedure should be explained to the child who is old enough to understand. If necessary, the child should be restrained or sedated. A local anaesthetic is used. The child is usually held in a sitting position, although with upper lobe involvement the prone or supine position may be more suitable.

Method

A 20 or 21 g needle is attached to an airtight 10 or 20 ml syringe containing a few drops of sterile saline. The tip is inserted as far as the pleural cavity. Pleural fluid is removed if present. If no pleural fluid is obtained, gentle suction is maintained for the remainder of the procedure and the lung is rapidly punctured to a depth of 3 or 4 cm. The needle should not remain in the lung for more than 2 or 3 seconds. During the procedure the child, if old enough, should be asked to hold his breath. The puncture is usually sealed with a drop of collodion.

After-care of the child

The child should be handled gently and returned to his bed. Half-hourly observations of vital functions should be carried out and any deviation from the normal reported immediately. The following complications could arise: pneumothorax (p. 379), which usually subsides without therapy and only rarely requires a chest tube and haemoptysis, which tends to be self-limiting.

Lung biopsy

Lung biopsy is a diagnostic procedure involving the removal of a portion of the lung, possibly for histological, immunological or other purposes. It is generally reserved for life-threatening or persistent pulmonary diseases when other methods have failed to identify the cause.

Two methods may be used. One method involves a surgical thoracotomy and the other is a closed lung biopsy which involves a small intercostal incision under local anaesthesia, followed by the passage of a cutting needle or trephine through the parietal and visceral layers of the pleura into the lung. The chief advantages of the closed biopsy are rapidity, simplicity, and the fact that it is relatively painless and can be repeated.

The preparation and care of the child is similar to that for lung puncture, but he needs to hold his breath in expiration for approximately 30 seconds.

Underwater seal drainage (Fig. 23.21)

Chest drainage is an important method employed in preventing and treating collapse of the lung. This may arise because of bronchial obstruction due to secretions or as a result of pressure on the lung by air, fluid, blood or pus. Although there are different methods required for the two causes, both types may occur together, e.g. pneumothorax causing partial collapse of the lung due to compression (passive) may be followed by inadequate bronchial drainage. Increased secretions cannot be absorbed causing an active collapse of the lung.

When fluid or air accumulate in the pleural cavity, the intrapleural pressure increases, the lung cannot expand and the compression of the lung causes it to collapse. The pleural cavity must then be aspirated or drained. When drainage is required, underwater seal drainage is used. The seal prevents entry of air through the drainage system and allows expansion of the lung. Air, blood or other exudate is drained.

Pleural drainage is undertaken for the following reasons:

1. Routinely after operation on the chest to prevent a tension pneumothorax:
   a. When lung tissue has been cut and air from the cut surface may continue to leak.
   b. To facilitate drainage when a large area may be expected to bleed in the post-operative period.
   c. To facilitate drainage when the oesophagus has been opened and there is possible contamination or leakage from the suture line.
2. To facilitate drainage after injury when a haemothorax or pneumothorax is present.
3. To relieve a tension pneumothorax following a spontaneous pneumothorax.
4. To relieve an empyema.

Equipment required

1. Large bottle (10 cm diameter) preferably with a measuring scale.
2. Known volume, e.g. 1 litre of sterile liquid.
3. Cork pierced with:
   a. Short angled tube.
   b. Long tube, diameter not less than 0.5 cm with 2.5 to 5.0 cm *under* the water level. This tube is attached to the chest drain by a suitable length of tubing, i.e. 75 to 100 cm.
   c. Spencer Wells forceps for pinching the tube when moving patient or changing the bottle.
   d. Adhesive strapping and safety pin, to prevent pull on the tube.
   e. Suction equipment with the vacuum set at about 10 mmHg. This promotes drainage from the pleural cavity and reduces paradoxical breathing. Paradoxical breathing results when the intercostal tube is attached to a fairly long piece of tubing to an underwater seal drain. The greater the 'swing' of water level in the tube, the greater is the amount of paradox (p. 366).

Uses of the bottle

1. As the lung expands, air is pushed out or blown out through the seal.

2. Any blood or secretions can be measured.
3. Movement of water level in the long tube indicate ventilation of the lung and that the tube is patent.

Method. The assembly of the apparatus is shown in Figure 23.21. The surgeon inserts a self-retaining catheter in the most dependent part of the cavity where drainage is to be effected. The catheter is kept firmly clamped until it is attached to the apparatus. When attached to the apparatus, the clamp is released and blood and other secretions will flow by gravity through the tube into the bottle. The glass or plastic tubing below the surface of the water forms a one-way valve that permits air to be forced out by the more positive pressure developed during expiration and prevents air from being taken in during inspiration. This is confirmed by bubbles escaping through the water during expiration and the column rising in the tube during inspiration. As the lung expands, the vacuum created draws the fluid only a short way up the glass tube in the bottle. When the lung occupies the whole of the hemithorax the difference in pressure in the pleural cavity between inspiration and expiration is small and the oscillation in the tube may be only about 2 cm. If, however, there is atelectasis with poor or non-expansion of the lung, the lung fails to fill the

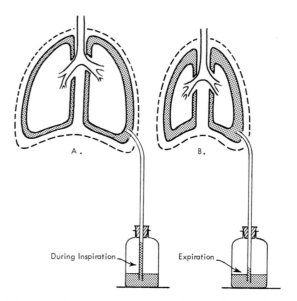

During Inspiration

Expiration

Fig. 23.21 Under water seal drainage. Note level of fluid in the tube during inspiration (A) and expiration (B).

space designed for it, and large fluctuations in pressure in the pleural cavity will occur on breathing. There will be a corresponding increase in the oscillations observed in the glass tube. The greater the height of the oscillation, the poorer the expansion of the lung. The height between the chest and the surface of the water seal should be sufficient to prevent water being drawn into the chest by maximum inspiratory effort. A strong inspiratory effort may produce a negative pressure equal to a 60 cm column of water. Therefore, a height of 100 cm is advisable.

Nursing care of the child

Careful positioning of the child is important, so that there is no pull on the tubing and no compression of the tubing. Adhesive tape can be attached to the tubing and pinned to the undersheet leaving enough tubing to permit some movement of the child. Forceps should always be available to clamp the tubing immediately should any emergency occur.

Any nursing procedure should be carried out by at least two nurses. When the bed linen has to be changed, two nurses should make the bed, while a third nurse holds the child and controls the tubing. Feeds can be given to the infant in the supine position which also allows maximal efficiency of the muscles of respiration. Care of pressure areas is important, since little change of position occurs voluntarily nor is it encouraged because of the danger of pull on the tube. The older child will need to be reassured and sedation may be required if restlessness is excessive. Physiotherapy is instituted early and breathing exercises are given.

Management of chest drainage

The drainage bottle should initially contain a predetermined volume so that measurement of the increase of level will give an accurate recording of the volume of drainage. It is usually connected to a low vacuum suction to promote satisfactory drainage (10 mmHg, 1.3 kPa). The following points should ensure satisfactory drainage:

1. The tube should be firmly fixed to the chest wall; there must be no leakage between the tube and the stab wound in the skin.

2. All connections must be airtight.
3. Milking of the tube from the chest and that leading to the drainage bottle should be carried out regularly to prevent blockage by a clot.
4. The drainage tube must be *clamped* periodically and disconnected from the connecting tube to allow blood to drain from the connecting tube to the bottle. A large pair of artery forceps is used and, to protect the tube, polythene tubing can be placed between the forceps and the tube.
5. Tubing should be prevented from kinking or constricting.
6. Allow sufficient length of tubing for movement of the child.
7. Tubing may be changed once in 24 hours.
8. It is essential that all members of the staff understand the dangers to the child should any part become disconnected. This could lead to air rushing into the pleural cavity and so to collapse of the lung.

The bottle should be maintained in a position at least 80 to 100 cm below the level of the chest; if it is raised higher, with vigorous inspiratory effort, the fluid could be sucked into the pleural cavity. If it is lifted above the level of the chest, fluid would enter the pleural cavity by siphonage.

Removal of the catheter

Oscillations may cease when the lung is fully expanded, or if the tube has become blocked with pus or blood. Clinical findings and X-ray will prove if it is the former. When the lung is fully expanded, the catheter is removed provided there is no accumulation of air within 24 hours. Whenever the oscillations stop the medical officer is notified. The method of removal of the tube depends on the method used for insertion. If the tube is held in position with a stitch, this has to be cut, the catheter is quickly removed and an airtight dressing applied immediately. Alternatively, a purse string suture may be used if no dressing is desired.

After-care of the child

This is concerned mainly with observation of breathing and ensuring that there is full expansion of the lungs. Gentle handling is important and any indication of breathing difficulty must be reported immediately.

Bronchoscopy

This is a direct vision examination of the trachea and the main bronchial tubes. It is not only an aid to diagnosis, but also a means of access to the lower reaches of the trachea and the main bronchi for biopsy and for the removal of foreign bodies in these structures.

Preparation of the equipment

Special bronchoscopes of varying sizes are used with suckers, or long biopsy forceps. The bronchoscopes contain light carriers; these have to be sterilised. A formalin cabinet can be used. A powerful sucker with adequate length of tubing from the suction bottle is essential. The bottle contains approximately 2 inches (5 cm) of water, to facilitate cleaning of the bottle. Instruments and batteries must be in working order. A specimen bottle may be attached to the equipment by means of a disposable sterile unit which fits on to a universal container. Apart from the operative equipment, it is essential to have resuscitation equipment available.

Preparation of the child

This procedure is carried out under general anaesthesia (see pre-operative preparation, p. 128).

The child is placed on the table, his head extended so that the trachea is in a straight line; his arms are placed straight at the sides, the hands resting below each buttock. He is covered with a cotton blanket.

After-care of the child

This examination may result in serious complications and it is, therefore, essential that the nurse should watch for any signs of difficulty in breathing. Respiratory obstruction may occur due to oedema of the lax subglottic tissue of the infant under 2 or 3 years of age. It is less likely to occur in the older child.

The anaesthetist may have to introduce an endotracheal tube or, in extreme cases if breathing is very difficult, a tracheostomy may be performed to provide an air entry to the lungs. While the child is unconscious, he is nursed in the lateral, head-low position to ensure drainage of mucus and saliva which otherwise may irritate the lung tissue. Suction must be available and used when necessary to clear the pharynx (see bronchial suction, p. 386). Until the effects of the general anaesthesia have abated and the cough and swallowing reflexes have returned, the child must be watched carefully. When consciousness has returned, the child is gradually moved to the upright position and encouraged in deep breathing. When the cough and swallowing reflexes have returned, fluids can be given slowly in small quantities. A croupette, or other apparatus, may be used to create a humid atmosphere if the child has difficulty in breathing following this examination. A difficult bronchoscopy may cause trauma to the mucous lining of the bronchial passages leading to swelling, inflammation and pneumonia.

Endotracheal intubation

Endotracheal intubation is the oral or nasal insertion of a soft, flexible, non-reactive polyvinyl chloride tube into the trachea. The aim is to establish and maintain a patent airway; to provide optimum ventilation; to permit the removal of secretions; and to prevent aspiration by sealing off the trachea from the digestive tract. The latter is achieved if a cuffed tube is used. It can be used to provide mechanical ventilation of the lungs over a prolonged period of time. Oro-tracheal intubation is the preferred route in an emergency situation. Later, it is often desirable to change to a naso-tracheal intubation for prolonged management. This has the advantage over the oro-tracheal route in that it facilitates care of the mouth and oropharynx.

The selection of the tube of the appropriate size is important and correlates best with the height of the child. Where it is impossible to obtain this measurement, it is based on the age of the child to be intubated. Endotracheal tubes are sized by both the internal diameter (mm) and external circumference (mm). Three sizes of tubes should be available for the use of an individual child. A resuscitation trolley should always have available a full range of tube sizes and a chart with the recommended tubes for age and intubation guide. For example, a new-born baby weighing less than 1 kg should have a tube with an internal bore of

2.5 mm and the insertion for nasal tube should be 11 cm, and for oral insertion 10 cm. Tube size and intubation length increase with age.

Insertion of the tube

Once the decision has been made to intubate the child, the stomach should be emptied to prevent vomiting and aspiration of vomitus (p. 509). The child is anaesthetised with ketamine 2 mg/kg given intravenously or 5 mg/kg given intramuscularly. Atropine and a muscle relaxant are also given. In some centres 100 per cent oxygen and halothane is preferred to intravenous anaesthesia.

The procedure is carried out by a skilled medical practitioner. The child is placed in the supine position with the head slightly extended to straighten the pharynx and the trachea. If oral insertion is decided on, a laryngoscope will guide the tube into the larynx and trachea. Most commonly, infants and young children are intubated with uncuffed endotracheal tubes to minimise tracheal compression injury which can lead to tracheal stenosis. This produces a variable amount of leakage around the endotracheal tube. Correct tube positioning is checked by observing chest movements and by auscultation during manual ventilation and it is finally confirmed by chest X-ray. The tube is then fixed stably to avoid the danger of accidental extubation. Various methods can be used but a harness construction is most suitable for infants and children.

Principles of treatment and nursing management

1. *Maintaining position of the child.* The position to place the child in will depend on his condition. Position of the head is important. Extreme flexion of the head in any direction should be avoided, and excessive movement of the head should be prevented as this can result in damage to the vocal cords and trachea. The direction of the tube should always follow the anatomical structure.
2. *Humidification.* The upper airway, and particularly the nasopharynx, is responsible for controlling the humidity and temperature of inspired air. The high blood flow of the nasal mucosa is an effective source of radiant heat for warming. The water saturation, if from inspired air, is provided by the mucous glands which line the nasal passages, trachea and bronchi. Whenever the normal humidifying and warming mechanisms are bypassed with an endotracheal tube or tracheostomy (p. 386) dry and cold air reaching the trachea, unless modified artificially, will impair mucociliary clearance and result in inspissated mucus. This leads to crust formation, which obstructs both artificial and natural airways, resulting in atelectasis and possible death from asphyxia.

A number of devices are available. The *humidifiers* are often inefficient. Least efficient are those which split air/oxygen mixtures into very small bubbles during their passage through water. Heating the water improves the humidification but there is always the danger of malfunction and overheating leading to damage to the upper airway. *Aerosol generators* generate water droplets in the form of a mist. The ultrasonic nebulisers use ultrasonic frequency waves (p. 382) to agitate the water, generating very fine water particles which are carried in the air/oxygen stream. When the secretions are very tenacious this type of nebuliser is helpful. However, care must be taken because of the possible danger of overhydration. This is particularly the case in small children with cardiac and renal disease. Another method which can be used is by instilling sterile saline 1 to 5 ml hourly. This can prevent drying and crusting of secretions in the airway.

3. *Aspiration of tube.* The artificial airway bypasses the glottis and thereby interferes with normal, effective coughing and the expulsion of mucous secretions. The tube and large airways are aspirated periodically using a sterile technique. An end-hole catheter is used to avoid suction damage to the lateral wall of the trachea, which could occur if a side-hole catheter is used. The diameter of the catheter is critical and should allow for smooth entry into the trachea without occluding the lumen, which could cause severe pulmonary collapse.

The catheter is inserted to maximum depth on alternate bronchi, suction being applied only during withdrawal over as short a period as practical (10 s) to prevent arterial hypoxaemia. The lungs are manually inflated with oxygen before and after each suction.

The heart rate is monitored during the suctioning and any bradycardia signifying hypoxaemia, should be followed by cessation of suction and the giving of oxygen. Suction pressure should be in the range of 10 to 15 mmHg (1.3 to 2 kPa).

4. Constant presence of the nurse is essential to observe the child and take immediate action if there is any interference with the integrity of the airway which may range from minimal obstruction by mucus to total occlusion. If suction does not relieve the obstruction the tube may have to be removed and a new one inserted. Measurement of vital functions will indicate the general state of the child.

5. General nursing management should include: cleanliness of the child; attention to pressure areas; providing adequate nutrition; and reassuring the anxious child.

6. *Support for parents.* Whenever possible the parents should be included in some aspects of care. Explanations should be given about the treatment and management of the child and they should be given the opportunity to give expression to their anxieties.

Prevention of complications
There are a number of potential complications associated with the use of the artificial airway. Since these may be life-threatening, careful observations and quick action will be necessary.

The importance of humidity has already been stressed in preventing blockage of the tube, but obstruction of the airway may also result from kinking of the tube.

The endotracheal tube may become accidentlally displaced. This is particularly dangerous when there is damage to the upper airway due to infection, e.g. in croup or epiglottitis, and reintubation is difficult. To prevent extubation, the tube must be fixed securely and care taken that the child does not remove the tube. Restraint may be required (p. 86). It is essential to check constantly the integrity and position of the airway and to identify the reason for the child's restlessness. The rest-

lessness may be due to hypoxaemia from underventilation.

Restlessness, pain and anxiety increase oxygen requirements and may be relieved by giving sedation. However, cardio-pulmonary function should be assessed before sedation is administered. Secondary infection of the lungs is always a problem and every effort should be made to prevent it by careful attention to aseptic technique.

Mechanical ventilation
This is used as a means of maintaining life when normal respiratory effort is inadequate. It seldom treats the original condition, but allows time for the condition to improve. The exception is pulmonary oedema, which is decreased by positive-positive ventilation. There are several types of ventilators in use and the one used in a paediatric unit must be able to ventilate efficiently any patient from an infant to an adult. Humidification is essential, but water overload in infants can be a real hazard.

The mechanism of artificial ventilation is to drive gas into the lungs via the airways using positive pressure from the machine. Alveolar pressure rises above atmospheric, which interferes with return of blood to the heart. During expiration the chest wall returns to its resting position, and the alveolar pressure falls to atmospheric. During this time, blood can return to the heart. If the cardiovascular system of the patient is normal, compensation occurs by a rise of venous pressure so that sufficient blood reaches the heart and the cardiac output is not reduced. If the circulating blood volume is reduced or low, compensation may be inadequate.

There are a variety of mechanical ventilators available for use in children. They are classified according to their method of control:

1. *Volume preset.* These are effective for use in children with abnormal lung mechanism. They are designed to deliver a preset volume of gas into the lungs irrespective of the resistance of the airway or compliance of the lungs.

2. *Pressure preset.* The pressure generated throughout the inspiratory phase is determined by the design of the ventilator and is unaffected by the physiological characteristics of the child's

lungs. The flow and volume which result are determined by airway resistance and lung compliance. An adequate gas volume can be delivered at low pressure provided inspiration time is long enough. This type of ventilator is used in the treatment of respiratory distress syndrome in infants.

3. *Time-flow preset.* This is another method of control. Time-flow preset ventilators, like pressure preset ventilators, afford the advantage of a rapid response time at rapid ventilator rates, with continuous flow intermittent mandatory ventilation capability. In this system the child may breathe spontaneously from a fresh gas source at low resistance while receiving active inflations from the mechanical ventilator at preset intervals with the same level of end-expiratory pressure.

Methods of ventilation

Intermittent Positive Pressure Ventilation (IPPV)
A ventilator delivers a mixture of oxygen and air above atmospheric pressure to inflate the infant's lungs rhythmically. This takes place intermittently to allow the child to exhale.

Positive End-Expiratory Pressure (PEEP)
In this instance, a ventilator exerts a few centimetres of positive pressure to keep the alveoli open slightly at the end of expiration, thereby facilitating gas exchange within these alveoli. PEEP may increase carbon dioxide retention and the possibility of pneumothorax.

Constant Positive Airway Pressure (CPAP)
This is the same as PEEP but is done while the infant is breathing spontaneously. The small amount of positive pressure exerted on the airways helps him to take the next breath.

Intermittent Mandatory Ventilation (IMV)
The child breathes mainly on his own, and the ventilator gives an occasional breath for him.

Weaning from the ventilator
The decision to wean a child from controlled ventilation will depend on the clinical state of the child. All vital functions should be steady, secretions should be minimal, blood-gas tension

should be maintained at a satisfactory level and the X-ray of the chest should show improvement.

Most children can be weaned by means of a T-tube adaptor and heated nebuliser connected to the child's tracheal tube. As the level of respiratory support is reduced during the weaning process, there are changes in the pattern of breathing and in the lung volumes which tend to produce small-airway closure and an increase in small-airway resistance. This can lead to atelectasis and a deterioration in gas exchange.

Careful observations of the vital functions are essential and if the child shows restlessness, tachycardia, cyanosis, hypotension and arrhythmias, then these are indications for resuming controlled ventilation. If the weaning period is stressful, then rest periods of full-time mechanical ventilation are important, especially at night.

If weaning is successful and there are no appreciable changes in the clinical state or blood-gas tension, then the child can be extubated. Humidified oxygen is administered at the same concentration as that given during the weaning period. It is important that the child is encouraged to cough and clear secretions, while taking slow, deep breaths as often as possible.

Throughout the period of weaning from the ventilator, the child should not be left alone. This is not only to observe and encourage him but also to allay any fears he may have regarding his ability to breathe.

Although the nurse's time will be taken up with monitoring the mechanical events, it must not be forgotten that the focus of attention should be the child, who is not only alive, but if conscious, will be very frightened. He should never be left alone and, whatever the age of the child, he should be given constant reassurance and encouragement. All nursing care should be carried out with understanding of the child's needs and, to cause least disturbance, two nurses should work together when lifting or position change is necessary.

Phrenic pacing
Patients with neurogenic respiratory failure usually require mechanical ventilation to maintain their respiratory function. It is now possible to induce respiration by means of a surgically implanted device which, when electrically stimulated by an

external transmitter and antenna, stimulates the phrenic nerve and causes the diaphragm to descend. The descent of the diaphragm allows air to flow into the lungs.

Indications for phrenic pacing

The success of phrenic nerve stimulation depends on normal function of phrenic nerves, lungs and diaphragm. Prior to insertion of the electrodes, the surgeon will ascertain that phrenic nerve stimulation can produce diaphragmatic contractions. Phrenic nerve pacing is valuable in: (1) a high cervical lesion; (2) ventilatory dependence: (3) chronic dysfunction of the respiratory control centre; and (4) a patient with a paralysed diaphragm.

Loss of involuntary respiratory control usually requires implantation of only one pacemaker to enable breathing during sleep. Loss of both voluntary and involuntary control requires implantation of two pacemakers, one for each phrenic nerve. To prevent fatigue of the diaphragm, each pacemaker is operated alternately.

Method of implantation

The procedure can be performed under local anaesthesia. The electrodes are implanted in the

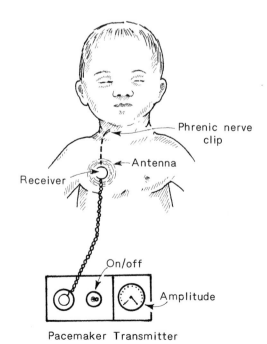

Fig. 23.22 Phrenic pacemaker.

neck around the phrenic nerve (Fig. 23.22). A subcutaneous tunnel is made for the electrode wires which attach to a receiver which is placed under the skin either in the subclavicular area or in the lower lateral rib cage. An antenna, which is attached to a pacemaker transmitter box, is placed on the skin overlying the subcutaneous receiver. Before completion, the phrenic pacemaker is tested to ensure its proper operation and activated to determine threshold and maximal diaphragmatic contraction.

Management of the child

Principles of management

The doctor will determine the transmitter setting and the specific pacing schedule. A ventilator must be available and ready for use if the child is totally dependent on respiratory support.

If the child is old enough then an explanation must be given and his co-operation obtained. The antenna is applied to the skin directly over the receiver and secured with adhesive tape. The child is placed in the position considered suitable, e.g. either lying flat or with the head of the bed elevated 30°. The pacemaker is activated after expiration. The abdomen is observed for respiratory movement and the doctor will listen for breath sounds. Throughout the initial pacing trials, the child is monitored carefully for signs of fatigue and decreased abdominal movement, signs of hypoxia, tachycardia and hypotension. The doctor should be notified if any of the above signs are present; phrenic pacing will be discontinued and the child attached to the mechanical ventilator.

When the pacing trial has been completed, the child should be told that he will be reconnected to the ventilator. The pacemaker will be turned off after the next expiration and the antenna removed and stored for the next pacing trial. The antenna site should be checked for redness.

When the child is on full-time pacing, it is important to keep the system dry to prevent minor electric shock and malfunction. The battery must be tested regularly to ensure that pacing continues without interruption. If the pacemaker fails to function and the battery is charged, then the fault may be with the antenna. Problems could also arise if the child is vomiting as this causes changes in intrathoracic pressure and may lead to aspiration during phrenic stimulation. It may be necessary to discontinue pacing during this episode.

Complications

Complications may arise if there is injury to one or both phrenic nerves, preventing the pacemaker from adequately supporting ventilation. There may be infection at the site of entry or there may be mechanical failure of the receiver due to seepage of body fluids into its electrical components. This can be identified by erratic pacing or sharp pain over the operative site. However, the pacer may fail without warning.

Preparation for home

When the child is ready to go home, the parents must be given the opportunity to participate in the care of the child. They must be shown and given a full explanation of the working of the pacemaker, how to identify malfunction and what action to take. They must be reassured that if they are worried about any aspect of care and management they can contact the hospital. The community services must be alerted and advised on the care of the child.

Chapter 24
Disorders of the cardiovascular system

The ability of every cell, tissue and organ to function is dependent upon receiving an adequate supply of nutrients and oxygen, and also on removing carbon dioxide and waste products formed in the tissues during the metabolic process.

The system responsible for those vital functions is the cardiovascular system which acts not only as the transport system, but also as an exchange system via the capillaries. The mechanism is provided by the heart which acts as a pump and by the blood vessels through which the blood and its constituents travel.

Development of the cardiovascular system

The cardiovascular system is the only system which has a specific function early in embryonic life. The cells must receive food and oxygen if they are to survive and develop. These materials are obtained from the mother, via the placenta. The blood vessels and blood cells arise from the materials derived from the mesoderm and by the time the embryo is 3 weeks old, blood vessels appear within the embryo proper.

As a pumping organ, the heart is essential in early embryonic life. In its early stages, there are four chambers which form a single tube and which develop into four separate chambers. These are necessary for separating the oxygenated and de-oxygenated blood coming from, and going to the lungs and the body circulation. In the embryo, this separation is not necessary, since the lungs are not functioning and very little blood passes through them.

However, by the end of the second month, the two ventricles have separated and the two atria have partially separated. This remains so until after birth when the foramen ovale closes. During intra-uterine life blood passes freely between the two cavities. Since the lungs are not functioning, it would otherwise mean that no blood enters the left atrium. Almost all the blood enters the embryo's heart through the right atrium into which the superior and inferior vena cava empty the blood. The opening between the two atria enables half of this blood to cross over to the left side and allows the pumping function of the heart to be divided between the powerful ventricles (Fig. 24.1).

Gradual changes also take place as the aortic arches develop, that is, from a single arch on either side going through various stages, leading to development of some and degeneration of others until the fourth arch becomes the adult aorta and the last arch becomes the pulmonary artery.

Regulation of heart rate

An interesting aspect of the embryology of heart tissue is that during each of its developmental stages, the parts of the cardiac tissue laid down have their own inherent rate of beating, even though the heart as a whole has not started to beat. Initially, the heart beat starts in the ventricular region, but during early development, the control of the heart beat is found to be in the sino-atrial region. Eventually, nerves and hormones begin to influence the heart rate, e.g. sympathetic and parasympathetic nerves, adrenalin, noradrenalin and thyroxin act on the pacemaker. The fetal heart rate usually ranges from about 135 to 150 beats per minute. This raised heart rate may provide the fetus with the high cardiac output necessary to meet its high metabolic requirements.

Fetal circulation (Fig. 24.2)

Physiologically, the fetal circulation is arranged in

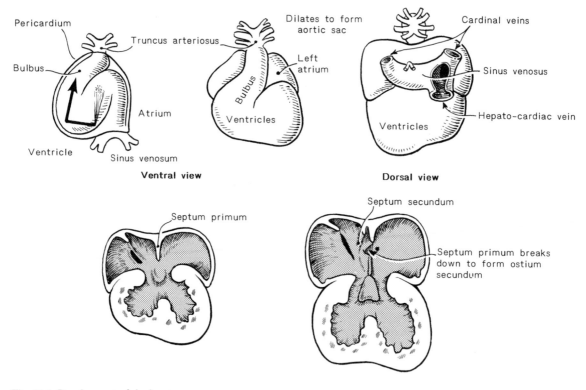

Fig. 24.1 Development of the heart.

such a way that it transports the most highly oxygenated blood to the brain and the heart.

The 'functioning' fetal lung is the placenta. The umbilical arteries convey very deoxygenated blood from the fetal tissues to the placenta. In the placenta the blood is oxygenated and it leaves in the umbilical vein about 80 per cent saturated with oxygen. This oxygenated blood travels to the liver where part of the blood passes directly via the *ductus venosus* into the inferior vena cava. The rest of the blood is distributed to part of the liver by offshoots of the umbilical vein, while the other part of the liver receives blood from the portal vein. Blood from the liver reaches the inferior vena cava by the hepatic veins. This mixture of blood is about 67 per cent saturated. The blood in the inferior vena cava enters the right atrium and as it passes into the heart, the blood is divided into two streams by the crista dividens. The major portion is directed from the inferior vena cava to the left atrium where it mixes with a small amount of pulmonary venous blood, while the smaller

amount enters the right atrium where it mixes with blood from the superior vena cava.

The crista dividens forms the rim of the foramen ovale. The blood from the left heart goes to the myocardium via the coronary vessels and to the head and upper extremities via the ascending aorta.

After leaving the right ventricle, the blood enters the pulmonary trunk, but because pulmonary resistance is higher than systemic vascular resistance, the blood bypasses the lungs via the *ductus arteriosus* and enters the descending aorta, which supplies the trunk and lower limbs.

Changes at birth (Fig. 24.3)

When the baby is born, the circulatory system has to convert from the intra-uterine situation to the postnatal state. In mechanical terms, this involves the closure and obliteration of shunting channels, the foramen ovale, ductus venosus and ductus arteriosus, and the removal of the umbilical arteries, the placenta-umbilical vein unit.

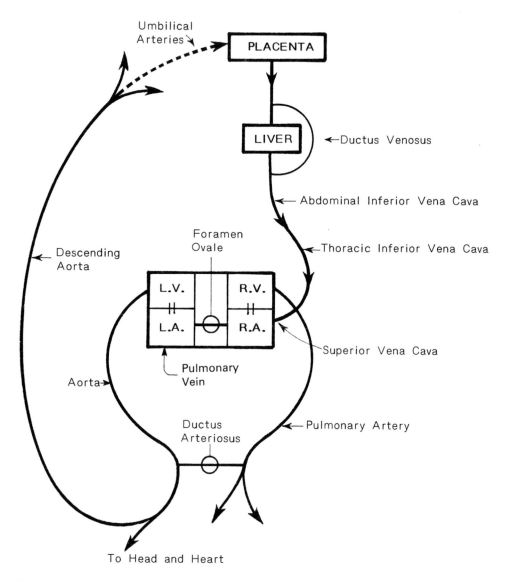

Fig. 24.2 Fetal circulation.

Foramen ovale

With the onset of breathing, which causes an expansion of the lungs, the pressure in the right side of the heart falls greatly because of the diminished pulmonary resistance and less blood flowing back to the heart via the inferior vena cava as a result of the removal of the placenta.

The free end of the foramen ovale closes from the left side like a hinged door. With the fall in pressure in the right atrium to below that of the left atrium, the valve closes. Obliteration of the foramen ovale is not effected for some weeks and so changes in pressure on either side of the valve may cause it to re-open. Occasionally, the valve fails to close and oxygenated blood and deoxygenated blood mix.

Ductus arteriosus

This vessel represents the most important vascular shunt in the fetal circulation. The ductus arteriosus shunts blood from the pulmonary artery to the descending aorta, thereby bypassing the lungs.

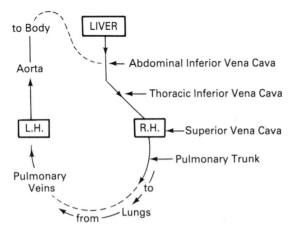

Fig. 24.3 Changes in circulation after birth.

During fetal life, pulmonary artery pressure is very high and greater than the aortic pressure, therefore, blood flow in the ductus is from the pulmonary artery to the aorta. Closure is said to be due to the increase in oxygen tension in the blood. Persistence of the duct is called *patent ductus arteriosus.*

Ductus venosus
The precise function of this duct is not fully understood, but it is suggested that it plays a part in the control of placental vascular resistance, especially during hypoxia. The duct closes during the first minutes after birth and anatomical closure is completed within 20 days of birth.

General structure and function of the heart

The heart and the roots of the great blood vessels are contained in a tough fibrous bag (fibrous pericardium) which is lined with thin membrane (serous pericardium). This serous pericardium is similar to pleura in both structure and function, i.e. it forms a bag with a space between the two layers. The serous layer adheres to the cardiac muscle. The space or cavity contains a thin layer of fluid. Excess fluid or blood is found in conditions such as pericardial effusion. Since the outer fibrous coat is tough and unyielding, any excess fluid will interfere with the pumping action of the heart.

The myocardium is the middle muscular layer. It is very specialised muscle, arranged in such a way that each muscle cell is separated by narrow interposed intercellular spaces. When one cell is excited, the excitation process spreads easily across to the other muscle cell.

The endocardium is a smooth, thin, glistening membrane which lines the chambers of the heart. It is continuous with the lining of the large vessels and by its reduplication it assists in forming the valves. Endocarditis can develop due to bacterial infection and when there is already congenital heart disease present.

The heart is divided into four chambers, right and left atria, and right and left ventricles. The thin-walled atria are separated from each other by an interatrial septum and the thicker-walled ventricles by the interventricular septum.

Atria and ventricles are connected by a fibrous atrio-ventricular ring. This ring is penetrated on the right side by the tricuspid valve and on the left by the mitral (bicuspid) valve. Chordae tendinae are attached to the free edges of the valve cusps and act like ropes.

On the right side, the pulmonary orifice is guarded by the pulmonary or semilunar valve. The pulmonary orifice leads from the ventricle to the pulmonary artery. A similar construction is found at the aortic orifice (aortic valve) which leads from the left ventricle to the aorta. These valves *open* at the onset of ventricular ejection and *close* when the relevant arterial pressure exceeds that of the corresponding ventricle, when it begins to relax. Closure of both atrio-ventricular valves causes the first heart sound and closure of the semilunar valves causes the second heart sound.

The function of the heart valves is to prevent fluid flowing in the wrong direction. When any valve is damaged by disease, there may be reflux of blood and characteristic 'murmurs' can be heard on auscultation.

The weight of the heart varies with the age of the individual. For example, at birth it weighs 20.6 g, at 1 year 43.0 g, at 5 years 90.0 g, at 10 years 145.0 g and in the young adult 245.0 g. In early life the heart lies somewhat higher in the chest than in later life. The apex beat in the newborn infant can therefore be heard in the 4th left interspace and after the age of 2 years the apical impulse is usually in the 5th left interspace (p. 104).

Nervous supply to the heart

The nervous control of the heart beat is effected by the parasympathetic and sympathetic nerves (Fig. 24.4) The parasympathetic nerve supply *slows* the heart beat. These fibres pass from the cardiac centre (a group of nerve cells in the medulla) and through the vagus nerve trunk, as preganglionic fibres, to the nerve cells in the heart muscle, where they synapse with ganglion cells which are found in the vicinity of the sino-atrial and atrio-ventricular nodes, in the atrium (right). Stimulation of the vagus reduces the rate of impulse generation by the sino-atrial node. It also reduces the rate of propagation of the cardiac impulse and diminishes the force of atrial contraction. Vagal stimulation does not influence contraction of the ventricular myocardium directly, since it does not innervate the ventricles.

The sympathetic nerve cells lie in the intermedial lateral horn of the upper five thoracic segments of the spinal cord. Sympathetic nerves eventually pass to nodal tissue and to the muscle of the atria and the ventricles. Sympathetic stimulation *increases* the heart rate and the force and speed of the myocardial contraction.

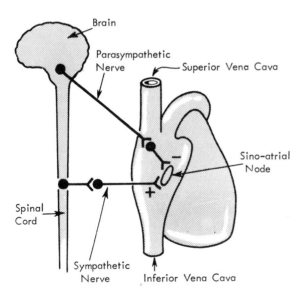

Fig. 24.4 Nervous control of the heart.

The action of the heart

The heart can be described as a double pump — it pumps blood to the lungs for oxygenation and it pumps blood through the blood vessels. The energy for this pumping action is derived from the contraction of specialised muscle tissue. As in skeletal muscle, there is a link between the biochemical breakdown of complex molecules and the mechanical contraction of the fibres. The link is provided by adenotriphosphate (ATP).

The contraction process is initiated by a wave of electrical depolarisation of the myocardial membrane. This process starts at the sino-atrial node which is situated at the junction of the superior vena cava and the free border of the right atrial appendix (Fig. 24.5). It has a rich capillary blood supply and is innervated by sympathetic and parasympathetic fibres. Since it initiates the heart beat it is called the pacemaker.

The impulse then spreads throughout the atria to the atrio-ventricular node, which is situated at the posterior and right border of the interatrial septum. From the atrio-ventricular node, it spreads to the bundle of His, which is found at the inter-ventricular septum where it forks, each branch passing under the endocardium of the ventricles, as the Purkinje fibres or tissue. This tissue differs from cardiac muscle, in that the fibres are larger and are richer in glycogen content.

The rhythmic contraction and relaxation of the myocardial muscle, in conjunction with the valvular system causes a unidirectional flow of blood through the heart. The amount of blood which passes through the heart each minute, (the *cardiac output*) depends on the contractile ability of the

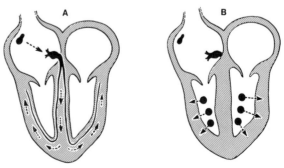

Fig. 24.5 A, Normal pathway of cardiac impulse. B, Ventricular fibrillation pathway.

myocardium and also on the state of the peripheral resistance.

Heart rate

The heart rate of the new-born infant is rapid and is subject to wide fluctuations, the average rate ranging from 120 to 140 beats per minute. During crying or other active periods this may increase to 170 beats per minute, while during sleep it may drop to between 70 and 90 beats per minute. As the child grows older, the average pulse rate becomes slower. Table 24.1 shows the average pulse rates at rest.

The rate of the heart beat is affected by:

1. Impulses from higher centres, e.g. emotion. In excitement the heart rate increases and sudden emotional shock produces slowing of the heart rate.
2. Respiration. In children normal breathing is associated with cardiac acceleration during *inspiration* and slowing during expiration. This is termed sinus arrhythmia.
3. Body temperature. A rise in body temperature leads to a rise in heart rate, conversely, a fall in body temperature leads to slowing of the heart rate.
4. Exercise. The heart rate increases progressively with increasing exercise.

Nervous and chemical factors also control the heart beat.

Table 24.1 Average pulse rates at rest

Age	Lower limits of normal	Average	Upper limits of normal
Newborn	70	120	170
1–12 months	80	120	160
2 years	80	110	130
4 years	80	100	120
6 years	75	100	115
8 years	70	100	110
10 years	70	90	110
12 years*	65	85	105
14 years	60	80	100
16 years	55	75	95
18 years	50	70	90

* Between the ages of 12 and 18 years, the figures are for boys, the pulse rates of girls being about 5 beats faster.

Nervous factors

Nervous control is achieved through baroreceptors which are responsible for reflex vagal tone. They are situated in the aortic arch, carotid sinus and right atrium. The baroreceptors respond as follows via the cardiac centre: a rise of right atrial and central venous pressure, i.e. atrial reflex, leads to *acceleration* of the heart rate; a fall of right atrial and central venous pressure leads to *slowing* of the heart rate, and a rise in blood pressure in the aortic arch or the carotid sinus causes *slowing* down of the heart rate, while a fall in blood pressure in these vessels, leads to *increased* heart rate.

Chemical factors

Adrenaline. This has a direct stimulating action on the heart, increasing the strength of ventricular contraction and heart rate.

Electrolytes. A rise in the *potassium* level in the plasma decreases the heart rate by relaxing the heart. If the level is high enough the ventricles go into irregular arrhythmia with a slow rate, while potassium depletion produces poor cardiac function. *Sodium* is an important extracellular electrolyte (p. 225). Sodium loss or depletion decreases cardiac output, while sodium retention increases it.

Calcium activates myosin (one of the contractile proteins) which is essential for the production of energy and for the contraction of the muscle. Low plasma calcium leads to diminished contraction, while calcium in excess produces strong contractions.

Oxygen. The role of oxygen should also be considered. The heart is very sensitive to any changes in oxygen. Oxygen lack is followed by coronary vasodilatation and in this way blood flow to the cardiac muscles is proportional to the metabolic requirements for oxygen by the muscle fibres. The mechanism in the feedback system involves the carotid and aortic bodies which contain specialised sensory receptors, sensitive to oxygen lack (chemoreceptors). Low oxygen concentration leads to reflex rise in arterial pressure, thus increasing oxygen flow.

The cardiac cycle

The period from the end of one heart contraction to the end of the next is called the *cardiac cycle*.

Each cycle is initiated by spontaneous generation of an action potential in the sino-atrial node. This travels rapidly through both atria to the atrio-ventricular bundle and into the ventricle. There is a slight delay of more than one-tenth of a second between the passage of the impulse from the atria to the ventricles. This allows the atria to contract ahead of the ventricles, pumping blood into the ventricles.

Two periods are recognised which are termed diastole (relaxation) and systole (contraction). The total time of the combined periods or cycle is 0.8 seconds. During each of these events there are pressure changes which can be recorded by a sphygmomanometer. The pressures measured are arterial pressures (p. 460). The blood pressure varies with the age of the child and is closely related to his height and weight. Significant increases occur during adolescence with many temporary variations until the more stable levels of the adult are attained. Exercise, excitement, coughing and straining may raise the systolic pressure in children as much as 40 mmHg to 50 mmHg above their usual levels. There are a number of factors responsible in maintaining blood pressure, but it is the heart which is of primary importance. Without the pumping activity of the heart, the blood pressure would be near zero. However, the pump has to be primed and this is effected by venous return which also affects cardiac output. Table 24.2 shows the normal blood pressure measurements for different ages.

The activity of the heart can be recorded by means of an *electrocardiogram* (ECG), which records the current and voltage waveforms associated with the contraction of the heart muscle. It is a recording of the electrical activity induced in the body fluids by the electrical impulses which spread through the heart during each cardiac cycle.

The electrocardiograph consists of three main deflections from the baseline:

1. The 'P' wave which is due to atrial depolarisation.
2. The 'QRS' complex which is due to ventricular depolarisation.
3. The 'T' wave which is due to ventricular re-polarisation (Fig. 24.6A).

The ECG represents the end-result of the electrical events which are highly complex. It is a useful diagnostic tool because it provides a clear pattern of overall electrical activity which can then be correlated with other signs of disease. In any individual the standard leads enable deductions to be made about heart rate, rhythm and electrical axis.

Since nerves and muscles may also be producing action potentials, it is essential to eliminate those as far as possible. The child should therefore be lying down and in a relaxed state.

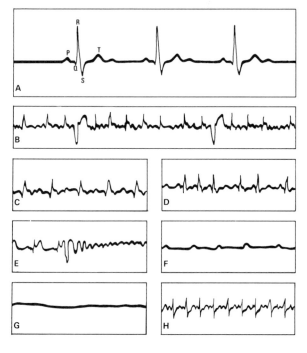

Fig. 24.6

Table 24.2 Normal blood pressure for different ages

Age	Mean systolic blood pressure	Mean diastolic blood pressure
Newborn	80	46
6–12 months	89	60
2 years	99	64
6–7 years	100	56
9–10 years	107	57
12–13 years	115	59
13–14 years	118	60

The first wave on a normal ECG trace is the 'P' wave; the second is the 'QRS' complex and the third wave is the 'T' wave (Fig. 24.6A). The P–R interval is measured from the beginning of the 'P' wave to the beginning of the 'R' wave. It represents the time for conduction of the impulse, which is to initiate ventricular contraction from its origin in the sino-atrial node to its arrival at the ventricles. In health it should not exceed 0.2 seconds, usually the interval is 0.16 to 0.18 seconds. In children it may be shorter, 0.12 to 0.14 seconds.

The 'QRS' complex is considered as a single entity and should not exceed 0.12 seconds. The final 'T' wave has an average duration of 0.27 seconds. The duration of the 'QRST' complex is therefore about 0.4 seconds.

If the paper speed is known, the heart rate can be calculated from the distance which separates two 'QRS' complexes. For example, if the paper speed is 25 mm/s and the two complexes (tips of 'R' waves are useful reference points) are separated by 12.5 mm, then the heart rate is 60 × 25/12.5 = 120 beats per minute.

The ECG is also an important way of diagnosing the precise nature of an abnormal heart rhythm. The following rhythms are commonly found.

Sinus rhythm

This is the normal rhythm which is due to impulses that originate in the sino-atrial node and travel the normal pathway. The 'QRS' and 'T' waves are regular and of constant shape. Each 'QRS' is preceded at a constant interval by a normal 'P' wave (Fig. 24.6A).

Sinus arrhythmia

The impulses arise irregularly at the sinus node. The rate increases in inspiration and decreases in expiration. There is an irregular sequence of 'P, QRS, T'.

Extrasystole

These are beats which arise from some region other than the sino-atrial node. Ventricular extrasystole is indicated by an abnormal 'QRS-T' wave and no 'P' wave. This is because these waves arise in the ventricles. The 'QRS' wave also tends to be prolonged.

Atrial extrasystole is not so easy to recognise; the 'QRS' wave is normal, but the 'P' wave is abnormal.

Tachycardia

This is a rapid heart rate. Paroxysmal tachycardia is the commonest type in infants. The heart rate is rapid and regular. Tachycardia arises at the sino-atrial node and is seen in pyrexia when the heart is normal. If it arises at an abnormal site, there will be a series of extrasystoles. In atrial tachycardia the 'QRS' complex appears normal; in ventricular tachycardia the 'QRS' complex is usually markedly abnormal (Fig. 24.6H).

Atrial fibrillation (Fig. 24.6B).

In this condition the normal electrical activity of the atria is replaced by impulses which arise at an extremely rapid rate (up to 500 to 600 per minute). This causes ineffective atrial pumping action. It also affects the ventricles since the atrio-ventricular node is bombarded at a high rate by atrial impulses. As only some of these impulses activate the ventricles, this leads to an irregular rate of ventricular contraction.

Ventricular fibrillation (Figs. 24.5 and 24.6F)

The electrical impulses arise in ventricular muscle and are associated with ineffective mechanical activity. This condition is rapidly fatal unless relieved by an electric shock (defibrillation — see p. 124) which should return the heart to a more normal rhythm.

Heart block (Fig. 24.6C and D)

In this condition there is an abnormality of the conducting tissue of the heart, so that the impulses are not conducted from the atria to the ventricles. The atrial beat is normal, but the ventricles must generate their own impulse, generally at a slower rate than that of the atria. If the rate is too slow, heart failure results (Fig. 24.6F and G).

The vascular system

When describing the heart it was stated that it contains four chambers, two atria, which although contractile, also act as reservoirs and two ventricles, which act as the pump proper.

The right atrium and ventricle receive blood which has returned from the tissues via the veins. The blood reaches the right atrium at a pressure slightly above zero. From the right atrium it is pumped into the right ventricle and from there into the pulmonary artery, which divides into many arterioles and then into pulmonary capillaries. (See pulmonary circulation.) The blood is oxygenated and then collected from the pulmonary capillaries by the pulmonary venules and veins, to be transported back to the heart into the left atrium and left ventricle.

The left ventricle has the function of pumping blood into the systemic circulation via the main distributing artery, the aorta. The aorta divides into arteries which supply all the various regional circuits. Every tissue is supplied with oxygenated blood as well as nutritive, immunological and hormonal substances.

The arteries undergo successive divisions and smaller branch arteries finally deliver the blood to vessels of between 500 and 100 μm in diameter, called arterioles. The arterioles divide and subdivide until they form capillaries which, in enormous numbers, permeate the tissues. They constitute a vast surface area and are extremely thin (one cell thick). This allows diffusion of nutrient substances to the immediate adjacent tissue cells and also allows them to take up carbon dioxide and waste products from the tissue cells. The capillaries distribute the blood to venules and from there to veins which return the blood to the right atrium. The return flow of blood is aided by the action of skeletal muscles.

The human circulation works as a constant pressure system. The level of pressure in the arteries is vigorously controlled and local flow to tissues is regulated by varying local resistance. When an increase in flow to any area is required, resistance to flow of blood in that area is lowered and more blood leaves the arterial system. The ability to control blood flow is in part dependent on the vessels themselves, which have distinctive anatomical features in different parts of the vascular system.

1. *The arterial vessels* consist of large elastic vessels, such as the aorta and its immediate branches. There are also large muscular distributing arteries, small arteries and arterioles. The arterioles are able to constrict due to the presence of vascular smooth muscle and nerves which control the diameter of the vessels.

2. *Capillaries* consist of a single layer of non-contractile endothelial cells. They are not innervated and they offer an extensive surface area for exchange of substances between blood and tissues. The flow rate is about 0.3 to 0.5 mm/s.

3. *Veins*. Smaller veins and venules have thinner walls than arterioles and are innervated, but less so than arterioles. Larger veins vary according to their position in the body. Some veins contain valves which permit flow only towards the heart; these are mainly in the legs.

Failure of the circulatory system may be either of central origin, i.e. when the heart fails to pump and the cardiac output is inadequate, or peripheral, i.e. when the heart is pumping normally but the output is inadequate because the central venous pressure is too low and the venous return to the heart is reduced. Examples are haemorrhage and severe burns, where plasma is lost across the walls of the damaged capillaries, or diabetic coma and severe vomiting and diarrhoea, where the volume of extracellular fluid is reduced.

Murmurs

Murmurs are noises which can be heard over various areas of the cardiovascular system where blood flow is turbulent, i.e. where the flow velocity is increased when passing through a narrowed part of a vessel. The turbulence causes the surrounding structures to vibrate and to generate the sound waves.

Murmurs are not harmful but are important signs in diagnosing defects in the heart and the circulation. Murmurs are not normally heard because the flow is usually laminar or streamline, but when there is (1) an increase in the blood velocity, as is found in anaemia or excessive thyroxine secretion; (2) an increase in the diameter of the vessel, as is found in aneurysm; and (3) a decrease in blood viscosity, as is found in anaemia, then murmurs are heard.

Diseases affecting the cardiovascular system

Diseases affecting the cardiovascular system can be

divided into those which are congenital or acquired.

CONGENITAL CARDIOVASCULAR ANOMALIES

The great majority of congenital cardiac anomalies result from arrested or distorted development of the heart during the early intra-uterine life, when the heart and the great vessels are formed from the primitive vascular tube. Anomalous defects are possible in one or more areas. The defects are classified as follows:

Cyanotic group

1. Without pulmonary hypertension:
   a. Tetralogy of Fallot (infundibular pulmonic stenosis, ventricular septal defect, hypertrophy of the right ventricle and dextroposition or 'overriding' or the aorta).
   b. Tricuspid atresia.
   c. Ebstein's anomaly (deformity and displacement of the tricuspid valve into the right ventricle).
   d. Total anomalous pulmonary venous drainage.
2. With pulmonary hypertension:
   a. Eisenmenger's complex (severe pulmonary vascular defects).
   b. Transposition of the great vessels.

Acyanotic group

1. With left to right shunts:
   a. Ventricular septal defect.
   b. Atrial septal defect.
   c. Patent ductus arteriosus.
2. With obstructive features:
   a. Isolated pulmonary stenosis.
   b. Aortic stenosis.
   c. Coarctation of the aorta.

General features and management

Acyanotic group. When the shunt defects are large enough to produce a significant pulmonary blood flow, there may be frequent respiratory infections, easy fatigue, dyspnoea on exertion and retarded physical development. If there is a severe obstructive defect, heart failure may result. In the new-born, there may be signs of heart failure and respiratory distress.

Cyanotic group. Cyanosis is present at birth; there is enlargement of the heart and liver, with pulmonary congestion. Cyanosis may also be due to peripheral circulatory failure and inadequate oxygenation of blood in the lungs.

Clubbing of digits. When clubbing and cyanosis localise in the toes alone it is said to be due to a reverse *patent ductus arteriosus* with blood flow going from the pulmonary artery to the aorta, joining the aorta below the level of take-off of the arteries supplying the upper extremities. Generally, cyanosis and clubbing reflect the presence of a right-to-left shunt, which permits unoxygenated blood to enter the general circulation by bypassing aerated pulmonary alveoli.

Peripheral cyanosis results from sluggish blood flow which permits greatly increased oxygen extraction by the tissues.

Correction of all congenital lesions is basically surgical if the defect is severe enough to result in disturbed haemodynamics and provided that irreversible complications have not occurred. Other forms of management include digitalisation, salt restriction, diuretics, oxygen therapy and appropriate antibiotics.

Before any surgery is undertaken it is important that the defect is identified. Several diagnostic procedures are performed and these are discussed in detail at the relevant section. Briefly, these involve the following:

1. Radiology of the heart and lungs. In children over 6 months of age the posterior-anterior film is taken with the child erect at a tube distance of 6 feet (1.83 m). In children under 6 months of age the film is taken with the infant lying down with the tube distance of 5 feet (1.52 m). The heart size and shape will be demonstrated.

   Lung vascularity is also assessed as it is of great importance in the diagnosis of congenital heart disease. When it is increased there must be a left-to-right shunt, resulting in an excessive flow of blood to the lungs. When it is decreased, there must be some obstruction to the flow of blood into the lungs.

   Occasionally, a barium swallow is used to confirm left atrial enlargement and to show the presence of coarctation of the aorta, aberrant arteries or a vascular ring.

2. Electrocardiography (p. 405).
3. Ultrasound cardiography (p. 463).
4. Cardiac catheterisation (p. 461).
5. Angiocardiography (p. 462).
6. Aortography (p. 463).

CARDIAC SURGERY

Many children with congenital heart disease will have some form of operation. The type of operation required will depend on the abnormality and the effect of the abnormality on the child. Where possible, the infant should be treated medically until it is evident that further improvement is not possible. Even a few weeks of satisfactory growth improves the prognosis.

Surgery may be 'palliative', aiming primarily to relieve the child's symptoms and prevent undesirable secondary effects, or 'corrective', where the lesion is repaired as completely as possible. Surgery of the heart can be extracardiac, that is surgery performed without opening the heart and limited to the vessels (for example, patent ductus arteriosus and coarctation of the aorta); or it can be intracardiac, which involves open-heart surgery. It is possible to open up a stenosed pulmonary valve without the use of cardiopulmonary bypass; this is achieved by inserting bougies through the right ventricular wall and breaking a way through the pulmonary valve.

Open-heart surgery requires a cardiopulmonary bypass, where cannulae are inserted into the right atrium (or both venae cavae) and the venous blood is sucked or allowed to drain into a heart-lung machine where it is oxygenated and then returned to the aorta by a pump which is capable of producing flows and pressures comparable to those in the normal circulation. The myocardium has to be protected while the heart's action is arrested and this is achieved by perfusing it with oxygenated blood. This method provides a safe period for about 3 hours, which is usually sufficient time for even complicated repairs.

Another method used is profound hypothermia, where the whole patient is cooled to 12 to 15°C. This allows the circulation to be stopped completely for up to 60 minutes. The heart ceases to function adequately at temperatures below about 27°C and therefore an extracorporeal circulation is required. In infants the initial cooling can be carried out by surface cooling and this shortens the period necessitating a bypass. This technique is useful for infants and there tends to be a lower incidence of post-operative pulmonary problems. This is probably because the lungs are unperfused for a much shorter time.

Types of operation

Blalock-Taussig procedure

This is a palliative operation designed to increase pulmonary blood flow. An anastomosis is made between the subclavian artery and pulmonary artery on the right or left side. If the subclavian artery is high up or the pulmonary artery is very small, a tube can be inserted between these two vessels to make sure there is adequate flow to the pulmonary artery. This anastomosis is preferred because it is easily closed at the time of complete repair and rarely results in distortion of the pulmonary artery.

Waterston operation

This is also a palliative operation performed on new-born infants. An anastomosis is created between the ascending aorta and right pulmonary artery. There is often kinking and narrowing of the pulmonary artery proximal to the shunt which requires patching at complete repair. It is also more difficult to close at the time of complete repair.

Pott's operation

This is also a palliative operation which is seldom used now. An anastomosis is made between the descending aorta and left pulmonary artery. This procedure often produces pulmonary hypertension and is difficult to close at the time of corrective repair.

Fontan operation

This is a palliative operation which is only possible if there is a right ventricle and pulmonary valve of adequate size. A conduit is inserted from the right atrium to the pulmonary artery. A modification of this procedure is to insert the conduit from the right atrium to the right ventricle, using the child's own pulmonary valve.

Banding of the pulmonary artery

This is a palliative procedure in infants with complex abnormalities associated with high pulmonary blood flow and pulmonary artery pressures at or near systemic levels. A piece of tape is tied around the pulmonary artery, tight enough to reduce the pressure beyond the band to about half that proximally. It helps by restricting blood flow through the lungs. It is also used when there are multiple ventricular septal defects and in complex lesions such as single ventricle.

Mustard operation

This is not strictly a corrective operation and many problems are associated with the long-term effect or ability of the right ventricle and tricuspid valve to support the systemic circulation. It is used for transposition of the great arteries. A patch is inserted to route the blood from the superior and inferior venae cavae into the left atrium through the mitral valve. Shrinkage of the patch leads to obstruction of the flow which requires further correction.

Tetralogy of Fallot (Fig. 24.7)

This is a common cyanotic malformation. It consists of infundibular pulmonic stenosis and a large ventricular septal defect, with secondary hypertrophy of the right ventricle and overriding of the aorta.

Pathological physiology

Moderate pulmonary stenosis allows adequate pulmonary flow to maintain near-normal peripheral arterial oxygen saturation for the first months of life. The slightly higher pressure in the left ventricle is balanced by the pulmonary stenosis, so that there is relatively little shunting of blood in either direction through the ventricular defect. As the infant grows, pulmonary flow cannot increase. Right ventricular hypertrophy increases and blood is

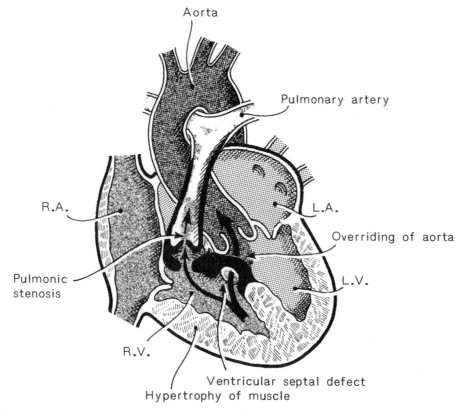

Fig. 24.7 Tetralogy of Fallot

shunted from the right to the left ventricle, producing cyanosis.

There are three clinical groups. Severely affected children get into difficulty early on due to the inadequate blood flow causing severe hypoxia. In the second group cyanosis develops more slowly, by about 2 to 3 years of age. There is limitation of exertion, and fatigue is the main problem. The mildest group can continue with minimal difficulty for some time.

Cyanosis is one of the outstanding features, but may not be present at birth. It is only when the ductus arteriosus closes in the first month of life that cyanosis presents. In infants who appear pink at rest, the first indication of some abnormality is the occurrence of a cyanotic attack. This may occur after crying, defaecation or feeding. The attacks are believed to be due to spasm of the muscle of the infundibulum. Clubbing of the fingers and toes is present by the age of 1 or 2 years. Dyspnoea occurs on exertion. The young child will play actively for a while and then sit or lie down. Older children are able to walk for short distances before stopping to rest. Squatting is a common feature and results in an increase in arterial oxygen saturation which will allow them to resume physical activity. Growth and development may be delayed.

Principles of treatment and nursing management

1. Investigations such as electrocardiography, echocardiography, cardiac catheterisation and straight X-rays, will be carried out. The cardiac catheterisation will reveal systolic hypertension in the right ventricle, while the electrocardiography shows evidence of right ventricular hypertrophy.

    Blood analysis such as red cell count and haematocrit levels will also be ascertained. These tend to be elevated. When the infant is iron-deficient the haemoglobin level may be normal or low but some polycythaemia is present.

2. Treatment of cyanotic attacks:
    a. Cyanotic attacks are believed to be associated with narrowing of the pulmonary artery due to infundibular spasm. The infant should be placed in the knee/elbow position; morphine (0.2 mg/kg) is given and these measures may terminate an attack. Other drugs such as propranolol or metaraminol may be given; the latter increases peripheral vascular resistance.
    b. Oxygen should be given and the acidosis which develops should be corrected by intravenous sodium bicarbonate.

3. Routine nursing care.

4. Providing adequate nourishment. Normal feeding if the infant is not too distressed, otherwise feeds may be given by spoon or by naso-gastric route. It may be desirable to give smaller feeds at more frequent intervals. Whatever method is used, the infant should not be allowed to become exhausted.

5. Careful observations of complications:
    a. Cerebral thrombosis is most common in severely cyanosed infants and young children and may cause hemiplegia. Since the haematocrit value tends to be high it is important that these children should be kept well hydrated to keep the viscosity of the blood within normal levels.
    b. The child may present with headaches, fever and a change in behaviour and this may be followed by vomiting and convulsions. This may be due to cerebral abscess.

6. In the management of the young child it is not necessary to restrict his activity since he tends to do this by squatting when required.

7. Preparation for operation. Routine preparation will be necessary (p. 128). It includes all the investigations mentioned on pages 461–3. The parents must be fully informed and their consent obtained. Since the child will probably initially be nursed in the intensive care unit it is advisable that parents are shown the unit and all the equipment which might be used for their child.

8. The choice of operation and the time it is carried out varies with the clinical severity of the abnormality, the size of the child and the evidence obtained by the various investigations. Some surgeons recommend total correction at all times, though generally it is agreed that palliative surgery should be carried out in the first year of life with total repair sometime before school age. The two usual procedures

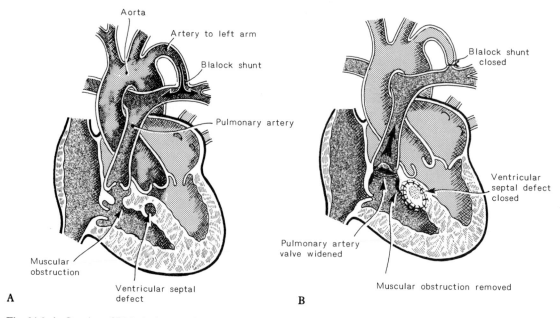

Fig. 24.8 A, Creation of Blalock shunt so that more blood can flow to the lungs. B, Total correction of the tetralogy of Fallot.

are Blalock-Taussig shunt (Fig. 24.8) and Waterston anastomosis (p. 409).

9. Post-operative care. The child requires constant care and this involves the following procedures:
 a. Assisted ventilation (p. 395).
 b. Oxygen administration (p. 382).
 c. Underwater seal drainage (p. 390).
 d. Intravenous infusion (p. 448).
 e. Monitoring of temperature, pulse, blood pressure and central venous pressure.
 f. Naso-gastric or oral feeding.
 g. Mouth and eye care.
 h. Wound care.
 i. Prevention of pressure sores. Since the child will be relatively immobile it is necessary to change his position at intervals. This will not only prevent formation of pressure sores but should also prevent pulmonary oedema.
 j. All routine care.
 k. Observations: recognition of complications:
  (i) Pleural effusion.
  (ii) Cerebral thrombosis.
  (iii) Haemorrhage, e.g. persistent drainage of blood from the drainage tubes.

  (iv) Heart block (this may occur due to injury of the conduction bundle). It may be necessary to implant an inter-pacemaker.
10. Support for parents:
 a. Recognition of anxiety and need to keep them informed of every stage of treatment and progress.
 b. Involvement in care for the child.
 c. Guidance regarding care of the child in the post-operative period.

Anomalous pulmonary venous drainage
Abnormal development of the pulmonary veins may result in their anomalous drainage into the systemic venous circulation. The abnormal entry may be into the right atrium, into the superior vena cava, inferior vena cava or one of their tributaries. The pulmonary veins may join a common trunk which enters the venous circulation via the portal vein, ductus venosus, etc. An atrial septal defect is usually present.

The condition may be partial when some pulmonary veins enter the right atrium, resulting in a left-to right-shunt, or total, when there is no venous connection with the left atrium and all the

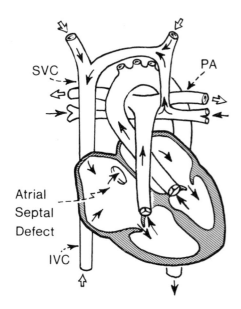

Fig. 24.9 Anomalous pulmonary venous return.
(SVC — superior vena cava; IVC — inferior vena cava;
PA — pulmonary artery.)

blood returning to the heart enters and mixes in the right atrium. Some of the blood passes into the right ventricle and pulmonary artery, the remainder passes through the atrial septal defect into the left ventricle (Fig. 24.9).

Clinical features
Failure to thrive is a common feature. The infant is cyanotic and becomes dyspnoeic on exertion. Congestive cardiac failure occurs early in life. The infant is extremely prone to respiratory infection and clinical signs of pulmonary oedema may be present. The electrocardiogram demonstrates right ventricular hypertrophy and the X-ray shows cardiac enlargement. Cardiac catheterisation reveals that the oxygen concentration is the same in the right atrium, right ventricle, pulmonary artery and femoral artery.

Principles of treatment and nursing management
1. Treatment of cardiac failure (p. 424).
2. Surgical correction must be carried out as soon as possible. The type of correction depends on the anomaly. For example, where the pulmonary veins drain directly into the right atrium, a patch of pericardium or Teflon is used to divert them through the atrial septal defect, which is enlarged if necessary. In some forms a wide, direct anastomosis is made between the confluence of pulmonary veins and the posterior wall of the left atrium. The operation is usually performed with either profound hypothermia or cardiopulmonary bypass.
3. Pre-operative preparation involves investigative measures and routine preparation (p. 128). Since the infant will probably be nursed in the intensive care unit initially, it is advisable that the parents are shown that department prior to the infant's admission to it. It is less traumatic for them if they are aware of the type of equipment used for their child.
4. Post-operative management. This involves both routine and specific care:
   a. Assisted ventilation (p. 395).
   b. Oxygen administration (p. 382).
   c. Underwater seal drainage (p. 390).
   d. Intravenous infusion (p. 448).
   e. Monitoring of temperature, pulse, blood pressure and central venous pressure.
   f. Naso-gastric or oral feeding.
   g. Mouth and eye care.
   h. Wound care.
   i. Routine care which includes pressure area care.
5. Observations and recognition of complications. For example, pulmonary oedema which may require positive pressure ventilatory assistance, haemorrhage, and heart block, which may require an external or internal pacemaker.
6. Support for parents:
   a. Recognition of their anxiety and fears and their need for adequate information.
   b. Encouragement to take part in nursing the child.
   c. Guidance regarding future care and continuous assessment.

Transposition of the great vessels
In the neonatal period this is the most common cyanotic defect in which the pulmonary artery arises from the left ventricle and the aorta arises from the right ventricle. The systemic circulation of oxygenated blood is therefore dependent on the presence of shunts between the two closed systems (Fig. 24.10).

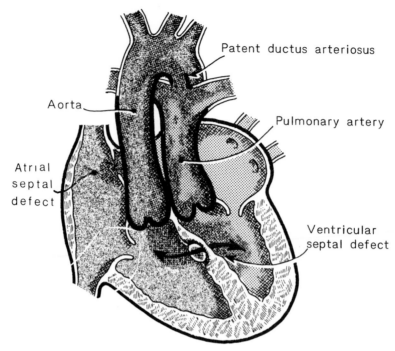

Fig.24.10 Transposition of the great vessels.

Pathological physiology

Most of the blood returned to the right atrium by the venae cavae goes directly into the aorta without being oxygenated. The pulmonary circulation is also largely through a closed circuit with pulmonary venous flow from the lungs returning primarily to the pulmonary artery. Ventricular defects, atrial defects and patent ductus arteriosus are common and produce bidirectional shunting of blood.

Clinical features

Cyanosis becomes progressively more severe soon after birth. Dyspnoea may be present at rest with subcostal recession, particularly during feeding. Clubbing of fingers may develop early in life. Failure to thrive and congestive cardiac failure occur early, frequently in the neonatal period and generally before the age of 4 months.

Investigations

1. Radiology. This shows that the pedicle of the heart is narrow and the heart itself looks like an egg on its side, the pointed part forming the apex of the heart.

2. Electrocardiography. The electrocardiogram shows right ventricular hypertrophy.
3. Cardiac catheterisation. This will reveal the pressure in the left ventricle, while angiograms will exclude the presence of a ventricular septal defect and patent ductus arteriosus. The pulmonary venous blood is usually fully saturated with oxygen but the aortic blood oxygen saturation may be as low as 16 per cent.

Principles of treatment and nursing management

1. Surgical correction. This involves intra-atrial correction (modified Mustard operation), by insertion of either Dacron or pericardium. This directs systemic venous blood to the mitral valve and ventricle and from there via the transposed pulmonary artery to the lungs. Oxygenated blood is pumped from the right ventricle into the aorta. Complications such as heart block and tricuspid valve incompetence, tend to occur.

   Another method used is balloon septostomy which aims at improving the mixing of blood between the two circulations and at lowering

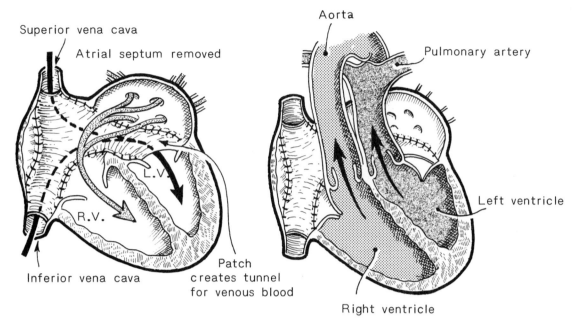

Fig. 24.11 Mustard operation changing the pattern of circulation entering the ventricles. Oxygenated blood flows into the aorta and deoxygenated blood flows into the pulmonary artery.

the left atrial pressure. A Rashkind double-lumen catheter is passed through the foramen ovale into the left atrium. The balloon is filled with radiopaque dye and pulled through the foramen rapidly so as to tear the atrial septum around the foramen. The procedure is repeated until there is no resistance when the balloon is pulled through and both atria have almost equal pressure. This procedure is not without risk and damage may be caused to the tricuspid valve, if the balloon is pulled through it (Figs. 24.11, 24.12 and 24.13).

An alternative operation is called the switch operation. The aorta and pulmonary artery are

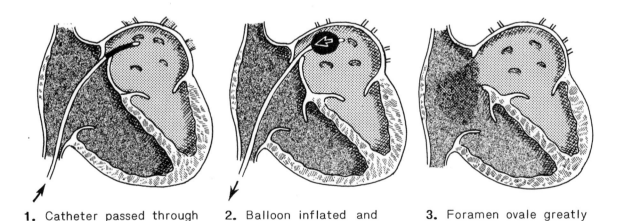

1. Catheter passed through foramen ovale

2. Balloon inflated and pulled through

3. Foramen ovale greatly enlarged

Fig. 24.12 Rashkind procedure. Balloon septostomy to allow a large amount of oxygenated blood to mix with deoxygenated blood.

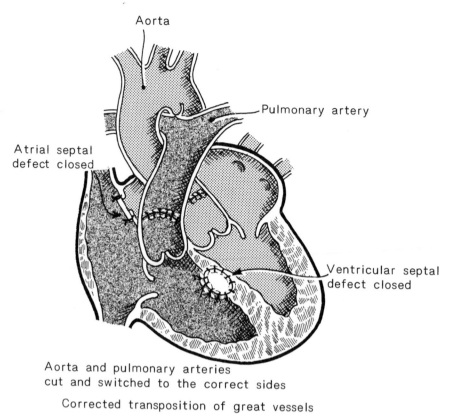

Aorta

Pulmonary artery

Atrial septal
defect closed

Ventricular septal
defect closed

Aorta and pulmonary arteries
cut and switched to the correct sides

Corrected transposition of great vessels

Fig. 24.13 Alternative operation, called the switch operation, for transposition of the great vessels.

cut across, switched to their correct sides and restitched (Fig. 24.13).

2. Pre-operative preparation involves investigative measures and routine preparation (p. 128). The condition must be fully explained to the parents and their consent obtained. Since the infant will be nursed initially in the intensive care unit, the parents should be shown the unit and the type of equipment which might be used.

3. Post-operative management. This involves both routine and specific care and is similar to that described on page 413.

4. Observation and recognition of complications such as pulmonary oedema, haemorrhage and heart block.

5. Support for parents. This includes recognition of their anxiety and a need to involve them in the care of their child. Clear and accurate information should be given regarding the child's present state and possible future developments.

Tricuspid atresia
In this condition the tricuspid orifice is absent and the right ventricle is underdeveloped.

Pathological physiology
There is a basic defect between the right atrium and ventricle, so that all blood entering the right atrium must cross an atrial septal defect, mixing with blood from the pulmonary veins. There are some variations, for example, a patent ductus arteriosus diverts some blood into the lungs or a ventricular septal defect is present which shunts some blood into the pulmonary artery (Fig. 24.14).

Clinical features
The infant is cyanosed from birth with dyspnoea during feeding. He fails to thrive, and there is early clubbing of fingers and periods of unconsciousness occur due to anoxia.

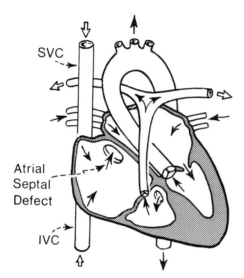

Fig. 24.14 Tricuspid atresia. (SVC — superior vena cava; IVC — inferior vena cava.)

Investigations

1. Radiology. This will show that the heart size is not increased. The vascularity of the lungs is diminished except in a group with a large ventricular defect.
2. Electrocardiography. This shows evidence of left ventricular hypertrophy.
3. Echocardiography. This demonstrates the presence of a single atrio-ventricular valve.
4. Cardiac catheterisation and angiography confirm the anatomical arrangement and demonstrate the size of the pulmonary arteries.

Principles of treatment and nursing management

1. The new-born or young infant whose foramen ovale is small and obstructuve will show some improvement from an atrial septostomy at the time of diagnostic catheterisation.
2. Surgical correction. If the infant is moderately or severely cyanosed, a Blalock-Taussig or Waterston operation will be required. When the pulmonary blood flow is excessive and heart failure occurs, banding of the pulmonary artery may help. A more definitive operation, i.e. Fontan operation, is now possible. In this operation a conduit is placed between the right atrium and pulmonary artery directly. The right atrium is then being used as the pumping chamber.
3. Pre-operative management. This includes both routine and specific. As in all cases of extensive surgical intervention, a full blood analysis is necessary; bacteriological swabs are taken and possibly prophylactic antibiotic cover given (p. 128).
4. Post-operative management (p. 413).
5. Monitoring of vital functions and observations of complications. For example, cardiac failure is associated with increased pulmonary blood flow.
6. Routine nursing care both in the immediate post-operative period and subsequently.
7. Support for parents. This includes recognition of their anxiety and relieving it by encouraging them to care for their child in a limited way. Providing accurate information about the treatment and results, and preparing them for the return home.

Patent ductus arteriosus (Fig. 24.15)
In this condition, the ductus arteriosus which normally becomes obliterated shortly after birth, persists.

Pathological physiology
Aortic blood flows throughout systole and diastole into the lower pressure pulmonary artery, flooding the lungs. The work of both ventricles is increased, but particularly that of the left ventricle which must supply a normal peripheral volume in addition to the shunted amount.

Clinical features
In the majority of cases, there are usually no symptoms in early childhood. When they appear there is slowly progressive exertional dyspnoea, followed by left ventricular failure or congestive cardiac failure. The child may be underdeveloped for his age.

Investigations

1. Radiology. This will show cardiac enlargement, particularly of the left ventricle. The pulmonary artery is of moderate size and there is an increase in the vascularity of the lungs.
2. Electrocardiography. This shows mainly

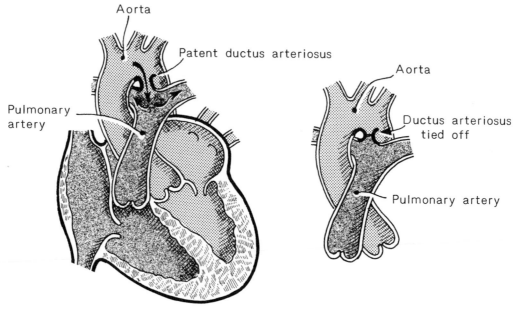

Fig. 24.15 Patent ductus arteriosus.

increased left ventricular activity, but there is also some increase in the right ventricle. However, there will be variations according to the size of ductus.

3. Cardiac catheterisation. This will be necessary if there is a large ductus.

Principles of treatment and nursing management
Surgical closure of the uncomplicated ductus is usually performed as soon as the diagnosis is made, irrespective of the child's age. Spontaneous closure is uncommon except in pre-term babies. However, if the baby exhibits symptoms of heart failure and respiratory distress, then initially attempts are made to control the heart failure.

1. Treatment of heart failure (p. 424).
2. Inhibition of prostaglandin activity by indomethacin. Prostaglandins have been demonstrated in high concentrations in the area of the ductus and are believed to play a part in maintaining the normal patency prior to delivery. If the infant has poor urinary output, hyperbilirubinaemia or bleeding disorder, these are contra-indications to indomethacin.
3. If surgical intervention is recommended then the child will be prepared for theatre as described on pages 128, 156.

4. Post-operative management. This includes care of the child with the following:
   a. Underwater seal drainage (p. 390).
   b. Intravenous infusion (p. 448).
5. Monitoring of vital functions.
6. Observations of complications, e.g. haemothorax, atelectasis and nerve injury.
   The phrenic nerve and laryngeal nerves may be damaged; the former may interfere with the action of the diaphragm.
7. Maintaining nutrition according to the child's age and needs.
8. Routine nursing care, including wound care.
9. Support for parents. As in all cases of serious illness, parental anxiety will be high. Accurate information about the condition and the possible outcome of surgery should be discussed with them. They should be encouraged to participate in the care of their child as far as that is possible. This will also prepare them and give them confidence to care for the child at home.

Coarctation of the aorta (Fig. 24.16).

Pathological physiology
This is an acute narrowing of the aorta near the

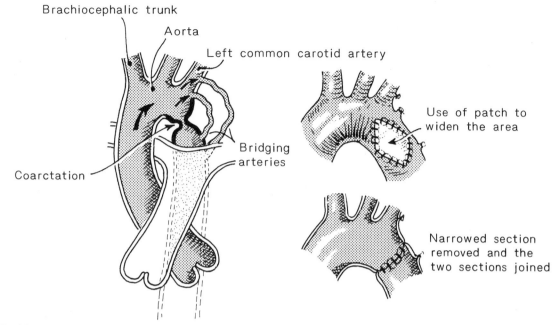

Brachiocephalic trunk

Aorta

Left common carotid artery

Coarctation

Bridging arteries

Use of patch to widen the area

Narrowed section removed and the two sections joined

Fig. 24.16

ductus arteriosus which may fail to close. Narrowing may occur in different positions, e.g. before, at or beyond the duct. The pre-ductal coarctation is not common but, if present, results in venous blood passing from the persistent duct into the distal aorta. Heart failure is likely. If the narrowing occurs at the opening of the duct, a significant lumen remains and the consequences are less severe. When the coarctation occurs beyond the ductus, enlarged accessory vessels feed the distal aorta. In this case symptoms and complications develop mainly in adult life.

Clinical features

Symptoms may appear later in childhood but can develop at any age. They are due to hypertension, decreased myocardial activity or deficient circulation to the legs. There is disparity in pulsation and in blood pressures between arms and legs. The femoral, popliteal and posterior tibial pulses are weak or may be absent, while the pulses of the arms and carotid vessels are full and bounding. Heart failure may be present.

Investigations

1. Radiology. In the new-born there will be a moderately enlarged heart and pulmonary congestion. In the older child the heart may appear normal, but left ventricular enlargement is frequently seen.
2. Electrocardiography. In the new-born, right ventricular hypertrophy is commonly seen, while in the older child the electrocardiography may be normal but, in severe lesions, there may be left ventricular hypertrophy.
3. Cardiac catheterisation, particularly in the new-born infant.

Principles of treatment and nursing management

New-born infant

The infant who is breathless with poor peripheral circulation, may also have oliguria or anuria. He may require ventilating (p. 395). Prostaglandins may be given to keep the ductus open, if possible, to perfuse the lower half of the body. An intravenous infusion will be set up to correct the acidosis. The infant is kept warm but must not be overheated. Any other biochemical imbalance such as hypoglycaemia and hypocalcaemia should be corrected. Surgical repair is performed using a modified operation. The aim is to enlarge the size of the aortic lumen, leaving an elongated scar rather than a circumferential scar. In this method there is less tendency for a stricture to redevelop with the growth of the child. There may be other abnormalities such as a ventricular septal defect, and this can be corrected at a later age.

The older child
Children who are symptom-free usually live a normal life. The discovery of a coarctation may be an incidental finding. Surgery is performed soon after it is diagnosed. Different types of operation are performed: (1) by removal of the narrowed segment and anastomosing the two cut ends; or (2) a patch is sewn into the aorta, which widens the narrowed part; or (3) excising within the aortic lumen and producing a gusset by bringing down the subclavian flap. The incision is a longitudinal one producing an elongated scar in which there is less tendency for a stricture to redevelop with the growth of the child.

1. Pre-operative management includes all the investigations and blood analysis and having the infant in particular in as good a state as possible (p. 156).
2. Post-operative management. This includes routine care of the child with specific care in relation to the following:
   a. Assisted ventilation (p. 395).
   b. Intravenous infusion (p. 448).
   c. Underwater seal drainage (p. 390).
   d. Urinary drainage and accurate fluid balance.
   e. Monitoring of vital functions: temperature, pulse, breathing, central venous pressure and blood pressure.
3. Observations of complications, e.g. haemo-thorax, due to bleeding from the chest wall or from the anastomotic point; abdominal pain, believed to be due to strong pulsatile flow entering the thin-walled arterioles in the mesentery; chylothorax, due to injury to the thoracic duct, when milky fluid is obtained by pleural drainage.
4. Routine and subsequent nursing care.
5. Meeting nutritional needs of the infant and child.
6. Support for parents. This includes recognition of their anxiety; providing accurate and clear information about the condition and any treat-ment given; allowing them to participate in the care of their child and giving them an opportunity to gain confidence in caring for their child in preparation for home care.

Endocardial fibro-elastosis
Two forms can be identified. In the *primary* form, the condition is usually present in the first two years of life. The cause is unknown but it is believed to be associated with infection of the myocardium.

Pathological physiology
The disease affects mainly the left ventricle and, less often, the left atrium. There is a thick, smooth glistening, white endocardium with involvement of the aortic and mitral valves. This leads to incompetence or stenosis.

Clinical features
The infant may be tachypnoeic from birth. Heart failure develops before 2 years of age and is often precipitated by a chest infection. The infant has dyspnoea and there is vomiting and failure to thrive.

Investigations

1. Radiology. This shows an enlarged heart.
2. Electrocardiography will show inverted 'T' waves.
3. Cardiac catheterisation.

Principles of treatment and nursing management

1. Treatment of heart failure. This is achieved by digitalisation (p. 424) and should be continued even if the symptoms disappear.
2. Diuretics may be given. For example, frusemide can be given either intramuscularly or intravenously.
3. Oxygen administration (p. 382).
4. Naso-gastric feeding (p. 512).
5. Placing the infant in a semi-upright position.
6. Measurement of apex heart beat; observation of rate and rhythm.
7. Routine nursing care.
8. Support for parents. This includes recognition of their anxiety and their need for information about the condition and the treatment. Where

possible they should be encouraged to help in the care of the child.

In *secondary* endocardial fibro-elastosis the condition is associated with some congenital heart lesions. For example, in coarctation of the aorta, ventricular septal defects and atrial septal defects.

Investigations
1. Echocardiography. This indicates the size of the shunt.
2. Cardiac catheterisation will show altered valvular function.
3. Electrocardiography. This will indicate myocardial damage.

Pathological physiology
When myocardial disease is associated with an atrial septal defect the raised left atrial pressure increases the left-to-right shunting and severe heart failure occurs.

Clinical features
These will include those associated with the cogenital defect, e.g. coarctation of the aorta, ventricular septal defect and atrial septal defect. Signs of heart failure will be evident (p. 424).

Principles of treatment and nursing management

1. Treatment of heart failure (p. 424).
2. Correction of defect.
3. Bed-rest. Ensure that the child is not isolated and that his physical and emotional needs are satisfied.
4. Oxygen administration.
5. Measurements of vital functions and recording these.
6. Provision of adequate and suitable nutrition.
7. Give support to the parents. Encourage them to participate in the nursing care of their child. Communicate with them and encourage them to express their anxiety.

ACQUIRED HEART DISEASE
The most common cause of acquired heart disease in children is that of acute rheumatism, though heart involvement occurs also in the course of other diseases, e.g. diphtheria, scarlet fever, influenza, poliomyelitis and meningococcal meningitis.

Acute rheumatic heart disease
Acute rheumatic heart disease is the consequence of rheumatic fever. The incidence of rheumatic fever has been decreasing. However, it is still responsible for cardiac changes in a small percentage of children.

The causative organism is the group A beta-haemolytic streptococcus and the mechanism by which it affects the changes is not clearly understood. There is evidence that the cell wall protein of the group A beta-haemolytic streptococcus contains antigens which react with membranes of the cardiac muscle cells and with the muscle coat of small arteries.

Lesions are found in the wall of the left ventricle, the interventricular septum, the mitral and aortic valves, the left atrium and pericardium and in the blood vessels of many organs.

Investigations

1. Radiology. This will show an enlarged heart.
2. Auscultation. A heart murmur will be heard. It can be due to mitral insufficiency.
3. The erythrocyte sedimentation rate is raised.
4. A rising antistreptolysin 0 titre is good evidence of previous streptococcal infection.
5. Electrocardiagraph. Prolongation of the P–R interval is good evidence of rheumatic involvement.

Clinical features
Symptoms occur between 10 to 12 days after streptococcal infection, usually a sore throat. The symptoms of rheumatic fever include polyarthritis, inflammation of the large joints with the pain moving from one joint to another. The child is pale and often sweats freely. Pyrexia may be present. The joints are swollen and warm and movement is painful. Carditis may be present without any joint manifestations, though fever, cough and dyspnoea will be present. Skin rashes often occur, particularly erythema marginatum and occasionally erythema nodosum. Subcutaneous nodules can be felt either over the occiput or on the extensor surfaces of elbows, wrists and fingers.

Principles of treatment and nursing management

1. Bed-rest is advisable but enforced immobility

is not necessary. If the child has painful joints a bed-cage will prevent bedclothes from aggravating the situation. If the child tends to be immobile, then a ripple mattress or sheepskin might help to prevent pressure on dependent areas.

2. Medication. Following throat swabs, benzathine penicillin G 600 000 to 1 200 000 units is given once intramuscularly or oral treatment with 250 to 500 mg penicillin at 8-hourly intervals is given for 10 days. If the child is sensitive to penicillin, erythromycin may be used.

Salicylates are specific in relieving joint pains. A dose of 120 mg/kg per day is given up to a maximum of 8 g/d. High dosage of salicylates can lead to salicylism when the child will complain of tinnitus, deafness, and there will be vomiting, headache and hyperpnoea. These symptoms can be relieved by either reducing the dose or withdrawing the drug. Steroids may be given when carditis is present; they are believed to cause a temporary remission when there is heart failure or complete heart block. Treatment for heart failure (p. 425).

3. Surgery is avoided in childhood because of the rheumatic activity. However, in some centres valve replacement has been performed in children who did not respond to conservative treatment.

4. Routine nursing care. Providing nutrition with emphasis on adequate intake of protein and vitamin C.

5. Measurements of vital functions, in particular of the apex heart beat. The sleeping pulse provides valuable information of cardiac involvement.

6. Educational programme according to the child's physical ability.

7. Graded increase of activity with careful observations of child's condition.

8. Support and guidance for parents. Information regarding the condition and treatment. Recognition of anxiety regarding the effects of the condition and guidance for future care, activity and schooling for the child.

Emphasising the importance of frequent follow-up examinations and the need to maintain antibiotic prophylaxis for at least two years if the child requires dental extractions. This is to prevent subacute bacterial endocarditis caused by the streptococcus viridans.

Acute myocarditis

The myocardium is the contractile tissue of the heart and any interference with its contractile power will reduce cardiac efficiency. Myocarditis is an inflammation or degeneration of the heart muscle, usually secondary to systemic infection. The common causes are beta-haemolytic streptococcal infection, diphtheria, poliomyelitis and other bacterial infections. The condition can occur at any age but appears most often in the first 7 years.

Clinical features

These include fever, anorexia, abdominal pain, cough and dyspnoea. The child becomes progressively ill with pallor and peripheral cyanosis. Tachycardia is out of proportion to the fever and cardiac rhythm is abnormal. In severe cases there is evidence of congestive cardiac failure.

Principles of treatment and nursing management

1. Drugs:
   a. Digitalis (digitalisation can be achieved by oral or intramuscular digoxin) Paediatric Lanoxin elixir 0.08 mg/kg/d may be given in four divided doses. After 24 to 48 hours a maintenance dose of 0.02 mg/kg/d may be given, twice a day (p. 426).
   b. Diuretics, such as chlorothiazide 25 mg/kg/d.
   c. Broad spectrum antibiotic to combat the primary infection.
   d. Corticosteroids may be given if the response to treatment is poor. There are, however, problems of salt and water retention which can aggravate the condition.
   e. Sedation. Restlessness is a common feature in cardiac failure (p. 424).

2. Routine nursing care. This includes:
   a. Administration of oxygen (p. 382).
   b. Feeding problems associated with dyspnoea.
   c. Maintenance of suitable position in bed (p. 110).
   d. Recording of apex heart beat (p. 104).

3. Support for parents:
   a. Recognition of anxiety and need to give adequate information.
   b. Guidance regarding care of the child, e.g. activity, mobility and schooling.
   c. Frequent assessments of the physical condition of the child.

Acute pericarditis

Acute pericarditis is usually associated with other disease processes. Although rheumatic fever is less common, the condition is associated with it and with other collagen diseases such as rheumatoid arthritis. Viruses such as group B Coxsackie, are the causative agents but the condition can occur without any obvious cause.

Inflammation of the pericardium is at times complicated by exudation of fluid into the pericardial sac (pericardial effusion). The fluid may be serous, purulent or haemorrhagic and this complicates congestive cardiac failure.

Clinical features and pathological physiology

Pain may be experienced when the outer surface of the lower part of the parietal pericardium is involved (the visceral pericardium is insensitive to pain). Changing position, e.g. to the sitting position, reduces the pain. Temperature is elevated and marked dyspnoea is present. Blood pressure shows high diastolic reading with a low pulse pressure. The low pulse pressure may be due to reduced left ventricular output due to the unyielding pericardium preventing normal filling of the left ventricle.

Principles of treatment and nursing management

1. If effusion is present, paracentesis may be performed, to remove the fluid. This involves introduction of a needle into the pericardial sac and aspirating the fluid.
2. Drugs:
   a. To treat the underlying cause, e.g. rheumatic fever (p. 421).
   b. To treat cardiac failure (p. 425).
   c. Corticosteroids.
3. Routine nursing care and specific measures:
   a. Position of the child, e.g. upright with head and back support to reduce dyspnoea.

b. Administration of oxygen (p. 382).
c. Observations of pulse variation and drug reactions.
d. Daily weighing, e.g. recognition of oedema.
e. Daily urine tests for protein.
4. Support for parents:
   a. Recognition of anxiety particularly during the acute stage of illness.
   b. Opportunities to participate in the care of the child.
   c. Adequate information about the condition, treatment and progress.
   d. Guidance regarding care at home, amount of activity, schooling and frequent follow-up visits to the outpatient department.
   e. Liaison between hospital, home and community services.

Bacterial endocarditis

This condition is often due to streptococcus viridans, but other organisms such as staphylococci, beta-haemolytic streptococci, etc. can cause the disease. In many instances, the predisposing condition may be rheumatic or congenital heart disease. It may also develop in children after surgical correction of the congenital heart defect.

Pathological physiology

The lesion is usually found on the valve cusps, but other areas can be involved. It consists of vegetation, composed of fibrin, leucocytes and bacteria. Parts of these vegetations can be carried by the bloodstream and may result in embolism in many organs, e.g. lungs, kidneys, brain and spleen.

Clinical features

There is often a history of predisposing heart disease. A child suffering from rheumatic fever might develop low-grade fever and anorexia. However, if the causative organism is streptococcus viridans, the temperature rises to about 39°C, while staphylococcal infection is indicated when the temperature is above 39°C. Pain in the chest, dyspnoea and haematuria may indicate renal embolism.

Principles of treatment and nursing management

1. Drugs. This depends on the causative organism and the result of the sensitivity tests to various antibiotics (see Table 9.2, p. 168).
2. Surgical correction of congenital lesion.
3. Correction of anaemia, if present.
4. Nursing care:
   a. Bed-rest and routine nursing care.
   b. Careful observations of pulse, respiration and colour (pp. 102–104).
   c. Sedation to allay restlessness.
   d. Care of the child during transfusion (p. 453).
   e. Oxygen administration (p. 382).
5. Support for parents:
   a. Adequate information of the condition and treatment of the child.
   b. Participation of nursing care.
   c. Guidance regarding home care, mobility and activity.

Cardiac failure

Heart failure can be defined as a state in which the heart fails to maintain an adequate circulation to satisfy the body's needs despite a satisfactory venous filling pressure. Myocardial function has become so seriously impaired that an adequate cardiac output can no longer be maintained even with the support of compensating mechanisms. These compensating mechanisms include an increased heart rate and an increased force of ventricular contraction in response to increased dilatation of heart chambers. Congestive cardiac failure can occur in both infants and children of all ages. Each will be considered separately.

Cardiac failure in infants

Congestive cardiac failure may be the result of various congenital heart defects and can occur in the early days or weeks of life. These include, amongst others, aortic valve atresia, transposition of the great vessels and ventricular septal defect with pulmonary hypertension.

Clinical features

The main non-cardiological cause of tachypnoea is lower respiratory tract disorders. Other causes can be cerebral abnormalities, acidosis from renal failure and metabolic disorders. Infants in heart failure are tachypnoeic with a breathing rate of more than 60/min at rest. There is intercostal and subcostal recession (p. 371) and the heart rate is greater than 180/min. They have difficulty feeding because they become breathless. Sweating is often seen from increased sympathetic activity to compensate for the reduced blood flow and from their high metabolic rate. Moist chest sounds may be due to infection but may also be due to left ventricular failure. Oedema is a late manifestation of heart failure, but a gain in weight despite poor food intake suggests fluid retention due to heart failure.

Investigations

1. Radiology. This will show an enlarged heart.
2. Electrocardiography. There may be a range of abnormalities depending on the underlying abnormality. An electrocardiogram should be recorded before digitalisation begins and again after 24 hours.

Principles of treatment and nursing management

1. Diuretics are given early. Frusemide is the drug of choice which can be given either intravenously or intramuscularly. The oral route can be used when the infant improves. Potassium loss can be avoided by giving potassium chloride or spironolactone.
2. Rapid and adequate digitalisation is important (p. 426); digoxin (Lanoxin) can be given intramuscularly in the sick infant but is otherwise given orally. Digitalisation is best carried out over 24 hours. The doses for infants/children are shown in Table 24.3.
3. Incubator care. High incubator temperature should be avoided as it increases oxygen requirements.
4. Position. The infant should be propped up.
5. Oxygen administration. If restlessness and cyanosis are present oxygen should be given at a concentration of 30 per cent (p. 382).
6. If the child is restless sedation should be given. Respiratory depressants should be avoided. Phenobarbitone is useful.
7. Feeding. Tube feeding is desirable if the infant is distressed. Clear fluids can be given

Table 24.3 Doses for children undergoing digitalisation

Age of child	Total digitalising dose given over 24 hours		Maintenance dose/24 hours	
	Oral	Intramuscular	Oral	Intramuscular
Pre-term or less than 1 month	0.04 mg/kg	0.03 mg/kg	0.01 mg/kg	0.01 mg/kg
1–24 months	0.06 mg/kg	0.04 mg/kg	0.02 mg/kg	0.015 mg/kg
2–10 years	0.04 mg/kg	0.03 mg/kg	0.01 mg/kg	0.01 mg/kg
After the age of 10, adult doses may be given				

first and, as he improves, milk feeds can be given. If he is able to suck then feeds should be offered by bottle. Prolonged sucking should be avoided and it may be better to offer smaller feeds more often.

8. Prevention of infection is important and any infection should be treated as it arises.
9. Daily weighing to determine retention of fluid.
10. Daily urine tests and accurate fluid intake and output recording.
11. Routine nursing regarding cleanliness and minimal handling (p. 110).
12. Support for parents. This is an anxious time for the parents. Where possible they should be allowed to help in the care of their child. Explanations should be given of the condition and treatment, and guidance given as to future management.

Cardiac failure in the older child

Left heart failure may occur in renal hypertension, aortic stenosis, mitral stenosis and patent ductus arteriosus, though right heart failure is more common. It may be caused by pulmonic stenosis, atrial septal defect, transposition of the great vessels and anomalous pulmonary venous drainage. The most common form of congestive cardiac failure involves both ventricles and is due to myocarditis, paroxysmal tachycardia or to pericarditis. When both sides fail together it is congestive cardiac failure.

Left-sided failure

The essential feature of left-sided heart failure is dyspnoea, i.e. excessive shortness of breath either on exercise or when at rest. The symptoms are due to pulmonary congestion which causes a reduction in pulmonary compliance (p. 367) and, therefore,

increases the muscular effort required to move air in and out of the lungs. Cough is troublesome and haemoptysis may occur due to rupture of congested pulmonary capillaries. pulmonary oedema is a serious complication of left-sided failure. The hydrostatic pressure in the pulmonary capillaries is raised and fluid is forced out into the pulmonary alveoli where oxygen uptake is interfered with. The elimination of carbon dioxide is also impeded but to a lesser extent.

Right-sided failure

This follows left-sided failure and chronic lung disease, but also the conditions mentioned above. In right-sided failure, there is engorgement of the systemic circulation and there is usually oedema of the body. This is partly due to raised venous pressure but also due to retention of salt and water.

Principles of treatment and nursing management

1. Bed-rest is essential with the child in the upright position, supported by pillows. The amount of mobility will depend on the degree of dyspnoea and weakness (p. 110).
2. Oxygen is important and should be given even if dyspnoea and cyanosis are absent.
3. Drugs:
   a. Digitalis (see below) (p. 426).
   b. Diuretics, to accelerate the removal of excess tissue fluids.
   c. Sedatives.
4. Diet. Low sodium, light diet.
5. Routine nursing care which should also include:
   a. Pressure area care, particularly if the child is oedematous and relatively immobile.
   b. Occupational therapy to suit his needs.
   c. Physiotherapy.

6. Support for parents. This should include guidance regarding care of the child both in hospital and at home. Co-operation between hospital, general practitioner, and home, with frequent reassessment. (See below on the social aspects of congenital heart disease.)

The use of digitalis

The most important part of treatment of congestive cardiac failure is rapid and adequate digitalisation. The action of digitalis is as follows:

1. In cardiac failure, it increases the force of the contraction of the myocardium, thereby increasing the cardiac output and decreasing venous pressure.
2. In arrhythmia, digitalis slows the conduction time between atrium and ventricle depresses the atrio-ventricular and sino-atrial node.
3. In atrial fibrillation, it slows the ventricular rate by prolonging the refractory period of the atrio-ventricular node.

Lanoxin (a solution of digoxin) is considered to be a stable solution, which can be measured accurately using the dropper provided. Lanoxin can also be given intramuscularly and intravenously; the latter route should never be used without electrocardiographic control.

When given orally it becomes effective 2 hours after administration and reaches its full effect after about 6 to 8 hours. It is rapidly excreted.

An electrocardiogram should be recorded before digitalisation begins and again after 24 hours. Digitalis must be administered in large doses in order to achieve tissue saturation. If the child is vomiting, the drug should be given intramuscularly. When digitalisation has been achieved, smaller doses will maintain saturation. There is an individual variation in the response to digoxin and the therapeutic dose is very similar to the toxic dose.

Signs of adequate digitalisation are:

1. Decreasing signs of cardiac failure.
2. Slowing of heart rate.

Before the drug is administered, the apex heart beat should be recorded (p. 104). If it is below the acceptable limit, as stipulated by the medical officer, the next dose may be withheld.

Digoxin toxicity. Toxicity is most commonly due to overdosage. Nausea, vomiting and diarrhoea are early symptoms of toxicity, but a cardiac arrhythmia may be the first sign. Paroxysmal atrial tachycardia with atrio-ventricular block may occur and if this is not recognised, atrial or ventricular fibrillation will occur if the digoxin is continued. Other toxic effects may include headache, excitement and disorientation.

Treatment of digitalis intoxication. The digoxin is stopped and this is usually sufficient to reverse the symptoms. It can be restarted after 2 or 3 days, using a lower dosage.

Serum electrolytes are checked. This is particularly important in relation to potassium ion. Digitalis and potassium have antagonistic pharmacological properties. Digitalis toxicity is more likely to occur when the potassium level is decreased. When a diuretic is given there is also a decrease of potassium and to prevent this potassium chloride 125 mg can be given to infants with a larger dose to older children.

Social aspects of congenital heart disease

It is important to recognise the anxieties and difficulties related to heart conditions. The problems of nursing these children, the difficulties in feeding and recurrent infections create a great deal of stress.

Explanations given by the doctor are often not fully understood and the nurse, both in hospital and in the community, should be able to simplify and clarify the situation. In the hospital setting, the nurse in charge should be present during the discussions so that she can interpret any terms used.

The child's general condition will mean that restrictions may be necessary and everyone involved should be aware of what the child can and cannot do. The child is usually able to deal with the physical limitation, e.g. during play he will stop and squat. This allows blood to flow in the aorta and provides oxygenated blood for the tissues. Other children show considerable sympathy and patience for these children.

Schooling. The educational programme should be as normal as possible. Teachers should be informed of the physical limitations of the child, particularly if he attends a normal school.

However, the more debilitated child may be better attending a special school for handicapped children. The local authority is also empowered to provide home tuition for those who cannot attend school, but can be cared for adequately at home.

Shock and peripheral circulatory failure

Shock can be defined as a state in which widespread areas of tissue are being damaged because of nutritive insufficiency. This insufficiency can be due to a defect in cardiac function or due to poor tissue perfusion. If cellular function is not improved, shock becomes irreversible and death will ensue even if the initial cause of shock is corrected.

Clinical features

Early signs of shock are: restlessness, confusion and thirst. The skin is pale, moist and cold. The nailbeds are cyanotic and local and peripheral oedema may occur; tachycardia and tachypnoea are present.

The new-born in shock appears pale and slightly grey, and in later stages there is a decrease in skin temperature, particularly of the extremities and there is a fall in blood pressure.

Causes of shock

Many apparently unrelated types of injury or disease may reduce venous return sufficiently to decrease cardiac output, but decreased cardiac output may be the primary cause. Each condition has its special pattern of disordered function, and basic disturbance indicating (1) deficient blood volume, (2) peripheral vasodilatation or (3) cardiac insufficiency which initiate alteration in body functions and compensatory mechanism which constitute shock and are recognised as the above features.

Principles of treatment and nursing management

The treatment of shock depends on its basic cause, however, the immediate treatment is as follows:

1. The child should lie flat in bed, legs may be elevated provided there is no respiratory difficulty.
2. The upper airway must remain clear and oxygen is administered. If the condition deteriorates it may be necessary to pass an endotracheal tube and to establish intermittent positive pressure breathing (p. 395).
3. Intravenous infusion to correct dehydration (p. 448).
4. Establishment of central venous monitor (p. 459).
5. Monitoring of arterial pressure, blood gases and arterial pH.

A. Hypovolaemic shock

This may be due to loss of whole blood, plasma or extravascular fluid, e.g. burns. Treatment aims to replace the loss:

1. Blood transfusion (p. 453).
2. Plasma replacement. Dextran is a good temporary volume expander and particularly useful when large amounts of plasma have been lost, e.g. in burns.
3. Fluid and electrolyte replacement in dehydration.

B. Cardiogenic shock

Cardiogenic shock is unusual in children. It may, however, occur with myocarditis, sepsis, in renal failure or following cardiac surgery. Outflow obstruction may be seen in congenital heart disease, with a tension pneumothorax or a pericardial effusion.

Bacterial toxins may damage the heart, or it may be damaged by lactic acid formed by the anaerobic metabolism in ischaemic tissues. Uncorrected metabolic acidosis can cause a severe impairment of cardiac function. This produces the vicious circle in which a reduction of cardiac output causes poor perfusion of peripheral tissues. This causes further acidosis and deterioration of cardiac function, which can be fatal.

Abnormal heart rate and rhythm can result in decreased cardiac output. This may occur during anaesthesia. Atrio-ventricular block may occur secondary to surgical trauma or injury to the conduction system. Treatment with prednisolone given intravenously or intramuscularly may be useful.

C. Biochemical disturbances

These interfere with cardiac output, e.g. acidosis, hypoxia and hyperkalaemia. Correction of these states will be necessary, e.g. sodium bicarbonate for acidosis and oxygen for hypoxia.

D. Toxic shock

This may be due to severe infections and circulatory bacterial toxins which result in peripheral collapse. Treatment will depend on treatment for the primary infection, and supporting treatment, such as fluid replacement, corticosteroids and drugs to raise the systolic pressure.

E. Anaphylactic shock

Mild allergic reactions presenting with urticaria are common. A number of allergens are known to cause reactions and these include drugs such as penicillin, local anaesthetics and contrast media for radiological investigations; immune sera, e.g. diphtheria, tetanus; blood transfusion; food allergies and insect stings. Severe systemic anaphylaxis is rare but, when it occurs, requires urgent treatment as it is life-threatening if there is laryngeal oedema, bronchospasm, shock and cardio-respiratory arrest.

Principles of treatment and nursing management

1. An adequate airway must be ensured; intermittent positive pressure ventilation should be given if necessary (p. 395).
2. Oxygen administration (p. 382).
3. Intravenous infusion should be set up (p. 448).
4. Adrenaline must be injected immediately. If the attack is severe it is given intravenously; in less severe attacks the adrenaline can be given subcutaneously. In anaphylactic shock there is extreme peripheral vasodilatation with moderate myocardial depression. Adrenaline will arrest the allergic process and is a peripheral vasoconstrictor as well as having inotropic properties, i.e. it affects the force of muscular contractions. Aminophylline is also given to relieve bronchospasms, if present. Piriton, an antihistamine, and steroids are given to ameliorate symptoms.
5. Constant nursing care must be given and vital functions monitored frequently.
6. Routine nursing care consisting of oral care and general cleanliness.
7. Accurate fluid balance measurements.
8. Support for parents during this anxious period.

It can be seen that the shock syndrome covers every facet of body activity and treatment will depend on the history and clinical features. The causes are wide and varied and the effect on the circulatory system will be in relation to the cause.

Chapter 25
Haematological disorders

The previous chapter discussed the cardiovascular system and the conditions which can affect its efficiency. The purpose of that system is to transport blood, the vital subtance on which the chemical life of the body depends. The materials for those chemical processes are carried to each cell by the blood and those which the cell discards are removed by the blood.

Blood consists of a fluid, the plasma, in which are suspended cells of different kinds adapted for special purposes. It is primarily a medium for the carriage of oxygen, nutrient materials, hormones and antibodies to the tissues. It removes carbon dioxide and other waste products from the tissues and eliminates them from the body.

Blood volume

The total amount of blood varies with age, sex, weight, body build and other factors. There is little variation in the blood volume of a healthy person over long periods, although each component of the blood is in a continuous state of flux.

For the new-born the blood volume is 85 ml/kg of body weight, while for the infant it is 80 ml/kg of body weight. In children, the mean blood volume is about 75 ml/kg of body weight and in adults it is 80 to 85 ml/kg of body weight.

Plasma

Plasma has a faint straw colour and consists of water (90 per cent), protein (fibrinogen, globulin, albumin 9 per cent), salts (0.9 per cent), glucose, urea, uric acid and creatinine, etc. Water is present primarily in order to dissolve the other substances and to give blood a degree of fluidity sufficient to allow it to move easily through the capillaries.

Plasma proteins

Two principal groups of plasma proteins are conventionally recognised: albumin and globulins. The globulin part is further subdivided into alpha, beta and gamma globulins and fibrinogen. Each of these plasma proteins have specific functions:

Albumin. This forms the greatest part of the total plasma proteins and has the lowest molecular weight. It is because of its size as well as its shape, that it passes more easily through the capillary wall than the other plasma proteins. Albumin is believed to be formed in the liver. In diseased liver therefore, less albumin will be found in the plasma. Plasma albumin is also mainly responsible for the osmotic effect of the plasma proteins and by virtue of that effect, fluid is retained in the blood capillaries. Any decrease in the level of plasma albumin leads to oedema. Loss of albumin occurs in diseases such as nephrosis.

Globulin. The globulins vary in size and are mainly produced in the liver, but gamma globulin is formed in the reticulo-endothelial tissue (i.e. group of system of cells found in the spleen, liver, bone marrow and lymph nodes), macrophages and lymphocytes.

The alpha globulins combine with bilirubin and play a part in the carriage of lipids and steroids.

The beta globulins also combine with substances like iron, lipid, steroids, etc. Prothrombin, necessary for clotting of blood, is a beta globulin.

The gamma globulins are the antibodies and are called immunoglobulins. Different types have been identified, each with specific functions (p. 240).

Fibrinogen (Factor I). This plasma protein plays a part in blood clotting. Absence of fibrinogen means that clotting does not occur.

The plasma proteins also act as buffers, that is they maintain acid-base balance by accepting hydrogen ions. They also contribute to the viscosity of the blood and have a transport function in that they combine with many chemical agents, for example, hormones, iron and copper, which are slowly released when required.

Plasma proteins are normally formed from food proteins, but in starvation they are formed from tissue protein. Plasma protein can also be synthesised from amino-acids, provided the 10 essential ones are present. These are as follows: leucine; isoleucine; methionine; phenylalanine; histidine; arginine; lysine; tryptophan; valine and threonine.

BLOOD CELLS

All blood cells have finite life spans and require constant replenishment from the haemopoietic tissues. Haemopoiesis or blood cell formation in the fetus is confined to the yolk sac in the first few weeks of gestation. From 6 weeks until 6 to 7 months of fetal life the liver and spleen are the main organs involved. They continue to produce blood cells until about 2 weeks after birth. However, the bone marrow is the most important site from 6 to 7 months of fetal life. After birth, haemopoiesis is confined to the bone marrow and, by the time of puberty, it normally only occurs in the femoral and humeral heads, and flat bones such as the sternum, ribs and vertebral bodies.

It is believed that a common stem cell gives rise to a series of progenitor cells for three main marrow cell lines, i.e. the erythroid, granulocytes and monocytes, and megakaryocytes.

Red blood corpuscles

Red blood corpuscles are formed in the red bone marrow. At birth all the long bones are filled throughout their length with red bone marrow. With increasing age the marrow becomes more fatty until by the age of about 20 years, only the upper ends of the femur and humerus contain red bone marrow. In the adult, red marrow also persists in bones of the skull, pelvis, vertebrae, sternum and ribs. Children have more red bone marrow than adults. The formed red blood corpuscles enter the bloodstream via the vascular arrangement of the bone. Examination of the bone marrow reveals different types of blood cells at different stages of development and this is also important for diagnostic purposes.

The red blood cell goes through various stages until fully developed. Stages I to III show active mitosis but by stage IV, mitosis has ceased. The fully developed red blood cell is a non-nucleated biconcave disc which contains haemoglobin. It is an elastic cell and can alter its shape when passing through narrow capillaries. This is important in relation to its function. In health, the average diameter is 7.3 μm, though at birth it is larger, approximately 8.4 μm.

Normal red cell count

The newborn infant's red cell count is very high (6 to 7M/mm^3). It falls rapidly in the first two weeks of life to near adult level (5M/mm^3) and maintains a relatively near adult value varying between 4.5 to 5M/mm^3 throughout childhood. The high red cell count is related to the high haemoglobin level in the fetus which falls gradually after birth. The life span of red cells is about 120 days. They then fragment and the fragments are taken up by the reticuloendothelial cells of the liver, spleen and bone marrow. Samples of blood show that both old and young red blood cells are present. This means that the total number is kept constant. In disease, the survival time of the red cells in the body is reduced when either the cells are abnormal or abnormal haemolysins are present.

Control of red blood cell production

Erythropoietic activity is regulated by the hormone erythropoietin, which is produced not only by the juxtaglomerular cells of the kidneys, but also probably by a direct effect of hypoxia on the bone marrow. The stimulus to erythropoietin production is the oxygen tension in the tissues of the kidneys. When anaemia occurs, or haemoglobin is unable to give up oxygen normally, erythropoietin production increases and stimulates erythropoiesis by: (1) increasing the number of stem cells committed to erythropoisis. In the chronic state there is anatomical expansion of erythroid tissue down the long bones and, in infants, the marrow cavity may expand into cortical bone, resulting in bone deformities; (2) increasing haemoglobin synthesis in red cell precursors; (3) decreasing maturation time of red cell precursors; and (4) releasing marrow reticulocytes into peripheral blood at an earlier stage than normal.

The red blood cells are destroyed by the reticulo-endothelial system. Haemoglobin is released, iron and globin are split off and bilirubin is formed. The iron is stored and released into the circulation for haemoglobin formation as and when required. Iron, vitamin B_{12} and folic acid are necessary for the formation of red blood cells. Absence of any of these leads to abnormal red blood cell formation.

Function of the red blood cells

The primary function of the red blood cell is to transport oxygen. Its efficiency as such depends on the quantity of haemoglobin it contains. This function will be interfered with if the haemoglobin level falls or if the volume of the red blood cell is altered. Lack of red blood cells or haemoglobin is called anaemia, while an excessive number of red blood cells is called polycythaemia.

Haemoglobin

Haemoglobin consists of the protein globin combined with the pigment haem. Haem is the iron part ferrous which becomes ferric when it is oxidised. Haemoglobin has the ability to combine loosely and reversibly with oxygen.

The functions of haemoglobin are: (1) it acts as an oxygen carrier and (2) it is partially involved in the transport of carbon dioxide and in the regulation of blood reaction.

Different varieties of haemoglobin occur in man:

1. Fetal haemoglobin (HbF). This type of haemoglobin is important for the fetus, because fetal blood can take up much larger volumes of oxygen than adult blood at low oxygen pressures. For example, at 20 mm oxygen pressure fetal haemoglobin is 70 per cent saturated and at 40 mm oxygen pressure it is 90 per cent saturated. In adults, at 20 mm and 40 mm oxygen pressure, the oxygen saturation is about 20 per cent and 70 per cent respectively.
2. Fetal haemoglobin disappears after 2 to 3 months and HbA (adult type) takes over.
3. Haemoglobin S (HbS) is associated with a severe anaemia called sickle-cell anaemia (p. 439).

Normal levels of haemoglobin. At birth the haemoglobin concentration is 23 g/100 ml and by 1 month it has fallen to about 10.5 g/100 ml which is below that of adult level. The level rises to 12. 5 g/100 ml by 1 year. The normal range in the young baby depends on his birth-weight, and the rate of decrease must be seen in relation to that weight.

One gram of haemoglobin when fully saturated combines with 1.34 ml of oxygen, therefore the haemoglobin concentration gives an indication of the oxygen carrying power of the blood. For example, haemoglobin level is 14.8 g, therefore, the oxygen power is $14.8 \times 1.34 = 19.8$ ml oxygen per 100 ml blood. This is the 100 per cent level. Lack of haemoglobin can occur due to excessive destruction of red blood cells and lack of iron, copper and amino acids, necessary for globin formation.

Blood groups

The membranes of the red cells have on their surface a group of agents that confer blood group specificity (i.e. that differentiate blood cells into groups). Most blood group substances are composed of carbohydrate linked to protein that determines the specific blood type. These substances are antigens capable of inducing the production of antibodies when injected into persons lacking the antigen.

More than 400 antigens can be recognised on the surface of human red blood cells. The more important systems include ABO, Rhesus, MNS and others.

ABO blood group system

Human beings can be divided into four main groups according to the presence or absence in their cells (and in certain tissue cells) of substances called ABO. The antigens A and B may be present singly or together (AB). The absence of both antigens gives group O. These genes are inherited as dominant characteristics, that is, when the gene is present the antigen is expressed. The A antigen is sub-grouped into A_1 and the weaker antigen A_2. Further sub-grouping is found in AB group, i.e. A_1B and A_2B. Naturally-occurring antibodies develop in the ABO system after the age of 3 months.

Blood in group A contains antibodies or agglutinates which, if mixed, will react against the agglutinogens of blood group B. The mixture will then clot. As a result, group A blood clots or agglutinates if given in transfusion to a group B recipient and vice versa. Agglutinin acting on agglutinogen A is called anti-A. Agglutinin acting on agglutinogen B is called anti-B. Group specific substance O does not normally act as an agglutinogen and there is no corresponding agglutinin or anti-O.

The agglutinin is found in the serum. Knowledge of blood groups is important when considering blood transfusions. The effects of transfusing blood of any group into the circulation of a member of another group can be worked out. Account need be taken primarily of the effect of the serum agglutinins of the recipient on the cells of the donor, although there are exceptions to this. If the agglutinins anti-A or anti-B are present in group O plasma in large amounts, they may agglutinate the recipient's cells after transfusion.

Table 25.1 is a table of blood compatibility and shows the effect of agglutinins on donor red blood cells. As a rule, blood selected for transfusion must be of the same ABO type as the recipient. In urgent situations, type O red blood cells may be used for patients of other blood types, or either A or B red blood cells may be used for AB recipients, but not both together.

Before any transfusion is given, however, it is essential that tests are done to determine the compatibility of the recipient and donor bloods. One major reason for this is the existence of the Rhesus (Rh) factors.

Rhesus (Rh) blood groups. The discovery of the Rhesus factors was made when red cells of the

Rhesus monkey were injected into rabbits. The rabbit responded by producing antibodies which agglutinated Rhesus red cells. When immunised rabbit's serum was tested against human red cells, agglutination occurred in 85 per cent of white men. These people were classified at Rhesus positive and their serum contained no Rhesus antibody. No agglutination occurred in 15 per cent and they were classified as Rhesus negative and their serum also contains no Rhesus antibody, except under certain conditions, e.g. when anti-D is induced.

There are several varieties of Rhesus antigen and of Rhesus antibody. The commonest Rhesus antigen is called D and its antibody is called anti-D. Those who possess it are called Rhesus D positive.

Blood group antigens are the result of the action of genes which are present in chromosomes. The gene corresponding to the antigen D is also called D; when D is absent from the chromosome, its place is occupied by the alternative form called d. A Rhesus gene is inherited by both father and mother. If gene D is carried by both sperm and ovum, the offspring is DD; if they carry D and d, the result is Dd and if both carry d, the result is dd. Both DD and Dd are Rhesus positive and dd is Rhesus negative (Fig. 25.1).

In individuals whose red cells contain no D agglutinogens, anti-D agglutinins are not naturally present in the plasma, but anti-D may be induced under the following conditions:

1. Transfusion of a Rhesus negative individual with Rhesus positive blood.
2. The presence of a Rhesus positive fetus in a Rhesus negative mother. (See haemolytic disease of the new-born, p. 437.) Cells from the fetus may pass across the placenta into the maternal blood forming anti-D which in turn destroys fetal red blood cells. Before a blood transfusion is given, it is therefore essential that both Rhesus and ABO tests are carried out.

White blood corpuscles (leucocytes)
The white blood corpuscles are divided into three groups:

1. Granulocytes — these include, neutrophils, eosinophils and basophils.

Table 25.1

Recipient (Agglutinins in serum)	Red cells of donor			
	AB	A	B	O
AB + no agglutinin (O)	−	−	−	−
A + agglutinin B	+	−	+	−
B + agglutinin A	+	+	−	−
O + agglutinins AB	+	+	+	−

+ sign indicates agglutination
− sign indicates no agglutination

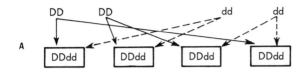

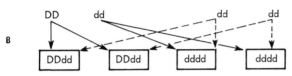

Fig. 25.1 Inheritance of Rhesus factor.
A. DD DD = homozygous Rhesus positive father.
   dd dd   = homozygous Rhesus negative mother.
   (All children are Rhesus positive.)
B. DD dd = heterozygous Rhesus positive father.
   dd dd   = homozygous Rhesus negative mother.
   (Some children are Rhesus negative.)

2. Lymphocytes, large and small types.
3. Monocytes.

White cells contain a variety of substances. For example, granulocytes contain histamine, and lymphocytes contain heparin. The granulocytes are phagocytes, that is they have the power to engulf and ingest foreign particles, such as bacteria. They contain enzymes which are able to dissolve the foreign particules.

Lymphocytes. These are smaller than granulocytes but have a large nucleus. They produce antibodies which react with the antigen of invading microorganisms. An increase in these cells is called lymphocytosis. During infection the lymphocyte count is increased and in leukaemia there may be an increase of lymphocytes due to uncontrolled production of lymphocytes. Some lymphocytes are formed in bone marrow, others in lymph tissue.

Monocytes. These are larger than the two previously mentioned white blood cells. Like the granulocytes, they are phagocytic cells.

White blood cell count
At birth 18 000/mm^3
At 6 months 10 500/mm^3
At 1 year 10 000/mm^3
2 to 12 years 9500 to 8000/mm^3
Adults approximately 7000/mm^3

Platelets
Platelets or thrombocytes are tiny fragments formed from the giant megakaryocytes in the bone marrow. Normally there are about 250 000/mm^3. At birth there are about 350 000/mm^3; these gradually decrease and by 2 years of age there are about 250 000/mm^3.

The functions of the normal platelets are concerned with (1) arrest of bleeding and blood clotting, (2) phagocytosis and (3) storage and transport of substances, such as histamine.

Haemostasis (arrest of bleeding) and blood clotting
Blood is normally fluid while circulating in the blood vessels, but clots when it escapes from the blood vessels. Clotting in the vessels is prevented by the action of enzymes (fibrinolytic enzymes) which rapidly remove any fibrin formed. In addition, plasma may contain a thrombin inactivator and cells of the reticulo-endothelial system may remove small quantities of activated clotting factors.

When a blood vessel is breached, blood escapes, provided the pressure within the vessel is greater than the pressure outside it. When the internal and external pressure becomes equal, bleeding will cease. This can occur if there is an accumulation of blood in the surrounding tissue, if there is a general fall in blood pressure or if there is local vasoconstriction. Bleeding also stops when a solid plug derived from blood forms. This is the most important mechanism and if it is defective bleeding will not stop, as in haemophilia.

The plug is formed initially by platelets collecting at the breach; later fibrin deposition occurs. The fully formed blood clot also contains red blood cells and leucocytes within the fibrin network. The essential reaction in coagulation of the blood is the conversion of the soluble protein fibrinogen into the insoluble protein fibrin by means of the enzyme thrombin. The mechanism is a complex one involving many blood clotting factors, which are mainly enzymes.

At least 12 different plasma components are concerned in the clotting process. These factors have been given the Roman numerals from I to XII. The numbers do not represent numerically the sequence of clotting, but the order in which they were discovered. Most of the factors are synthesised in the liver.

The general pattern of blood clotting is that one

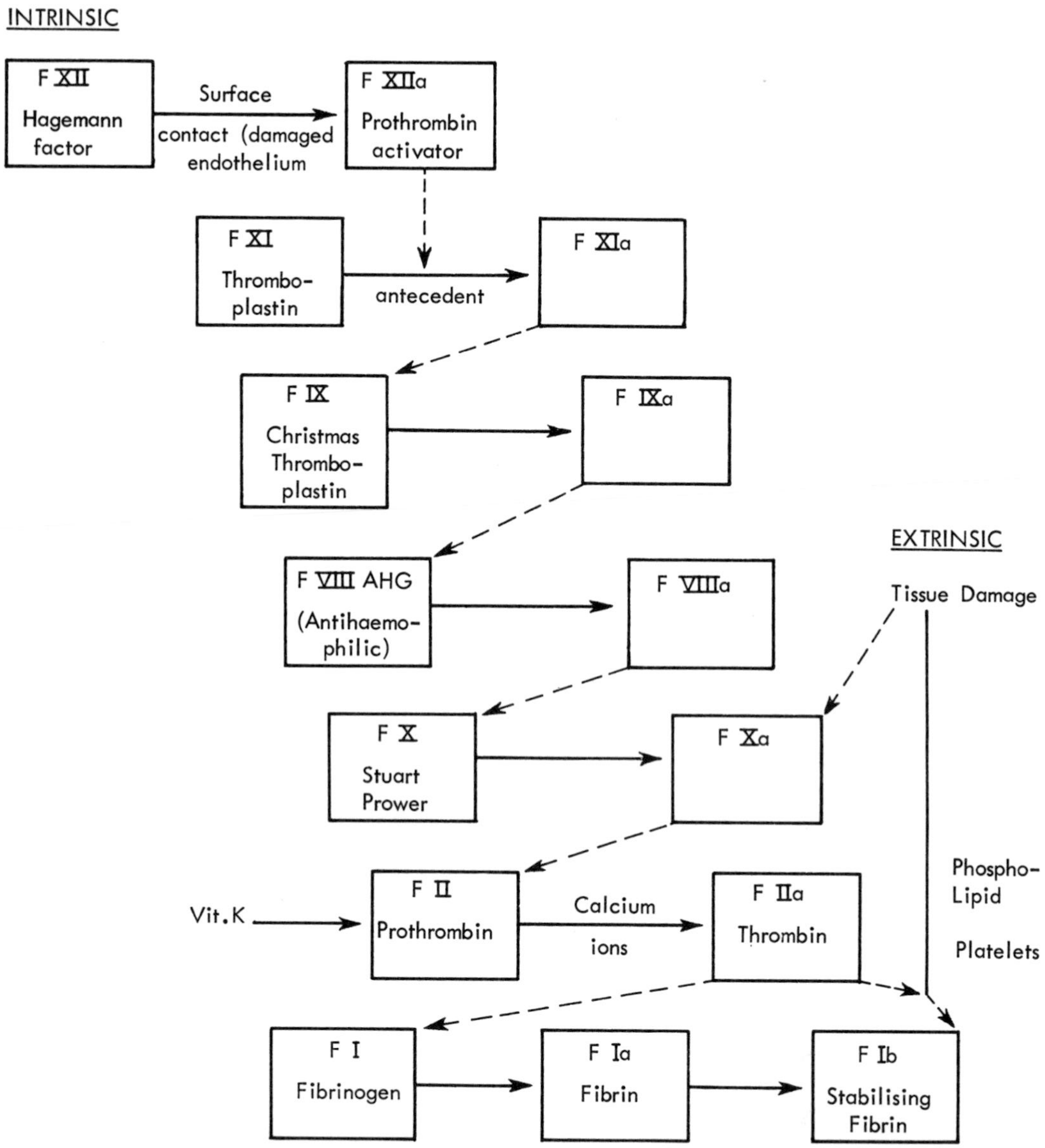

INTRINSIC

Fig. 25.2 Mechanism involved in coagulation of blood.

factor is converted enzymatically into an active form which in turn can activate a factor along the chain.

The clotting mechanism contains two further divisions, intrinsic and extrinsic. The extrinsic division joins the intrinsic at the Factor X stage. The intrinsic mechanism involves factors which are found in the plasma; the extrinsic mechanism depends on damaged tissue which liberates Factor III (tissue factor) which, in the presence of Factor VII activates Factor X. It is a faster system than the intrinsic one. Calcium ions (Factor IV) are involved at several points in both intrinsic and extrinsic clotting mechanisms (Fig. 25.2).

Diseases of the blood

Diseases of the blood involve most of the constituent parts of the blood. Each disease presents with specific features, including problems with the number of blood cells and structural variations which affect cell function. Diseases of the following blood constituents will be discussed below: red blood cells; white blood cells, platelets and plasma proteins.

THE ANAEMIAS

This is the general term to describe the illnesses associated with a reduced level of circulating haemoglobin. Anaemia may be the result of a number of causes — blood loss, excessive destruction of red cells, lack of iron — to name a few of the major ones.

Iron-deficiency anaemia

This is the most common of the anaemias. Iron is a necessary element in the formation of haemoglobin, therefore deficiency of iron will influence the amount of haemoglobin available. (See p. 431 regarding the function of haemoglobin.)

Several factors can result in iron-deficiency anaemia. In the infant it has been found to be due to prolonged milk feeding, both human and cow's. The full-term infant is born with a small store of iron which, when used up, is not readily replaced. Milk does not contain adequate amounts of iron, therefore, replacement from that source is inadequate particularly in the first 5 months. The rapid growth rate of the infant also means a proportional increase in haemoglobin mass. The smaller the infant, the greater the growth rate, and therefore the increase in haemoglobin mass is correspondingly larger.

Absorption of iron is also low and therefore the store of iron is quickly depleted. In addition, any blood loss in the neonatal period may be from the umbilical cord, or may be due to haemorrhagic disease of the newborn. Infection further aggravates the anaemia.

In the older child from about 10 months onwards, there may be anaemia due to inadequate diet and anaemia of steatorrhoea due to malabsorption.

Clinical features

Pallor may be the only early sign. The child tires easily and is listless; weakness and irritability appear later. If severe anaemia is long-standing it will interfere with growth. There may also be heart murmurs and enlargement of the spleen.

Iron is necessary for blood formation, and in particular, haemoglobin. When iron is deficient, the red blood cells are hypochromic microcytic and there may be a reduction in the number of red blood cells.

Principles of treatment and nursing management

1. Iron is the specific therapy and is given orally. In most cases the anaemia can be corrected at the rate of 1 per cent Hb per day. It may be given as ferrous gluconate in tablet form, as a syrup or as ferrous sulphate. Iron may also be given intramuscularly as Imferon, an iron-dextran complex. If the severely anaemic child suffers an infection, a blood transfusion would be given to raise the haemoglobin level rapidly.
2. Provision of an adequate dietary iron. Good sources of iron include liver (though children often do not like liver), meat, peas and eggs.
3. Treatment of infection and elimination of any underlying defect.
4. Routine nursing care related to the age of the child.
5. Guidance to parents if the treatment is to be continued at home. This should also include advice regarding the child's nutritional needs.

Hypoplastic anaemia

Congenital hypoplastic anaemia is associated with decreased haemoglobin, reticulocytes and occasionally white blood cells. The bone marrow shows deficiency of erythroblasts and it is believed that this form of pure red cells anaemia is a genetically transmitted condition in which there is a defect in red blood cell formation.

Bone marrow depression can also develop if large doses of chloramphenicol are given, though in some instances, permanent and potentially fatal aplastic anaemia may occur even after small doses.

Clinical features

Pallor is a presenting feature. Irritability is marked when the anaemia is severe.

Principles of treatment and nursing management

1. Treatment is based on bone marrow examination and blood analysis.

2. Blood transfusions are given when required.
3. Drugs:
   a. Corticosteroids such as prednisolone is usually given and in some cases, the response is good.
   b. Desferrioxamine, the iron-chelating agent is given with each transfusion and intramuscularly between transfusions. This is given to delay the development of haemosiderosis with the typical appearance of muddy, bronze skin pigmentation.
4. Routine nursing care.

Aplastic anaemia

Aplastic anaemia can be defined as a 'physiological and anatomical failure of the bone marrow which leads to a marked decrease or absence of blood forming elements in the marrow'. It is characterised by reduced red cell production due to replacement of the red cell production element in the marrow by hypocellular fatty tissue. It may also affect megakaryocytes leading to neutropenia and thrombocytopenia. The aplastic state may be contitutional (hereditary) or acquired.

Constitutional. This is also termed Fanconi's aplastic anaemia and it is considered that the inheritance is autosomal recessive. The chromosome shows structural abnormalities which include chromatid exchanges and breaks. It is often associated with other physical abnormalities, e.g. skeletal deformities, abnormal pigmentation.

Acquired aplastic anaemia. This form can be associated with exposure to infection or can be related to some specific toxic substance or have no specific cause and is said to be 'idiopathic'. Drugs such as 6-mercaptopurine and methotrexate cause marrow depression but this can be reversed once the drug is stopped. Chloramphenicol is a well-known causative agent.

Investigations

1. Blood analysis.
2. Bone marrow aspiration (p. 457).

Clinical features

The features usually appear in boys between 4 and 7 years of age and in girls between 6 and 10 years of age. There are however, some reported cases of infants and 2-year-old children when purpura may be present.

Pallor, purpura and haemorrhage are features and there is greater susceptibility to infection. Other associated abnormalities such as hypigmentation of the genitals, nipples and upper trunk, etc. are found in Fanconi's syndrome. The second type is similar but the age incidence is 3 to 7 years.

Principles of treatment and nursing management

1. Blood transfusion (p. 453).
2. Antibiotics to combat infection.
3. Prevention of cross-infection and early recognition of infection. (See reverse barrier nursing p. 250.)
4. Drugs. Specific therapy with androgens and corticosteroids. (Androgens encourage protein anabolism and growth, however, there are side-effects, e.g. hirsutism, deepening of voice etc.)
5. Marrow transplanation in acquired aplastic anaemia (problem of graft rejection).
6. Routine nursing care.
7. Support for parents. Recognition of anxiety and need to give clear and adequate information about the condition, treatment and progress. Opportunities to participate in nursing the child and guidance for home care.

HAEMOLYTIC ANAEMIAS

'Haemolysis' means disintegration of red blood cells. Hence this type of anaemia occurs when red blood cells are lost from the body faster than they can be replaced by the bone marrow. In childhood haemolytic anaemia may be due to (1) congenital defects in the production of red blood cells, or haemoglobin or both, e.g. hereditary spherocytosis, thalassaemia and haemoglobinopathies; (2) acquired defects in the red blood cells or their environment, e.g. due to the toxic substances (physical and chemical agents), infections, radiation, specific antigen-antibody reactions, etc.

Hereditary spherocytosis (acholuric jaundice)

This condition is inherited as a Mendelian dominant and is characterised by the presence in the peripheral blood of erythrocytes which are both smaller in diameter than normal erythrocytes and, at the same time, more spherical. The basic defect in this condition seems to be abnormal permeability of the cell membrance to sodium ions, with the result that the cells become swollen by excess intracellular fluid and electrolytes. The cells are abnormally fragile when exposed to hypotonic saline. This is an important diagnostic test. The major part of haemolysin of the abnormal red cells takes place in the spleen.

Clinical features
This disease does not present quite so readily in the neonatal period, though it can cause haemolytic jaundice. It appears more commonly during later childhood with pallor and lassitude. Jaundice and highly-coloured urine are not often present, but the spleen is enlarged.

Investigations

1. Coomb's test.
2. Bone marrow aspiration (p. 457).
3. Blood analysis.

Principles of treatment and nursing management

1. For the young infant, blood transfusions are given and folic acid is given until a splenectomy can be performed. Splenectomy does not affect the underlying defect but most patients have complete remission from the haemolysis and anaemia.
2. Splenectomy:
   a. Pre-operative preparation, routine and includes, preparation for blood transfusion (p. 128).
   b. Post-operative care, routine (p. 131).
3. Nursing care:
   a. Routine.
   b. Preparation for bone marrow aspiration and care during and after the procedure (p. 457).
   c. Care of the child receiving blood (p. 453).
4. Support for the parents. Recognition of their anxieties and the need to give full information and guidance about the condition, treatment and care of the child.

ABO haemolytic disease of the new-born
(erythroblastosis fetalis)
Jaundice in the neonate can be due to a number of causes, e.g. Rhesus disease, congenital infection, vitamin E deficiency in pre-term infants, etc. In some babies jaundice is due to ABO incompatibility produced by maternal antibodies.

Pathological physiology
The fetus possesses an A or B antigen which is absent in the mother, while the mother's serum contains anti-A or anti-B agglutinins. It has also been found that the ABO haemolytic disease affects those infants whose mother's blood group is 'O'. The bilirubin level is raised and when it reaches 350μmol/l, then complications appear.

Toxicity of bilirubin
Bilirubin interferes with cellular metabolism by uncoupling oxidative phosphorylation (an energy mechanism concerned with the formation of water in the cell) and inhibiting haem synthesis. The degree of cell damage depends on the concentration of bilirubin in the interstitial fluid. Fat cells tolerate bilirubin better than brain cells and may be due to the slower metabolism of fat cells. Liver damage may be partly due to bilirubin.

Clinical features
Jaundice occurs within 24 hours of life, but may appear later in mild forms of the disease. The condition is not confined to second or subsequent pregnancies as in the case of Rhesus disease, but also affects the first-born.

Sufficiently large bilirubin accumulation may result in brain damage due to deposition of bilirubin in the basal ganglia and brain stem nuclei (kernicterus). Early symptoms of kernicterus in term infants are lethargy, poor feeding and vomiting; opisthotonos, upward deviation of the eyes, convulsions and death may follow. Later in childhood, survivors may manifest the typical late triad of choreo-athetotic cerebral palsy and sensorineural hearing loss. There may be perceptual-motor handicaps and learning disorders.

Principles of treatment and nursing management
The treatment depends on the gestational age of baby and the bilirubin level:

1. Exchange transfusion (p. 454). This will be indicated when the bilirubin level is high and

to prevent it rising to higher dangerous levels, and when the haemoglobin level is low.

2. Phenobarbitone therapy. Phenobarbitone influences the metabolism of bilirubin in the liver by causing enzyme induction of glucoronyl transferase and related enzymes concerned with bilirubin excretion. Phenobarbitone administered to the mother for 2 weeks before the delivery of the baby, or to the infant after birth, results in lowering of the serum bilirubin level. However, phenobarbitone causes depression and drowsiness and other enzyme-inducing drugs are currently being tested.

3. Phototherapy. Exposure of the jaundiced infant to light from the blue-violet and yellow-green parts of the spectrum causes progressive photo-oxidation of fat-soluble bilirubin, first to biliverdin, and then to a series of water-soluble derivatives which are excreted in the bile and urine. Although this treatment is considered effective, there are some complications associated with it. These include:
   a. Red cell damage.
   b. Severe anaemia.
   c. Development of kernicterus in sick, pre-term infants.
   d. Damage of the retina.

   The infant is nursed in an incubator with his eyes covered to prevent damage to the retina. It is also possible to use a special shield between the light source and the infant to prevent ultra-violet rays passing through. The blindfold can be achieved by placing a non-irritant material on the eyes and holding the pads in position with a 'tubegauz' hood. Phototherapy may be given continuously or intermittently, for a minimum of 12 hours at varying light intensities. When feeding the infant, the light should be switched off and the blindfold removed. The light should also be switched off when blood is taken for bilirubin determination, since the bilirubin in the syringe and collecting tubes may photooxidise rapidly.

4. Routine nursing care.

5. Support for parents. The infant is probably admitted soon after birth and the mother may not see her child until she leaves the maternity hospital. The condition must be explained to both parents and every opportunity given to them to nurse the infant. This is important so that 'bonding' can develop and mother and infant begin to build that close relationship so necessary for both.

Haemoglobinopathies

In this type of haemolytic anaemia the primary defect is in haemoglobin synthesis, in which the erythrocytes are abnormally prone to haemolysis. The most important of these conditions are thalassaemia (Mediterranean anaemia) and sickle cell anaemia.

Thalassaemia (Cooley's anaemia)

Thalassaemia is a relatively common anaemia in persons of Mediterranean stock, particularly those from Italy, Sicily, Cyprus and Greece.

The primary defect is a genetically determined quantitative defect of haemoglobin synthesis, i.e. impaired production of certain globin chains in particular, the beta chain, though the alpha chain can also be affected. The condition may be either homozygous (alpha chain thalassaemia) which is lethal *in utero*, causing hydrops fetalis, or heterozygous (beta chain thalassaemia) which is a relatively benign condition.

Clinical features

Major form (homozygous). Both parents are carriers of the 'trait'. The symptoms present in the first year of life and are secondary to the anaemia; jaundice of varying degrees is present and the spleen and liver are enlarged. Pathological fractures and skeletal changes occur. The child has a mongoloid appearance due to the thickening of the facial bones. The facial bone changes are due to long-standing hyperplasia of the bone marrow.

Principles of treatment and nursing management

1. Repeated blood transfusions whenever the haemoglobin levels falls below 6 g/100 ml (p. 453).
2. Splenectomy when the spleen becomes so large as to produce discomfort.
3. Routine nursing care and specific care in relation to the treatment, e.g. care of the child having a blood transfusion. Most of the affected children die before reaching adulthood and

each episode will bring its nursing problems until terminal care is reached.

4. Support for parents. Frequent admissions to hospital and blood transfusions create anxiety and tension within the family. Sympathy and understanding of their problems are necessary and guidance should be given regarding the care of the child. Parents should be encouraged to participate in every aspect of care.

Children with thalassaemia major require repeated blood transfusions which lead to iron overload. To remove this excess iron, desferrioxamine is given either intramuscularly or intra-venously. This method is now being replaced by a subcutaneous battery-operated micropump infusion. The treatment is given at home by the parents who have received training and are competent to perform this procedure.

A butterfly needle is inserted deep into the subcutaneous tissue of the anterior abdominal wall or the thigh and is held in position with Micropore adhesive (Fig. 25.3). The motorised infusion unit is held in a special bag and the syringe is attached to the syringe driver. The calculated dose is injected over a period of 6 to 8 hours, the flow being controlled by the regulator or rate setter on the syringe driver. Care should be taken to ensure that the 9 volt battery is functioning before commencing the treatment.

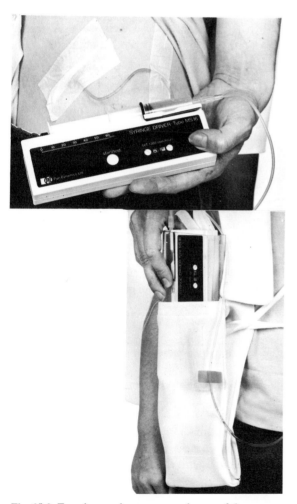

Fig. 25.3 *Top,* shows subcutaneous anchorage of the butterfly needle and syringe driver attachment. *Bottom,* shows the carrier for the syringe driver used during subcutaneous administration of desferrioxamine.

Sickle cell disease

In this condition the red blood cells contain an abnormal form of haemoglobin (HbS) with abnormal beta chains. As a result, they take on bizarre shapes (sickling) when their oxygen tension is reduced. This change of shape is due to a physio-chemical change in the haemoglobin molecule. This renders the cell abnormally liable to destruction in the spleen. The sickled cells become impacted in the capillaries, particularly organs where the oxygen tension is low. This leads to infarction in various organs like the spleen, intestine, bones, kidneys, heart, lungs and brain. The condition is interesting in that people having the sickle cell trait are not affected by the falci-parum malaria.

Clinical features

Sickle cell anaemia often presents in the first year of life with pallor, listlessness and mild jaundice. In some cases there is fever, headache, joint involvement, abdominal pain and tenderness, convulsions or meningism and localised paralysis. Nutrition is affected and there is interference with growth and development.

Principles of treatment and nursing management

1. There is no specific treatment and severe anaemia requires blood transfusions.
2. Pain is relieved with analgesics and rest in bed is essential.

3. Infections are treated when they occur with a suitable antibiotic.
4. Dehydration and acidosis is corrected.
5. Nursing care is aimed at careful observations, relief of pain and discomfort; care of the child with a blood transfusion (p. 453) and maintenence of fluid chart. A ripple bed might ease the pressure on the painful joints.
6. Routine nursing care.
7. Support for parents. Recognition of their problems and need to give support during acute episodes. Guidance regarding care of the child at home.

HAEMORRHAGIC STATES
Clinical haemorrhagic states may be due to:

1. Defective clotting mechanism.
2. Defective capillary contractility.

The condition may manifest itself either as excessive and/or prolonged bleeding from relatively minor trauma or as spontaneous haemorrhage into the skin or internal organs.

THE PURPURAS
In these conditions there is a tendency to spontaneous haemorrhages, usually beneath the skin, from various mucous membranes and in internal organs. Purpura is a common clinical phenomena in childhood and is due to a number of conditions.

The principal pathological factors are capillary defects and thrombocytopenia, sometimes both being present. In most cases the purpura is symptomatic of another disease. It is due to decreased capillary resistance in acute infections such as menigococcal (and other) meningitis, septicaemia, bacterial endocarditis, etc. It can also be present in scurvy, uraemia and snake-bite.

Purpura in the new-born
The main causes of purpura are: trauma, maternal thrombocytopenia, haemolytic disease, septicaemia, syphilis, toxoplasmosis, galactosaemia, etc. Petechiae occur particularly after severe anoxia, and are found especially over the head, neck and shoulders. Retinal haemorrhages are found in many newborn babies, particularly those born by vacuum extraction.

Henoch-Schoenlein purpura (anaphylactoid)
This condition is associated with infection. In most cases there is a history of a preceding sore throat or respiratory infection. In some cases it is possible to identify the beta-haemolytic streptococcus, but in the majority of cases, no organism is isolated and it is believed that a virus antigen-antibody reaction is present. Bleeding and clotting time, platelet count and capillary fragility tests are normal.

Clinical features
There are commonly petechiae on the extensor surface of the limbs and around the buttocks. It is frequently associated with effusion into joints and with abdominal pain. There is often bleeding from the bowel. It is often complicated with nephritis and haematuria.

The rash appears first as small separate urticarial lesions both visible and palpable. These soon become dusky red or frankly purpuric and do not fade on pressure.

Principles of treatment and nursing management

1. There is no specific treatment, but if the beta-haemolytic strepococcus is isolated, penicillin is given.
2. If it is due to glomerulo-nephritis, the relevant treatment is given (p. 532).
3. Severe abdominal pain is relieved with a pain-relieving drug, e.g. morphine.
4. Routine nursing care.
5. Specific care:
   a. Bed-rest.
   b. Daily specimen of urine (protein and blood).
   c. Accurate fluid charting (intake and output).
   d. Ripple mattress and cage to keep bedclothes off the child's limbs.
   e. Observations of evidence of bleeding from the intestines or kidneys.
   f. Diet suitable for the condition, e.g. fluids or light diet.
6. Support for parents. Understanding of their anxiety; need to give guidance regarding care of the child in hospital and at home.

Thrombocytopenic purpura

Idiopathic thrombocytopenic purpura is the most common type in childhood. It is associated with mucocutaneous bleeding and haemorrhages into tissues. There is a deficiency of circulating platelets, though there are adequate numbers of megakaryocytes in the marrow.

The disease often appears to be related to sensitisation by viral infections. For example, diseases such as rubella, or viral respiratory infection precedes the appearance of purpura. It is believed that an immune mechanism is involved.

Clinical features

The onset is frequently acute either following an infection or without antecedent illness. Bruising and generalised petechiae occur. Haemorrhages in mucous membranes may be prominent and nosebleeds are often severe and difficult to control. The most serious complication is intracranial haemorrhage. Although there may be considerable internal bleeding, the child does not feel ill.

Investigations

1. Blood count, e.g. platelet count may be below 40 000/mm³.
2. Bleeding time, e.g. platelet deficiency causes prolongation of bleeding time.
3. Clotting time: this is usually normal.
4. Bone marrow puncture (p. 457).

Principles of treatment and nursing management

1. Transfusion of platelets concentrate when there is bleeding into the central nervous system (p. 453).
2. Steroid therapy and blood transfusion to achieve remission.
3. Routine nursing care.
4. Specific nursing care.
   a. Prevention of trauma.
   b. Bed-rest during the petechial stage.
   c. Observations of fresh bruises, epistaxis, and signs of internal bleeding.
5. Splenectomy. This may be necessary in some children where medical treatment has not produced any improvement or where there is deterioration in the condition. However, it is contra-indicated if the number of megakaryocytes in the bone marrow is decreased.
6. Pre-operative preparation (p. 128):
   a. Routine.
   b. Blood transfusion (p. 453).
7. Post-operative care:
   a. Routine (p. 131).
   b. Observations of vital signs, e.g. blood pressure.
   c. Continuation of blood transfusion. (Care of child, see p. 453).
8. When splenectomy has failed, as in chronic thrombocytopenia, immunosuppressive therapy with azathioprine 3 to 6 mg/kg/d may be of value.
9. Support for parents. This is an anxious time for the parents and they should be kept informed of the treatment and response to the treatment. Guidance should be given during home care so that they know what features to expect and what action to take. Full co-operation between hospital, general practitioner and home is essential and arrangements may have to be made for special schooling.

BLOOD CLOTTING DEFECTS

Deficiency of plasma clotting factors

Bleeding from this cause may occur as a genetically determined deficiency of a single factor. The factors include the following: haemophilia (Factor VIII), Christmas disease (Factor IX) and vitamin K deficiency (found in liver disease).

Vitamin K deficiency

Pathological physiology

Vitamin K is a fat-soluble vitamin and its deficiency leads to a lack of other factors produced in the liver. Factor VII is the first to be affected, followed by Factors II, IX, and X. Malabsorption of vitamin K is the cause, but it can also occur in the new-born, when the deficiency arises partly from metabolic immaturity of the baby's liver and partly from the fact that the intestinal bacteria, which synthesise some of the body's vitamin K, have not yet become established. This leads to haemorrhagic disease of the new-born.

Clinical features

The presenting sign is bleeding but it varies in severity. The infant may pass frank blood per rectum or may pass melaena. He looks pale with signs of shock. There may also be haematemesis, vaginal bleeding, bleeding from the umbilicus and from the skin.

Investigations

1. Blood analysis.

Principles of treatment and nursing management

1. Intramuscular or intravenous administration of vitamin K_1 (phytomenadione 2 to 5 mg).
2. Where blood loss is excessive, a blood transfusion of fresh blood is given.
3. Routine nursing care.
4. Specific nursing care:
   a. Incubator care (p. 181).
   b. Care of the infant during blood transfusion (p. 453).
   c. Observations of bleeding.
   d. Preventation of infection.
5. Support for parents. Full explanation should be given about the condition and the infant kept under medical supervision, i.e. follow-up visits will be necessary. Parent participation is desirable.

Haemophilia

Pathological physiology

Haemophilia is a recessive, sex-linked, genetically determined condition (Fig. 25.4) in which there is deficiency of Factor VIII, the anti-haemophilic globulin. Only males are clinically affected, but females may act as carriers. However, it is theoretically possible that the union of a haemophilic male and a carrier female can give rise to children, of whom one in four is a haemophilic female. It was previously thought that this gene combination was lethal, but a few cases of true female haemophilia have now been recognised. Generally, the children of a normal male and a carrier female are on average 50 per cent normal, 55 per cent carrier females and 25 per cent haemophilic males.

The children of a haemophilic male and a normal female are 50 per cent normal males and 50 per cent carrier females.

Investigations

1. Clotting time, which will be prolonged (normal clotting time is 5 to 10 minutes).
2. Thromboplastin generation test (may reveal inefficient formation of thromboplastin due to lack of anti-haemophilic globulin).

Clinical features

These vary greatly in severity and many cases are mild. Bleeding is common from nasal or oral mucous membranes or from lacerated or damaged tissues. Bleeding occurs in the joints, where it may penetrate the capsule and spread widely, or in the genito-urinary tract, skin and muscles. There may be dangerous and persistent bleeding after circumcision, or tonsillectomy if these operations are performed before the diagnosis has been made. A blow may result in a massive haematoma on any part of the body and repeated haemarthroses may lead to crippling.

Principles of treatment and nursing management

1. Arrest of bleeding. This is achieved by increasing the concentration of anti-haemophilic globin, which is lacking. A rapid transfusion of fresh blood or freeze-dried fresh plasma is given and repeated frequently to maintain haemostasis. Another method of treatment is by the use of 'cryoprecipitate' (p. 449).
2. Arrest of local bleeding, e.g. tooth socket or laceration of skin. Sutures should be avoided and a pressure bandage can be applied. Powdered thrombin is the haemostatic agent which is applied to minor wounds. A venesection must never be performed and the femoral and jugular veins should never be used for venepuncture.

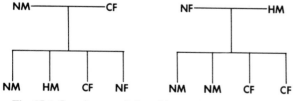

Fig. 25.4 Genetic transmission of haemophilia.

3. Treatment of haemarthroses. In addition to the treatment mentioned, bed-rest and temporary immobilisation is important, using a plastic or plaster back slab.
4. Sedation and analgesics may be given for relief of pain.
5. Routine nursing care.
6. Specific nursing care:
   a. Gentle handling is essential while he has swollen and painful joints.
   b. Care of the child while receiving transfusions (p. 453).
   c. Prevention of injury during ward activity.
   d. Observation of further episodes of bleeding.
7. Support for parents. It is important that both the parents and the child should recognise the limitations which this condition imposes and to organise the child's life in such a way that minor injuries are less likely to occur. He should, however, be encouraged to lead as normal a life as possible. The school authority must be informed of the child's condition and guidance given on the action to be taken, should bleeding occur. The child should also wear an identity disc indicating that he is suffering from haemophilia. Special facilities for holidays may be available so that the child can enjoy activity with other children under supervision.

Advice should be given to the parents on the type of toys to give to the young child, e.g. soft, cuddly toys without any sharp parts. Cooperation between hospital and home is essential and episodes of bleeding should be treated without delay.

Treatment can also be given at home with close liaison between home and hospital. Older children may be trained to give themselves Factor VIII intravenously, and for younger children, parents may be trained to give the injection. This is usually performed twice a week. A nursing member of the haematological team visits the home to provide help and give support.

There are two other diseases which are similar to haemophilia.

Christmas disease or haemophilia B
This rather rare disease is due to deficiency of Factor IX (Christmas factor, so-called after the first patient in Britain to undergo investigations for it) and inability to form thromboplastin. It is a sex-linked recessive disorder, affecting males.

The clinical features are similar to haemophilia and the treatment consists of giving transfusions of fresh frozen plasma or freeze-dried Factor IX. Nursing care is the same as for haemophilia except that home care involves only one transfusion per week.

Von Willebrand's disease
This is an autosomal dominant disorder, with a prolonged bleeding time. It is due to defective platelet function where there is also a mild reduction in the level of Factor VIII. Bleeding of the mucous membrane and haematuria are features of the condition. The replacement therapy is the same as in haemophilia.

THE LEUKAEMIAS
These are generalised proliferative malignant disorders of the blood-forming tissues, usually involving the leucocytes. Leukaemia can be either acute or chronic, however, in childhood, the acute form is more common, affecting mainly children between the ages of 1 and 5 years.

Leukaemias are regarded as a cancer of the blood-forming organs, but it is not possible to isolate the cause of this condition. Some forms of leukaemia, in some animals, are due to viruses, but there is no evidence of this in man. Environmental factors such as exposure to X-rays, radioactive substances and certain chemicals may be associated with these diseases. The most common types of leukaemia in childhood are lymphoblastic, stem cell, monocytic and myeloblastic.

Pathological physiology
Leukaemia is believed to begin as a local proliferation of neoplastic cells, arising in the bone marrow and lymph nodes (where the lymphocytes are mainly formed) or in the spleen, liver and thymus. These neoplastic cells are then disseminated through the bloodstream to lodge in blood-forming tissues where they continue their proliferative activity, infiltrating many body tissues, e.g. bones and kidneys. The blood picture shows immature cells. These are most often lymphocytes

and sometimes myeloblasts. The total white cell count is often raised between 20 000 to 30 000/mm³ (normal cell count is 8000 to 11 000/mm³) and only rarely to a very high figure. In some cases the white cell count is within normal limits, while in others, it may be abnormally low. The condition is confirmed by bone marrow puncture showing:

1. Gross leukaemic infiltration by immature or abnormal white cell precursors.
2. Decrease in erythropoietic activity (red cell formation).
3. Disappearance of megakaryocytes, i.e. absence of platelets.

All forms of leukaemia are invariably fatal, but spontaneous remissions, lasting for a short time, can occur. Untreated children die within a relatively short period from the time of diagnosis. In those children who receive treatment, the life span is prolonged by the use of a variety of drugs. The response to the chemotherapeutic measures varies and depends on factors such as the degree of infiltration and the number of lymphoblasts in the blood stream.

Clinical features

The initial signs and symptoms may include fever, anaemia, bleeding, weakness, bone or joint pain with or without swelling. Purpura is common and the liver and spleen are enlarged. If there is infiltration into the central nervous system, signs of meningitis may be present (p. 308). The cerebospinal fluid contains increased protein and decreased glucose. There also appears to be some relationship between leukaemia and Down's syndrome (Mongolism).

Investigations

1. Bone marrow puncture (p. 457).
2. Blood analysis.
3. Lumbar puncture (p. 312).

Principles of treatment and nursing management

1. Bacteriological investigations. These are primarily to determine the presence and types of microorganisms present so that they can be eliminated. The aim is to have a pathogen-free environment since the child will be on immunosuppressive drugs and resistance to infection will be low. Swabs are taken from the throat, nose, vagina, rectum, skin and hair. Swabs from these areas are taken again at frequent intervals during the treatment.
2. General measures:
   a. Antibiotics to treat infections, a broad spectrum antibiotic is given in combination with drugs like gentamicin and vancomycin.
   b. Anti-fungal drug, e.g. nystatin is given to prevent fungal infection while the child is receiving antibiotics.
   c. Transfusion of fresh whole blood or packs of platelets concentrate if thrombocytopenia is present (p. 453).
3. Specialist treatment of *acute lymphoblastic leukaemia*. This consists of specific drugs to induce or re-induce remission.
   a. Prednisolone. This is a synthetic steroid which is a more potent anti-inflammatory agent than hydrocortisone or cortisone but has less sodium and water-retaining effect. The dose is 40 mg/m²/d given orally over 3 weeks and is gradually reduced to stop in week four. It produces haematologic remissions.
   b. Vincristine. This is a cytotoxic drug which interferes with mitosis. The dose is 1 to 1.5 mg/m² and is given once weekly intravenously for three injections. This drug cannot be given over a prolonged period, because of its toxic effect on neuromuscular tissue leading to pain, muscle wasting, parasthesia and constipation due to bowel dysfunction. To prevent constipation methylcellulose is given.
   c. Allopurinol is given to prevent damage to the nephron by accumulation of uric acid.
      To maintain remission, i.e. when there is less than 5 per cent marrow blast cells, the following drugs may be given:
   d. Methotrexate. This is an antimetabolite which acts as a folic acid antagonist (folic acid induces the maturation of megaloblasts to normoblasts). The dose is 20 to 30 mg/m², given orally on 2 days per week. Toxicity produces mouth ulcers and intestinal ulceration with bleeding. Methotrexate

is also given intrathecally to prevent leukaemic infiltration of the central nervous system. The dose varies with the age of the child, e.g. 1 to 2 years old 8 mg; 2 to 3 years old 10 mg, and over 3 years old 12 mg.

e. 6-Mercaptopurine. This is a purine analogue which will produce a haemotological remission. In most cases there are no toxic manifestations, but occasionally, abdominal pain or mouth ulcers may occur. Severe toxicity produces bone marrow depression. This drug may be given instead of methotrexate and when clinical, peripheral blood and marrow remission is obtained.

f. Cyclophosphamide. This is a nitrogen mustard derivative. It is used if the child is resistant to other agents. It depresses bone marrow activity and may also cause alopecia and haemorrhagic cystitis.

g. Remission can be prolonged by giving asparaginase 6000 units/m^2 intramuscularly nine times over 21 days.

4. Specialist treatment of *acute myeloblastic/monocytic leukaemia*:

a. Daunorubicin. This drug interferes with DNA synthesis. The dose is 55 mg/m^2/d, given intravenously on the first day.

b. Cytosine arabinoside. This drug interferes with DNA synthesis. The dose is 70 mg/m^2/d and is given intravenously on the first, second, third, fourth and fifth day.

5. *Meningeal leukaemia.* This serious complication develops in at least 50 per cent of children with lymphoblastic leukaemia. Children should be treated prophylactically with intrathecal methotrexate once per week. The purpose of this treatment is to destroy unwanted cells which are more sensitive to radiation than healthy tissue. If the child develops symptoms of central nervous system involvement, e.g. headache and vomiting, then methotrexate should be given intrathecally, twice weekly. In order to eliminate residual leukaemic cells from the nervous system (brain and spinal cord) the skull is irradiated. This may result in temporary loss of hair. It is given as 10 fractions of 180 Rads over 2 weeks.

6. Maintenance therapy. The child is given maintenance therapy for about three years. He is given daily oral 6-mercaptopurine approx. 75 mg/m^2/d; once-weekly oral methotrexate 20 mg/m^2/week and monthly intravenous vincristine which is followed by a seven-day course of oral prednisolone 40 mg/m^2/d in divided doses. The dosage is adjusted to keep the total white cell count between 2000 to 3000/mm^3. The duration of the treatment is about three years, when all chemotherapy is stopped.

Not all patients benefit from this treatment and one of the hazards of administration of immunosuppressive drugs is pneumocystis carinii and other forms of pneumonitis.

7. Nursing management:

a. Reverse barrier nursing (p. 250).

b. Adequate nutrition with sterilised food according to the needs of the child.

c. Prevention of infection, i.e. no one with an infection should nurse the child, and the technqiue of reverse barrier nursing should be understood by all the staff. If a laminar flow is used, the principle of its function should be understood by all the staff and other children should be prevented from breaking the barrier. Regular air specimens must be taken to test the efficiency of the system.

d. Careful observations of the body functions, e.g. temperature, as an indication of infection or effect of drug therapy; pulse and respiration rate; stools, for presence of blood or constipation; urine, amount and presence of blood; skin, appearance of petechiae; mucous membrane, for the presence of ulcers or thrush; complaints of abdominal pain and vomiting, the former as an indication of liver damage, the latter indicating involvement of the central nervous system.

e. Routine nursing care with the barrier system.

f. Preparation for home during remission. As soon as the cell count and marrow picture are near normal levels, the child will be able to go home. The parents will be interviewed by the medical officer and guidance will be given regarding continuation of drug therapy, activity, schooling, and follow-up visits to the outpatient clinic.

8. Support for parents and child:
   a. Child. Recognition of problems of isolation and the need to have physical and emotional support; the need for play and other forms of occupation during the isolation period. Loss of hair can cause a great deal of unhappiness. The child, if old enough, and the parents should be warned that this can happen but that the child will be given a wig. They should be reassured that the hair will grow back again in about three months but that it may be of different colour and texture.
   b. Parents. Recognition of their anxiety and their need to play an active role in caring for the child; understanding of their fears and their need to discuss them particularly with the medical staff; while in hospital, to provide them with some measure of peace and quiet so that they can relax a little and obtain some relief from the tensions in the ward.
9. Terminal care (p. 125).

Procedures relating to the cardiovascular system

Venepuncture

This procedure is carried out by the doctor and is performed for the following reasons:

1. To obtain a specimen of blood for:
   a. Biochemical investigation, e.g. estimation of blood urea.
   b. Bacteriological investigation to culture bacteria.
   c. Estimation of erythrocyte sedimentation rate.
2. To inject substances into the bloodstream; e.g. iron, glucose, saline, blood and opaque media.

Requirements

1. Dressing pack.
2. Mediswabs or cleansing solution.
3. Syringes; sizes according to the purpose required, e.g. 2 ml for erythrocyte sedimentation rate; 5 ml for culture.
4. Needles of appropriate sizes.

5. Appropriate containers for the blood.
6. Water-repellent sheet.
7. Disposal bag.
8. Sterile gloves, if there is a high risk of viral hepatitis.

Preparation of the child

If the child is old enough the procedure should be explained to him. It can be quite difficult to restrain a struggling child and it might be necessary to have adequate assistance so that the procedure can be performed with the minimum of trauma. It is often difficult to find a suitable vein and to penetrate one so that the procedure may take longer than usual.

The nurse places a water-repellent sheet over a pillow and places the child's arm in the supine position, applying pressure over the area above the elbow joint. This tends to distend the vessel with blood, and makes penetration easier. As soon as the doctor has withdrawn the needle, the nurse releases her grip, and applies a swab and pressure over the puncture. If a drug or other substance is to be injected the nurse will release the pressure over the elbow area as soon as blood enters the syringe. When the injection is completed, pressure is applied over the punctured site until there is no oozing from the puncture. This prevents loss of the substance injected and also prevents the formation of a haematoma.

Fontanelle tap

This is a method of obtaining blood from an infant during the first year of life when the anterior fontanelle is still patent. A short thick needle is inserted into the posterior midline of the anterior fontanelle to reach the longitudinal sinus. The requirements are the same as for venepuncture, except that the needles are short and thick with a short bevel.

Preparation of the child

Shaving of the head should only be undertaken if the doctor requests it. The infant is wrapped in a sheet or light blanket and the crown of the head is held level with the edge of the table. Light flexion of the head may be necessary and any movement of the head must be prevented. (Fig. 25.5). As soon as the needle is withdrawn,

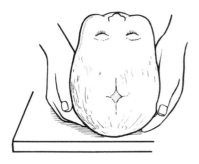

Fig. 25.5 Fontanelle tap. (Note the position of the child.)

the head is raised quickly and firm pressure is applied to the punctured site. The infant is only returned to his cot when oozing of blood or serum has stopped.

Puncture of the jugular vein
This is another method by which blood may be obtained from a small child. The position the child has to adopt will frighten him, so that constant reassurance will be necessary. The requirements are the same as for the venepuncture.

Preparation of the child
A pillow is placed on the edge of the table and the child is placed with his head on it, turned to the side, and well extended over the edge of the table. It is important that the head does not move during the procedure, but crying will distend the vein, facilitating entry into the vein (Fig. 25.6).

As soon as the doctor removes the needle, pressure must be applied to the puncture site while

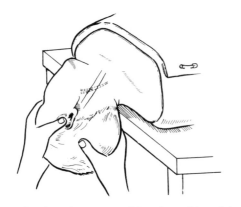

Fig. 25.6 Jugular vein puncture. (Note the position of the child's head.)

the child is in the sitting position. While applying pressure, the child is comforted and when no further oozing occurs, the pressure is released and the child can be returned to his bed.

Puncture of the femoral vein
This is also a useful method for obtaining blood in infants and small children, but it is not without danger to the child. The femoral artery and vein lie in close proximity and it is easy to puncture the femoral artery. Care must be taken to prevent infection by ensuring that the inguinal and perineal regions are clean. The requirements are the same as for venepuncture.

Preparation of the child
The child's napkin must be changed and the napkin area cleaned. The child is placed on a flat, firm table with a water-repellent sheet beneath his buttocks. The legs are abducted and held firmly to prevent any movement. After the needle is withdrawn, firm pressure must be applied for 3 to 5 minutes. When bleeding has stopped, a clean napkin is placed in position and the child returned to his cot. Half-hourly inspection of the puncture site is essential to ensure that bleeding has not recommenced or that a haematoma has not formed.

Arteriopuncture
Arteriopuncture is performed in studying blood-gases concentration and haemoglobin saturation. It may also be performed to measure arterial blood pressure when an arterial cannula is introduced to monitor arterial blood pressure directly. The radial, brachial and temporal arteries can be used, and the umbilical artery is useful in the immediate neonatal period.

Requirements
1. Dressing pack.
2. Appropriate syringes (these must be airtight) and stopper or cap.
3. Needles. Nos. 23 to 25 scalp vein needles or a cannula.
4. Heparinised solution.

Preparation and care of the child
The preparation is the same as for a venepuncture.

When the specimen of blood has been obtained, firm pressure must be applied to the punctured site for 5 minutes. Half-hourly inspection of the site is essential to ensure that bleeding has not recommenced. If the child has received anticoagulant medication, pressure will have to be maintained until bleeding stops and frequent inspections made, to ensure that no further bleeding has occurred.

If the arterial blood sample is for pH estimation, the syringe containing the blood must be immersed in ice, to prevent a significant fall in the pH of the blood. If the blood samples are for estimation of blood gases, the syringe must be capped immediately to prevent room air from entering, giving a false analysis.

Intravenous administration of fluids, electrolytes and nutrients

The initiation of an infusion is primarily the responsibility of the medical officer, however, the nurse plays an important part by preparing for the procedure, assisting during the procedure and caring for the child during the administration.

The objectives of intravenous therapy should be understood so that the child will be able to receive the necessary substances safely and with a minimum of discomfort. The objectives are as follows:

1. To maintain or replace body stores of water, electrolytes, vitamins, proteins, carbohydrates and fats. This may be necessary if the child is unable to obtain these substances by the normal route or when normal digestive functions are impaired. Dehydration and loss of electrolytes occur very rapidly in infants suffering from severe vomiting and diarrhoea, toxaemic shock, intestinal obstruction and malabsorption syndrome.
2. To restore acid-base balance in conditions such as diabetic coma where ketoacidosis causes a severe lowering of the pH of the blood.
3. To replace blood and plasma loss.

The types of fluids which can be given depend on the condition for which they may be required. These include the following:

1. *Isotonic fluids.* These are fluids which have the same osmotic pressure externally as that found across the semi-permeable membrane within the cell, e.g. normal saline 0.9 per cent and dextrose 5 per cent in water. Isotonic fluids are given in hypotonic dehydration.
2. *Hypotonic fluids.* These fluids have a lower osmotic pressure than extracellular fluid, causing cells to expand or swell, e.g. sodium chloride 0.45 per cent. Hypotonic fluids are given in hypertonic dehydration.
3. *Hypertonic fluids.* These fluids have a higher osmotic pressure than that of extracellular fluid, causing cells to shrink, e.g. dextrose 5 per cent in saline. Hypertonic fluids may be given to supply fluid and calories.
4. *Blood related fluids:*
   a. Whole blood. This consists of red cells, white cells, platelets and plasma. It is used to replace blood loss.
   b. Red blood cells. Concentrated red blood cells are given to patients who require only this component, e.g. in the treatment of anaemia and when there is risk of circulatory overload. Red blood cells can be separated by centrifuging whole blood and removing the plasma. Red blood cells may be frozen and stored at very low temperatures for long periods of time before they are used.
   c. White blood cells. At the present time, the neutrophil polymorph (granulocyte) is in greatest demand for therapeutic purposes. Granulocytes are given to patients who have insufficient of their own, or whose granulocytes do not function. They are also given when there is infection, or to cover a period when there is a strong possibility of infection, e.g. post marrow transplant. Granulocytes can be collected by centrifugation or by filtration.
   d. Platelets. These are given to patients in the treatment of thrombocytopenia, to stop bleeding or when the platelets do not function. Platelets are obtained by centrifugation of whole blood and can be stored for 2 to 3 days under controlled conditions.
   e. *Plasma components.* Plasma may be given whole or may be fractionated into a variety of components. *Fresh whole plasma* may be used to replace various coagulation factors.

It is usually stored as frozen fresh plasma (FFP). The congulation factors keep well at −20°C.

Freeze-dried whole plasma may be used to replace fluid loss following severe burns or haemorrhage until cross-matched blood is available.

Cryoprecipitate is obtained from fresh plasma which is frozen and then slowly thawed at 4°C leaving a precipitate rich in Factor VIII (the anti-haemophilic factor). Once extracted it is frozen and stored until required. It goes rapidly into solution when warmed to 37°C when it is suitable for immediate use.

Freeze-dried coagulation factors are obtained from fresh plasma and are used in the treatment of haemophilia (Factor VIII) and Christmas disease (Factor IX).

Albumin can be used to induce diuresis in a hypoproteinaemic patient who is not responding to diuretics.

Fibrinogen. Freeze-dried fibrinogen can be used in patients whose fibrinogen is abnormal.

5. *Plasma expanders.* These are used to improve the circulating blood volume, e.g. dextran.
6. Parenteral nutrition (triple feeding).

Methods used in the administration of intravenous therapy
The needle or catheter may be introduced either as a puncture, i.e. venepuncture, or as a 'cutdown', i.e. venesection. Some of the requirements vary in each method but the control, maintenance and nursing management are the same in both methods.

Venepuncture
A needle or cannula is inserted via the skin directly into a vein. It is used whenever possible, but difficulty may be encountered in infants and young children, especially if they are in a collapsed state or severely dehydrated.

Requirements

1. Dressing pack.
2. Sterile dressing towels.

3. Skin cleansing lotion.
4. Intracath or needles as requested.
5. 5 ml syringe.
6. Normal saline.
7. Appropriate administration set.
8. Air inlet, if required.
9. Bottle holder, if required.
10. Splint.
11. Bandage and adhesive tape.
12. Tubegauze or limb restrainers.
13. Intravenous stand and Ivac pump (if available).
14. Prescribed bottle or plastic container of fluid.

Preparation of the child
A simple explanation should be given to the older child if he is well enough. This will help him to understand what is going to be done and how he can co-operate during the administration of the fluid. It is particularly important to impress upon him the necessity of keeping his arm straight. If the child is very apprehensive, a sedative may be given. The clothes are removed from the arm and the child is placed in the position of greatest comfort, with his arm resting on a pillow. A prepared splint of the correct size is applied to the arm, taking care that the adhesive tape is not applied too tightly which might constrict the blood vessels and interfere with the circulation of the injected fluid (Fig. 25.8).

The doctor then inserts the needle or intracatheter and the filled and prepared giving set is attached to the needle or catheter. A swab is placed over the needle insertion and held in position with a strip of adhesive tape; care must be taken not to encircle the limb and constrict the circulation.

Scalp vein puncture
This method is used for infants up to 6 months of age. The superficial scalp veins in infants are more prominent, thus permitting easy entry into the vein and thereby avoiding the necessity of using larger veins for venesection which may be required at some later date.

Requirements (as for venepuncture)

1. Dressing pack (swabs, cotton wool, gallipots, dissecting forceps).

2. Scalp vein needles, various sizes.
3. Intracatheter and syringe.
4. Intravenous infusion set.
5. Adhesive tape (cut into 10 to 12 cm narrow strips).
6. Bandages, arm restraints or tubegauze for mitts.
7. Prescribed bottle or plastic container with solution.
8. Intravenous stand.

Preparation of the child

It may be necessary to shave the infant's hair at the area chosen for the puncture. The temporal veins on either side are most frequently chosen. The infant is wrapped in a shawl or small sheet and the arms are restrained. If the child is restless, sedation may be prescribed and should be given 30 minutes before this procedure is due to begin.

The infant's head is held gently but firmly to one side, with the prepared side uppermost. The doctor inserts the needle and fixes it in position as shown in Figure 25.7. A certain amount of movement is permissible, but the infant should not be allowed to become restless.

Venesection

When fluids are urgently required and difficulty is encountered in entering a vein by venepuncture, a vein must be exposed surgically. A small incision is made into the vein and a cannula or polyethylene tubing inserted. In infants, the site chosen is usually the internal saphenous vein of the lower limb and it has the advantage that it can be used two or three times if necessary. In older children, the median basilic vein of the upper limb is the usual one of choice.

Requirements

1. Infusion stand, prescribed bottle or plastic container with solution.
2. Dressing pack.
3. Appropriate administration set.
4. Venesection equipment, e.g. Bard-Parker handle and blades, fine dissecting forceps, aneurism needle, probe, fine-pointed scissors, two pairs mosquito foceps, Spencer Wells forceps, needle holding forceps and skin suture needles.
5. Skin cleansing lotion, e.g. Betadine and methylated spirit.

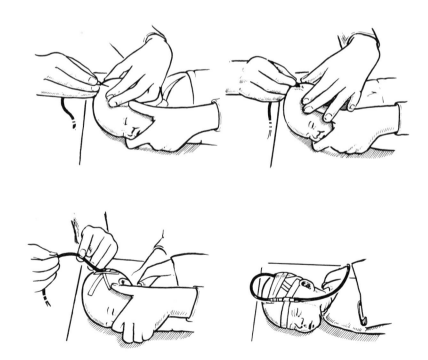

Fig. 25.7 Scalp vein infusion.

6. 4/0 catgut atraumatic suture; 3/0 black silk atraumatic suture.
7. 2 ml syringe and needles No. 21 and 23. } For local anaesthesia
8. Mediswabs and gauze swabs.
9. Local anaesthesia.
10. Gowns and masks.
11. Splint, bandages, adhesive tape, tubegauze or limb restrainer.
12. Ivac pump (if available).

If the infusion is for a baby receiving small amounts of fluid half-hourly, or when drugs are being given, the following will be required:

Heller's valve.
Three-way adaptor and 10 or 20 ml syringe.

Preparation of the child
An explanation should be given to the older child if he is able to understand it and it should be emphasised that he must keep his limb in the position it is placed and only limited movement will be possible. The smaller child or the very ill child may become restless and it is advisable to sedate him before the procedure is carried out.

The nurse prepares the splint, which should be of the correct size, and if the lower limb is to be used, she straps the splint to the limb exposing the inner malleolus. (Fig. 25.8). Care should be taken

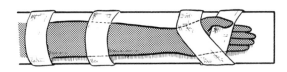

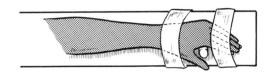

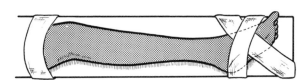

Fig. 25.8 Immobilisation of arm and leg. (Note the position of adhesive tape.)

not to constrict the blood vessels, which might interfere with the circulation of the fluid injected. The splint is then tied securely to the bed. The other leg is immobilized by applying a limb restrainer and fixing it to the bed. Whatever type of limb restraint is used, it is essential to ensure that it is not constricting the limb and should allow limited movement. A woollen sock may be put on this foot and a light cover may be placed over the limb to keep the extremities warm.

After the doctor has inserted the needle or cannula, sutured the skin and applied a dressing, the child is made comfortable. A small cage may be placed between the bedclothes and the limb.

Nursing care of the child
1. *Position of the child.* The position the child is placed in will depend on his general condition. He may be sitting upright, supported by pillows or semi-recumbent. His position should be changed to prevent respiratory complications.

2. *Care of pressure areas.* Since the child tends to remain in the same position for fear of moving his limb, he will require frequent changes of position to avoid interference with the blood supply at the pressure areas. The napkin is changed frequently and the buttocks washed in the normal manner. Infusion of fluids has a diuretic effect and the infant may pass frequent and larger amounts of urine. The older child will require routine pressure area care (p. 94).

3. *Care of the mouth.* While the infusion is in progress, oral fluids may be discontinued. Salivary secretions may be diminished or suppressed therefore care should be taken to ensure that the mouth is kept moist and clean (p. 96).

4. *Routine nursing care,* e.g. bathing, hair care, etc. will be carried out with modifications to suit the situation (Ch. 5).

5. *Observations of the infusion.* (a) *Rate of flow.* The amount of fluid to be given will be prescribed by the medical officer and should be written on the fluid chart. The rate of flow must be checked frequently. There are a number of factors which effect the rate of flow and which should be considered when there are variations, for example, *pressure gradient,* i.e. the difference between two levels in a fluid system; *friction* due to interaction between the fluid molecules and the vessel wall;

height of column of fluid (the higher the column of fluid the more rapid will be the rate of flow, and the lower the column of fluid, the less rapid will be the rate of flow); and *fluid viscosity* (the thicker the fluid, the slower will be the rate of flow).

(b) *Calculation of the rate of flow.* Each infusion set is metered to deliver a certain amount of fluid over a given time and it is important to read the instructions on each set. However, the rate of flow can be calculated by timing the rate of flow for 1 minute. The following formula can be used:

$$\frac{\text{Drops}}{\text{per minute}} = \frac{\text{Total volume infused} \times \text{drops per ml}}{\text{Total time for infusion in minutes}}$$

Example: 40 ml of dextrose 5 per cent to be given in 1 hour (set indicates 60 drops per (ml)

$$\frac{40 \times 60}{60 \text{ min}} = 40 \text{ drops per min}$$

Complications of intravenous therapy

1. *Leakage at the site of the insertion.*

(a) This may be due to fluid entering the tissues. The first indication of this may be the presence of oedema surrounding the site of insertion. For this reason it is important that the insertion point should not be bandaged over but should be covered loosely with a sterile swab. An older child may complain of pain and the rate of the infusion flow may be decreased. The doctor should be notified at once and if the infusion is to be continued, the nurse will have to prepare for another venesection or venepuncture. Meanwhile, the infusion should be stopped to prevent further infiltration.

(b) It may be due to faulty connection which should be remedied by the doctor. However, nurses are now permitted to change infusion sets provided they have been trained to do so. Each hospital will have its own policy and standard, but the overall aims and objectives are that the procedure should be carried out aseptically and to prevent air from entering the vein. Aseptic technique is essential and the cannula should rest on a sterile field before the set is attached to it. Fluid must run through the new infusion set to force air out before the set is attached to the needle or cannula.

(c) The infusion may stop due to blockage of the needle or cannula. The medical officer is notified immediately and preparations made to remove the blockage. The following equipment should be prepared.

1. Bowl for normal saline.
2. Normal saline.
3. 5 ml or 10 ml syringe.
4. Sodium citrate.
5. Dressing pack.
6. Adhesive tape.

(d) The rate of flow may be decreased or stopped for a variety of reasons. For example, spasms of the vein due to mechanical irritation, such as that caused by the needle or cannula, or cold, or abnormal position of the limb or constriction of blood vessel by tight adhesive tape.

2. *Pyrogenic reaction.* The child may show signs of reaction due to infection. The following features might indicate infection from the infusion when they occur about 30 minutes after the start of the infusion:

1. Sudden increase of temperature with shivering.
2. Sudden increase in pulse rate.
3. Nausea and vomiting.

The medical officer should be notified at once; the infusion will be discontinued and the necessary treatment given to combat the infection. The infusion equipment and the solution must be retained for further laboratory investigation to determine the cause of the contamination and the type of organisms.

Maintenance of accurate records

An accurate fluid balance chart must be kept. This chart must contain all the measured amounts of fluids given and all output. The fluid container must never be allowed to empty completely, so the level of fluid in the container should be watched constantly. When renewing a fluid container, it must be checked by two people to ensure that the correct fluid is given. A record must be made of this event on the fluid chart, stating the time the change has been made and signed by the person who changed the container.

Completion of the intravenous infusion

When the infusion has been completed, the nurse prepares the following equipment:

1. Dressing pack.
2. Skin cleansing lotion.
3. Stitch scissors and dissecting forceps.
4. Bandage and adhesive tape.

The infusion is discontinued by closing the control clip and, using aseptic technique, the needle or cannula is removed. The area is cleaned and a sterile dressing is applied. The splint is removed and the child is made comfortable. Stitches are usually removed on the fifth day.

If the infusion had been via a venepuncture, it is necessary to apply pressure over the punctured site once the needle or cannula has been removed. This is necessary to avoid oozing and loss of blood with the formation of a small haematoma.

Blood transfusion

In general, there are two main reasons for blood transfusion:

1. To restore the volume of circulating blood as in haemorrhage or when blood has to be replaced due to loss during a long and extensive operation.
2. To provide some cellular or protein component which is deficient in the patient, e.g. red blood cells as in hypochromic anaemia and platelets in thrombocytopenia. (See p. 448 for blood and blood related fluids.)

In the UK blood is obtained from donors by the Regional Blood Transfusion Services who group it and distribute it to the various hospitals. To help to identify the different blood groups an international colour code is used for the bottle label: yellow for A; pink for B; white for AB; blue for O.

Blood is further coded for Rhesus grouping. Thus Rhesus negative blood has red lettering and a red vertical stripe, and Rhesus positive blood has black lettering without a vertical stripe.

Storage of blood

It is essential that bottles of blood are stored in a refrigerator with a controlled temperature of 4°C. It can be stored for up to 21 days and when it is required it can be kept for up to 3 hours in an insulated box after it is issued from the blood bank. Blood must not be warmed or frozen.

Cross-matching

Before blood is given to a child, it is essential to cross-match his blood with that of the donor's. This entails placing the red cells of the donor with serum of the patient and then examining for agglutination. About 5 ml of blood will be required.

Checking the bottle or packs

The label on the bottle must be checked carefully before the blood is given to the child. The label must contain the child's name, ward, blood group and Rhesus type (see code above). Blood and blood products must be regarded as potentially dangerous substances and great care must be taken to ensure that the correct bottle of blood is given to the correct child.

Requirements are as for venepuncture or venesection with the additional equipment of a blood transfusion giving set.

Care of the child

Basically the care of the child is similar to that given during administration of fluids. However, careful observations and supervision will be necessary to recognise any adverse effects and to take the appropriate action.

Signs of transfusion reactions

Transfusion reactions may be either non-haemolytic or haemolytic.

1. *Non-haemolytic reactions.* These include pyrexial and allergic reactions to the transfusion fluid, circulatory overload, air embolism and septicaemia from contaminated fluid. The signs include: rise in temperature; rigor; rise in pulse rate and urticaria and increased central venous pressure.

2. *Haemolytic reactions.* These result from the destruction of either donor or recipient cells. The following signs would be found: tachycardia; tachypnoea; rigor; headache; nausea and feeling cold; jaundice and convulsions and renal failure.

As soon as a reaction is recognised the doctor must be notified and the transfusion discontinued.

The bottle/pack, giving set and any equipment used must be retained and sent for bacteriological investigation. Even if there has been no reaction to the transfusion, the pack and giving set are retained for 24 hours after the completion of the transfusion. It is also important to change to a fresh giving set whenever the transfusion is preceded or followed by an infusion of dextrose solution, or to ensure that the blood transfusion follows or precedes that of sodium chloride 0.9 per cent. Red blood cells tend to agglutinate in a high concentration of dextrose and such cells may then be haemolysed in the patient.

On completion of the transfusion, details of the transfusion are entered on a special form and any untoward reactions can then be traced without difficulty.

Exchange transfusion

The reason for this treatment is to prevent the accumulation of high levels of circulating bilirubin. High levels of bilirubin cause kernicterus; the infant may die or suffer permanent brain damage. This condition is found in infants suffering from erythroblastosis (p. 437). Exchange transfusion is also the treatment for ABO incompatibility or other haemolytic conditions when the serum bilirubin rises to levels of 20 to 25 mg per 100 ml. In exchange transfusion most of the circulating antibody and affected erythrocytes are removed and replaced by fresh donor blood which is Rhesus negative and of the same blood group as the infant.

Requirements

1. Special exchange transfusion pack, containing, bowl, instruments, cord ligatures, three-way stopcock, swabs, cotton wood balls.
2. 2 × 20 or 10 ml syringes and needles No. 21.
3. 2 ml syringe.
4. Blood administration set.
5. Flask of sodium chloride 0.9 per cent.
6. Jaques catheter F.G. 14, 1 feeding catheter to use as marker.
7. Umbilical catheter F.G. 6 and 9.
8. Sodium bicarbonate 8.4 per cent (for first exchange only).
9. Calcium gluconate.

10. Adhesive tape.
11. Skin cleansing lotion.
12. Antibiotic spray for cord stump.
13. Intravenous stand.
14. Limb restrainers.
15. Baby warmer.
16. Resuscitation trolley, oxygen and suction.

Preparation of the baby

The infant is nursed in a warm environment, either in an incubator or a cot. The umbilical stump is kept moist with saline packs to prevent drying and shrivelling. The infant is weighed and measured and the gastric contents are aspirated. When the temperature is stabilised and the infant's blood has been cross-matched, he is prepared for the transfusion with his limbs restrained.

Technique and care of the infant during procedure

The umbilical vein is identified, but if there is any difficulty in finding it, a small incision is made above the umbilicus and the vein is cannulated. The blood is warmed to 37°C and an ambient temperature of 28° to 30°C is maintained to prevent hypothermia. A total volume of 160 to 180 ml/kg weight is used in aliquots of 20 ml via a two-way syringe. During the procedure, an accurate record is kept of the amount of blood withdrawn and replaced, the time of withdrawal and replacement, and any observations made. This includes recording the apex heart beat, body temperature, breathing rate and signs of difficulty in breathing. Administration of drugs must be entered stating the amount and time the drugs have been given.

Type of blood used

The infant is given Rhesus negative blood which is compatible with the baby, if this is possible, without incompatibility with the mother's serum. The donor blood is cross-matched with the mother's serum to exclude incompatibility from a second maternal antibody outside the Rhesus system.

Example:

a. Baby's blood group is A and mother's is A, therefore, donor blood group A Rhesus negative is given.

b. Baby's blood group is A and mother's is O, therefore, donor blood group O Rhesus negative is given. In this case, there is a danger that O group blood will contain anti-A which will react with the baby's A cells.

After-care of the infant

After completion, the cannula may be left in position and is covered with a sterile swab, ready for another transfusion should the bilirubin level be increased after subsequent blood tests. The infant is placed in an incubator and oxygen is given for a prescribed period. Fluids may be withheld for a period of 4 to 6 hours. The infant's general condition must be observed carefully and his apex heart beat, breathing rate and rhythm and temperature recorded hourly for the first 4 hours.

Dangers of exchange transfusion

1. Acidosis due to acid-citrate-dextrose anticoagulant. Sodium bicarbonate is given to combat the acidosis.
2. Hyperkalaemia due to loss of cell potassium which increases with the age of the blood. The condition can be avoided if the donor's blood is less than 4 days old when it is used.
3. Hypercalcaemia due to calcium binding by the citrate of acid-citrate-dextrose. It can be prevented by giving 1 ml of 10 per cent calcium gluconate.
4. Hypothermia. This can be prevented by maintaining an ambient temperature of about 28 to 30°C.
5. Hypoglycaemia may be present already before the transfusion is commenced, particularly in the pre-term infant.
6. Bacteraemia can be prevented by using aseptic technique throughout.
7. Portal vein thrombosis.

Intra-uterine transfusion

This procedure is not performed in a paediatric setting and is included because it is of interest to the paediatric nurse. This method is only employed when the Rhesus disease is of such severity that the baby would die *in utero*. It also carries a high element of danger to the unborn baby and the placenta because of the possibility of trauma.

The principle is that red cells injected into the fetal peritoneal cavity are slowly absorbed into the circulation via the lymphatics. Fresh group O Rhesus negative blood, compatible with the mother's serum is given. The blood is 'washed' to remove immunocompetent lymphocytes to prevent host reaction.

Intravenous nutrition

This form of feeding is necessary in the following situation and conditions:

1. Malnutrition — Due to inability to take food or
2. Starvation — adequate amounts of the essential food factors or when food is not available.
3. Catabolic states. When tissue proteins are used to repair damaged tissue or where disease prevents normal absorption, assimilation and use of protein, e.g. Crohn's disease, ulcerative colitis, major intestinal resection, gastro-intestinal fistula and severe burns.
4. Malabsorption syndrome (p. 500).
5. Prematurity (when the umbilical vein is used).

In these and other conditions such as coma and renal failure, food is provided intravenously. The food is in pre-digested form given as amino-acids, sugars and fats. There are, however, *contrindications* for this form of nutrition and these include:

1. Uraemia.
2. Liver disease.
3. Thrombocytopenia.
4. Hyperlipaemia.

The following solutions are available:

1. *Amino-acid solutions* (these are synthetically produced and are similar to the protein in egg, fish and meat). Vamin, Aminoplex 14 and 5, Aminosol 10 per cent, FreAmine, Amigen. Amino-acids must be given slowly, otherwise they cannot be absorbed by the tissues and are lost in the urine.
2. *Carbohydrate solutions.* Dextrose 20 or 50 per cent provides energy, but there is a danger of hyperglycaemia and therefore the urine must be

tested 4-hourly. If the blood sugar level rises too high, insulin can be given. Insulin is believed to be reducing the catabolic mechanism. Fructose and sorbitol can be given. They are converted to glucose, but are not so useful in ill patients.
3. *Fat.* Fat emulsions provide a concentrated form of energy. The fat emulsions consist of fat particles similar to milk.
4. Fluid and electrolytes, minerals and vitamins.

Method

The bottles each contain their specific solution and they are run in concurrently:

1. Amino-acid infusion is given slowly and continuously throughout the 24-hour period.
2. Y-connector tubes and Ivac pumps with multi-channel taps are used. This allows several bottles to be used at the same time.
3. Medication can be added to the burette chamber.

Routes

The infusion should be given into a large vein, since smaller veins can be damaged.

1. *Peripheral vein.* A scalp vein needle can be used, but the needle must be changed every 24 hours to prevent phlebitis. There is also the problem of finding enough veins for resiting the infusion and the trauma to the child because of frequent punctures.

2. *Superior vena cava.* A catheter is passed into the superior vena cava or the right atrium via the external or internal jugular veins or by using the subclavian vein. This allows fast flow of fluid and dilutes irritating solutions. There is, however, a risk of infection and major venous obstruction as well as cardiac arrhythmia.

3. Using a fine Silastic catheter and passing it from a scalp vein into the superior vena cava and the right atrium. A No. 16 butterfly needle should be used. The route of the catheter is checked radiologically.

Dangers of intravenous nutrition

1. Infection via bottles, cannula, etc. (the tip of the cannula should be sent to the bacteriology department when it is withdrawn). Specimen of urine, stools and swabs from the skin should be taken routinely to determine the presence of any pathogenic organisms and to institute the necessary treatment as soon as possible.
2. Fluid retention. An accurate fluid intake and output chart must be maintained so that renal function can be estimated.
3. Dehydration. This can occur due to rapid infusion of dextrose causing diuresis, i.e. renal diuresis.
4. Hypoglycaemia. This may occur when insulin is given to combat the hyperglycaemia.
5. Liver and renal insufficiency, i.e. inability to metabolise and eliminate the nutritional substances.
6. Impairment of bone marrow function.

Principles of treatment and nursing management

1. Routine nursing care.
2. Specific nursing management:
   a. Care of the child receiving intravenous infusion (p. 448).
   b. Fluid chart.
   c. Four-hourly urine testing for sugar and acetone.
   d. Observations of vital functions, e.g. temperature, pulse and respiration to detect infection, overload and respiratory difficulty.
   e. Oral care (p. 96).
   f. Limb movements are essential to prevent muscle wastage due to long periods of immobility.
3. Support for the parents, particularly when long-term care is required with repeated episodes of intravenous feeding, e.g. in chronic diarrhoea in young children. Recognition of parental anxiety for the child and the need to allow the parents to take some part in his care. The tube may be occluded and left in position and the child may be allowed home. The parents will require guidance on the care of the catheter, feeding of the child and there should be effective liaison between home, family doctor and the hospital.

Problems of infants

1. If the infant has been on intravenous feeds for

a long time, he may be unable to suck when oral feeds are resumed. Dummies can be used as these stimulate saliva and initiate sucking. This presents a problem of infection by unclean dummies.

2. Resumption of oral feeds. This should be a gradual process and may be started with 30 ml of 5 per cent glucose in N/5 normal saline, given 2- to 3-hourly. He may then be given Pregestimil, a pre-digested food which is easier to assimilate. As more oral feeds are given, intravenous feeds are decreased until oral feeds meet the infant's nutritional requirements.

Subcutaneous infusion, or hypodermoclysis

This method of giving fluid to correct dehydration and electrolyte loss, is used for an infant when a small quantity is required, which cannot adequately be given orally, and the intravenous method is considered unnecessary. It is also a useful method when another venesection is not considered desirable. Only isotonic or approximately isotonic fluids should be administered by this route. The flow of fluid should be carefully regulated and should not be too rapid, since overdistension of the tissues is painful.

Hyaluronidase. This is a tissue enzyme which is a spreading factor causing breakdown of the collagen fibres in tissues, thus permitting the fluid to spread over a much wider area and, therefore, be more readily absorbed.

Requirements

1. Dressing pack.
2. Intravenous administration set.
3. Y extension set with clamps.
4. Sterile water.
5. Ampoules of hyaluronidase.
6. 2 ml and 10 ml syringes, needles G21 and 25.
7. Gauze swabs (to cover the two needle insertions).
8. Skin cleansing lotion.
9. Adhesive tape, limb restrainers.
10. Infusion stand.

Preparation of the child

The infant or small child is suitably restrained and the chosen site is exposed. These sites may be: scapulae, axillae, abdominal wall and the anterior aspects of the thighs. It is important to recognise that there are problems associated with using the axillae, since it is difficult to restrain the arms and the needles may be pushed too far into the tissue. When the subscapular region is used, the infant lies on his abdomen, and the needles are inserted just below the lower border of each scapula.

Method

Two nurses are required, one to perform the procedure and the second to assist and comfort the child. Aseptic technique must be used (p. 139).

The apparatus is assembled, and fluid is run through the giving set to expel air. When air has been expelled, the flow is stopped and the needles are placed on a sterile field. Hyaluronidase is prepared and one ampoule is usually divided between two sites.

The skin area is cleaned and dried and the needles are inserted approximately two-thirds of their lengths at an angle of 15°. The needles are covered with sterile gauze and held in position with adhesive tape. When the fluid is flowing at the prescribed rate, the hyaluronidase is injected into both ends of tubing just above the needles. The rate of flow must not exceed the rate of absorption and induration should not be allowed to develop. Some oedema may be present, but this should be soft and obviously dispersing. The areas should be neither unduly red nor blanched. The rate of flow can be altered as desired and, if necessary, one side may be stopped until the fluid has dispersed. A careful record must be maintained of the amount of fluid given.

While the infusion is in progress, it is not essential to stay with the child, provided he is adequately restrained. However, it is essential to make regular observations of the infusion sites and any leakage or induration must be reported.

On completion of the infusion, the flow is stopped, the needles are withdrawn and a small gauze dressing can be applied to the punctured sites. All restraints are removed and the child is left comfortable.

Bone marrow puncture

This procedure is indicated to aid diagnosis of blood dyscrasias such as leukaemia and reticuloendotheliosis, and to obtain cultures. A small amount of juice is withdrawn from the iliac crest, sternum or the tibia. The tissue is examined for cellular structure or to isolate bacteria.

Preparation of the child
This is a painful and unpleasant procedure. Sedation is usually given before the procedure is due to begin and some small children are given rectal Pentothal, in which case full pre- and post-operative care should be followed (pp. 128 and 131).

Requirements

1. Dressing pack.
2. Additional gallipots, sterile hand and dressing towels.
3. Sterile gloves.
4. Masks and gowns.
5. Skin cleansing lotion.
6. 2 ml syringe, needles (for local anaesthesia).
7. 20 ml syringe and bone marrow puncture needles.
8. Local anaesthesia.
9. Wound sealing aerosol and Micropore.
10. Slides, two to three watch glasses.
11. Fine-toothed dissecting forceps.
12. Fixing fluid.

Technique and care of the child
The child is placed on a table with the bone to be punctured, uppermost, for example:

1. Sternum. The child is placed in the recumbent position.
2. Crest of the iliac. The child lies in the recumbent position with the pelvis slightly raised on the side to be punctured.
3. Tibia. In small infants a splint may be applied to the limb to give adequate support in order to avoid fracture of the bone. This may occur when force is applied during the needle insertion.

When the skin has been cleaned, the needle and stillette are introduced into the bone, using a boring action. The stillette is removed and marrow is aspirated with the syringe.

When sufficient juice has been obtained, the needle is withdrawn and firm pressure is applied to the puncture, to prevent bleeding. A wound seal is applied and the child is returned to his bed. If a basal anaesthetic has been given, the child is treated as any post-operative unconscious child. Half-hourly pulse recordings are necessary for the first 4 hours, in case of bleeding. Although complications are rare, infection of the bone can occur leading to osteomyelitis.

Bone marrow transplantation
Bone marrow transplantation is used clinically in children suffering from a variety of conditions including severe aplastic anaemia, refractory leukaemia or congenital immunodeficiency syndromes. If it is performed for leukaemia then it is usually for myeloid type when the child is in his first remission, while for acute lymphoblastic leukaemia it is performed when the child is in first and subsequent remissions. The transplantation procedure itself is simple and involves aspiration of a quantity of nucleated marrow cells from the donor by multiple aspirations, filtering and then infusing intravenously into the recipient.

For a transplant to be successful and prevent graft-versus-host disease it is essential that the recipient is matched with a compatible donor. Compatibility is determined by two tests: human leucocyte antigen typing and mixed lymphocyte culture results. Human leucocyte antigen is the major histocompatibility complex, so named because the complex is easily identified and tested in white blood cells. The locus (where the human leucocyte antigen genes are located on a chromosome) is on chromosome 6. Four separate loci are present: HLA (human leucocyte antigen) — A, B, C and D.

Each individual inherits one HLA-A, B, C and D gene from the mother and one from the father. The number of possible combinations in an offspring is four, and the chance of two non-twin siblings being identical in HLA composition is 25 per cent (one in four). Identical twins mirror each other genetically and will always match.

Types of transplants
There are four basic types of bone marrow transplants: syngeneic (those that have identical genotypes); HLA-matched allogeneic (being of the

same species but antigenically distinct, e.g. non-twin siblings); HLA-mismatched allogeneic (this allows transplantation of non-histocompatible marrow using lectin separation which removes harmful mature T-lymphocytes from the donor's marrow by agglutination); and autologous transplants, where the patient's own marrow is frozen and stored for reinfusion as an autograft following chemotherapy and radiation, which destroys the underlying malignancy.

Preparation for bone marrow transplant

1. A Hickman line is established using the internal jugular vein or cephalic vein. This line is used for intravenous administration of drugs and marrow transplant.
2. The child will be nursed under neutropaenic regime (reverse barrier nursing).
3. Radiotherapy is given for total body irradiation.
4. Drugs such as Mesnum and cyclophosphamide are given. Mesnum inactivates the breakdown of cyclophosphamide and this is helpful in preventing haemorrhagic cystitis.
5. Full explanation to parents and child (if he is old enough to understand). The parents must understand what the treatment consists of and the possible complications which may arise. If the donor is a sibling then he/she too must be reassured, particularly if pain is anticipated.

Post-transplant management

1. The child will be kept under the laminar flow up to 21 days until the white blood cells are normal.
2. Strict neutropaenic regime is maintained.
3. General supportive measures will be taken, e.g. platelets may be transfused to prevent spontaneous haemorrhage.
4. Skin care is important and a foam mattress may be useful.
5. Drug therapy will be continued. To prevent graft-versus-host disease, methotrexate is given intermittently.
6. Observations of complications:
   a. Graft-versus-host disease. This will be characterised by fever, exfoliative dermatitis, hepatitis, diarrhoea, vomiting and abdominal pain.
   b. Graft rejection with exacerbation of symptoms and overwhelming infection.
   c. Blood pressure measurements are usually done twice daily to identify development of hypertension.
   d. Swabs should be taken from the intravenous line for bacteriological tests.
7. Support for parents. Parents will be very anxious, particularly about the possibility of infection and rejection of the graft. Even if the graft has been successful they will be worried about a relapse. Because of the emotional stress that this situation causes, a multi-disciplinary approach is helpful. The service of a psychiatrist may be required if the anxiety interferes with life. Home care is very valuable and requires a good supporting service either via the hospital service or in co-operation with the community services.

Central venous pressure
Central venous pressure measurements are valuable as a guide to the adequacy or otherwise of fluid replacement. They measure the competence of the right side of the heart to accept and expel the blood returned. They also provide an index of right atrial filling pressure. The normal range is usually accepted to lie between 6 and 12 cm H_2O, relative to the midaxillary line with the patient lying in the horizontal position, or to a line horizontally backwards from the sternal angle if the patient is not horizontal. Central venous pressure is low when the cardiac output is inadequate due to underfilling of the peripheral circulation (shock), and tends to be high when the primary cause is cardiac impairment.

Requirements
As for venepuncture or venesection fluid administration plus a saline manometer, additional tubing and a three-way adaptor.

Method

1. The cannula is inserted into the subclavian vein and the three-way adaptor is attached to the cannula, tubing to the manometer and to the infusion set. The manometer zero mark must be level to the line described above. Open tap to the manometer.

2. The fluid is allowed to run in at the prescribed rate (an infusion may cause a significant increase in venous pressure if more than 20 ml per minute is given). The fluid in the column falls until it balances the central venous pressure in the superior vena cava. Allow the fluid level to settle and read it off in centimetres of water.
3. Turn the stopcock to allow the fluid to flow into the vein. (It should be noted that some oscillation takes place with respiration and the mid-point of the swing should be taken as the level.)

Determination of arterial blood pressure

Blood pressure means the lateral pressure exerted by blood on the arterial walls. It depends on the force of ventricular contractions, arterial wall elasticity, peripheral resistance, and blood volume and viscosity. Blood pressure is measured in millimetres of mercury using a sphygmomanometer and a stethoscope, and generally refers to the arterial pressure in the brachial artery. In any individual, arterial pressure is not constant, but subject to variation over short intervals of time.

The measurement of blood pressure is of diagnostic value and is indicative of progress or deterioration in certain conditions such as shock, head injury where there is increased intracranial pressure, kidney or heart disease. In the child, hypertension may occur in blood loss due to an overcompensating mechanism. When a fall in blood pressure occurs, it is sudden and dramatic. Excitement and struggling will increase the systolic pressure by as much as 50 mmHg above the usual level. Two pressures are measured:
1. Systolic, which is the higher one, due to contraction of the heart muscle.
2. Diastolic, which is the lower one and is the pressure exerted on the arterial walls by the blood during rest, i.e. non-contractile phase (p. 404).

Requirements

1. Sphygmomanometer with the required size of cuff. Approximate cuff width can be determined as follows:

New-born   2.5 cm
1–24 months   5 to 8 cm
2–10 years   9.5 cm
Over 10 years   12 cm.
2. Stethoscope.

Method

The procedure should be explained to the older child. It is not painful but can be uncomfortable if extended or frequent measurements have to be made. Arterial pressure is greatly affected by emotional factors and it is therefore important that the child is in a state of physical and mental rest. It is also important to select the correct size of cuff in relation to the size of the child and the amount of fatty tissue present. For example, if the arm is very obese, greater cuff pressure will be needed to compress the tissues and occlude the artery. This will result in higher pressure measurements, but can be overcome to some extent by using a wider cuff. This is not possible in infants and young children, since a wider cuff would extend beyond the elbow and make auscultation impossible.

The child is either lying flat or semi-recumbent. The arm should be relaxed in a position of abduction and slight flexion. The armband or cuff is wound round the upper arm above the elbow, covering about two-thirds of the surface area of the upper arm. The sphygmomanometer must be placed on a flat surface and is viewed with the meniscus at eye level. The artery pulsation in the antecubital fossa is located by palpation, and the stethoscope is placed gently over it. The bag is inflated rapidly until it is just sufficient to obliterate the pulse. The point at which the pulse disappears is noted. The pressure in the cuff is released slowly (at 2 mm/s). The point at which the first Korotkoff sound is heard (phase I) is the systolic pressure. As pressure is further reduced, the sound becomes loud and sharp (phase II). This is followed by phase III when a softer, blowing sound is heard. With further deflation a muffled sound (phase IV) will be heard to be followed by silence (phase V). Some controversy exists as to which phase represents actual diastolic pressure. Latest data indicate that it lies between phases IV and V. If phase IV is prolonged, both pressures should be recorded.

It is important to remember that erroneously high values can be obtained if the cuff is too narrow, and low values are obtained if the cuff is too wide. Once a reading has been obtained then the cuff is removed. However, for frequent readings the deflated cuff may be left in position.

Method of measuring the blood pressure of an infant
In the infant the procedure is usually carried out by the doctor. If an electronic blood pressure monitor is not available, the 'Flush' method can be used. The equipment is the same as for older children, with the addition of a crepe bandage.

Method
A small sphygmomanometer cuff is applied to the forearm or lower leg, just above the wrist or ankle. A crepe pressure bandage is wound round the hand or foot starting distally and the cuff is then inflated. When the bandage is removed, the limb will be white. The pressure in the cuff is slowly reduced and the point noted on the sphygmomanometer, at which the blood re-enters the limb causing flushing. This method has the disadvantage of providing only the mean pressure.

Blood pressure monitor
Systolic and diastolic blood pressures are recorded by electronic devices. Readings may be taken automatically on a 2-minute or a 4-minute cycle or whenever it is considered necessary. Such equipment is of immense value for obtaining accurate measurements and causes the least disturbance to the very ill child.

Measuring arterial blood pressure by cannulation
Arterial cannulation is employed in order to measure and record the systolic and diastolic pressure continuously. A cannula is introduced into the radial, brachial or femoral artery and the arterial blood pressure measurements are recorded on the appropriate chart.

Care must be taken to ensure that the cannula does not slip out of the vessel, as this could lead to arterial bleeding. The cannula must also be kept patent by syringing with a small amount of heparinised saline at regular intervals and as instructed by the medical staff. The arterial cannula can also be used to obtain arterial blood samples for acid-base and blood-gas determinations. There may be interference with accurate pressure recording, which may be due to the deposition of a clot in the cannula. If this is suspected the doctor must be notified and it is an indication that the cannula should be syringed with heparinised saline to ensure its patency.

Cardiac catheterisation

Cardiac catheterisation is performed to aid or confirm diagnosis of lesions of the heart and the greater vessels. A radiopaque catheter is introduced into a vein under fluoroscopic guidance and passed into the right atrium, right ventricle and the pulmonary artery. It is more difficult to study the left side of the heart, but it is possible to estimate the pressure in the left atrium, by pushing a catheter through the right side of the heart and 'wedging' it in a small pulmonary artery. The left atrial pressure is thought to be reflected by this wedge. A catheter may also be introduced into the femoral artery and pushed back until it enters the left side of the heart. Trans-septal catheterisation can also be used, when a catheter is passed into the right atrium and a hollow needle is passed up through the catheter and is used to puncture the atrial septum. A second catheter is then passed through the needle into the left side of the heart.

Cardiac catheterisation is useful in obtaining the following information:

1. Oxygen concentration in each chamber, e.g. abnormal concentrations will be found in atrial and ventricular septal defect, when there is mixing of venous and arterial blood.
2. Pressure in each chamber. An abnormally high pressure in a ventricle or atria indicates obstruction to the outflow of that chamber, e.g. as in pulmonary stenosis.
3. Measurement of cardiac output.
4. Calculation of the flow of blood in cardiac shunts.
5. Provides intracardiac electrocardiographic and phonographic information.

Preparation of the child
A simple explanation should be given to the older child. It should be recognised that a more detailed description of the operation can be very frightening for the child. Sedation may be given the night before the operation and is repeated 1 hour before the scheduled operation. The child should be prepared for a general anaesthetic. Food and

drink is withheld to prevent vomiting and the danger of aspiration.

The operation and its complications will have been discussed with the parents and the consent form must be signed before the child leaves the ward.

Technique

The child lies supine on the X-ray table, which has an image intensifier, television camera and 16 mm cine camera. Electrodes are placed on the limbs and are connected to the electrocardiographic oscilloscope and a direct writing recorder. The activity of the heart can then be recorded continuously. The right leg or left arm is then splinted and a local anaesthetic given in preparation for a venesection. The radiopaque catheter, which is approximately 80 to 100 cm long, is introduced, under fluoroscopic guidance, into the right saphenous or femoral vein, along the inferior vana cava or, if the left basilic vein is used, along the superior vena cava into the right atrium, right ventricle and then into the pulmonary artery. With the tip of the catheter at various sites in each chamber and vessel, the other end is connected via the cuvette of a direct reading oximeter and a catheter (umbilical type) to a Statham gauge electromanometer which measures the pressure wave in that position. The Statham gauge is connected to a direct writing recorder which provides a permanent record. It is also connected to an oscilloscope where the pressure recording can be seen by the cardiologist as he manipulates the catheter.

At each site a specimen of blood is drawn via a 5 ml glass syringe through the catheter into the cuvette, which rests on a magnetic stirrer over which a photoelectric cell is passed. Immediately the oxygen saturation of the blood at this site has been recorded, the blood is returned to the child via the cardiac catheter. A record is kept of the oxygen concentrations and the site from which these were obtained.

Throughout the catheterisation the catheter is kept patent with 5 per cent dextrose in quarter strength physiological saline which is heparinised. A careful record must be made of the amount of fluid infused. After each oxygen analysis, the cuvette is washed through before the next specimen is obtained.

After-care of the child

When the examination has been completed and the catheter has been removed, the child is gently returned to his bed or incubator, if he is a small infant. Temperature, pulse and respiration are monitored every 15 minutes until they are stable. Observations should include signs of haemorrhage and arrhythmias. Contamination of the wound may occur, particularly if the saphenous vein has been used. A Chiron bag can be applied to collect any urine or faeces passed. The child is usually placed in an oxygen-rich environment for a period prescribed by the doctor. The peripheral pulses should be checked and the temperature of the extremity felt, to determine signs of arterial insufficiency.

Complications of cardiac catheterisation

Cardiac catheterisation is not without risk to the child and includes some of the following complications:

1. Development of arrhythmias, vasospasm and syncope.
2. Injury to the myocardium.
3. Thrombophlebitis of the vein used for catheterisation.
4. Perforation of the great vessels of the heart.

Angiocardiography

This is an X-ray study of the heart and is useful in the diagnosis of cardiac anomalies. The open-ended catheter used for the catheterisation is withdrawn, and a special catheter with six perforations close to the tip is inserted. This type of catheter eliminates the risk of damaging the endocardium when injecting the contrast medium under high pressure and prevents catheter recoil.

Technique

A test injection of the contrast medium is given during catheterisation. The catheter tip is introduced into that part of the heart or vessel where a defect is suspected and where most information will be obtained.

A stainless steel syringe is filled with the contrast medium and all air is expelled. The amount of contrast medium used depends on the weight of the child. The pressure of the injection is regulated by a pneumatic pump and depends on the site of the catheter and the nature of the defect. The cine camera records the passage of the fluid through the heart chambers and the great vessels.

Aortography

This is performed in much the same way as an angiography; the medium is injected under pressure into the ascending aorta, the catheter having been advanced into the aorta via the femoral or brachial artery.

After-care of the child

When the examinations are completed, the child is returned to the ward and kept warm. Observations should include pulse and respirations measurements to exclude adverse reactions. The pulse rate should be recorded half-hourly and any handling of the child should be carried out as gently as possible.

Echocardiography

Echocardiography is a very useful non-invasive technique. It is painless and safe to use and can be repeated as often as necessary. It is valuable in diagnosing single ventricle, overriding aorta, atretic valves, hypoplasia of the left heart, and truncus arteriosus. It can also be used in diagnosing pericardial effusion and myocardial disease. It can be used in assessing the progress of lesions before and after surgery and following the insertion of prosthetic valves.

No preparation is necessary but a simple explanation should be given to an older child.

Erythrocyte sedimentation rate

Normally the red blood cells do not show much tendency to aggregate on standing, with the result that sedimentation is slow, but in certain conditions they run together very readily to form rouleaux which sediment quickly. The speed of sedimentation rate is expressed in millimetres (mm) per hour and its chief value is in estimating the progress in cases of rheumatic fever or when an inflammatory process is present.

Method

2 ml of blood is added to 0.5 ml of 3.8 per cent sodium citrate. It is well mixed and is then sucked up into a graduated Westergren tube to the zero mark and the tube is clipped into position on a special rack. The distance fallen by the red cells is read at the end of 1 hour and sometimes repeated after 2 hours. Normally, the erythrocyte sedimentation rate is below 10 mm per hour.

Care of the child with an electronic pacemaker

In the healthy heart the rate of contractions is controlled by the sino-atrial node, forming the intrinsic pacemaker. The timing impulse normally spreads from the sino-atrial node to the atria and the ventricles, where most of the contractile force is generated. If the conducting pathway is blocked, the ventricles contract at their own natural rate which is only about half the normal beats per minute and is not enough to sustain the normal activity of the body.

To overcome this problem, an electronic pacemaker can be inserted to stimulate the heart muscle. The pacemaker consists of a pulse generator which is driven by a long-life lithium battery delivering small electrical impulses via two connecting wires to the heart. The pacemaker, enclosed in a plastic shell, is very small and is stitched to the subcutaneous tissue, usually over or near the heart, in the region of the ventricles. The rate is selected by the surgeon before the device is implanted.

A temporary external pacemaker may be required following open-heart surgery in order to maintain an adequate heart rate and rhythm. Permanent pacing is indicated when rhythm disturbances produce excessively slow heart rates, and particularly those associated with the occurrence or risk of ventricular standstill.

Methods of pacing

Most pacing wires are inserted transvenously using subclavian, cephalic or jugular veins. The tip is positioned in the right ventricle under X-ray control. The generator is then implanted in the pectoral region. When a heart block is noted at the start of the operation it may be possible to suture permanent pacing wires to the epicardium, and the generator is then implanted in the abdominal wall. In atrial disease, it may be better to pace the right atrium, although this tends to produce greater problems.

Types of pacemakers
Various electronic circuits are available to provide a variety of pacemaker function. Those which are commonly used include:

1. Ventricular inhibited pacemakers, which are 'shut off' when the patient's heart rate is higher than that of the pacemaker, thereby avoiding competition between the pacemaker and the patient's own rhythm.
2. Programmable ventricular pacemakers can be altered by an external device to change the pacing rate or strength of the stimulus. The increased rates available may be useful in children, and by setting the strength of the stimulus just above the minimum required, excessive drain on the battery can be avoided.
3. Atrial pacemakers are similar to ventricular pacemakers but require a more sensitive circuitry to detect spontaneous atrial activity to enable them to switch off when the patient's own atrial rate is high enough.
4. Atrio-ventricular pacemakers require a connection both in the right atrium and right ventricle. They pick up the atrial activity and generate a corresponding impulse to stimulate the ventricle so that they allow the ventricular rate to vary with exercise in a more physiological way. These are mainly used in complete atrio-ventricular block but are also able to provide a regular standby mode if atrial activity ceases.
5. Paroxysmal supraventricular tachycardia can be interrupted by using a specialised pacemaker, which senses the tachycardia. This leads to a short series of impulses being delivered to the atrium, which stops the tachycardia.

Pacemakers come in two types: *fixed-rate*, which fire continuously without regard to the patient's heart rate; and *demand*, which sense the patient's heart rate and fire accordingly. Where continuous stimulation is dangerous, it is safer to use a *demand* pacemaker, which picks up the natural impulse from the sino-atrial node and delivers it to the ventricles. The rate is therefore regulated by the patient's own nervous system. The device is usually bigger and is placed on the child's back supported by a harness during the waking and active period.

Complications of pacemakers
Complications depend on the surgical approach, e.g. endocardial placement could lead to thrombus and embolus formation. Infection presents a problem and requires the removal of the system and reinsertion of a new one. During and immediately following the insertion, ventricular ectopics and, rarely, ventricular fibrillation may occur, but these tend to settle within hours or days. The wire may become dislodged or break due to stretching from growth of the child. This presents with a real problem and frequently requires the introduction of a new system before the generator battery fails.

Principles of treatment and nursing management

1. Initially, the apex heart beat is recorded hourly and when the rate remains satisfactory, either the apex heart beat or radial pulse beat is recorded 4-hourly.
2. Observations:
   a. Recognition of battery failure and its effect, e.g. bradycardia, pallor, clammy skin and the child becomes agitated.
   b. Regular checking of the battery. A screwdriver and a spare battery must always be available. Nurses should know how to change a battery. This applies to an externally placed device.
   c. When the child has an externally placed pacemaker, the leads are checked to ensure that they are connected.
   d. Leads are attached to the skin with adhesive. This may present problems, particularly if the child's skin is sensitive to the adhesive. This might be overcome if a slightly larger piece of adhesive is kept on the skin to serve as anchor for the lead-retaining adhesive.
   e. When the controls are readily accessible, the child might be able to manipulate these, changing the rate. It is, therefore, essential to check that the rate setting has not been altered.
3. Night control (demand pacemaker). The pacemaker is removed from the child's back and placed at the side of the bed, with the leads left in position. The child usually sleeps in the upright position.

4. Bathing. It is essential to keep the leads dry and, to ensure this, it is safer to wash rather than bath the child.
5. Follow-up clinics. Once the child is able to go home, the parents will be shown how to observe and care for him and how to check his pulse rate and rhythm. Because of the potential problems, patients require regular follow-up at clinics where the rhythm and various pacemaker parameters can be checked. If the patient lives a long way from such a centre it may be possible to make these checks using a special transducer with a telephone link to the pacing centre.

Chapter 26
Disorders of the alimentary tract, liver and pancreas

This chapter discussions disorders affecting the alimentary tract, liver and pancreas. The disorders may be due to some structural abnormality or infection of the various structures.

The function of the alimentary tract is to digest and absorb the food ingested and eliminate that which the body does not require. Any interference with any of its functions will have profound and characteristic effects. The liver, as the largest and metabolically the most complex organ of the body, if damaged, will have serious biochemical consequences, while disorders of the pancreas will affect both digestive processes and the chemical control of sugar in the body.

ALIMENTARY TRACT

Mouth

The mouth is the first part of the digestive tract. The walls of the mouth cavity are structured to serve the functions of mastication, salivation, swallowing, tasting and speaking. The mouth is bounded on either side of the cheeks formed by the buccinator muscles; its roof is the palate which separates it from the nose and upper part of the pharynx; and the tongue forms the greater part of the floor.

The palate consists of two parts: the anterior or bony part and the posterior part which consists of mucous membrane and is called the soft palate. In the fetus the cavities of the mouth and nose are one; later they are divided by the palatal processes which meet in the midline. Persistence of a separate palate is often associated with a similar rift in the upper lip (cleft lip and palate, p. 471).

There are three pairs of salivary glands (parotid, mandibular and sublingual). Salivary glands secrete saliva via ducts into the mouth. The glands are innervated by both parasympathetic and sympathetic fibres, the former being more important. Saliva contains water, mucin (which acts as a lubricant), and ptyalin, an amylase which initiates digestion of starch. The pH of saliva is below 7 at low secretory rates, and increases as the rate of salivary formation increases.

The function of saliva is mainly mechanical. It assists mastication and swallowing, aids speech, and also has antiseptic action.

Secretion is provoked by the taste or thought of food. Salivary secretion is decreased during fever, illness and salivary gland disorders (p. 96).

Sucking, biting and swallowing are activities of the mouth. The infant's mouth is capable of forming a seal around the nipple or teat. The seal must be airtight if the baby is to suck. In the young infant the tongue is firmly opposed to the palate, therefore he can only breathe through the nose.

The saliva does not contain starch-digesting enzyme amylase for the first three months and therefore foods like cereals should only be introduced from 3 months of age.

Tongue

The tongue of the new-born is relatively short and broad. Taste buds are present on the papillae and the suckling response is increased by sweet substances. The tongue occupies the oral cavity and is attached directly to the epiglottis in the larynx. The epiglottis is situated quite high and this allows it to make direct contact with the soft palate. Three cleft-like spaces form the structures in the mouth, which allow fluids to pass into the pharynx. The elevation of the larynx directs the opening of the larynx into the nasopharynx so that the infant can breathe freely while fluid is passing into its pharynx. This is important since the new-born infant is a nose breather.

Table 26.1 The primary and permanent teeth

Primary teeth							
	Molar	Canine	Incisor	Incisor	Canine	Molar	
Upper jaw	2	1	2	2	1	2	
							20
Lower jaw	2	1	2	2	1	2	

Permanent teeth								
	Molar	Premolar	Canine	Incisor	Incisor	Canine	Premolar	Molar
Upper jaw	3	2	1	2	2	1	2	3
									32
Lower jaw	3	2	1	2	2	1	2	3

Teeth

Man is provided with two sets of teeth, which appear at different periods of life. The first set are the *primary* or deciduous teeth which are temporary and erupt through the gums during the first and second years. The second or permanent set replace the primary teeth and these start to erupt about the sixth year of life. By the age of 25 all the permanent teeth are present, with the possible exception of the third molar teeth or wisdom teeth.

There are 20 deciduous teeth and 32 permanent teeth (Table 26.1).

Teeth are of different sizes and shapes, but in any tooth there are three parts — the crown (visible above the gum), the neck (covered by the gum), and the root (held in the socket of the bone). Covering the crown is the enamel, which when intact, resists bacterial action. Cementum covers the neck and root and surrounds the dentine layer. This is a dense material resembling bone. The inner part of the tooth is the pulp cavity which contains nerves and blood vessels.

Oesophagus

The oesophagus is a muscular tube. It measures 8 to 10 cm from the cricoid cartilage to the cardiac part of the stomach. It doubles its length during the first 3 years after birth. Thereafter the growth rate is slower until it reaches the adult length of 23 to 30 cm.

The average diameter at birth is 5 mm with a less pronounced curvature than in the adult. The narrowest part is where the oesophagus joins the pharynx. This area is easily injured with probing instruments such as bougies or catheters.

The oesophagus descends and enters the abdominal cavity through an opening in the diaphragm (oesophageal hiatus). After about 1.25 cm, it opens into the stomach through the cardiac orifice. Just above this orifice is a circular layer of muscle called the cardiac sphincter. This muscle is capable of strong contraction and sometimes goes into spasm or achalasia (cardiac achalasia).

Disorders of the oesophagus include structural defects like oesophageal atresia and stenosis, infection, achalasia, oesophageal hiatus hernia and reflux.

Stomach

All the subdivisions of the adult stomach are present in the stomach of the fetus before birth. The capacity of the stomach is between 30 and 35 ml at birth and increases to about 75 ml by the second week of life; at the end of the first month it is about 100 ml, while the average stomach capacity of the adult is 1000 ml.

The mucosa and submucosa of the new-born infant are relatively thicker than they are in the adult. The number of gastric glands in the new-born is about 2 million, while in the adult it is over 25 million. Acid secretion begins before birth and proteolytic activity is also present, but at a lower level than that found after 2 to 3 months of age.

The musculature of the stomach is only moderately developed at birth and the peristaltic activity (contractions of the stomach) is poorly developed.

As the infant grows, the stomach develops until it has all the features of the adult stomach. These include the *main gastric glands* which secrete hydrochloric acid and mucus. The mucus covers the lining of the resting stomach and protects it by

preventing damage to the mucosa by acid digestion. The peptic cells contain pepsinogen (a
protein) which is converted to the enzyme pepsin
which acts on protein. The main gastric glands
also secrete a mucoprotein (called the intrinsic
factor) which combines very firmly with dietary
vitamin B_{12}. Rennin, an enzyme which curdles
milk, is found in the gastric juice of young children. Its function can also be performed by
pepsin.

Pyloric glands, found in the greater and lesser
curvature, secrete mucus which is alkaline and
protective to the surface on which the chyme
moves during digestion.

Cardiac tubular glands, are found at the oesophageal end of the stomach. These secrete mucus
and protect the gastric mucosa surrounding the
oesophagus. (Important in hiatus hernia.)

The prime function of the stomach is to prepare
the food for intestinal digestion, to break it up,
add fluid to it and, when it has been reduced to
a semifluid consistency, to pass it on to the
duodeum.

Small intestine

The small intestine is subdivided into the
duodenum, jejunum and ileum. Its length at birth
is about 300 to 350 cm. It increases about 50 per
cent during the first year of life and by adulthood
it measures about 6 metres.

The duodenum is the shortest part (7.5 to
10 cm) and its diameter is about 1 to 1.5 cm.

The intestinal wall is divided into several layers:
mucous, submucous, muscular and serous
(peritoneal).

The mucous membrane contains the following
structures:

1. Circular folds which run partially or
completely around the interior of the small intestine. These vary in size and number along the
small intestine. In the lower part of the ileum they
are small and only a few, if any, are present. They
serve to increase the absorbing surface of the
intestine.

2. Intestinal villi, which are finger-like processes
and project from the inner surface of the intestine,
consist of the following: epithelial covering
through which absorption takes place; smooth
muscle fibres; a lymph vessel (lacteal) which transports fats and a plexus of blood vessels fed by an
arteriole (Fig. 26.1).

The villi are larger and more numerous in the
duodenum and jejunum than in the ileum. These
villi are the absorbing units of the intestine. The

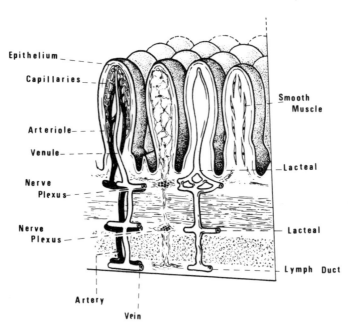

Fig. 26.1 Intestinal villi (normal).

smooth muscles are ceaselessly contracting and relaxing rhythmically during digestion. This causes shortening and lengthening or swaying movements of the villi. Damage to the villi interferes with absorption and is one cause of the malabsorption syndrome.

Openings of minute tubular glands which secrete intestinal juice are found at intervals between the villi. Brunner's glands, which are found in the first part of the duodenum, secrete an alkaline juice rich in mucus, which protect the mucosa against damage by the acid chyme of the stomach.

The other intestinal juice is also alkaline containing mucus and two enzymes (enterokinase and amylase). Certain other important enzymes are present in the lining cells of the intestine. Jejuno-ileo insufficiency can occur in conditions such as excision of the small intestine, gastro-colic fistula and gluten-sensitive enteropathy.

Maldevelopment of the small intestine may occur, e.g. atresia, re-duplication, malrotation and persistence of the vitalline duct connecting to the terminal ileum (Meckel's diverticulum).

Large intestine
The large intestine runs from the ileocaecal valve to the anus. It is described in five parts: the caecum, the ascending colon, the transverse colon, the descending colon and the sigmoid colon.

The caecum is the blind end of the ascending colon and is shaped like a pouch. The ileum enters it from the side and is guarded by the ileocaecal valve. The appendix, largely containing lymphoid tissue, is attached to the caecum at its base, and is a common site of inflammation (appendicitis).

The ascending colon, transverse colon and the descending colon form roughly three sides of a square and appear to enclose the small intestine, while the sigmoid colon becomes continuous with the rectum. In the new-born, the upper part of the rectum is usually directed to the right and the lower part descends vertically. At the lower end of the rectum is the anal canal which is about 2 to 3 cm long (in the infant it is relatively longer than in the adult) and it opens to the exterior through the anal orifice which is surrounded by the internal and external anal sphincter muscles.

The walls of the large intestine, like those of the small intestine, consist of mucous, submucous, muscular and serous (peritoneal) layers. There are no villi in the large intestine and its glands do not secrete digestive enzymes.

Functions of the large intestine
The large intestine secretes mucus, which facilitates the easy passage of the faeces and passes on the unabsorbed fraction of ingested iron, calcium and phosphate. Absorption of water, salt and glucose takes place in the large intestine.

Faeces
The faeces are derived partly from the ingested food, but mainly from the intestinal secretions. Faeces of the new-born is meconium, a thick mucous-green material consisting of intestinal debris. As the infant begins to feed, the faeces change in colour and consistency. Increase in faecal fat is found in coeliac disease, congenital fibrocystic disease and infantile steatorrhoea.

Movement of the alimentary tract
Wave-like movements occur along the alimentary canal. These waves (peristalsis) are found in the oesophagus and involve the Auerbach plexus. Swallowing initiates peristalsis, which also occurs in a different form in the stomach, in the upper part of which the peristaltic waves begin.

Movement of the small intestine is said to be of two kinds: peristalsis and segmentation. In peristalsis, the chyme is passed along the small intestine by a series of frequent and very rapid waves which carry it a little distance along. Each wave is followed by a resting period. In segmentation, a small portion of the small intestine becomes divided into a number of small segments by a series of constrictions. Segmentation causes no forward movement of the contents but it helps to mix the chyme with the intestinal juices and therefore aids digestion. It also brings the chyme into intimate contact with the villi and therefore aids absorption; it helps to squeeze blood and lymph out of the bowel and aids their return to the thoracic duct.

In the large intestine rhythmic variations occur which do not propel the contents onwards, but serve to mix them and so aid absorption of water. After each meal a gastro-colic reflex is set up. This initiates a brief, powerful peristalsis which drives the contents onwards. The normal rectum is empty, except immediately before defaecation.

Disorders of movement of the alimentary canal will hold up or block its contents. Some of these disorders are due to local degeneration of cells of the Auerbach plexus (Hirschsprung's disease), spasm of the pyloric sphincter leading to hypertrophy of the sphincter, or paralytic ileus (mechanical obstruction).

LIVER

The liver is the largest gland in the body and has many and varied functions. It consists of lobes which are subdivided into lobules. Each lobule is made up of branching columns of liver cells which are often indistinct and tissue-like, without distinguishable cell walls. The cells are supplied with blood from the portal vein and hepatic artery and blood is removed by the hepatic veins. The hepatic capillaries have no specific endothelial wall but ramify between the hepatic (liver) cells. There is therefore intimate contact between blood and liver cells. This is an ideal arrangement as the liver has to transform or modify many of the constituents of the blood.

Bile is formed in tiny vacuoles in the interior of the hepatic cells and is discharged through fine canaliculi into the bile capillaries. From the bile capillaries, the bile is transported via the bile duct into the gall-bladder, where it is stored.

The failure of some or all of the many functions of the liver may have widespread effects. A number of these effects seriously alter the composition of the extracellular fluid and the brain is particularly sensitive to these changes. The functions of the liver are as follows:

1. It modifies and makes harmless chemicals which would otherwise accumulate and poison the body.
2. It is the sole significant source of plasma albumin. In liver disease, there is a fall in the plasma albumin level.
3. Glucose is synthesised to glycogen in the liver and when the blood glucose level falls, stored glycogen is converted back into glucose and released into the blood. The liver, therefore, has an important role in maintaining a normal blood glucose level.
4. The liver secretes bile. Bile salts are essential for the digestion and absorption of fat, because they emulsify fat into small, water-soluble particles. This enables lipase (an enzyme) to act on fats and facilitate absorption.
5. The liver forms and destroys red blood cells.
6. It is the most important central organ of metabolism.

In the new-born, the liver appears to be structurally mature, but it is functionally immature. For example, it cannot handle bilirubin efficiently because of enzyme deficiency. It also does not allow vitamin K to function normally because of lack of other factors.

PANCREAS

The pancreas is a dual organ which consists of two types of tissue. The externally secreting alveolar tissue forms pancreatic juice and the internally secreting tissue (islets of Langerhans) forms insulin.

The composition of pancreatic juice varies with the rate of secretion; it contains the following substances: sodium bicarbonate which makes it markedly alkaline; sodium and potassium; chloride and enzymes (alpha-amylase) and lipase and proteolytic enzymes such as tripsinogen and chymotrypsinogen. Ribonuclease and deoxyribonuclease are also found; these split nucleic acids into nucleotides.

Pancreatic juice is an important part of the digestive process. Its secretion is regulated by nerves (vagi) and hormones (secretin and pancreozymin). The former responds to intake of food and the latter responds to the acid gastric contents emptying into the duodenum. Some diseases of the pancreas prevent pancreatic juices being formed or being available for digestive purposes, e.g. fibrocystic disease of the pancreas.

The islets of Langerhans provide the endocrine functions of the pancreas. There are up to 2 million islets which vary in diameter from 20 to 300 μm and which contain two main types of granular cell: alpha cells and beta cells. The alpha cells secrete glucagon which *raises* blood glucose. The beta cells secrete insulin which *lowers* blood glucose. Both cells are placed side by side, separated only by pericapillary spaces through which glucagon could readily be transported to act on the beta cells and promote secretion of insulin. The islets have a rich blood supply which drains into the portal vein. Both glucagon and insulin reach the liver in high concentration and exert profound effects there before they enter the systemic circulation to act elsewhere.

The functions of *glucagon* are to promote *glycogenolysis* (that is the conversion of glycogen to glucose mainly in the liver) and to stimulate gluconeogenesis (that is the formation of glucose or glycogen from non-carbohydrate sources, e.g. amino-acids, lactate and glycerol).

Insulin circulates in the blood plasma bound to a beta globulin. It is a protein and is destroyed by the proteolytic enzymes of the alimentary tract. For this reason it has to be given by injection when it is prescribed for treatment of diabetes mellitus. Insulin is an important hormone and deficiency or absence leads to a series of interconnected metabolic disturbances, e.g. metabolism of carbohydrate, fat, protein, electrolytes and water which have repercussions in most body systems.

The fundamental function of insulin is to promote the entry of glucose into certain cells (e.g. skeletal muscle, cardiac muscle, adipose tissue cells). Decreased entry leads to an intracellular glucose deficiency with an increased extracellular glucose (hyperglycaemia). Insulin prevents lipogenesis (i.e. mobilisation of fat) from adipose tissue and it is necessary for protein synthesis preventing protein breakdown. (See diabetes mellitus p. 281).

PERITONEUM

The peritoneum is the serous membrane lining the abdominal and pelvic cavities. It encloses the viscera, though some are only covered on their abdominal or pelvic surfaces. The peritoneum, like the pleura, consists of two layers which are in contact, the parietal layer and the visceral layer. The space between the layers is called the peritoneal cavity. The peritoneum follows the coils of the intestine and is thrown into folds and curves. These folds are called the mesentery. The peritoneum carries blood vessels, lymphatics and nerves to and from the bowel, and provides an important protective function, although it is also subject to inflammation (peritonitis).

Disorders of the alimentary tract

These disorders involve not only the structure but also the function of the digestive system. They include both abnormal formation of the structures as well as acquired abnormalities and disordered functions due to infection and trauma. It is not possible to include all the conditions and only those more commonly found will be considered. Also there are many conditions of other systems which partially manifest themselves in the alimentary tract.

Since nutrition is vital for the child, this aspect of nursing presents both a problem and a challenge to the nurse. Each child is an individual and will respond in his own way; this makes it difficult to provide solutions to all the different problems which the nurse will meet. It is hoped, however, that some of the ideas presented can be modified to suit individual needs.

DISORDERS OF THE MOUTH

Cleft lip and palate

Both conditions will be discussed together since they are so closely connected. They are developmental anomalies which are believed to occur in approximately one in 1000 births. There is no clear cause but it is thought that they are associated with family history and there is thus a greater risk of occurrence in children whose parents suffer from such abnormalities.

The deformities are usually divided into three groups:

1. Pre-alveolar cleft, in which the lip or lip and nostril are involved (fourth degree).
2. Alveolar cleft, where the cleft involves lip, alveolar ridge and usually the palate (third degree).
3. Post-alveolar cleft, in which the cleft is confined to the palate only (first and second degree). (See Fig. 26.2.)

Cleft lip (Fig. 26.3)

Varying degrees of malformation may occur, from a slight notching of the lip margin right or left of the midline, to a complete cleft running up to the nostril. There are further variations of this defect involving the palate.

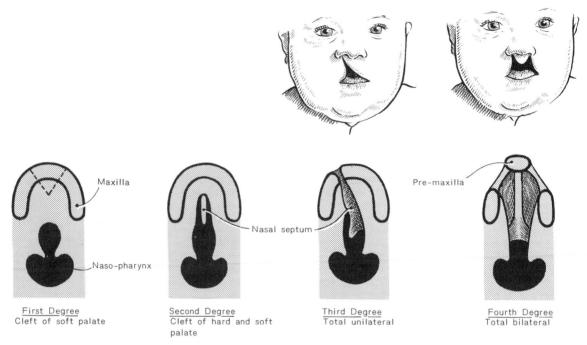

Fig. 26.2 First, second, third and fourth degree cleft lip and palate.

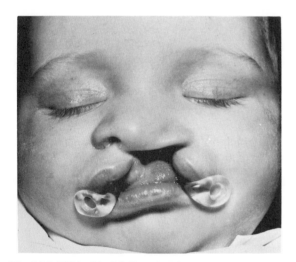

Fig. 26.3 Child with cleft lip and cleft palate. (Prosthesis for cleft palate shown.)

Principles of treatment and nursing management
The aims are to restore anatomical structure, correct the disfigurement and enable the child to have normal function in relation to swallowing, breathing and speech. These aims are achieved by surgical intervention and the operation is usually carried out when the child is about 3 months old, though in some centres it is carried out soon after birth.

1. Pre-operative care:
   a. Establishment of feeding, Feeding may be difficult at first but this will depend on the degree of deformity. In mild cases, it may be possible to breast feed the infant; otherwise bottle feeding may be easily established. If bottle feeding presents difficulty for the infant, he can be spoon fed, being allowed to suck from the spoon. If no cleft palate is present then little or no difficulty should be encountered; otherwise the infant will have problems not only with swallowing but also with sucking, since a complete palate is necessary for teat manipulation and sucking. Regurgitation of milk via the nose introduces another problem which is not without danger. Inhalation of milk must be prevented and suction equipment must be available at all times. The need to establish a good feeding pattern is essential to ensure that the infant is in a good physical state,

is gaining weight and is not anaemic. Anaemia should be corrected if, and when, it occurs.

b. Antibiotic cover is given to ensure that the post-operative period is not endangered by micro-organisms, already present, or introduced during the operative and post-operative period.

c. See general pre-operative preparation (p. 128).

2. Post-operative care:

a. See routine (p. 131).

b. Specific management.

Immobilisation of arms is an important aspect of nursing care. This is to prevent the infant from touching the stitch line (p. 86).

Sedation. A crying infant may increase tension on the stitch line. Although the tension is often reduced by applying a device, such as Logan's bow (Fig. 26.4), nevertheless some sedation may be advisable.

Dressing of stitch line. The stitch line is usually left uncovered and cleanliness is maintained by dabbing the area with sterile water or saline after each feed. Stitches are removed between the fifth and the eight day.

Feeding. Feeding can commence as soon as the infant is conscious and swallowing reflexes have been established.

If malalignment of the dental arch is present, an orthodontal plate will be inserted. This serves two functions: (1) it helps improve alignment of the arch by the time the baby is 3 months old and ready for lip repair, and (2) sucking is facilitated.

Cleft palate

Surgery is generally undertaken before the child begins to speak.

Clinical features

Feeding and speech will be difficult. Regurgitation of feeds presents problems of breathing, and inhalation of milk can lead to irritation of lung tissue and repeated upper respiratory infection. The palate is necessary for feeding and phonation. Surgical closure is undertaken by the time the child is 15 months old.

1. Pre-operative care:

a. This aims at establishing satisfactory feeding in the infant. A prosthesis is made to close the cleft to permit feeding without regurgitation of milk (Fig. 26.5).

b. The child is admitted 1 or 2 days prior to operation to accustom him to the hospital

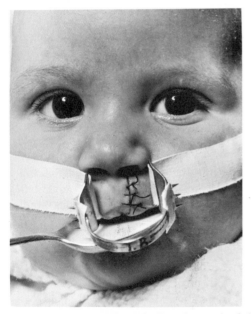

Fig. 26.4 Logan's bow and spoon feeding after repair of cleft lip.

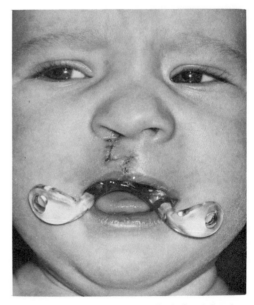

Fig. 26.5 Repaired cleft lip and prosthesis for cleft palate.

environment. Where possible, the mother should be resident with the child to decrease the trauma.

    c. Antibiotic cover should be given and any existing infection should be cleared before the operation.

    d. Routine pre-operation preparation (p. 128).

2. Post-operative care:

    a. Routine post-operative care (p. 131).

    b. Specific care.

Immobilisation. The arms should be restrained to prevent damage to the repair (p. 86).

Nutrition. The immediate post-operative diet should consist of clear fluids, e.g. glucose drinks. Normal diet once established should consist of soft food to be followed by sterile water. Hard foods and sweets should not be given for two or three weeks following the operation.

Removal of stitches. This is usually undertaken in theatre under sedation between the eighth and tenth day.

Speech therapy. If speech is not developing satisfactorily speech therapy will be given. This is initiated by a trained speech therapist. Since the amount of treatment or training to be given by a speech therapist will be limited, the main burden will fall on the mother. Therefore both mother and child should take part in these sessions with the speech therapist so that the mother can continue the therapy at home. With conscientious training it should be possible for the child to achieve a level of speech which will enable him to communicate freely and easily with others by the time he starts school.

Oral thrush

This is an infection of the mouth by the *Candida albicans.* In the new-born infant, it may occur as a result of monilial infection in the mother, but it may also be a complication of hypoparathyroidism or of continued antibiotic therapy.

Clinical features

The lesions appear as white patches on the mucous membrane of the mouth. They look like milk flakes but can not be removed. The infant becomes anorexic and refuses feeds, and he may vomit and have loose stools.

Principles of treatment and nursing management

1. Use of anti-fungal drug, e.g. nystatin 100 000 units/ml given after feed.
2. Use of gentian violet 0.5 per cent in water. This must be freshly prepared or evaporation of water will leave a concentrated solution which can cause ulceration. When gentian violet is used, the infant's arms should be immobilised to prevent him from placing his hands in his mouth. Since gentian violet causes severe staining, clothes should preferably be older ones which are at least washable, if not disposable. The treatment usually lasts about 3 days.
3. Routine nursing care.

Acute stomatitis

In this condition, the mucous membrane of the mouth is inflamed and ulcerated. The great majority of cases are caused by a dermotrophic or neurotropic virus which is probably transmitted by direct contact with skin or mouth lesions.

Clinical features

The child appears to be acutely ill with a temperature of 38 to 40°C. The gums are quite red and swollen and bleed easily. Numerous vesicles may form and rupture, leaving greyish sloughs and ulcers. Vesicles develop on the palate, tongue and gums. Since this is very painful, the child is unable to eat and may have difficulty in drinking.

Principles of treatment and nursing management

1. There is no specific drug therapy.
2. Nursing care:

    a. Care of the mouth (p. 96). For the young child this involves gentle cleaning of the mouth and removal of any food particles. Solution of potassium chlorate 60 mg three times a day seems to afford some relief.

The older child is able to rinse out his mouth with saline and this should be done frequently. Sedation helps to relieve the discomfort and facilitates the swallowing of fluids.

    b. A fluid chart should be maintained to record both intake and output.

    c. Immobilisation of arms may be necessary to prevent the young child touching the sore area (p. 86).

d. Gradual introduction of soft diet when the mouth lesions improve.

e. Routine nursing care.

Pierre-Robin syndrome (micrognathia)

This anomaly may be associated with a wide cleft of the soft and hard palates. Primarily it is due to hypoplasia of the mandible. The tongue is poorly fixed and tends to fall back into the gap, interfering with feeding and breathing.

Clinical features

The severity of the symptoms is related to the degree of displacement of the tongue. The principal difficulties are severe inspiratory stridor, cyanotic attacks and feeding difficulties. It is particularly dangerous in the new-born infant.

Principles of treatment and nursing management

1. Surgical intervention and correction:
   a. Tracheostomy may have to be performed in severe cases to relieve the obstruction to breathing (p. 386).
   b. Repair of cleft palate. As the baby grows older, the shape of the mandible improves and the palate is repaired at about 15 months.
2. Nursing management:
   a. Position of the infant. The infant should be nursed in the prone position. This tends to keep the tongue forward and thereby prevents obstruction to breathing. The infant may be placed on a frame.
   b. Feeding. This always presents a problem and the most suitable position should be found to ensure that the infant can feed without breathing difficulties. Feeds may be given by naso-gastric tube or by spoon. Another method which may be helpful is 'orthostatic' feeding whereby the infant is fed in the upright position. The teat is pressed against the upper alveolus and held sufficiently away from the lower alveolus to make him strain forward with his lower jaw to grasp the teat.
   c. Suction equipment should be available during feeding and at all other times to prevent inhalation of milk.
   d. Routine nursing care.

3. Guidance for parents. The parents should be shown how to handle and feed the infant and before returning home the mother should feel confident in her ability to do so. Close medical supervision will be necessary and the parents should be encouraged to contact the hospital if they are worried.

DISORDERS OF THE OESOPHAGUS AND STOMACH

The new-born infant may be born with oesophageal abnormalities. These include congenital oesophageal atresia, stenosis or duplication.

Congenital atresia of the oesophagus
(Fig. 26.6)

This is generally in the form of tracheo-oesophageal fistula. In 95 per cent of cases the oesophageal pouch ends blindly and the lower pouch communicates directly with the back of the trachea. The two oesophageal ends are separated by about one or more centimetres (Type A).

Other variations include Type B, where the lower oesophagus has no connection with the trachea, the lower pouch is very short and protrudes only slightly above the diaphragm; Type C, where only the upper pouch communicates with the trachea; and Type D, where both oesophageal segments communicate with the trachea.

About 30 per cent of children have associated anomalies such as congenital heart disease and malformations of the anus and rectum.

Clinical features

Characteristic findings are seen in the early hours of life and diagnosis should be made before the first feed is given.

1. Excessive salivation, i.e. saliva tends to dribble from the mouth in the form of froth.
2. If feeding is attempted, there will be gagging and coughing.
3. Breathing difficulties and cyanosis.
4. There will be feeding difficulties with some aspiration of feeds leading to aspiration pneumonia. However, this may not be evident until 2 or 3 days after feeding has begun.
5. Pneumonitis due to damage from reflux of gastric juice through the lower pouch.

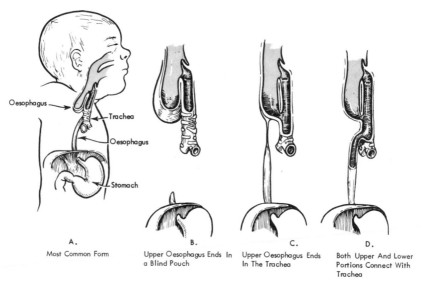

Fig. 26.6 Atresia of the oesophagus.

A.
Most Common Form

B.
Upper Oesophagus Ends In a Blind Pouch

C.
Upper Oesophagus Ends In The Trachea

D.
Both Upper And Lower Portions Connect With Trachea

Confirmation of diagnosis

1. Whenever the abnormality is suspected, the patency of the oesophagus is investigated. For this purpose a special radiopaque catheter is passed via the mouth into the oesophagus. Care must be taken to ensure that the catheter does not curl up in the oesophageal pouch, giving the appearance of having passed into the stomach. If an atresia is present, the catheter will be arrested 10 to 12 cm from the alveolar margin.

2. X-ray examination. With the radiopaque catheter in position an X-ray will then be taken. Rarely, contrast media is instilled via a small urethral catheter. This will outline the blind oesophageal pouch. A lateral film is also taken to demonstrate, if possible, the presence of a fistula. During this examination the infant should be lying prone and the medium aspirated on completion of the examination. If a tracheo-oesophageal fistula is present, as in approximately 90 per cent of cases, the X-ray will demonstrate air in the stomach.

Principles of treatment and nursing management

1. Pre-operative care:
   a. General neonatal pre-operative nursing care (p. 156).
   b. Constant nursing presence.
   c. Warmed humidity to help keep secretions fluid. The infant is in danger of choking, should secretions be allowed to build up in his throat. Oral and naso-pharyngeal suction will be required, probably at hourly intervals. It is sometimes necessary to aspirate the mucus more frequently, perhaps even half-hourly, but suction done too often may actually encourage secretions and would necessitate handling the infant more often.
   d. To aid drainage of secretions a Replogle tube, which is a catheter with a double lumen, is inserted into the base of the blind pouch, or to the back of the throat, and the main lumen is attached to continuous suction at a level of approximately 5 cm water.
      To keep the secretions moist and to keep the opening at the end of the catheter clear, 0.5 ml of water is inserted half-hourly through the side arm of the tube.
   e. Nursing the infant in the prone position is another method which can be adopted to allow more satisfactory 'drainage' of secretions, preventing them from entering the lungs. However, he should be repositioned regularly, partly from side to side, to aid circulation and lung expansion.

f. If the diagnosis has not been made shortly after birth, some degree of lung damage may be present and physiotherapy can help to loosen deep secretions. This can be done with a battery-operated toothbrush padded with gauze which is moved over the infant's chest. More vigorous physiotherapy is not normally required.

g. Antibiotics will be ordered if a chest infection is present.

h. Blood-gas analysis may be ordered.

2. Operation. Surgery is performed via a right thoracotomy. The aim is to divide the tracheo-oesophageal fistula, close the trachea and unite the two segments of oesophagus. While the anastomosis is being performed a fine tube — normally size 6 FG — is passed through one nostril, across the anastomosis and into the stomach. The chest is closed with underwater seal drainage to the pleural cavity.

Sometimes the gap between the ends of the oesophagus is too wide for a primary anastomosis to be done, and one alternative which may be considered is the creation of an oesophagostomy. This consists of the proximal oesophagus being brought out in the neck, allowing drainage of pharyngeal secretions and helping to prevent aspiration pneumonia.

When a primary anastomosis is not achieved, a gastrostomy is performed to enable feeding.

3. Post-operative care: primary repair of oesophageal atresia and division of tracheo-oesophageal fistula.

a. Routine post-operative neonatal care (p. 131).

b. Constant nursing presence while the baby is acutely ill.

c. Clamps will have been applied to the chest catheter in theatre, so that a closed system is achieved, and immediately on return to the ward the underwater seal system, as described on page 390, is correctly joined up. Only then are the clamps released and the fluid checked to be fluctuating. The bottle is secured at a level lower than the infant's chest. The tubing must always be clamped when any prolonged procedure is being carried out, to prevent reflux of fluid. A dated marker is placed at upper level of the fluid in the bottle, stating the amount of fluid used. It is then possible to determine how much additional fluid, i.e. drainage, is in the bottle after a period of 24 hours. The distal tubing and bottle are changed daily, under strict aseptic conditions. An hourly record is kept to show whether the underwater seal system is fluctuating and whether it is draining. The colour and consistency of the fluid are recorded.

d. Some infants are nursed on mechanical ventilation for 24 hours post-operatively. On return from theatre the system is checked and the settings recorded. Thereafter the machine settings are recorded hourly.

It may only be necessary to give oxygen via a head box, with a high level of warmed humidity.

e. Respirations, apical heart rate and body temperature are recorded. Initially these measurements are made hourly but approximately 8 hours post-operatively they may be charted 2-hourly then 4-hourly, as the infant's condition allows. The incubator or radiant heater temperature is also recorded.

f. Oral and nasal suction and endotracheal suction, if a tube is in place, are performed immediately on return from theatre. Great care must be taken that the pharyngeal suction catheter is not inserted further than the level of the anastomosis as it could cause a breakdown of the suture line. The surgeon should be asked to state a safe length for the catheter to be passed and a measure should be taped in a conspicuous place as a warning that a longer insertion may endanger the baby's recovery.

g. Reflux of stomach contents up the oesophagus could cause breakdown of the anastomosis; the stomach is therefore kept empty by the transanastomotic naso-gastric tube being kept on free drainage and aspirated hourly. Until the anastomosis is healed it is unsafe to risk the trauma of passing further catheters; therefore the existing catheter should be as secure as possible. This can be done by putting a little adhesive tape at each side of the nose, and then putting an atraumatic suture through the naso-gastric tube and securely knotting the thread. Each end of the thread is then placed over the tape and secured by a further piece of adhesive. The suture also acts as an ideal marker, from which it can be seen whether the tube has slipped.

h. The baby is placed in a slightly 'head up' position and is initially turned 2-hourly then, as his condition allows, less frequently to avoid disturbing him unduly. Repositioning, usually from side to side, will aid lung expansion.

i. Intravenous fluids are checked on return from theatre, then hourly. Blood urea and electrolyte levels will determine the type of fluids given.

j. The wound and underwater seal dressings are checked hourly for 12 hours, for any indication of leakage.

k. Physiotherapy with a toothbrush (see p. 477) is not normally done until 24 hours after operation, and the infant's condition will determine its frequency.

l. Antibiotics may be ordered.

m. A post-operative chest X-ray will check the position of the underwater seal drain.

n. Blood gases will be checked regularly to determine the amount of oxygen necessary. A PO_2 monitor may also be used.

By the second post-operative day, 5 ml of glucose water may be given hourly via the nasogastric tube which is connected to a syringe barrel and elevated. The naso-gastric tube is aspirated 2-hourly prior to feeding and some fluids tested for acidity to confirm its presence in the stomach. Accurate records are kept. Some infants are given total parenteral nutrition for varying periods, perhaps a week, post-operatively while others may have intravenous fluids discontinued earlier in the post-operative period. Milk feeds of 10 ml hourly are gavaged but a check on the urea and electrolyte balance will indicate whether there is a need for the infusion to be retained. Unless there are contra-indications, oral feeding is commenced approximately 10 to 14 days after operation following a barium examination or a 'trial' feed of water. Some surgeons will request removal of the naso-gastric tube while others

favour retaining it until the infant is sucking well and no complications have arisen.

Oxygen may be discontinued after 24 hours but humidity will be continued for a few days to keep pharyngeal secretions moist. By the third or fourth post-operative day humidity may be stopped and pharyngeal suction should not be necessary any more than 4-hourly, following physiotherapy.

The chest drain is removed as early in the post-operative period as possible; usually when the lung is fully inflated and it is obvious that drainage has stopped and there is no evidence of a recurrence of the tracheo-oesophageal fistula. It should be removed by an experienced member of staff, along with a competent assistant. Firm pressure is applied over the drain site as it is removed so that air will not enter the pleural space, and a chest X-ray will confirm that this is the case. An occlusive dressing is kept in place for 2 days.

Wound sutures are removed approximately 8 days post-operatively. A routine renal ultrasound is done to rule out the presence of renal abnormalities and if there are no complications the infant will go home about two to three weeks following operation. The parents will be advised to provide normal care for the child. However, they should also be told how to identify the onset of complications and it must be stressed that medical aid should be sought if they occur.

4. Complications:

a. The first indications of a leak at the level of the anastomosis may be a rise in respiratory rate, then apical heart rate. If the leak is severe the distal oesophagus may have to be closed and an oesophagostomy formed from the proximal oesophagus. A gastrostomy is performed.

b. If the tracheo-oesophageal fistula recurs, some mucus or feed may be seen in the chest catheter or tubing. Feeds will either be completely stopped and the baby given total parenteral nutrition for a period, or feeding may continue via the naso-gastric tube by continuous drip, to minimise reflux. Further operative treatment may, however, by required.

c. Approximately a third of these babies have some narrowing at the level of anastomosis and this should be considered if they do not feed well or if they choke whilst feeding. Oesophagoscopy and dilatation of the stricture is necessary.

d. Wound or chest infections are treated with antibiotics and, where appropriate, by physiotherapy.

Nursing care following oesophagostomy and gastrostomy

1. Routine post-operative neonatal care (p. 131).
2. The oesophagostomy is exposed and gently cleaned with dry, sterile cotton wool as necessary (Fig. 26.7).
3. Immediately following operation the gastrostomy tube is left on free drainage and aspirated hourly. Feeding is started on the first post-operative day when the tube is attached to a syringe barrel and elevated.
4. The gastrostomy dressing is changed daily.
5. Approximately one week after operation the infant will start to have sham feeds. These are given at the same time as gastrostomy feeds and consist of the baby being fed orally and the feeds being discharged through the oesophagostomy so that, while his stomach is filling up, he is learning to suck and swallow. Care must be taken to keep the skin around the oesophagostomy intact, therefore after sham feeding it

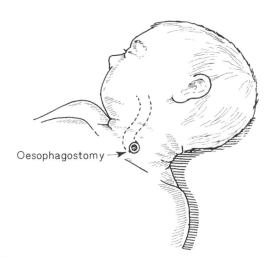

Oesophagostomy →

Fig. 26.7 Oesophagostomy stoma.

must be cleaned and dried carefully. A barrier cream may be of value.

6. During the time the infant is in hospital, his parents will have been given opportunities to feed him and to care for the skin around his oesophagostomy and gastrostomy. When the baby is thriving and his parents are confident in caring for him he will be allowed home.

Delayed primary repair

Another early method of treating the baby who is unable to have a primary repair of oesophageal atresia, is to leave the proximal pouch intact, applying continuous suction. Eventually the infant may be able to cope without continuous suction, by dribbling excess secretions from his mouth. Daily oesophageal bougienage is performed and it is hoped that this, along with the infant swallowing, will help to enlarge the proximal pouch.

The distal end of the oesophagus may be stretched if bolus feeds are given via a gastrostomy tube which is spigotted between feeds. Regular barium studies will indicate growth of the oesophagus and this, along with the infant's general condition, will determine the best time for surgery.

Generally, a delayed primary repair between the proximal and distal oesophagus may be done at 6 months to 1 year of age. Other common methods of repair are:

1. Gastric tube replacement. A 'tube' is formed from the fundus of the stomach and is anastomosed to the proximal oesophagus.
2. A segment of colon is placed between the two ends of the oesophagus or between the upper end of the oesophagus and the stomach.
3. Gastro-oesophagostomy. Another method which has been attempted is for the stomach to be brought up the posterior mediastinum and anastomosed to the proximal oesophagus.

Following the above procedures recovery may be complicated by a leak at the anastomosis which usually heals spontaneously. When feeding has been established the gastrostomy tube is removed.

Achalasia of the cardia (cardiospasm)

In this condition the oesophagus is dilated, hypertrophied and lengthened, but there is no apparent mechanical obstruction. It is not a common condition.

Clinical features

The child has difficulty in swallowing: feeds are regurgitated and there is retrosternal discomfort. The diagnosis is made by radiography (barium swallow).

Principles of treatment and nursing management

Treatment consists of: (1) relieving the cardiospasm with anti-spasmodic drugs (which do not give permanent relief); and (2) surgery, e.g. Heller's operation, in which the hypertrophied muscles are divided. This operation is similar to Ramstedt's operation for pyloric stenosis (p. 481).

1. Medical treatment. The anti-spasmodic drug is given before the feed.
2. Surgical treatment:
   a. Pre-operative preparation (p. 128).
   b. Post-operative care:
      (i) Routine (p. 131).
      (ii) Specific: feeding can be commenced when consciousness has been reestablished, starting with fluids and gradually introducing semi-solids.
3. Routine nursing care.
4. Support for parents. Explanation about the condition and participation in nursing. Recognition of anxiety during the acute phase.

Cardio-oesophageal chalasia

'Achalasia' means failure to relax. 'Chalasia' means relaxation. It is used here to denote abnormal action of the cardio-oesophageal sphincter, which leads to persistent relaxation of the sphincter causing vomiting. The cause is unknown.

Pathological physiology

The oesophagus fills with gastric contents when the stomach is compressed or when the head is lowered. This can be demonstrated with a barium swallow.

Clinical features

1. Vomiting. The baby vomits soon after birth. Vomiting is effortless and occurs frequently, either during or immediately after each feed.

2. The infant fails to gain weight and there may be evidence of weight loss. If severe enough, there may also be dehydration and malnutrition.

Investigations

1. Barium swallow. This shows the barium flowing freely up the oesophagus (see above).
2. Serum studies, e.g. calcium level may be lowered and alkalosis may be found due to loss of gastric juices.

Principles of treatment and nursing management

1. Position of infant. The infant is nursed in the sitting position. Care must be taken to ensure that the baby is well supported, either in a padded chair or with pillows.
2. Feeds may be thickened by adding cereals. If the feed is given by bottle, the teat hole should be enlarged to allow easy flow of feed. This enlarged-hole teat should be used only for thickened feeds and not for normal milk feeds, as the young infant cannot control a rapid flow of milk and may inhale the milk.
3. Correction of dehydration if present.
4. Accurate recording of the amount of feed taken, and if vomiting occurs, the amount vomited and the type of vomiting.
5. Routine nursing care.
6. Support for parents. The mother should be given the opportunity to nurse and feed her baby. Once feeding is established with minimal vomiting, then the baby can be nursed at home. Guidance and full explanations should be given to enable the mother to care for her child.

Congenital hypertrophic pyloric stenosis

This is common condition which occurs more frequently in males than in females and is usually diagnosed between the ages of 3 and 6 weeks.

The pattern of inheritance is polygenic (due to the actions of several different genes) and there is an increased risk in siblings and the offspring of affected children.

Pathological physiology

The smooth circular muscle fibres of the pylorus hypertrophy giving rise to a mass about the size of a small nut (about 20 × 15 mm). The mucosa

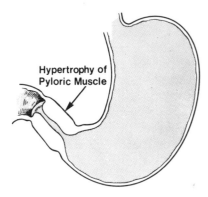

Fig. 26.8 Pyloric stenosis.

is pushed inwards decreasing the pyloric lumen which is further reduced due to oedema produced by forcing the food bolus through the lumen. Constriction of the lumen at the distal end of the stomach causes the stomach to become dilated. There is also some hypertrophy of the muscular coat of the stomach (Fig. 26.8).

Clinical features

Vomiting is the earliest sign. At first it is non projectile but as the obstruction progresses it becomes projectile. There is loss of weight or failure to gain weight and the infant is eager to feed.

Repeated vomiting leads to constipation and decreased stools, decreased urinary output and signs of dehydration with loss of electrolytes. Alkalosis develops and urinary chlorides are decreased or absent.

Investigations

1. Test feeding. This consists of giving the infant a feed. The infant lies with the abdominal area exposed while feeding, and the doctor inspects the abdomen and observes the passing of peristaltic waves during and after feeding. These waves may be seen passing from left to right across the epigastrium. Visible gastric peristalsis is not regarded as a positive diagnostic feature, palpation of the tumour being a more positive test. If there is any doubt the diagnosis is confirmed radiologically.
2. Barium meal. A small quantity of barium will show a narrowed pyloric canal, with indentation of the duodenum.

3. Serum studies. Sodium and pH are increased, while serum chloride and potassium are decreased.

Principles of treatment and nursing management

1. Medical treatment. This takes longer and consists of daily gastric lavage and oral administration of Eumydrin, given 20 minutes before each feed.
2. Surgical treatment. This is the most common form of treatment.
   Pre-operative care includes:
   a. Correction of dehydration.
   b. Gastric lavage 4 hours before the operation, leaving naso-gastric tube in position.
   c. Conservation of body heat.
   d. Pre-medication.
   e. If a local anaesthetic is given, the infant is immobilised, e.g. bandaged on a 'T' splint or Velcro splint.
   f. Prevention of infection (isolation).
   The operation used is 'Ramstedt's pyloromyotomy'. A longitudinal incision is made through the serous and muscular layers, without involving the mucosal layer.
3. Post-operative care:
   a. Maintenance of body heat.
   b. Prevention of infection.
   c. Establishing feeding. Feeding is started 3 to 4 hours after operation. Small quantities of glucose saline are given at half-hourly intervals for 2 hours and then milk feeds are started. Small feeds, approximately 30 ml per feed are given and these are gradually increased until the infant receives the required amount.
   d. Wound care. Provided there is no obvious infection the wound is not disturbed until the stitches are removed, usually on the tenth day.
   e. Preparation for home. To prevent cross-infection, the infant is sent home as soon as feeding is successfully established. The mother is given clear instruction on handling the infant, e.g. feeding and bathing, and told not to disturb the dressing (the would should be inspected before sending him home) and a date given to bring the

infant back for removal of stitches and reassessment.

4. Routine nursing care.

Hiatus hernia

The term hiatus hernia implies that part of the stomach protrudes through the oesophageal hiatus into the chest. Normally, the junction of the oesophagus and stomach is situated below the hiatus of the diaphragm leaving a short length of oesophagus within the abdominal cavity. Two types of hernia are recognised in infancy:

1. Sliding hiatus hernia. In this type, a portion of the stomach is drawn upwards above the diaphragm by the oesophagus which appears to be shorter than normal.
2. Para-oesophageal hernia. The oesophagus is of normal length and a part of the fundus of the stomach is prolapsed alongside it.

In both types there may be reflux of gastric contents leading to oesophagitis, dysphagia, haematemesis and melaena.

Clincal features

Vomiting occurs early in infancy though occasionally the onset of vomiting may be delayed. Vomiting is often copious and projectile and may occur during or shortly after feeding. The vomitus may contain blood and mucus. The infant presents with loss of weight or inability to gain weight.

Investigations

The condition is confirmed by barium swallow and fluoroscopy. A positive faecal occult blood test is also strong evidence of the presence of a hiatus hernia. An oesophagoscopy is also often performed to assess the degree of oesophagitis and stricture formation.

Principles of treatment and nursing management

1. Medical treatment. The aim is to prevent reflux of gastric contents. This can be achieved to a certain extent by nursing the baby in the sitting position at an angle of 60° or more both by day and by night. Frequent small feeds may help to reduce vomiting in small infants. Gaviscon, an alginate/antacid compound can be given after meals and at bedtime. A similar preparation can be mixed into the feeding bottle. Since it would increase the sodium content of milk feeds, it is preferable to use a sodium-free preparation such as Asilone.

2. Surgical treatment:
   a. A gastrostomy may be performed to rest the lower part of the oesophagus.
   b. Repair of defect. This varies with the age of the child. A gastropexy (surgical fixation of the stomach) may be performed in children under 12 months, combined with tightening of the hiatus, provided there is no stenosis present. In the presence of stenosis, or in children over the age of 12 months, a more extensive operation is required. The oesophagus is mobilised to ensure an adequate length within the abdomen and is then retained by a Nissen fundoplication, in which the body of the stomach is wrapped around and sutured in front of the oesophagus.

3. Pre-operative preparation (p. 128).
4. Post-operative management:
   a. Immediate care (p. 131).
      (i) Care of the child with underwater seal drainage (p. 390).
      (ii) Care of the child receiving intravenous infusion (p. 448).
      (iii) Observation of wound.
      (iv) Observations of vital functions.
   b. Nutrition:
      (i) Gradual introduction to oral feeding.
      (ii) Observations regarding sucking, swallowing and retention of feed.
   c. Repeated dilatation if a stricture is present.
5. Routine nursing care.
6. Support for parents:
   a. Recognition of the difficulties and feeling of revulsion due to the frequent vomiting with its associated offensive odour which necessitates constant washing.
   b. Satisfying the need for information regarding the condition, treatment and progress.
   c. Participation in nursing the child.

Diaphragmatic hernia

This is a congenital abnormality which occurs during the complex developmental process. If it occurs during the early stage, there is free communication between the pleural cavity and the abdomen. During the later stages of development a pleural sac will be present consisting of both membranes.

The most common herniation is in the left posteriolateral part of the diaphragm.

Clinical features and pathological physiology
The severity of the symptoms depends on the degree of herniation of the abdominal organs into the chest and the degree of displacement of the lungs. It also depends on the presence or absence of intestinal obstruction. In relation to the above there may be evidence of dyspnoea and cyanosis. Vomiting will be present due to the presence of intestinal obstruction.

Investigations
The condition can be confirmed by (a) chest X-ray which will show a portion of the gastro-intestinal tract in the thorax, and (b) X-ray examination of the gastro-intestinal tract.

Principles of treatment and nursing management

1. Pre-operative care:
   a. Routine neonatal pre-operative nursing care (p. 156).
   b. Constant nursing presence.
   c. Naso-gastric drainage will help to keep the stomach deflated. The tube should also be aspirated hourly.
   d. An endotracheal tube will probably be passed to prevent further expansion of abdominal viscera. Intermittent positive pressure ventilation (p. 395) may be necessary.
   e. Prophylactic antibiotics may be prescribed.
2. Operation. Operation is normally performed through an abdominal incision and the herniated gut is pulled down from the chest and out through the abdominal incision, allowing the diaphragmatic defect to be repaired. The spleen or part of the liver may be in the chest and these are replaced in the abdominal cavity. A left underwater seal drain is inserted into the left pleural cavity. Many surgeons favour the idea of bilateral chest drains as there is a danger of contralateral pneumothorax occurring.

3. Post-operative care:
   a. Routine neonatal post-operative care (p. 131).
   b. Constant nursing presence.
   c. If the infant has been under 24 hours old at operation he will probably require intermittent positive pressure ventilation for approximately 18 hours after he returns from theatre, but this, of course, depends on his condition.
   d. Confirm that underwater seal systems are correctly connected and are checked hourly (p. 390).
   e. Sterile water, 0.5 ml, is instilled hourly via the endotracheal tube prior to suction. Sterile gloves are worn. Oral and nasal suction is also done hourly.
   f. Respirations, apical heart rate and body temperature are recorded hourly, then less frequently, as the infant's condition allows.
   g. Hourly suction and drainage of a naso-gastric tube will help to keep the stomach empty.
   h. Intravenous fluids and the infusion site are checked hourly. Blood urea and electrolytes will be checked.
   i. Hourly to 2-hourly repositioning. Care must be taken not to dislodge the endotracheal tube during this procedure. Ideally it should be done by two nurses. The infant's head is kept in a straight line with his body and a small piece of linen rolled up under his neck will help to maintain the position of the tube.
   j. Dressings are checked hourly for 12 hours, for any indication of leakage.
   k. Physiotherapy may be ordered shortly after operation and will be continued 4-hourly.
   l. Antibiotics may be prescribed.
   m. Blood gases will determine the amount of oxygen necessary.

Approximately 12 hours after ventilation has been discontinued the infant may be extubated and the tip of the endotracheal tube is sent for bacterial culture. Oxygen therapy with high, warmed humidity is continued after spontaneous respirations are established.

The underwater seal drain on the unaffected

side will normally be removed approximately 48 hours after operation because the risk of contra-lateral pneumothorax is markedly decreased as the lung on the affected side expands. The drain on the side of the defect will be removed when the lung is fully expanded and this normally takes place between the second and fifth post-operative day. Removal of the drain will be followed by a chest X-ray to ensure that the lung remains inflated. The intravenous infusion may be stopped approximately 2 days after operation if the baby is tolerating naso-gastric feeds. Some infants with this condition have a degree of malrotation of gut following repair, therefore any vomiting must be reported.

Naso-gastric feeds will probably be continued for a week or more, when the infant should be able to cope with feeding orally and shows no signs of respiratory distress.

If his mother feels she can cope, the infant may go home after two or three weeks, as long as he is feeding well, gaining weight and his chest X-rays are satisfactory.

VOMITING

Vomiting is a common symptom throughout child-hood and may be associated with a wide variety of diseases of all degrees of severity. It is a reflex action which is co-ordinated in the medulla oblongata, whereby the contents of the stomach are forcibly expelled through the mouth. Vomiting may be associated with food poisoning, disease of the digestive tract, intracranial disease, drugs and toxins produced by bacteria.

Vomiting in infancy

Vomiting in the first 24 to 48 hours of life is usually due to swallowed blood or liquor amnii. If vomiting persists, consists of green material and is associated with abdominal distension, then it is suggestive of intestinal obstruction.

Vomiting of mouthfuls of milk is fairly common, especially in breast-fed infants. It does not interfere with satisfactory weight gain and is generally due to the swallowing of air. In bottle-fed infants, this can be due to the hole in the teat being too small so that more air than milk is swallowed. The infant does not appear to be ill, there is no elevation of body temperature and there is no associated diarrhoea.

Vomiting due to infection. Nasal obstruction from rhinitis makes feeding difficult and leads to air swallowing and vomiting. This can be relieved by the instillation of nose drops, e.g. 1 per cent ephedrine in physiological saline, before each feed. Other infections which are associated with vomiting include gastroenteritis, meningitis and respiratory infections.

Vomiting due to obstruction. In infancy this may be due to pyloric stenosis when it is projectile and forcible, or due to intestinal obstruction or hiatus hernia.

Rumination. Rumination can be defined as the regurgitation of partially digested food. This is said to be a habit which allows the infant to obtain a measure of oral gratification by voluntarily bringing back into his mouth some of his feed, which he partly vomits and partly chews. When observing the infant he can be seen to curl his tongue into a funnel and milk is regurgitated along it by rhythmic back and forward movements of his mandible.

The reason for this behaviour is not clear, but it is considered a psycho-neurosis of infancy associated with some emotional disturbance. The treatment is often difficult and nursing management demands a great deal of patience and skill. The emphasis is on preventing regurgitation and several methods may have to be attempted. For example, feeds may be thickened with cereal, after which he should be propped up to a sitting position. He should be prevented from placing his fingers or fists into his mouth by some means of immobilisation. This causes a great deal of frustration to the infant. Some doctors sedate the infant, but this is not often successful. His attention should be diverted and he should be given a great deal of affection, e.g. he could be lifted out of his cot for feeding and cuddling. It is sometimes difficult to cuddle an infant who frequently regurgitates his feeds with the attendant unpleasant odour, and so every effort should be made to keep the infant clean and fresh. Rejection must be avoided however difficult it may be. Fortunately regurgitation tends to stop when the infant begins to stand unsupported.

Older children

Vomiting in older children is associated with conditions similar to those in infants. These include obstruction or infection of the digestive tract or a general infection, in fact, almost any disease with fever at the onset. Vomiting may also be associated with disease of the central nervous system, e.g. tumours, oedema and acute meningitis.

Cyclic vomiting. This is also known as the periodic syndrome. It comprises severe attacks of vomiting lasting from 12 to 72 hours which may result from psychological or emotional causes. The attacks may be precipitated by upper respiratory infection or emotional disturbances. Recovery is spontaneous and after the attack, the child seems well and active. However, in severe cases the child becomes dehydrated and his breath has the sweet smell of acetone, which is also contained in the urine.

Principles of treatment and nursing management

1. Treatment of the cause:
    a. Antibiotics for infection.
    b. Surgical intervention for intestinal obstruction.
    c. Drugs, such as promazine hydrochloride, to stop the vomiting.
    d. Intravenous infusion to correct fluid and electrolyte imbalance (p. 448).
2. Nursing management:
    a. Accurate recording of vomiting, e.g. time, type and amount.
    b. Administration of oral fluids and maintenance of accurate fluid chart.
    c. Care of the child receiving intravenous infusion (p. 451).
    d. Psychological support. The nurse's role is a supportive one when vomiting occurs and requires self-discipline and control.
        The child suffering from cyclic vomiting, tends to be sensitive and intelligent and every effort should be made to approach the child with sympathy and understanding.
3. Routine nursing care.
4. Support for parents. Parents will be anxious and require support in caring for the child. They should be encouraged to talk about their problems, particularly when the cause is unknown or when it is thought to be due to psychological causes. In the latter case, it should be emphasised that over-protection should be avoided and that the child should also be encouraged to communicate his fears and anxieties.

Peptic ulcers

Acute gastric or duodenal ulcers may occur in the neonatal period and infancy following acute stresses such as severe respiratory distress. In later childhood acute peptic ulcers may occur in association with severe stress situations such as burns and meningitis. They may also be related to steroid therapy. Chronic peptic ulcers are seen mainly in children from school age upwards.

Clinical features

In the neonatal period and infancy they can present with bleeding, perforation or obstruction. In later childhood there may be severe bleeding with haematemesis or melaena. In chronic peptic ulcers there is abdominal pain which can be relieved by alkali, food or vomiting.

Investigation

1. A straight radiograph will reveal free gas in the peritoneal cavity.
2. In less acute cases, and in infants, lipiodol (radiopaque substance) is given and the ulcer can be seen by fluoroscopy, while in older children a barium meal is given.
3. Fibre endoscopy is a very useful diagnostic technique where radiological investigations are inconclusive.
4. Examination of faeces for blood.

Principles of treatment and nursing management

1. Medical treatment. This consists of rest in bed, a bland diet, an antacid and anticholinergic drugs. The aim is to promote healing by neutralising the gastric juices. Meals should be taken regularly. To relieve pain and inhibit acid secretion an H_2 receptor antagonist cimetidine, 20 to 40 mg/kg of body weight per day, can be given for four to six weeks.

2. Surgical intervention. If a perforation has occurred this must be closed. Blood loss is replaced early since such a loss is not well tolerated (p. 453). Mechanical obstruction is relieved by posterior gastro-jejunostomy where the jejunum is sutured to the stomach providing a second outlet for gastric contents. Vagotomy may also be carried out to reduce gastric secretions and movements.

   a Routine pre- and post-operative care (pp. 128 and 131).

   b. Specific measures include:

     (i) Intravenous feeding (p. 455).

     (ii) Gastric suction to remove fluids and gas (p. 509).

     (iii) Gradual introduction of feeds (oral).

     (iv) Careful observation of vital functions.

     (v) Care of wound and drains (if present).

     (vi) Fluid intake and output chart.

3. Routine nursing care.

Gastroenteritis or infective diarrhoea and vomiting

The term gastroenteritis is widely used to describe patients who have developed acute diarrhoea and/or vomiting. The term implies that there is an inflammatory process in the stomach and intestines. This is not necessarily the case, however, as in some conditions such as cholera or those produced by *E. coli*, the gastric and intestinal mucosa tend to be structurally normal.

The condition is one of the major health problems in the world today and carries an appreciable mortality and morbidity. This is particularly the case during infancy, and the malnourished infant is very vulnerable. In Britain the incidence and mortality have decreased markedly but it remains among the five most common causes of hospital admission in children.

Pathophysiology

Certain bacterial species elaborate exotoxins that impair intestinal absorption and can produce excessive secretions of electrolytes and water. These include both cholera and *E. coli* enterotoxin. Other *E. coli* species, some *Shigella* and *Salmonella* penetrate the mucosa of the small bowel or colon and produce microscopic ulceration. Vomiting and diarrhoea may follow non-bacterial food poisoning. Viruses are the major pathogens in this country. Rotavirus is the commonest, but other viruses such as ECHO viruses, Coxsackie viruses, reoviruses and adenoviruses have also been identified as causative agents in diarrhoeal disease.

Diarrhoea and vomiting are the essential features which lead to dehydration, due to extracellular fluid loss and electrolyte imbalance. Acid-base balance is affected, leading to acidosis (p. 230). Both types of dehydration can be seen, i.e. hypotonic and hypertonic dehydration (p. 230).

Clinical features

The onset is sudden with vomiting and diarrhoea. The stools are large in volume, watery in consistency and usually grassy-green in colour. Vomiting may be slight or frequent and the infant is restless and unable to sleep. The anterior fontanelle is depressed. Initially he is reluctant to drink but he later becomes thirsty and drinks eagerly, though vomiting often.

The greater the degree of dehydration the more irritable he will be, due to brain cell damage. The fontanelle, eyes and abdomen are sunken and the skin turgor is poor, i.e. it wrinkles abnormally when lifted between thumb and forefinger. The extremities are cold and may look cyanosed. Metabolic acidosis is produced by the loss of sodium and potassium in the stools and this is reflected in rapid breathing. When the loss of body weight exceeds 10 per cent of the body weight, the infant's condition is critical. This is due to oligaemia and peripheral circulatory failure. There is also fever. Other systems may be involved, e.g. the nervous system, leading to convulsions.

Principles of treatment and nursing management

1. Treatment depends on the degree of dehydration. *Mild dehydration.* It is possible and preferable to treat the child at home, provided that efficient medical care can be provided:

   a. Withdrawal of milk feeds which are replaced by a glucose-electrolyte mixture (Dioralyte).

b. Fluids should be given 2-hourly during the day and 4-hourly during the night, and continued for 24 hours.

c. After 24 hours milk feeds are restarted, when small amounts are given (15 ml of half-cream milk) every 4 hours with saline between feeds.

d. As the milk feed is increased, the amount of the glucose-electrolyte mixture is correspondingly decreased.

e. Sucrose is only added when stools have become formed.

Moderate dehydration. In this case, the clinical features are well established and the infant should be hospitalised:

a. Withdrawal of milk feeds.

b. Replacement of fluid and electrolyte deficits and correction of acid-base disorders. This is based on clinical assessment, or on records of recent weight loss. Replacement may be either orally or intravenously and will depend on the diarrhoeal loss of water and electrolytes.

c. Care of the infant on intravenous therapy (p. 448).

d. Biochemical investigation and clinical observation to determine electrolyte state.

e. Gradual introduction of oral fluids to determine ability to retain fluids.

f. Gradual introduction of milk feeds as described for mild dehydration.

g. Removal of intravenous cannula and care of the wound.

h. Daily weighing and collection of urine (daily tests).

i. Routine nursing care.

Severe dehydration. The infant is extremely ill with circulatory failure:

a. Intravenous infusion of suitable electrolyte solution and carefully graded fluid intake.

b. Plasma infusion to replace decreased plasma volume.

c. Correction of metabolic acidosis by intravenous administration of 8.4 per cent sodium bicarbonate with reassessment of acid-base state.

d. When fluid and electrolyte state has been corrected, milk feeds are gradually reintro-duced as described for mild dehydration.

e. During the acute phase, the infant is nursed in an incubator. Oxygen is given and the infant is observed carefully, since reduced serum potassium levels produce changes in cardiac activity, and a rapid increase in potassium level carries the risk of cardiac arrest.

If the infant suffers from hypertonic dehydration, careful observations are essential. The features to look for are convulsions, lethargy and circulatory failure. Both fluid and electrolyte replacement must be monitored carefully. The fluid chart must be accurately maintained and the rate kept as recommended.

2. Routine nursing care:

a. Administration of drugs, mainly antibiotics to combat the infective agent. If vomiting is severe, suitable drugs, such as chloramphenicol or streptomycin, can be given parenterally.

b. Isolation of infants (preferably in a cubicle) and understanding of the process of cross-infection and its prevention.

c. Care of the infant's buttocks. Loose stools cause redness and excoriation of skin. The infant must not be left lying in wet or soiled napkins. The napkin area is washed gently and a protective cream can be applied. Leaving the buttocks exposed is a good method of encouraging healing.

d. Inspection and care of infant's mouth.

e. Support for parents. If there is evidence of lack of understanding with regard to infant care, the mother should be encouraged to stay with the child. Nursing care can then be supervised and help given. It should be remembered, however, that many infants suffering from gastroenteritis do so despite good infant care, and parents should not be blamed for the existing state.

f. Preparation for return home. As soon as the infant's feeding regime has reached the level for his age and needs, and when there is a satisfactory weight gain and there is no vomiting or loose stools, he should be allowed home. The parents will be asked either to attend the outpatient department or to contact their general practitioner to assess the infant's progress.

DISORDERS OF THE SMALL AND LARGE INTESTINES

Disorders of the small and large intestines can be considered as those due to abnormal development and those which are acquired. There are a variety of abnormalities and only the more common ones will be discussed.

ATRESIA OR STENOSIS OF THE INTESTINE AND COLON

Atresia denotes a complete block, while stenosis indicates narrowing of the intestinal lumen and these can involve any part of the intestine and colon. The abnormality is caused by arrested development of portions of the tract during the second and third months of fetal life.

Duodenal atresia

This atresia is often distal to the ampulla of Vater. Bile enters the duodenum at the ampulla and therefore when vomiting occurs it contains bile. When the obstruction is above the ampulla of Vater, the vomitus consists only of gastric contents.

Investigations

1. X-rays of the abdomen show a 'double bubble' pattern. When obstruction is incomplete, small amounts of air in the lower bowel may be present.
2. A barium enema may demonstrate associated malrotation.

Clinical features

Vomiting starts soon after birth and becomes progressively worse with subsequent feeds. The stools may look like normal meconium, but on examination, do not contain stratified epithelial cells. Demonstration of epithelial cells indicates patency of the bowel. As dehydration increases, there will be fever. A body temperature of 39°C is indicative of peritonitis due to rupture of the atresia. The abnormality is often found in Down's syndrome babies.

Principles of treatment and nursing management

1. Pre-operative care:
   a. Routine neonatal pre-operative care (p. 156).
   b. Correction of dehydration which is not usually severe, as the diagnosis should be made early.
   c. Naso-gastric tube on free drainage and hourly suction.
2. Operation. A duodeno-duodenostomy or duodeno-jejunostomy relieves the obstruction and the remainder of the gut is examined as further obstructions are occasionally present. A gastrostomy may be performed and a fine transanastomotic tube is passed into the jejunum.
3. Post-operative care:
   a. Routine neonatal post-operative care (p. 131).
   b. Hourly aspiration of the gastrostomy tube which is on free drainage.
   c. Intravenous fluids are continued until feeding by tube is established.

Continuous transanastomotic feeding at a maximum speed of 1 ml per minute is started 24 hours post-operatively, commencing with dextrose and gradually changing in amount and consistency until, at approximately 7 days post-operatively, full-strength milk is being given. To maintain fluid and electrolyte balance the gastric aspirate can be replaced through the transanastomotic tube and this may eliminate the need for intravenous therapy being continued. It is not unusual for large volumes of aspirate to be obtained for some time post-operatively, up to weeks in some instances, as the dilated stomach and proximal duodenum take time to return to normal function. When it decreases, gastrostomy suction is performed less frequently and alternate feeds are given into the stomach for 24 hours. Oral feeding is gradually introduced before removal of the transanastomotic tube, followed 2 days later by the gastrostomy tube. The infant's weight is carefully monitored.

4. Support for parents. This is an anxious period for the new mother and every opportunity should be taken to involve both parents in the care of the infant. Support will be extensive to

begin with but gradually, as the infant's condition improves, this support can be decreased until the parents, particularly the mother, can handle the child.

When the child is ready to go home, the parents will be given an outpatient appointment so that regular assessments can be made of the child's progress.

Duodenal stenosis
In this condition, the lumen of the duodenum is narrowed and the infant vomits and fails to gain weight. Investigation, treatment and nursing management are as for duodenal atresia.

Jejuno-ileal atresia or membrane
In this section of the intestine, the tube has failed to develop.

Clinical features
Vomiting which starts on the first day of life contains bile and has a faecal odour. Stools are absent or scanty and the abdomen is distended if the infant has swallowed amniotic fluid or if he has been fed. Dehydration is evident and the body temperature is elevated.

Investigatiions
Straight X-rays are usually adequate for diagnosis.

Principles of treatment and nursing management

1. Pre-operative care:
   As for duodenal obstruction. See page 488.
2. Operation. As the bowel proximal to the obstruction is grossly dilated an oblique end to side anastomosis is performed.
3. Post-operative care:
   a. Routine neonatal post-operative care (p. 131).
   b. A naso-gastric tube is left on free drainage and aspirated hourly.
   c. Intravenous therapy is continued until feeding is established. After 24 hours, 5 ml glucose water will be given hourly and the naso-gastric tube aspirated 2-hourly. Any bile aspirated may be replaced. When the bile staining has stopped and the naso-gastric aspirate volume lessens, milk feeding

is gradually introduced. As long as the infant is feeding well, passing normal stools and gaining weight, he may be discharged home about two weeks post-operatively.
4. Complications. Diarrhoea, probably due to sugar intolerance (p. 197), occasionally occurs following introduction of milk feeding. A low lactose feed should be used and the infant is usually able to recommence normal feeding after some weeks.

Meconium ileus
This is a common cause of intestinal obstruction in the neonatal period. The condition is part of a widespread disturbance affecting the pancreas and the mucus-secreting glands of the alimentary and respiratory tracts. The mucus-secreting glands of the alimentary tract are altered, their secretion is diminished in amount and is thick and sticky. As a result of the altered pancreatic physiology, that is reduced enzyme secretion, the meconium in the lower ileum is dark, putty-like, very sticky and causes obstruction. Absorption from the bowel is reduced leading to abdominal distension. There is wasting of the body. Since there are also changes in the tissue of the respiratory tract, the child is also prone to respiratory disturbance and recurring infection.

The middle or lower ileum if often distended above the area of the obstruction. This may produce volvulus (twisting of the intestines) and may perforate. If perforation occurs, this can lead to meconium peritonitis.

Investigations
Radiography. This reveals distended loops of small intestine with fluid levels and bubbles of air.

Clinical features
Vomiting starts soon after birth, the abdomen becomes distended and there may be visible peristalsis. Electrolyte disturbance is a feature which presents many problems during and after the operation.

Principles of treatment and nursing management

1. Mild cases. Occasionally these respond to enemata, gastric lavage and pancreatic enzymes.

2. Surgical intervention. In acute intestinal obstruction, resection of the affected part and a double ileostomy are performed. The proximal ileostomy is used for decompression of the bowel above; the distal ileostomy is used for instillation of pancreatic enzymes and washing out of the terminal ileum and colon. The ileostomy is closed within two to three weeks.

3. Pre-operative care:
   a. Routine neonatal pre-operative care (p. 156).
   b. Intravenous fluids may be necessary if the infant has been vomiting for some time.
   c. A naso-gastric tube is left on free drainage and is aspirated hourly.
   d. Abdominal girth is measured and recorded as an increase may indicate some deterioration.
   e. Antibiotics will be ordered.

4. Post-operative care:
   a. Routine post-operative neonatal care (p. 131).
   b. Intravenous therapy is maintained.
   c. The naso-gastric tube is left on free drainage and is aspirated hourly, initially.
   d. Observation of ileostomy colour is made hourly to ensure that a good blood supply is maintained. Sterile paraffin gauze is placed over the stoma (p. 153).
   e. High, warmed humidity may be ordered.
   f. Positional changing is done 2-hourly.
   g. Physiotherapy is carried out 4-hourly.

When the ileostomy becomes active an appliance is placed over the stoma. The skin should be completely clean and dry and a protective adhesive sheet or fluid is placed around the stoma. It is possible, subsequently, for the infant to be immersed in a bath while the adhesive remains in place. The adhesive, along with the appliance itself, must fit snugly around the stoma to prevent leakage (p. 153).

Material will be discharged from the ileostomy after 24 hours then, after a few days, practically all stools will be passed per rectum.

On the first post-operative day, small glucose feeds will be given and the naso-gastric tube aspirated 2-hourly. When the feeds are being well absorbed, milk will gradually be introduced. Pancrex is usually given orally as soon as milk feeding is commenced (p. 506). High humidity, if used, is gradually reduced over a number of days.

A sweat test will be done before the infant is discharged home. This will be of no value until the baby born at term is at least 2 weeks old as, under this age, babies do not normally sweat. Good support and counselling must be given to the parents and there should be careful follow-up domiciliary supervision. Particularly with a first affected infant, emphasis should be placed on the importance of genetic counselling.

Malrotation

Other conditions which cause intestinal obstruction in the new-born include *malrotation*. This is due to arrested development which leads to lack of attachment of the mesentery to the posterior abdominal wall. This results in twisting of the caecum and obstruction of the duodenum or it can lead to volvulus of the mid-gut. It involves the small intestine and the twist may be anything from half a turn to two complete turns. This causes obstruction at the duodeno-jejunal junction and in the transverse colon.

Clinical features

Vomiting is an important feature; the contents of the vomitus indicate the area where the obstruction is, e.g. duodenal obstruction leads to bile-stained vomiting. Incomplete or intermittent obstruction may allow some stools to be passed and these may be blood-stained. Vomiting causes dehydration and there may be fever associated with the dehydration.

Investigations

The diagnosis is confirmed by radiographic examination.

Principles of treatment and nursing management

1. Pre-operative care:
   a. Routine pre-operative neonatal care (p. 156).
   b. Intravenous infusion if necessary, although most infants with malrotation are in good general condition and will not be dehydrated.
   c. Naso-gastric suction hourly, with free drainage of the catheter.

d. Abdominal girth will be measured and recorded, as an increase may indicate deterioration.
2. Operation. Operation consists of dividing the peritoneal bands which are causing the obstruction and replacing the large bowel in the left side of the abdominal cavity and the small bowel in the right side.
3. Post-operative care:
    a. Routine neonatal post-operative care (p. 131).
    b. Intravenous infusion (p. 448).
    c. Gastric suction (p. 509).
    d. Drainage and wound care (p. 142).
    e. Feeding regime following gradual introduction of oral fluids.
4. Routine nursing care.
5. Support for parents (as for duodenal atresia) (p. 488).

Exomphalos

An exomphalos is a type of abdominal hernia, the protrusion occurring through the umbilicus. When the exomphalos is small the infant is likely to be otherwise normal at birth and it is sometimes possible to correct the defect without operation. The umbilical cord is rotated and the gut gradually compressed into the abdominal cavity. Adhesive strapping is then placed over the umbilicus and retained for approximately one week. Larger lesions often occur in low-birth-weight infants who may also have other congenital abnormalities.

The hernial sac may contain part, or whole, of the liver as well as bowel. To further add to the problem, the sac may be ruptured. This is dealt with in the same manner as gastroschisis (p. 492).

Principles of treatment and nursing management

1. Pre-operative care (sac intact):
    a. General neonatal pre-operative care (p. 156).
    b. A naso-gastric tube is passed to help keep the bowel deflated. It is put on free drainage and aspirated regularly.
    c. Intravenous therapy will be started if there is a major defect.
    d. A photograph may be taken.
2. Operation. The aim is to return the prolapsed gut into the peritoneal cavity and repair the umbilical defect. Some infants will require further operative treatment at a later stage, to repair a residual hernia and it may be necessary to do a 'staged' repair at six-monthly intervals.

However, in some instances it is not possible to achieve the aim of the operation and the contents of the sac are enclosed in a sheet of Silastic-coated Teflon (Fig. 26.9). The subsequent care of these infants will be discussed under 'Gastroschisis' (p. 492).

3. Post-operative care (repaired defect):
    a. Routine neonatal post-operative care (p. 131).
    b. Constant nursing presence may be required.
    c. Oxygen may be ordered for the first 24 hours and blood-gas analysis will be done.
    d. When the hernial sac has been large there may be some degree of respiratory embarrassment, due to the increase in abdominal contents pushing the diaphragm upwards. It is important to note the infant's respirations and colour. Nursing in a 'head up' position may minimise this problem but these infants may require a period of assisted ventilation (p. 395).
    e. The naso-gastric tube is left on free drainage and is aspirated hourly. It is not uncommon for atresia or malrotation of gut to occur in these infants; particular emphasis is therefore placed on the amount and colour of aspirate obtained.
    f. The abdominal girth is measured regularly as any increase may indicate the onset of further problems, e.g. malrotation.
    g. Intravenous therapy will be maintained. Initially this may be in the form of dextrose saline but some infants may then require a period of total parenteral nutrition (p. 455) as they will be unable to absorb alimentary feeds. This may be continued for some weeks and, if a central venous line is used, any abnormality in temperature, deterioration in colour, or lethargy in a usually fairly active infant should be reported immediately as these signs may indicate infection.

When naso-gastric secretions are free of bile, small amounts of dextrose can gradually be introduced before milk is eventually attempted.

It should be made clear to the parents of the infant who has a large exomphalos that treatment is likely to be prolonged, as in some instances it is many weeks before he is well enough to be discharged home.

Gastroschisis

This is an abdominal wall defect, adjacent to and usually to the right of the umbilicus, which allows the bowel to prolapse through. Due to the reaction of the prolapsed gut to liquor, it may become grossly thickened. Unlike an exomphalos, this defect never has a covering sac.

Principles of treatment and nursing management

1. Pre-operative care (gastroschisis and ruptured exomphalos):
   a. Routine neonatal pre-operative care (p. 156).
   b. Constant nursing presence.
   c. Heat loss may be excessive as the prolapsed gut greatly increases the surface area, therefore particular attention must be paid to maintenance of body temperature.
   d. The prolapsed gut is covered with warm, sterile soaks and sterile towels.
   e. A naso-gastric tube on free drainage and regular suction with a syringe will help to keep the bowel deflated.
   f. Intravenous therapy may be established (p. 448).
   g. Oxygen therapy will probably be necessary (p. 382).
   h. Antibiotics are prescribed.
   i. A photograph may be taken.
2. Operation. The aim is to return the viscera to the abdominal cavity and close the abdominal wall.

   However, as with a large exomphalos, this is not always possible and a staged approach has to be adopted.

   The abdominal defect is enlarged, and a pouch is made using material such as Silastic-coated Teflon. This is sutured to both sides of the wound and then joined together, enclosing the prolapsing gut.
3. Post-operative care (gastroschisis and ruptured exomphalos): If the defect has been repaired the post-operative care is similar to that of the repair of the large exomphalos which has been enclosed in a hernial sac.

   However, the post-operative care of the

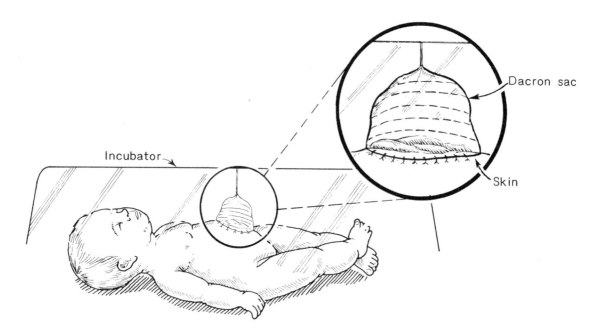

Fig. 26.9 Dacron sac enclosing abdominal contents.

infant who has required the application of a Silastic 'pouch' is as follows:

a. Routine neonatal post-operative care (p. 131).
b. Constant nursing presence.
c. Oxygen may be required and blood-gas analysis will help to determine the amount necessary.
d. Some infants may require a period of assisted ventilation (p. 395).
e. The naso-gastric tube is left on free drainage and is aspirated hourly. As with the infant who has had repair of a covered exomphalos, the amount and colour of aspirate must be very carefully noted.
f. Intravenous therapy is dealt with as in post-operative care of the repair of exomphalos (3e).
g. The Silastic pouch is sprayed with an antibiotic or iodine-based preparation 6-hourly, as it is important to prevent infection.
h. A thread may be attached to the apex of the pouch and loosely anchored above, for example to the roof of the baby warmer or incubator. This helps to prevent movement of the pouch which could create tension on the stitches holding it to the muscle.

From the first post-operative day, the pouch is reduced in size daily. This is done by the surgeon compressing the gut into the abdominal cavity then inserting a line of sutures along the pouch, underneath the previous suture line (Fig. 26.9). At approximately 7 to 12 days after operation the infant will return to the theatre to have the defect repaired. Post-operative care is then given as for the infant who has had primary repair (p. 492).

Hirschsprung's disease

Hirschsprung's disease, also called congenital aganglionic megacolon, is a congenital absence or diminution of the parasympathetic ganglion nerve cells in the mesenteric plexus of the distal colon.

Since there are reduced or no ganglion cells, peristalsis does not takes place in the affected area. The section is usually narrow but the intestine above is hypertrophied and dilated. There may also be mucosal ulceration in the new-born. Faecal material cannot pass along the narrowed section, resulting in abdominal distension and obstruction.

Genetic factors are probably involved. There is an increased familial incidence of the disorder. In the common short segment type, the incidence is five times greater in males than in females and the chance of a male sibling of an affected child also having the disease is one in 20. In the long segment type the sex incidence is equal and the chance of a sibling being affected is one in 10 irrespective of sex.

Clinical features

Most present in the first week of life. The remainder present as cases of chronic constipation increasing in severity with the child's age.

In neonatal cases there may be a history of passage of meconium although this is often delayed for 3 or more days. The abdomen becomes distended, there is visible peristalsis and increase in bowel sounds. With continuing obstruction there is bile-stained vomiting. Periods of diarrhoea alternating with constipation are not uncommon. The child fails to thrive. When it is complicated with enterocolitis the child will pass large, offensive stools containing blood.

In older children there is usually chronic constipation with anorexia and failure to thrive. The abdomen is distended and faecal masses are felt in the abdomen. The rectum is found to be narrow on digital examination and may contain a small amount of normal faeces.

Investigations

1. Radiological examination will reveal abnormality of the colon following a barium enema. Plain radiographs will show dilatation of the colon above the aganglionic segment.
2. Rectal biopsy. This is performed under general anaesthetic. It involves obtaining either a sample of muscle coats of the rectum for examination for the presence of the ganglion cells of Auerbach's plexus or a more superficial biopsy obtaining mucosa and submucosa for examination of Meissner's plexus. When a deep biopsy is performed, there is a danger of adhesions and infections of the deep tissues.
3. Anorectal manometry. In this test a balloon is

placed in the rectum and inflated. Normally the inflation of a balloon inhibits the internal anal sphincter. In Hirschsprung's disease this inhibitory effect is absent and, if the balloon is in aganglionic gut, abnormal rectal waves can be identified. It is a simple test but both false positive and false negative results may be obtained in the neonatal period.

Principles of treatment and nursing management

Mild variety

1. Laxatives, saline washouts and olive oil enemata. (Water must not be used because of the danger of water absorption leading to water intoxication. This is due to rapid diffusion of water into the circulation from the dilated intestine.)
2. The child should be admitted to hospital only when faecal impaction causes obstruction.
3. Careful follow-up and supervision with eventual surgical intervention.

Confirmed cases with moderate and severe symptoms

1. Surgical intervention. This consists of the removal of the obstructing aganglionic segment of bowel. The operation of recto-sigmoidectomy is performed by a pull-through technique and can be achieved by a one-stage, two-stage or three-stage procedure. In the two-stage and three-stage procedure, the recto-sigmoidectomy is preceded by a colostomy. The colostomy is closed in the two-stage procedure.
2. Pre-operative preparation:
   a. Colonic lavage (p. 521).
   b. Antibiotics.
   c. Intravenous infusion (p. 448).
   d. In-dwelling naso-gastric tube (p. 509).
   e. Routine pre-operative care (p. 128).
3. Post-operative management:
   a. Routine (p. 131).
   b. Wound care.
   c. Care of colostomy (p. 153).
   d. Observation. Abdominal distension, colostomy function, peritonitis, paralytic ileus and increased temperature.
4. Support for parents. Even a temporary colostomy can be difficult to accept. Parents must learn how to handle the child with a colostomy, what observations to make, how to cleanse the stoma and how to apply the colostomy bag. By the time the infant is ready to go home the parents should feel confident in caring for the child. There would be close medical follow-up with frequent visits to the hospital. The community services will also provide guidance and support while the child is at home.

Intussusception

Intussusception is the invagination of a portion of the intestine into an adjacent more distal section of the intestine (Fig. 26.10). The cause is generally not known, but in young children the greatest incidence is between the fourth and eighth month, when there is a change to a more solid diet which may alter peristalsis. Increased peristaltic activity may initiate intussusception. Sometimes a definite mechanical factor can be found to be responsible for initiating the invagination. There are other possible contributing causes, such as Meckel's diverticulum (a duct arising from the ileum which closes at the umbilical end but remains open at the intestinal end), or polyps or cysts in the intestine.

Classification

The classification is based on the location of the intussusception:

1. Ileocaecal: the ileum invaginates into the ascending colon at the ileocaecal valve.
2. Ileocolic: the ileum invaginates into the colon.

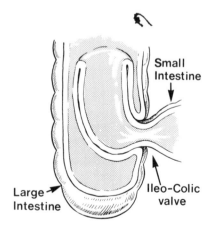

Fig. 26.10 Intussusception.

3. Colocolic: the colon invaginates into the colon.
4. Ileo-ileo: the small intestine invaginates into the small intestine.

Clinical features

The child is usually healthy and the onset is sudden. He suddenly screams loudly, drawing up his knees as if in extreme abdominal pain. The attack ceases suddenly and the child falls asleep. The attack is repeated after varying lengths of time. If the attack has been severe or prolonged, the child will be pale, listless and perspiring freely. Vomiting is not conspicuous but he may vomit after each bout of colic. Rectal examination reveals a trace of blood on the examining finger. The pulse is rapid and soft and the temperature subnormal.

Investigations

X-ray examination of the abdomen shows a step-like appearance.

Principles of treatment and nursing management

1. Reduction of intussusception may be done by colonic injection of saline, air or barium. This method is not often employed since there is a risk of perforation, however, small, and there is no guarantee of a successful reduction.
2. Surgical reduction:
   a. Pre-operative care:
      (i) Routine (p. 128).
      (ii) Indwelling naso-gastric tube (p. 509).
      (iii) Correction of dehydration (if present).
   b. Reduction of intussusception by direct vision, keeping the intestines warm with hot saline. This also helps to reduce oedema.
   c. Intravenous plasma should be available in case of collapse.
   d. If the intussusception is not reducible, resection and primary anastomosis will be necessary.
3. Post-operative management:
   a. Routine (p. 131).
   b. Incubator care for the small infant (p. 181).
   c. Administration of oxygen (p. 382).
   d. Continuation of intravenous fluids.
   e. Antibiotics.
   f. If an ileostomy has been performed, suction drainage is applied to the ileostomy tube

until continuity of the bowel has been restored. (See care of stoma p. 153).
   g. Observation of vital functions.
   h. Wound and drain care.
4. Routine nursing care:
   a. Feeding should be re-established as soon as possible, i.e. when there is cessation of vomiting and peristaltic activity is satisfactory.
   b. Bathing and handling.
5. Support for parents. The amount of support necessary depends on the general state of the child and the operative measures taken. The child's condition should be fully explained and reassurance given. Once the child's general condition has improved the parents can participate in nursing him.
6. Preparation for home. Once the intussusception has been successfully reduced, and the wound healed, the child can return home. There should be a follow-up period in case the intussusception recurs. This has been found in about 2 per cent of patients (Dennison, 1974).

Acute appendicitis

Acute appendicitis is the most common surgical emergency in childhood. The appendix is attached to the caecum. It varies in structure, length and position in different individuals. In childhood, the appendix of the majority is not straight but shows angular bends and twists. When inflammation occurs there is an accumulation of purulent exudate within the lumen and an obstruction occurs. The blood supply is reduced, blood vessels are damaged and gangrene occurs early in the disease. Fluid enters the peritoneal cavity and bacterial activity is increased from the inflamed but intact appendix, or from a perforated appendix.

Appendicitis is rare in the first year of life but becomes more common from the second year onwards.

Clinical features

The onset is sudden with colicky pain in the umbilical region. This is followed by vomiting. The pain moves to the right iliac fossa where it becomes a persistent ache. Temperature is raised, but rarely above 40°C and the child looks ill.

Although constipation is more common, diarrhoea, if it occurs, may be quite severe.

The diagnosis is confirmed by gentle palpation of the abdomen which reveals consistent tenderness and involuntary rigidity in the right iliac fossa. If peritonitis develops, there will be rapid deterioration in the child's condition. There is high fever, a rising pulse rate, dehydration, ketosis and distension due to paralytic ileus.

Principles of treatment and nursing management

1. Removal of the appendix.
2. Pre-operative preparation:
    a. Routine (p. 128).
    b. Urine tests for protein and sugar.
    c. Intravenous infusion, if necessary.
    d. Antibiotics.
    e. Indwelling naso-gastric tube (p. 509).
3. Post-operative care:
    a. Routine care (p. 131).
    b. Gastric suction (p. 509).
    c. Oxygen, particularly if paralytic ileus is present (p. 382).
    d. Continuation of antibiotic therapy.
    e. Wound and drain care.
    f. Feeding (if no gastric decompression), bland fluids, initially and, if there is no vomiting, gradual introduction of soft and light diet.
    g. Observation for complications. These include intestinal obstructions, paralytic ileus, respiratory complications, wound infection, faecal fistula and peritonitis.
       Peritonitis is a serious complication which is indicated when there is diffuse tenderness and 'board-like' rigidity with abdominal distension. There is fever and an increased pulse rate. Treatment consists of intravenous infusion to correct fluid and electrolyte loss, surgery to remove the source of infection, and antibiotic treatment.
4. Physiotherapy. Deep breathing exercises and gradual mobilisation.
5. Preparation for home. Stitches are removed on the 8th to 10th day and the child can return home. Guidance should be given to parents on how to increase activity gradually during the convalescent period and, if of school age, when he may return to school.

Necrotising enterocolitis

This is a serious inflammatory disorder of the intestinal mucosa. It usually occurs in sick preterm infants and in infants who have had an indwelling umbilical catheter or an exchange transfusion.

The cause is unknown but the disorder may be due to (1) a defect in the immunological system since infection is generally with the usual intestinal flora, and (2) bowel ischaemia, due to perinatal asphyxia, when blood is diverted away from the intestine.

Bottle-fed infants may be more susceptible because the milk feeds lack antibodies and macrophages, which are obtained from colostrum, and which protect the bowel mucosa against bacterial invasion.

Clinical features

The infant, usually several days old, becomes suddenly ill with abdominal distension and vomiting, and passes stools containing blood.

Investigations

X-ray shows linear lucent shadows which are produced when gas from the bowel lumen enters into the submucosal or subserosal layer of the bowel wall.

Principles of treatment and nursing management

The aim is to rest the intestines and encourage healing.

1. Oral feeds are discontinued.
2. Intravenous infusion is commenced to replace fluid and electrolytes.
3. Intravenous feeding (p. 455).
4. Insertion of a naso-gastric catheter to allow free drainage (p. 509).
5. Antibiotics to combat the infection.
6. Routine nursing care which might include incubator care.
7. Observations for complications, such as perforation and stenosis:
    a. Increased abdominal distension.
    b. Vomiting.
    c. Increased pulse rate.
    d. Dyspnoea.
    e. Decreased urinary output.
    f. Increase in body temperature.

8. Preparation for operation — routine and specific (p. 156).
9. Surgery. Resection of the necrosed segment and anastomosis.
10. Post-operative management:
    a. Routine (p. 131).
    b. Intravenous infusion (p. 448).
    c. Blood transfusion (p. 453).
    d. Gastric suction (p. 509).
    e. Charting of fluid intake and output.
    f. Antibiotics.
    g. Gradual introduction of oral fluids and feeds.
    h. Care of the wound and drains.
11. Support for parents. This involves understanding of their anxiety particularly during the acute phase, and giving reassurance regarding the disorder. Participation in nursing should be encouraged as soon as the infant's condition makes this possible. This is important, since the mother may not have nursed her child and may be apprehensive about doing so. When oral feeding is established and progress is maintained, the mother will be able to assume greater responsibility for the care of the infant so that she will gain confidence in handling him.

DISORDERS OF THE RECTUM AND ANUS

A perineum without an anal opening is described as 'imperforate'. However, most malformations of the anus or rectum communicate by a fistulous track with either the urinary or genital systems. Anal and rectal anomalies and associated malformations are due to arrested development in the 7th and 8th week of fetal life.

Anorectal anomalies are classified according to type and method of treatment:

1. Those which consist of high anomalies, e.g. anorectal agenesis, with or without fistula and rectal atresia.
2. Those which consist of intermediate anomalies, e.g. anal agenesis (with or without fistula) and anorectal stenosis.
3. Those which consist of low anomalies, e.g. at the normal anal site (covered anus) and at the perineal site (anterior perineal anus).

There are also sexual differences (Fig. 26.11).

Clinical features

In most of these anomalies the new-born baby presents with intestinal obstruction. The following signs would be indicative of some abnormality:

1. Absence of anal opening.

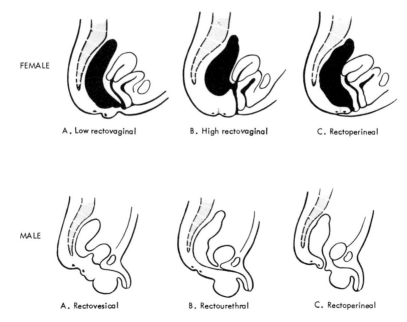

FEMALE

A. Low rectovaginal   B. High rectovaginal   C. Rectoperineal

MALE

A. Rectovesical   B. Rectourethral   C. Rectoperineal

Fig. 26.11 Anorectal anomalies (female and male).

2. Meconium coming from an abnormal orifice.
3. Vomiting, with abdominal distension.
4. Difficulty in defaecation, e.g. passing ribbon-like stools as in stenosis.
5. Perineum bulges but the napkin is not stained with meconium. This occurs when the infant cries and strains.

Investigations

1. X-rays. These demonstrate the presence of gas in the bowels.
2. Radiopaque dye is introduced into the urinary tract, e.g. a micturating cysto-urethrogram will demonstrate recto-urinary communication and urinary abnormalities.

Principles of treatment and nursing management

1. Colostomy is necessary in the neonatal period for rectal deformities. *Rectal deformities* cause more problems because of the associated abnormalities. If the nervous tissue is not too involved, continence may be obtained but a large percentage of these patients lack complete control.

   In *anal deformities* the prognosis is better and continence can be achieved by the majority of these children.
2. Dilatation of anal or rectal stenosis. Parents may be taught how to continue dilatation (digital dilatation) at home for periods up to several months.
3. Pre-operative care:
   a. Routine (p. 156).
   b. Indwelling naso-gastric tube (suction) (p. 509).
   c. Intravenous infusion (p. 448).
4. Post-operative care.
   a. Routine (p. 131).
   b. Continuation of gastric suction.
   c. Care of the child during intravenous infusion (p. 451).
   d. Care of colostomy stoma (p. 153).
   e. Wound care.
   f. Antibiotics.
   g. Feeding. When the naso-gastric tube has been removed and intravenous infusion has been discontinued, oral feeding can be reestablished.

h. Observations for complications, e.g.:
   (i) *Anal strictures* may develop after anoplasty or rectoplasty. The new anus must be dilated regularly for several months.
   (ii) Sloughing of the rectum. This occurs due to ischaemia.
   (iii) Abscess formation.
   (iv) Recurrent fistulas.
   (v) Complications of the colostomy, e.g. prolapse of the colon, stenosis or intestinal obstruction.
   (vi) Urinary complications, e.g. urinary incontinence and urinary tract infection.
5. Routine nursing care.
6. Support for parents. Parents must be fully informed of the condition of their child. As soon as his condition improves, they can take part in nursing him. Help and guidance should be given to them regarding any special procedures. However, they should be introduced to these procedures gradually. The emotional shock of such abnormalities takes some time to overcome, but with time and patience they will be able to take over their parental function.

Constipation

Constipation is defined by the consistency of the stool, not the frequency of defaecation. The stool consists of small, hard dry balls. In infancy stools may occur one to three times per day and breast-fed babies may not have a bowel movement for as long as 5 days and not be constipated. Older children will not report failure of bowel movements and may become constipated.

Mechanism of constipation

The normal rectum is empty most of the time, except when a mass reflex of the colon passes faeces into the rectum once or twice each day. The distension stretches the muscles and stimulates pressure receptors. These provide the stimulus in the afferent arc of the defaecation reflex. The urge is felt and the efferent arc causes contraction of the rectum and relaxation of the sphincters; evacuation is completed with the aid of contractions of the muscles of the abdominal wall.

In acute constipation, the rectum retains its tone and defaecation is readily produced by the stimulation of a laxative, suppository or enema.

In chronic constipation, the rectum is not empty and its wall is chronically overstretched, so additional oncoming faeces neither reach it nor stretch the rectum further. The sensory receptors do not respond, the rectal wall is flaccid and is unable to contract effectively.

When the stool is not passed soon after it enters the rectum, water is absorbed and the stool becomes harder. The harder the stool, the more difficult and painful its passage. This produces cracks and fissures in the anal mucosa, which make it more difficult for the child to defaecate.

Predisposing factors

1. Too early stress on toilet training, e.g. the toddler may react to the regime and refuse to co-operate. Usually little training is necessary.
2. Dietary, e.g. lack of cellulose fibres to promote peristalsis.
3. Organic obstruction, e.g. anal stenosis or Hirschsprung's disease.
4. Neural lesions, e.g. spinal trauma.

Principles of treatment and nursing management

1. Investigation of cause. This may be carried out as an outpatient.
2. Re-establishment of normal habits of defaecation, e.g. attention to diet, extra fluids, etc.
3. Treatment of organic obstruction.
4. Emptying of rectum by:
   a. Digital disimpaction, followed by —
   b. Olive oil enema, followed by soap and saline or disposable enema (p. 520).
   c. Colonic lavage (p. 521).
   d. Suppositories (p. 174).
   e. Laxatives. These help to soften the stool; they are given daily for several weeks and adjustments are made to the dose according to the consistency of the stools.
5. *Observation of faecal soiling*. Chronic constipation is the most common cause. The faeces passed are soft and escape around the impacted faecal mass and through relaxed anal sphincters. *Encopresis* is the term used when there is faecal soiling without constipation or neuro-genic basis. The cause is considered to be a functional abnormality of psychological origin.

The treatment here aims at clearing the rectum, establishing normal habits and treating the underlying emotional disturbance.

Anal fissure

Anal fissure is the most common cause of rectal bleeding. It is generally confined to infants and toddlers. There is a history of constipation with pain on defaecation. The outside of the stool is streaked with blood, the bleeding occurring during or just after defaecation. The child cries when defaecating and often refuses to do so.

On examination, the fissures can be easily seen, either midline posteriorly or as multiple radiating fissures of varying depths.

Principles of treatment and nursing management

1. When the child refuses to sit on a potty or cries when defaecating, it is essential to investigate the reason. It is so easy to assume that he is obstinate and to force him to sit on a potty when there is good reason for his refusal.
2. Softening of stools. This can be achieved with a mild laxative and generally this is all that is necessary. In older children, the fissure is anaesthetised and digital dilatation is performed twice a day. In some children cauterisation may be necessary or the fissures are excised and the anus stretched under general anaesthesia.
3. Guidance to parents in handling the child. Crying on defaecation may continue for some time after the fissures have healed. The child will need a great deal of patience, love and understanding to help him to overcome the fear of pain.

Rectal prolapse

Rectal prolapse is not uncommon in toddlers. The prolapse may be partial, when the mucous membrane only is prolapsed, or complete, when there is protrusion of the entire rectal wall. There are a number of factors which are said to cause a prolapse.

1. Straining at stool by a child who is constipated, though diarrhoea too can be a cause of prolapse.

2. Complete prolapse occurs in the marasmic, debilitated child.

Clinical features

The prolapse rolls out painlessly during defaecations and usually returns spontaneously. The mucosa may become injured while it is prolapsed and may cause some bleeding.

Principles of treatment and nursing management

1. Treatment of the cause. Constipation is the commonest cause. (See treatment for constipation).
2. The child should not use a potty as this assumes a squatting position which stretches the pelvic floor and the anal sphincters. An adult type of toilet is probably better. There should also be a limit on the time he is allowed to sit on the toilet.
3. The prolapse is replaced by gentle pressure with cotton wool moistened with warm water. The buttocks may be strapped with adhesive. However, since repeated removal of adhesive would cause excoriation of the skin, strips of adhesive are placed lengthwise on each buttock and one strip is then placed crosswise on the vertical strips. The cross-band is pulled firmly across these bands holding the buttocks together. When the child defaecates, the cross-band only needs to be changed.
4. Injection of a sclerosing agent. This treatment is used for stubborn cases which do not respond to more conservative measures. The substance used is phenol 5 per cent in almond oil; 0.5 ml is injected into the submocosa at three equally spaced areas. This causes some fibrosis and a contraction on the wall of the rectum.
5. In some cases it may be necessary to resort to a circumferential perianal stitch (Thiersch operation).
6. Guidance for parents. A rectal prolapse is rather frightening and the parents should be reassured. They should be shown how to replace the prolapse and guidance given on the measures possible to prevent a prolapse.

The malabsorption syndrome

The majority of conditions causing malabsorption involve the small intestine. The small intestine in children varies in length, but this length and its mucosal surface area must be sufficient to ensure that absorption is adequate. Its impaired motility or change in its structure may interfere with the peristaltic function (i.e. transport of food bolus and the mixing of this food with pancreatic juices and bile) and thereby lead to malabsorption.

Other causes of malabsorption are, for example, (1) altered bacterial flora which interferes with vitamin B complex and K synthesis, (2) impairment of portal venous return, (3) anoxia, (4) lack of pancreatic secretions, and (5) biliary abnormalities.

Coeliac disease (gluten enteropathy)

Coeliac disease is a specific disease entity associated with abnormal jejunal mucosa. The condition usually presents between the ages of 6 and 18 months and is of varying severity.

Pathological physiology

This is a hereditary congenital disorder caused by sensitivity to the gliadin fraction of gluten, a cereal protein found in wheat and rye, and to a lesser extent in barley and oats. Gliadin, acting as antigen, combines with antibodies to form an immune complex in the intestinal mucosa that promotes the aggregation of K-lymphocytes. In some way these lymphocytes cause mucosal damage with loss of villi and proliferation of crypt cells. It is also believed that a primary deficiency of an intracellular peptidase results in accumulation of a toxic peptide which causes cell damage and villous atrophy. Examination of mucosal specimen shows villous atrophy. The mucosa are flat and devoid of normal villi (Fig. 26.12). Other cases show abnormally short, broad and thickened villi.

Clinical features

Diarrhoea is an early feature. Initially it may be intermittent and may simulate an intestinal infection. Subsequently, it is continuous with characteristic large, bulky, frothy, pale and offensive stools. Growth is retarded due to the malabsorption of nutrient substances. The abdomen becomes distended because of carbohydrate fermentation and the buttock and thigh tissues become wasted.

The child is miserable and unhappy and cries

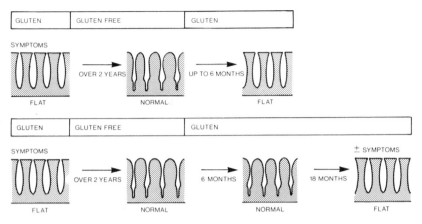

Fig. 26.12 Flattened villi due to gluten (showing normal appearance of villi when on gluten-free food).

a great deal. There may also be vomiting, constipation and abdominal pain. Other features of malabsorption include iron-deficiency anaemia and evidence of vitamin B complex deficiency. Calcium deprivation leads to osteoporosis and delayed ossification.

Investigations

1. Faecal fat content. A 3-day collection of stools is obtained when the child is given a diet containing a known amount of fat (30 to 40 g/d). This will show diminished absorption (under 90 per cent; normal absorption is 90 to 98 per cent of ingested fat) (p. 517). Daily output of fat in excess of 4 g indicates steatorrhoea.
2. Impaired carbohydrate absorption:
   a. The D-xylose absorption test is reliable in children. Five grams of D-xylose is given and a 24-hour collection of urine started. If it contains less than 25 per cent of the dose, malabsorption is indicated.
   b. Oral glucose tolerance test. A flat oral glucose tolerance curve is obtained (if given intravenously a normal curve is obtained).
3. X-ray:
   a. Bones. This will show osteoporosis.
   b. A barium meal and follow-through will show changes in mucosal pattern.
4. Duodenal or jejunal biopsy. Peroral intestinal biopsy is a reliable test but there is a small risk of haemorrhage or perforation (p. 516).
5. Blood analysis.

Principles of treatment and nursing management

1. *Diet* should be gluten-free. In the United Kingdom, all wheat flour has been excluded. Bread and biscuits made from gluten-free wheat starch are commercially available.
2. Adequate intake of vitamins, particularly vitamin D.
3. Correct anaemia. Oral iron preparation is given but if the child fails to respond, intramuscular iron can be given. If serum folate is low, folic acid is prescribed.
4. Support for parents. The condition is fully explained to the parents. They are issued with a list of foodstuffs which contain gluten and are therefore forbidden, and those which are gluten-free and permitted. The dietician should give them recipes for home baking of gluten-free bread, biscuits and cakes. The diet should be continued for at least five years when gluten-containing foods may be gradually introduced. Some children may have to remain permanently on a gluten-free diet. It should be emphasised that if the diet is relaxed or broken too soon, then relapses can occur. It can be quite a problem to maintain strict supervision at all times, particularly if other children or misguided neighbours give gluten-containing foods to the child.

Crohn's disease (regional enteritis)
This disease is a chronic inflammatory disorder affecting the full thickness of segments of the bowel.

The cause in unknown, but it is believed that genetic factors are involved. The terminal ileum is frequently involved, but other areas in the small and large intestine may be affected. Changes in the tissue include inflammation and thickening; the serosal surface is grey with scattered pale lymphoid nodules, the mucosal surface may show scarring and abscesses may also form.

Clinical features

Crohn's disease may affect children of all ages, including the neonate. There is failure to thrive, mild fever, moderate anaemia and a high ESR. Diarrhoea and abdominal pain are often late symptoms. Nutritional disturbances and deficiencies are present, due to extensive disease affecting the small intestinal mucosa. Malabsorption of vitamin B_{12} and bile salts are frequently involved, since their specific absorption sites are often affected. Despite the lack of vitamin B_{12} children do not tend to suffer from megaloblastic anaemia, but lack of bile salts leads to steatorrhoea. Loss of protein from the intestines leads to hypoproteinaemia and oedema. There is also intense psychological stress and this increases the severity of the symptoms.

Investigations

1. Barium studies of small and large intestines.
2. Sigmoidoscopy. This may show a characteristic 'cobble-stone' pattern; the mucosa may be very red and oedematous with scattered ulcers.
3. Rectal biopsy. This shows changes in the mucosa and crypt abscesses.

Principles of treatment and nursing management

1. Medical treatment. This is intended to suppress the symptoms:
   a. Rest in bed for a period.
   b. High protein, low residue diet.
   c. Correction of nutritional deficiencies, e.g. iron, folic acid, vitamin B_{12}.
   d. Control of pain and diarrhoea, e.g. administration of codeine phosphate. If the pain is severe, relief can be obtained by giving atropine (0.02 mg/kg) intravenously.
   e. Corticosteroids and corticotrophin are effective early in the disease.
   f. Parenteral nutrition and withdrawal of oral feeding. This allows the intestines to rest (p. 455).
2. Surgical treatment. This may be necessary for acute complications such as perforation, haemorrhage or obstruction. If the rectum is involved, proctocolectomy and ileostomy may be carried out (p. 153).
3. Nursing management in relation to:
   a. Medical treatment.
   b. Surgical treatment.
   In both instances the child will require a great deal of support to overcome or to manage the underlying depression. A great deal of patience and understanding will be required to deal with fluctuating moods. The parents too will need help and understanding during the child's long periods of ill health. Daily routine should include school and play periods and care should be taken to ensure that the child is kept occupied and does not get bored. The older child will have a need to talk and the nursing staff should find time to listen.
   c. Careful observation of vital signs, particularly of frequency, consistency and contents of stools.
   d. If surgical treatment is required, this will involve:
      (i) Pre-operative preparation: routine blood transfusion (p. 128).
      (ii) Post-operative care: routine, intravenous infusion, stoma care (p. 131).
4. Support for parents. The condition of the child produces a great deal of anxiety in the family. Throughout the treatment the parents should be kept informed of any changes in the treatment and the reasons for them. When the child is allowed home, contact with the hospital should be maintained and there should be cooperation between home, hospital and community services.

DISORDERS OF THE LIVER

The liver is the largest gland in the body and has a wide range of functions (p. 470). During fetal life it is an important haemopoietic organ, but at birth or near birth it takes over functions which were previously carried out by the placenta. This includes bilirubin excretion. Abnormal functions of the liver include:

1. Impaired cell function, e.g. decreased uptake of bilirubin and failure of bilirubin conjugation in the cells.
2. Impaired synthesis of proteins, fats and carbohydrates, e.g. there may be hypoglycaemia as a result of the liver's inability to produce glucose from non-carbohydrate sources; there may be generalised muscular wastage due to abnormal protein synthesis and there may be defective formation of various clotting factors.
3. Impairment of hormonal metabolism and failure to detoxicate toxin.
4. Hepatic fibrosis impedes blood flow through the liver so that portal venous pressure rises (portal hypertension).

Liver cell failure
The liver contains a variety of cells with different functions and the clinical manifestations of hepatic failure are widespread. The mature liver has a large functional reserve and considerable recuperative powers. Damage must be extensive before evidence of hepatic failure manifests itself.

Liver cells can be damaged by infections of a variety of organisms. Viruses, bacteria, fungi, protozoa and helminths may be responsible for an infectious process involving the liver. Drugs, toxins and metabolic diseases must also be considered as being implicated in liver cell damage. Drugs and toxins may interfere with bilirubin metabolism or have a direct toxic effect on the liver cells.

Jaundice
Jaundice is the clinical manifestation of defective hepatic function. It is a yellow discolouration of the skin and sclerae from the accumulation of the bile pigment bilirubin. However, jaundice may occur from causes other than defective hepatic function: for example, haemolytic anaemia where there is excessive red cell breakdown and when there is biliary obstruction outwith the liver.

Jaundice occurs when the body is unable to excrete bilirubin as rapidly as it is formed. It can be clinically detected when the concentration of bilirubin in the plasma exceeds about 35 μmol/l (2 mg/100 ml).

Bilirubin is formed within the cells of the reticuloendothelial system from the haemoglobin of degenerating red blood cells. A small amount is also formed in the liver from the breakdown of compounds other than haemoglobin. It is an insoluble waste product which must be converted to water-soluble forms for excretion. It is normally removed from the blood by the liver, becoming in the process conjugated with glucuronic acid and thereby water-soluble. In this form it is able to pass through the renal glomerular capillary membrane. Disorders of bilirubin metabolism can result in jaundice.

Persistent neonatal jaundice
Persistent jaundice in the first months of life has many causes and may be classified according to whether the raised serum concentrations of bilirubin are predominantly conjugated or unconjugated. In the unconjugated type the concentration of conjugated bilirubin is not raised, whereas in conjugated hyperbilirubinaemia the concentration of conjugated bilirubin is raised. Causes of unconjugated hyperbilirubinaemia include Rhesus and ABO incompatibility, hereditary spherocytosis, septicaemia, cephalhaematoma, hypoxia and many other conditions.

In the new-born infant bilirubin production may be twice that of the adult as a result of shortened red blood cell survival, increased turnover of haem-containing enzymes and from ineffective erythropoiesis. Hepatic uptake of bilirubin may be impaired and other liver cell function may be inefficient. There may also be persistent jaundice without hyperbilirubinaemia and this is found in breast-fed babies. Although the reason for this is not clearly understood, it may be due to inhibition of bilirubin excretion by fatty acids and perhaps by some actions of prostaglandins. If the jaundice is associated with breast feeding and the serum bilirubin levels are greater than 290 μmol/l, then breast feeding should be discontinued for 24 to 48 hours.

Neonatal hepatitis
Most cases of prolonged neonatal obstructive jaundice are due to neonatal hepatitis caused by viruses such as echovirus, rubella virus and Coxsackie B

virus, which are capable of passing through the placental barrier to the fetus.

Clinical features
The infant is jaundiced; the urine is dark and the stools are pale. He is lethargic and is too sleepy to feed and his liver is enlarged.

Investigations
1. Blood analysis.
2. Urinalysis.
3. Liver function tests.
4. Liver biopsy.

Principles of treatment and nursing management

1. Routine nursing care. Feeding, bathing, etc.
2. Chemotherapy:
   a. Bile acid binding substance and phenobarbital.
   b. Supplementary vitamins in water-miscible form.
   c. Antibiotics.
3. Pre- and post-operative care for liver biopsy (pp. 128 and 131).

Infections of the liver

A variety of agents can be responsible for infections affecting the liver. These can be viruses, parasites and bacteria. Vital infections are due to viruses A, B and specific viruses such as cytomegalovirus, yellow fever virus and influenza virus A and B, Varicella-Zoster virus and others. The latter viruses are believed to be implicated in Reye's syndrome which consists of an encephalopathy and fatty degeneration of viscera including the liver. Bacterial infections include pyogenic abscesses of the liver due to *Staphylococcus aureus*, haemolytic and non-haemolytic streptococci, *E. coli* and others. Parasitic infections include toxoplasma gondii, hydatid disease and abscess formation by the amoeba *Entamoeba histolytica*. Acute viral hepatitis is a common and important worldwide disease. It involves two distinct types of viruses which cause diffuse hepatocellular inflammatory disease.

Hepatitis type A

This form of hepatitis is more common in children than hepatitis B. There are seasonal variations, the majority of cases occurring in the late autumn and the first half of winter. Transmission is generally by the faecal/oral route, but some epidemics have been caused by contamination of water and food. The incubation period is 15 to 50 days.

Clinical features
The illness tends to be mild. Prior to the onset of jaundice there can be marked anorexia, nausea, vomiting, abdominal pain, mild diarrhoea and pyrexia. Children under 3 years of age frequently do not have jaundice. Bile appears in the urine just before the onset of jaundice and may last 7 to 10 days.

Investigations

1. Biochemical and virological studies.
2. Blood analysis.
3. Urine test for bile.

Principles of treatment and nursing management

1. Bed-rest is important until bile pigments have disappeared from the urine.
2. Nutritional needs. Diet in the acute phase should include an adequate fluid and carbohydrate intake. As the condition improves protein and a low fat intake is provided.
3. Constipation may be a problem and can be relieved by giving saline laxative.
4. As he recovers greater activity is possible.
5. Routine nursing care.

Hepatitis B

The B virus is associated with a wide spectrum of liver disease but is not so common in children in this country. However, there are circumstances in which infections can occur. These include transplacental or perinatal infections; infections can occur in children with disorders of immune function, e.g. leukaemia, and there is a risk to children with haemophilia who require multiple transfusions with blood or blood products.

The virus can be transmitted by parenteral route as well as by the oral route. The incubation period varies from 50 to 180 days. A very small proportion of children who aquire the virus become persistent carriers of the hepatitis B antigen. This presents a serious problem and precautions must be taken when collecting and testing blood samples. Each hospital authority will have clearly stated policies regarding method for collection and disposal of blood and used equipment.

Clinical features
Some similarity can be identified to hepatitis A. It is more likely to affect adolescents and adults. There may be rashes and arthritis. Increase in body temperature is usually mild. There is usually anorexia, nausea and vomiting and the disease is frequently moderate to severe. The degree of jaundice present also varies but is not as prolonged as in hepatitis A.

Investigations

1. Various tests for detecting hepatitis B surface antigen.
2. Blood analysis.
3. Urine tests.

Principles of treatment and nursing management

1. Isolation and prevention of cross-infection.
2. Limitation of activity.
3. Meeting nutritional needs. In the mild or moderately severe case a well-balanced diet should be given.
4. Observations of complications such as fulminating hepatitis, where massive necrosis of liver parenchyma occurs (see hepatic failure).

Hepatic failure
Hepatic failure is a complex clinical syndrome associated with severe impairment of liver function. It can occur during the course of an acute hepatitis complicated by extensive necrosis of liver cells, or it may represent chronic liver disease. The cause can be infection such as viral hepatitis type A, or drugs such as paracetamol or some hypersentivity to drugs.

Clinical features
The jaundice of hepatic failure is due mainly to impaired liver cell function. There is decreased uptake of bilirubin by the liver cells and failure of bilirubin conjugation within the cells. There is impaired synthesis of proteins, fats and carbo-

hydrates. There may be hypoglycaemia as a result of the liver's inability to produce glucose from non-carbohydrate sources. There is evidence of brain involvement and children show disturbed behaviour and mania. Intellectual function deteriorates and consciousness may be disturbed. Hyperventilation and hyperpyrexia are features in the terminal stage. Bleeding may occur due to disturbance in coagulation. As the jaundice deepens, the liver shrinks in size, there is abdominal pain and vomiting may occur.

Investigations
Blood analysis. Serum transaminases are often increased; serum albumin levels tend to be low; blood sugar level is frequently low and the child may be alkalotic. The blood ammonia level is often markedly increased and is believed to be the cause of the neuropsychiatric manifestations.

Principles of treatment and nursing management

1. Intravenous infusion (p. 448).
2. Blood transfusion — either frozen plasma or whole blood.
3. Provision of adequate calories; reduction or withdrawal of dietary protein to minimise the production of ammonia.
4. Administration of enemas and magnesium sulphate to minimise absorption of ammonia.
5. Suitable antibiotic.
6. Care of the acutely ill child (p. 107).
7. Support for parents. Recognition of their needs; participation in nursing care; explanation of the condition and treatment.

Biliary atresia
The cause of this condition is uncertain, but it is suggested that it may be due to a destructive inflammatory process. The most common abnormality found is complete atresia of all extrahepatic biliary structures, e.g. bile ducts.

Clinical features
The infant is jaundiced soon after birth. The stools are pale and the picture is similar to neonatal hepatitis. If the condition is not treated, the liver becomes enlarged, the heart becomes involved and there are signs of fat malabsorption.

Investigations

1. Blood serum analysis.
2. Liver biopsy.

Principles of treatment and nursing management
The aim is to establish a pathway for the bile, otherwise the prognosis is poor, death occurring within 2 years of life.

1. Surgery. An opening is made at the porta hepatis in the liver in an attempt to enter a major intrahepatic duct; the hole in the liver can be anastomosed to the end of a segment of the jejunum.
2. Pre- and post-operative care (pp. 128 and 131).
3. Routine nursing care.
4. Support for parents. The parents should be interviewed by the surgeon and the condition explained. They should be encouraged to handle and nurse the child and, since the prognosis is often poor, they will require a great deal of emotional support.

DISORDERS OF THE PANCREAS
The pancreas assumes two distinctive roles:

1. Exocrine activity which is the manufacture and excretion of pancreatic juice containing proteolytic, lipolytic and amyolytic enzymes. The functions of these enzymes are to break down protein, fat and carbohydrate. The pancreatic juice also adjusts the reaction of the duodenal contents, i.e. makes it alkaline.
2. Endocrine activity, i.e. the production of insulin and glucagon. Disorders of the pancreas can be congenital and acquired and include infections, cysts and tumours, as well as embryological malformations and cystic fibrosis.

Acute pancreatitis
There are a number of causes of acute pancreatitis in childhood which include, trauma, drugs, metabolic (hypercalcaemia) and genetic disorders. The pancreas may be damaged by haemorrhage, sepsis and necrosis.

Clinical features
Abdominal pain is present and there may be shock and renal failure due to plasma loss. Electrolyte disturbance may be severe and these may be reflected in the electrocardiogram. The urine may contain sugar and albumin.

Principles of treatment and nursing management

1. General routine nursing care:
   a. Gastric aspiration (p. 509).
   b. Intravenous infusion to correct fluid and electrolyte imbalance (p. 448).
   c. Relief of pain.
   d. Drugs to reduce pancreatic activity, e.g. propantheline bromide.
   e. Antibiotics to combat secondary infection.
2. Support for parents.

Cystic fibrosis of the pancreas
Cystic fibrosis is an inherited disease transmitted as an autosomal recessive trait. One in 20 of the population will be heterozygotes, and the likelihood of two heterozygotes mating can be estimated to be about one in 400. It is a multiorgan disease characterised by chronic lung disease, pancreatic insufficiency, liver dysfunction and increased concentrations of electrolytes in sweat. There are abnormally viscid mucous secretions and susceptibility to thermal stress. The disease is usually recognised in infancy or early childhood.

Pathology and pathophysiology
Nearly all exocrine glands are affected but in varying distribution and degrees of severity. The underlying metabolic defect is still unknown but cell studies have demonstrated a number of abnormalities, e.g. increased activity of the lysosomal enzyme α-glucosidase and increased concentrations of acid mucopolysaccharides.

The glands involved fall into three types: (1) those that become obstructed by viscid or solid material in the lumen (pancreas, intestinal glands, intrahepatic bile ducts, gall-bladder, submaxillary glands); (2) those that produce an excess of normal secretions (tracheobronchial and Brunner's glands); and (3) those that are histologically normal but secrete excessive sodium and chloride (sweat, parotid, and small salivary glands). Duodenal secretions are viscid and contain an abnormal mucopolysaccharide. In adulthood, the male reproductive organs are affected with maldevelopment of the vas deferens, resulting in aspermia. Some women are unable to conceive due to viscid cervical secretions, but many women with cystic fibrosis have been able to carry pregnancies to term.

The pulmonary lesion is believed to begin with diffuse obstruction of the small airways, due to abnormally thick mucous secretions. As the disease progresses further changes occur due to superimposed bacterial infection resulting in chronic bronchitis and bronchiectasis. Eventually the larger airways become filled with purulent and viscid secretions. Organisms such as *Staphylococcus aureus* and *Haemophilus influenzae* are found early in the disease, while *Pseudomonas aeruginosa* is often isolated later in the disease. As the pulmonary lesion advances, bronchial walls thicken, bronchogenic abscesses form and the hilar lymph nodes enlarge. Death usually results from a combination of respiratory failure and heart failure known as cor pulmonale.

Clinical features

Since several organs show pathological changes there are a variety of symptoms. The pattern of the disease seems to be faily constant. In about 10 per cent of cases the illness can be recognised in the neonatal period in the form of meconium ileus (p. 489). Respiratory infection is an early sign in infancy and this does not respond readily to antibiotic therapy. There is fever and dyspnoea with subcostal recession. The infant has spasms of coughing which lead to vomiting and interfere with feeding.

As the child gets older, the respiratory picture becomes that of bronchiectasis with purulent sputum. There is increased emphysema and clubbing of fingers. An essential feature of all cases is the presence of semi-formed, greasy, bulky and excessively offensive stools. After the first year of life, these stools occur in association with abdominal distension and wasting of tissue. Occasionally there may be rectal prolapse but it usually rectifies itself with dietary treatment and surgery is rarely necessary.

Clinical evidence of vitamin deficiencies may be present involving vitamins A, D, E and K; the last manifests itself in intracranial or cutaneous bleeding in infancy. Excessive sweating results in loss of fluid and electrolytes and this can occur during hot weather or fever. If it is not corrected it will lead to hypovolaemia, dehydration and circulatory failure.

Diabetes mellitus occurs as the child grows older. This is due to increasing encroachment on the islet cells as the pancreatic lesion progresses. It is generally mild and easily controlled.

Investigations

1. Examination of stools for tryptic activity. In cystic fibrosis of the pancreas this enzyme is absent. Presence of fat globules in stools is a useful test (p. 517).
2. Duodenal intubation. Duodenal juice is obtained to demonstrate absence or diminished trypsin (p. 516).
3. The sweat test is the most definitive test (p. 267). Na and Cl levels above 60 mmol/l denote cystic fibrosis provided at least 100 mg of sweat is obtained.

Principles of treatment and nursing management

1. Control of lung infection. The staphylococcus is the causative organism. Antibiotic treatment is usually permanent and this presents problems of resistance to antibiotics. Examples of useful drugs are: tetracycline (25 mg/kg/d), cloxacillin (50 mg/kg/d) and cephalosporin.
2. Relief of coughing and decreasing viscous sputum:
   a. Croupette (particularly at night), inhalation of 10 per cent propylene glycol in 3 per cent sodium chloride solution.
   b. Ultrasonic nebuliser.
3. Physiotherapy. This is important —
   a. To obtain proper drainage by postural drainage (p. 377).
   b. For deep breathing exercises.
4. Oxygen therapy is often indicated to maintain adequate arterial oxygen tension during acute exacerbations. Home care often includes oxygen administration, particularly at night, and has been found to relieve recurrent morning headaches.
5. Diet. The child should receive a protein-rich diet (about 6 g per kg) and the intake of fat should be low.

6. Extra salt is required because of the losses in sweat. During hot weather, the salt intake should be 2 to 3 g per day in addition to the dietary intake. Excessive loss of sodium chloride leads to peripheral circulatory failure (p. 225).
7. Pancreatin supplements like Pancrex V forte powder 0.5 g for infants and young children, increasing to 2 g by the age of 2 years. This is given immediately before meals, mixed with water or fruit juice. In older children six to 10 tablets are required with each meal. Cotazym or Nutrizym are other pancreatin supplements which can be given. Each of these preparations contain protease, amylase and lipase.
8. Vitamins in a water-miscible base.
9. Routine nursing care plus:
   a. Care of buttocks; with excessive loose stools, the buttocks become sore (p. 115).
   b. Feeding is a problem, particularly during the spasms of coughing. Tube feeds may have to be given.
   c. If sweating is excessive, the child will require frequent baths and changes of personal and bed clothes.
10. Support for parents. The condition should be explained fully to the parents and genetic counselling is advised. Crises are particularly anxious times for them, but full support, guidance and understanding of their problems and difficulties are essential at all times. When the child is nursed at home the community services should be utilised, e.g. a Croupette and nebuliser should be made available. The parents should be shown how to invert the child and achieve maximum postural drainage. Arrangements should also be made for regular physiotherapy and frequent follow-up periods.

INTESTINAL PARASITES

The more common parasites affecting children in the United Kingdom are tapeworm, threadworm and giardiasis.

Tapeworm

The child may become a host by ingesting imperfectly cooked beef containing the worm. The worm is about 6 metres long and has about 2000 segments; however, there are also worms found in pork and fish which can infect man.

Clinical features
Each of the different worms affect specific tissues. Abdominal pain may be present and the segments are passed in the stools.

Principles of treatment and nursing management

1. Rest in bed.
2. Diet. A soft, fat-free diet is given for 48 hours.
3. Medication, e.g. niclosamide.
4. Routine nursing care.
5. Examination of stools.

Threadworms

The male worm is about 3 mm in length and the female, which looks like a piece of thread, is about 10 mm in length. The female lives in the colon and the eggs are laid when the female passes out of the anus. The ova after ingestion hatch in the small intestine. The initial infection may be from contaminated water or uncooked foodstuffs.

Clinical features
The most common symptom is an itchy anus. The child scratches and the area becomes sore. Reinfestation also occurs from the child's contaminated fingers. Thread-like worms can be seen in the anus and in the faeces.

Principles of treatment and nursing management

1. Cleanliness of perianal skin.
2. Prevention of scratching (pyjama trousers should be worn to prevent reinfestation).
3. Treatment of the whole family. The drug used is either piperazine, Pripsen or Viprymium (as a single dose).
4. Guidance for parents. The condition should be explained to the parents and advice given on prevention, i.e. personal hygiene and adequate food preparation.

Giardiasis (lambliasis)

Giardia intestinalis is a common intestinal parasite in the United Kingdom. The portal of entry is the mouth and the parasite inhabits the upper small intestine, causing mucous diarrhoea, abdominal pain and weight loss. Diagnosis is by finding cysts in the stools.

Principles of treatment and nursing management

1. Drugs like metronidazole or quinacrine are given.
2. Bed-rest during symptoms of abdominal pain and diarrhoea.
3. Guidance for parents. The condition should be explained to the parents and advice given on prevention, i.e. personal hygiene.

Procedures relating to the digestive system

Lubrication of oesophageal and gastric tubes

It is not a pleasant experience to swallow a tube and the majority of children will object strongly. It is nevertheless possible to pass a tube successfully and safely, provided the tube is firm and moist. It is recommended that the tube is either moistened or lubricated with a water-soluble jelly. The reasons for this are as follows:

1. Lubricants which have an oily base, e.g. liquid paraffin, are associated with lipoid pneumonia when these are inhaled. The older child also finds the taste unpleasant and retching is a common feature.
2. Lubricants such as liquid paraffin may well have a considerable aperient action if the tube has to be passed at frequent intervals.

When lubrication is necessary, KY jelly is satisfactory. It is water-soluble and has no known harmful effects. If a rubber tube is used and it is soft, the tube can be placed in iced water to make it firmer; the water acting as lubricant. Plastic tubes may be too firm and these can be placed or dipped in warm water to make them softer.

Oesophagoscopy

This is a direct vision examination of the oesophagus. It may be carried out:

1. In an effort to recover a foreign body which has become lodged in the oesophagus.
2. As an aid to diagnosis, or to determine progress in the presence of dysphagia, or suspected disease of the oesophagus.

3. To dilate the oesophagus when there is a stenosis.

Oesophagoscopes or endoscopes of varying sizes are used. The procedure is usually performed under general anaesthesia in the operating theatre.

Preparation of the child
Routine pre-operative care (p. 128).

After-care of the child
There may be some degree of dysphagia afterwards and, if present, fluids are given in small quantities more frequently. Small frequent milk drinks will help to alleviate pain if there is an oesophagitis. It is also preferable to have the child propped up as soon as possible to prevent reflux of gastric juices up the oesophagus. These would cause considerable irritation and pain.

If there has been difficulty in removing a foreign body, resulting in injury to the mucosa of the oesophagus, sterile fluids are given.

Gastric aspiration

Gastric aspiration is performed to relieve the stomach and small intestines of gaseous distension and fluid content. It may be performed for the following reasons:

1. As part of the treatment for mechanical obstruction, e.g. intussusception, volvulus or atresia of a section of the digestive tract.
2. When paralytic ileus is present.
3. For pre-operative preparation prior to surgery of the digestive tract.

Inhalation of regurgitated stomach contents constitutes a danger to any child. This danger is increased when there is some form of intestinal obstruction. Gastric intubation and aspiration of contents is essential and the tube is left in position and unclamped to allow free drainage of fluid or gas.

Paralytic ileus or paralysis of the intestinal muscles is associated with various conditions. It provides as effective an obstruction to the onward passage of bowel content as the mechanical type. A paralytic ileus may develop following an accident or after abdominal surgery when handling of the intestines leads to cessation of its peristaltic activity. Other causes of paralytic ileus include reduction in serum potassium and uraemia leading to interference with smooth muscle contraction.

Preparation of the child

An explanation should be given to the older child. The younger child will require to have his arms restrained until he is used to the tube and is no longer likely to pull it out.

Requirements

1. Tube (Ryle's or oesophageal) size 9 to 12 FG or 4 to 6 EG. (The size must not be larger than that which can be passed comfortably via the nose.)
2. Lubricant (see above).
3. Dressing pack.
4. Thread (if required).
5. Adhesive tape.
6. Spigot (if required).
7. Syringe (10 ml).
8. Blue litmus paper.
9. Bowl for aspirate.
10. Bowl with sterile water to rinse the syringe.
11. Collecting bag (for continuous drainage).
12. Protection for child and tissues.

Method for passing naso-gastric tube (Fig. 26.13)

Two nurse are required; one to perform the procedure and the other to hold and comfort the child. Both should wash and dry their hands. The child should lie comfortably in bed with one or more pillows. The child's nostrils are cleaned with moist cotton wool and dried. The tube is measured from the nape of the nose to the tip of the xiphisternum. It is moistened and passed approximately 2.5 cm to 8 cm beyond the measured point or until the aspirated material flows freely. Force should not be used and the other nostril should be used if there appears to be any obstruction. To check whether the tube is in the stomach:

1. Aspirate the contents of the stomach with a 10 ml syringe and test with litmus paper. It should give an acid reaction if it is gastric content.
2. Alternatively, place a stethoscope over the epigastrium and inject a small amount of air. The air entering the stomach can be heard with the stethoscope.

When the tube is correctly positioned, it is strapped on the cheek.

Observations during the above procedure

1. When passing the tube, the infant's or child's colour should be normal and he should be able to breathe without any difficulty. Retching or gagging often occurs but should not produce cyanosis. Should coughing occur accompanied by cyanosis and breathing difficulty, the tube must be withdrawn immediately. Since the tube is very fine, it is possible for it to enter the trachea, producing the above symptoms.
2. There may be difficulty in passing the tube. Force should never be used. The fact must be reported. It may be due to fibrous narrowing of the oesophagus.
3. It is important to examine the mouth of the child or infant to ensure that the tube has not curled up at the back of the throat.

Method of aspiration

The gastric contents are aspirated with a 10 ml syringe and the aspirate is measured. Aspiration is continued until the stomach is empty. The tube is then left open and allowed to drain into a drainage bag.

Gastric suction can also be achieved by using either electric or wall suction. Suction must not be too strong, a vacuum of 12 mmHg (1.5 kPa) is considered satisfactory. Strong suction could

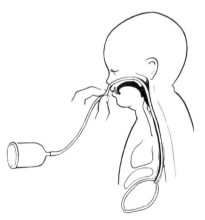

Fig. 26.13 Naso-gastric catheter in position. Note the tip of the catheter at the end of the oesophagus.

damage the gastric mucosa if the eye of the tube rests against the wall of the stomach.

Gastric lavage

Gastric lavage or stomach washout is performed for the following reasons:

1. In cases of poisoning, in an effort to remove and dilute the poison.
2. Where there is irritation of the gastric mucosa due to causes other than poisoning, e.g.:
   a. Gastroenteritis.
   b. Mucus swallowed during the process of birth.
   c. In the infant with an upper respiratory infection where irritation is due to the swallowing of infected material.
3. To cleanse and empty the stomach prior to operation on the stomach or upper part of the digestive tract. A gastric lavage may also be necessary when an emergency operation has to be performed, to ensure that the stomach is empty.
4. For diagnostic purposes. To assess the amount of residue present, or to obtain gastric washings; the latter is necessary to obtain sputum for bacteriological examination. Young children tend to swallow sputum.

Requirements

1. Dressing pack, litmus paper, lubricant, 10 ml syringe and sterile water.
2. Oesophageal catheters, sizes according to age. For small infants — No. 15 FG or 8 EG, for the older child — No. 20 to 24 FG or 12 to 14 EG.
3. Nutrient funnel, tubing and a connecting tube.
4. Flask containing the required solution, e.g. sodium chloride. The strength of the solution depends on the age of the child. For example, infants under 2 months sodium chloride 0.225 per cent; for children between 2 months and 2 years, sodium chloride 0.45 per cent and for children over 2 years, sodium chloride 0.9 per cent.

   The solution should be at a temperature of 37.2°C and to achieve this, the flask can be placed in a bowl of warm water.

5. Lotion thermometer.
6. Water-repellent sheet to protect the child.
7. Floor protection (if required).
8. Pail or basin for return flow of solution.
9. Measure of the residue. A measure is also useful to ensure that the returned fluid is accurately measured.
10. Vomit bowl and tissues.
11. Disposal bag.
12. Split pressure tubing 5 cm in length should be available to slip on to the oesophageal tube. The split tubing is placed between the teeth to prevent biting the oesophageal tube and is to be preferred to the use of a mouth gag.

Preparation of the child

Two nurses should always carry out this procedure and each must be aware of the dangers which might present themselves.

The child, if old enough, should have an explanation of what is about to happen. The child should be placed in the lateral position and should be effectively restrained. If the child is struggling, more assistance will be required. The infant is best placed in the sitting position, supported and restrained by one nurse.

Principles of the procedure

1. Recognition of danger of regurgitation of fluid. This may easily lead to aspiration into the lungs. Weak and unconscious children are more likely to regurgitate. Should regurgitation occur, the child should be inverted, the funnel lowered and the fluid syphoned back. The catheter is removed and the airway cleared by using suction.
2. Knowledge of the capacity of the stomach at different ages (p. 512). Great care should be taken not to overload the stomach.
3. Understanding of the reasons for the procedure and the type of solution to use, e.g. certain poisons require specific antidotes.

Method

The catheter is introduced as described on page 510, but it is not fixed to the child's face.

When the catheter is in position, it is held by the assistant. The funnel is attached to the tubing and connecting rod and these are connected to the oesophageal tube. The funnel is lowered to collect the residue which is emptied into a graduated measure. This is proof that the catheter is in the stomach. If there is difficulty in syphoning fluid back, a small amount of sterile water can be introduced as this often establishes return flow.

The lavage can then proceed by introducing the required amount of solution. When the funnel is almost empty, it is lowered to collect the return flow. The amount instilled should also be returned. The lavage is continued until the return fluid is clear, or until the ordered amount of fluid has been used. For small infants this may only amount to 600 ml. The returned fluid is kept for inspection and, if necessary, for analysis.

This is not a pleasant procedure and the child will require gentleness and should be comforted before he is returned to bed.

ARTIFICIAL FEEDING
There are various methods of feeding by artificial means. The two most common are oesophageal and gastric tube feeding (gavage) (1) in which the catheter is withdrawn immediately after completion of the feed, and (2) in which the catheter is left in place and the child is fed intermittently or continuously.

Temporary oesophageal and gastric gavage
The catheter is passed either through the nose or mouth into the stomach or to the lower end of the oesophagus. The catheter is withdrawn on completion of the feed.

This method is used when it is considered unwise to leave a fine oesophageal catheter in position, or when regular artificial feeding is not necessary. It is useful when nursing infants with the following conditions: prematurity, if the infant is unable to suck or becomes easily exhausted when sucking; exhaustion in infants suffering from congenital heart disease accompanied by heart failure, and in acute respiratory diseases. However, it is not considered desirable in premature infants where repeatedly passing a catheter via the nose could lead to irritation and trauma.

It is best to pass the catheter only as far as the end of the oesophagus as this is less irritating to gastric mucosa and therefore less likely to cause vomiting. If gastric tube feeding was carried out at 3- or 4-hourly intervals over a long period of time, there might be a danger of injury to the gastric mucosa by repeatedly hitting the same point on the greater curvature on the stomach.

Requirements

1. Dressing pack, thread, adhesive tape, litmus paper.
2. Sterile water.
3. Oesophageal catheter (connection, if required).
4. Nutrient funnel or 20 ml syringe.
5. Feed (if pre-packed feed, heating is not necessary); prepared feed should be warmed to 37.2°C.
6. Food thermometer.
7. Water-repelled sheet.
8. Disposal bag.

Method
The catheter is introduced as described on page 510. When the catheter is in position, it must be held carefully and the feed is given slowly. The rate is determined by the condition of the child. A guide for an infant is that it should take as long to give as the child would normally take to feed by bottle.

The capacity of the stomach to accommodate food or fluid increases with age. The following table is a guide as to the capacity of the stomach in the first year of life:

At birth	30–36 ml
1 week	39–45 ml
2 weeks	60–90 ml
4 weeks	75–90 ml
3 months	100–135 ml
6 months	135–180 ml
1 year	225–270 ml

When the feed has been given, the tubing is firmly nipped and removed. There is a danger that the child may start to retch while the catheter is removed and this can lead to vomiting. Observations of the child's reaction will be the best guide in deciding whether the catheter should be withdrawn quickly or slowly. In some units, it is policy to introduce about 15 ml of sterile water before withdrawing the catheter. This ensures that the catheter is free of milk when it is withdrawn and therefore there is less danger of milk being inhaled.

The child should be placed in the position most comfortable for him, but it is safer to maintain the upright position, if that is possible. He should be comforted once the procedure is completed.

Continuous or intermittent oesophageal and gastric gavage

This method is used when it is necessary to give feeds very slowly and to prevent trauma to the nose by frequent insertion and withdrawal of the catheter. It is useful when the child is debilitated or has received extensive injury. A very fine oesophageal or polyvinyl tube is used. This causes no irritation and may be left in position for one or two weeks. However, it is desirable that the catheter is changed every 4 to 6 days to prevent infection since milk is a good media for bacterial growth.

Feeds can be given very slowly and are, therefore, more readily tolerated. The debilitated older child may have artificial feeding during the night, the catheter being clamped by day, allowing him to take food normally. This method is also used for the unconscious child. In deep coma, the cardiac sphincter is relaxed and allows the contents of the stomach to rise into the oesophagus, leading to regurgitation and aspiration of feed. In these cases it is essential, therefore, to give only small amounts very slowly.

Preparation of the child
Where possible, an explanation should be given. It may also be necessary to restrain the child's arms. The older child is placed in the semi-recumbent position, and the unconscious child in the right lateral position with the head of the bed raised 30°.

Requirements
The requirements are the same as for temporary tube feeding with the following additions:

1. Disposable intravenous giving set, or similar apparatus.
2. For infants and small children, a 60 ml nutrient funnel and two pieces of connecting tubes, and a connecting rod.
3. Clamp.
4. Infusion stand.

Method
The catheter is passed as described on page 510. The intravenous set is connected to the flask and the air is expelled from the tubing. The end of the intravenous set is connected to the oesophageal catheter and allowed to drip in slowly. The rate of flow is adjusted according to the amount of feed to be given. The rate of flow should be constant and care taken not to increase the rate suddenly. If an open funnel is used, it should be approximately 30 cm above the child's head. The funnel should be covered with a sterile swab to prevent contamination. The apparatus is removed when the total amount of feed has been given and a new one is attached.

Throughout the procedure, the child must be observed carefully for signs of regurgitation of feed and inhalation of feed. In intermittent naso-gastric feeding the catheter is left in position for some time. Before commencing the feed it is essential to verify that the catheter is patent and that it is in the stomach. The method of testing is the same as that used for determining the position of the catheter initially. However, when the catheter is left down there is a tendency for it to become blocked. This blockage can be cleared by instilling sterile water approximately 15 ml, or by aspirating it with a syringe. If the blockage cannot be cleared, a new catheter must be inserted.

When the feed has been given a small amount of sterile water, about 15 ml, is introduced and the catheter is closed, either with a spigot or by replacing the plastic cap.

If the patient is a small infant it is useful to fit a tubegauze cap on the infant's head and to keep the catheter in place beneath it. This will enable the infant to move his head without danger of pulling the tube out. The hands can be enclosed in mittens but it is essential to check frequently to ensure that the infant's fingers are *not* constricted.

Mouth care is important when the normal means of feeding is not utilised. For a discussion on the method see page 96.

Naso-duodenal/jejunal feeding

This form of feeding is considered useful in pre-term infants and permits high intake rates of fluid and nutrients from the first 2 or 3 days of life.

The equipment is the same as for naso-gastric feeding, except that a silicone radiopaque duodenal catheter is used. It has a metal olive at its tip and is 125 cm long (Vygon 5 FG).

Method

The tube is inserted, via the nose, into the stomach as for naso-gastric feeding. Its position is confirmed by testing a specimen of aspirate for acidity with litmus paper. The tube is then inserted a further 12 cm into the stomach and secured to the forehead with adhesive tape. To facilitate passage of the tube through the pylorus, the infant should be placed horizontally on his right side. Gradually, the tube is inserted further by 1 cm until the tube is in the desired position. To confirm that the tube is lying in, or beyond the duodenum, the content is aspirated. The aspirate should be stained yellowish-green giving an alkaline response when tested with litmus paper. Radiographic confirmation of the tube's position is necessary before a milk feed is introduced. The tube is then secured to the infant's forehead and the proximal end can be attached to an extension set and connected to a syringe pump, or other suitable pump, which gives a constant continuous low-volume infusion.

Gastrostomy feeding (Fig. 26.14)

A gastrostomy is an opening into the stomach through the abdominal wall into which a catheter is passed. The skin is invaginated (as in an unspillable inkpot) to prevent leakage of gastric content around the catheter. The catheter is inserted for 5 to 7 cm, depending on the size of the child, and is stitched into position.

This method of feeding is necessary when there is some obstruction to the normal route, e.g. stricture or atresia of the oesophagus. The catheter is kept in position and is changed every few weeks or when necessary.

Requirements

1. Nutrient funnel.

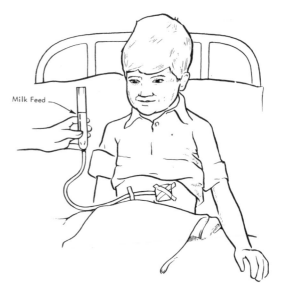

Milk Feed

Fig. 26.14 Gastrostomy feeding. Note position of the nurse's hand, holding funnel.

2. 30 cm length of tubing (if required).
3. Container with feed (if it is to be warmed, the temperature should not exceed 37.2°C).
4. Food thermometer.
5. Sterile water.
6. Towel.

Method

When the feed is given for the first time, the procedure should be explained to the child, provided he is old enough to understand. Subsequent feeds are usually readily accepted and anticipated, the older child often participating with his own feeding.

The child is made comfortable in the position he finds most acceptable either in bed or sitting in a chair. The nurse washes and dries her hands assembles the apparatus, and then checks the temperature of the feed. A towel is laid under the gastrostomy catheter, the spigot is removed, and the connection is attached. A small quantity of water is run into the catheter and if there is no obstruction to its flow, the feed is given slowly.

The funnel should be kept just about the level of the abdomen and the flow is controlled by raising or lowering the funnel (Fig. 26.14). If the child is destressed, or retching, the feed will come up the funnel, and for this reason the funnel should always be only half-filled. When the child has recovered, the feed can be continued to run in slowly. After the feed has been given, the tube is cleared with a small quantity of water and the catheter is closed with a spigot or a plastic cap.

After-care of the child

The child should be moved gently and remain in the upright position after the feed has been given. Oral hygiene is essential. He may be permitted to suck something pleasant during feeding, not only to give him satisfaction but also to stimulate the gastric juices.

Care of the wound

The dressing around the gastrostomy catheter is changed as necessary. It is considered as a surgical dressing, and not part of the feeding procedure. Observations of the wound should include recognition of leakage of gastric contents and the presence of bile. The latter indicates that the catheter has passed through the pylorus into the duodenum and may require action, e.g. the catheter may be withdrawn slightly or removed and re-passed.

Gastric analysis (augmented histamine test)

The gastric mucosa secretes gastric juice throughout the 24 hours, the amount varying with the age of the child. The rate of secretion is not constant, nor is the level of acidity. In the new-born infant gastric acidity is relatively high but falls rapidly in the first 10 days and then rises gradually to adult levels at 12 years.

Average normal gastric juice contains a high concentration of hydrochloric acid, organic material including mucin, enzymes, and inorganic constituents such as sodium, potassium, magnesium, chloride and other salts. It also contains the important intrinsic factors required for the absorption of vitamin B_{12}.

Tests are performed to determine the presence of hydrochloric acid and the degree of acidity of stomach contents. There are different types of tests but the one most frequently used is the augmented histamine test. When gastric and duodenal ulcers are suspected these can be readily confirmed by straight radiographs or fluoroscopy.

Requirements

1. Flask marked 'fasting juice'.
2. Labelled specimen flasks (four).
3. 20 ml syringe.
4. Ryle's catheter and spigot.
5. Dressing pack.
6. Flask of normal saline — temperature 37.2°C.
7. Mediswabs, 2 × 2 ml syringes and needles No. 25 gauge.
8. Adhesive tape and safety pin.
9. Litmus paper.
10. Histamine acid phosphate (increases gastric secretion).
11. Anthisan (antihistamine).
12. Vomit bowl and disposable towel.
13. Disposal bag.

Method

The test is performed on a fasting stomach, and the procedure should be explained to the child. Books and toys should be available during the procedure and some attempt should be made to prevent the tantalising sight of food. Younger children should have their arms restrained and with some children it may be necessary to sedate them.

The catheter is introduced as described on page 510. The position of the catheter is checked radiologically; it should be at the greater curvature. Throughout the procedure, the child is kept lying on the left side in a semi-upright position:

1. Collect a fasting specimen and put into the flask marked for that purpose.
2. The stomach is washed out with normal saline until the returned fluid is clear. The 20 ml syringe is used for that purpose.
3. Minute 0. 'Basal juice' is aspirated; a suction pump may be used at a suction pressure of 10 to 15 cm of water.
4. Minute 40. Anthisan is given intramuscularly; amount according to doctor's written instruction.
5. Minute 60:
   a. 'Basal' collection is discontinued. The amount aspirated is measured and retained.
   b. Histamine is given subcutaneously according to written instruction.
   c. Specimen 'A' is obtained.
6. Minute 80. Collection of specimen 'B' is started.

7. Minute 100. Collection of specimen 'C' is started.
8. Minute 120. Collection is completed.

At the end of the collection, the catheter is removed. A mouthwash can be given to the older child followed by a light meal, and the infant is given a feed.

Throughout the procedure it is important to watch the child carefully for any signs of reaction. Medical aid should be summoned if there are any signs of flushing, faintness or headache.

Duodenal intubation

This procedure is carried out as an aid to the diagnosis of fibrocystic disease of the pancreas, when some doubt exists with all other tests. It is most conveniently performed under fluoroscopic control.

Duodenal fluid is normally clear and watery; it may be colourless or of varying shades of yellow, depending on its bile content. It is alkaline in reaction containing the enzymes trypsin, amylase, and lipase. In fibrocystic disease mucosis and fibrosis of the glandular tissue occur, leading to deficiency or absence of pancreatic enzymes in the duodenal juice. For practical purposes the fluid need only be tested for the presence of trypsin. A very low amount or absence of trypsin is indicative of the disease.

Requirements
As for passing a naso-gastric tube with the addition of:

1. Ryle's or duodenal catheter.
2. 20 ml syringe.
3. Six to 10 test tubes.
4. Bowl containing ice to keep the specimen cool.

Method
The child is fasted from 10 p.m.; the infant is given a 6 a.m. feed but the 10 a.m. feed is omitted. An explanation should be given to the older child but it may be necessary to restrain his arms at least until the catheter has been passed. The infant is sedated prior to this procedure. He is wrapped in a cotton blanket to restrain his arms. The right lateral semi-recumbent position is suit-

able as this appears to aid gravitation of the catheter into the duodenum.

Suction is applied either with the syringe or continuous suction at a controlled pressure is applied to the duodenum. The aspirated fluid is collected into ice-cooled tubes or flasks each containing equal quantities of glycerol.

When duodenal juice has been obtained (this should be alkaline) the catheter is removed and the child is made comfortable and given a feed or meal.

Jejunal biopsy

In this procedure, tissue from the jejunum is obtained for histological examination. Examination of the tissue may reveal flat mucosa which is devoid of normal villi and is therefore indicative of coeliac disease (p. 500).

Requirements

1. As for passing a naso-gastric catheter with the addition of a special Crosby catheter.
2. 20 ml syringe.
3. 2 ml syringe and needles No. 25.
4. Jar for specimen.

Preparation of the child
If the child is old enough, a simple explanation should be given. He should be fasted for at least 8 hours and sedation is given prior to the commencement of the procedure. The child is taken to the radiology department where the catheter is passed. To assist the catheter to gravitate into the duodenum and jejunum the child is placed on his right side.

The procedure is performed by the medical officer and the nurse's function is to maintain the child's position.

After-care of the child
The child is made comfortable and nursed in bed for the rest of the day. Fluids only are given when the child is conscious. Clear fluids are given initially and are later followed by milk drinks. A light diet can be given the following day.

This procedure carries a small risk of haemorrhage or perforation and it is therefore essential to observe the child carefully. The pulse rate is recorded half-hourly for the first 4 hours. Any vomit must be kept for inspection and the presence of blood reported immediately. Complaints of pain in the epigastric region should also be reported immediately and any stools passed are tested for faecal occult blood.

Faecal fat excretion

Raised fat excretion is a reliable index of malabsorption but it does not indicate the cause. The test is carried out to determine the fat content in faeces. Normal faecal fat varies with different age levels. From 2 to 6 months, the total faecal fat is 0.3 to 1.3 g per day; from 6 months to 6 years, it is 0.33 to 1.8 g per day. A daily output in excess of 4 g per day indicates steatorrhoea. It is not necessary to measure the intake of fat accurately but an estimate should be made using food tables of the fat in the diet. In young children, the fat comes from milk, butter, eggs and cheese.

However, it is important that all the stools passed for 3 consecutive days, are collected. If any stools are discarded a fresh collection must be started. If stools are passed irregularly and days are missed the collection should be extended for a fourth or fifth day.

Stool collection

1. All stools passed per 24 hours are put in one container and marked with the name of the child, date and day of collection.
2. Polythene sheets can be used inside the potty or bedpan to collect the stools. In infants, the napkin may be lined with a polythene sheet which should be changed frequently to prevent sore buttocks. In some units, the infant is sat on a special chair and the stools are collected in the pan placed underneath the chair.

Examination for tryptic activity

This examination is carried out when the child presents a history of loose stools. Specimens of faeces are sent to the biochemical department where they are analysed for tryptic activity. Trypsin is a protealytic enzyme which is one of the pancreatic enzymes. Tryptic activity may either be absent or diminished in fibrocystic disease of the pancreas.

D-xylose absorption tests

These are valuable tests for malabsorption syndromes, e.g. ideopathic steatorrhoea.

1. Urinary xylose excretion test

The child is fasted overnight. At 7.30 a.m., the child is asked to empty his bladder. The urine is discarded. He is then given 5 g of D-xylose in 100 ml of water. During the next hour he is given another 150 ml of water when he wants it. Urine is collected for 5 hours after the xylose is given and sent to the laboratory. In the healthy child, at least 1 g is recovered in the urine.

2. One hour blood xylose method for infants and children under 30 kg

This test is of value in young children suffering from coeliac disease. The rate of absorption is abnormal when the mucosa is abnormal.

Method

1. The child should be fasted for at least 6 hours.
2. He is given a drink of 5 g of D-xylose in 100 ml of water (the time is noted).
3. Exactly 1 hour later, doctor takes off 1 to 2 ml of venous blood and puts it into a standard fluoride (blood sugar) tube.

Result

A 1 hour blood level above 20 mg/100 ml (1.3 mmol/l) is normal and below 20 mg/100 ml (1.3 mmol/l) is abnormal.

Liver biopsy

This procedure is performed in children suspected of suffering from cirrhosis of the liver, prolonged jaundice, particularly neonatal jaundice, Wilson's disease, suspected liver disease without jaundice and others. It is contra-indicated in the presence of clotting defects, hydatid disease (because of the danger of risk of dissemination and anaphylactoid shock) and vascular tumours of the liver.

Technique

A special liver puncture needle is inserted into the liver, passing between the lower ribs. As the needle passes through the liver tissue, it cuts a long core of tissue which remains in the barrel of the needle. The specimen of liver tissue is placed in normal saline or absolute alcohol and sent to the laboratory.

Requirements
1. Dressing pack, containers with cleansing lotions and normal saline.
2. Two Menghini liver biopsy needles with obdurator.
3. 20 ml glass Leur-lock syringe.
4. 2 ml, 10 ml disposable syringes and needles.
5. Scalpel and blade.
6. Drapes and sterile hand towels.
7. Jar for liver tissue.

Preparation of the child
The child is prepared for a general anaesthesia and a simple explanation should be given.

Care of the child
Throughout the procedure and following it, careful observations are necessary. The child's pulse and respiratory rate should be monitored in recognition of possible complications such as haemorrhage. After the procedure, the child is nursed in the upright position supported by pillows. The punctured site should be examined for any discharge and, should it occur, pressure can be applied over the site.

Barium swallow and meal
These examinations are carried out to aid diagnosis when there is a suspected abnormality of the digestive tract. The following are some of the conditions which may be diagnosed by findings after a barium swallow or meal: hiatus hernia; oesophageal stricture or diverticulum; oesophageal varices; pyloric stenosis; peptic ulcers and hairballs in the stomach.

Principles involved
Barium sulphate is an opaque medium, which is non-toxic and is not absorbed. Because of its opacity to X-rays, it clearly shows the size, position and shape of the stomach, together with the character of peristaltic waves. The rate at which barium leaves the stomach and any irregularities of contour caused by ulceration or new growth will be visible.

Preparation of the child
The child should have no food for 4 hours prior to the examination. Suitable clothes should be worn without pins or buttons. Since the examination takes place in dim surroundings the child may be frightened. He should be accompanied by either a nurse he knows and likes or by his mother and the examination should be explained to him. The mixture may be prepared in the ward or in the X-ray department and it is given by bottle or by cup, depending on the child's age.

Method
1. Barium swallow. The barium is given to drink while the lights are dimmed and the child is in position on the table. The progress of the barium is watched on the X-ray screen and permanent films are taken as required.

2. Barium meal. As soon as the barium has been swallowed, its progress is watched on the screen and films are taken at suitable moments. Its passage through the digestive tract is followed at intervals and subsequent X-rays are taken. The whole examination may take 2 or 3 hours. Metoclopramide 5 to 10 mg may be given orally 5 to 10 minutes before the barium is given to speed the gastric emptying.

Gastrografin. This is a contrast medium for radiological ingestigation of the gastro-intestinal tract. It may be given orally, or as an enema. It is an aqueous solution and is much more rapidly dispersed than barium, reaching the colon in a small infant in under 1 hour. It is therefore of value in suspected obstruction and in intestinal atresia.

Very small quantities are required. In an infant weighing 3.2 kg 10 ml given orally will reach the rectum in 45 minutes. When it is given rectally a greater amount is required and the medium is diluted as 1 in 4 parts of water.

Investigations for tracheo-oesophageal abnormality
Examinations are carried out when there is a suspected tracheo-oesophageal fistula with or without oesophageal atresia or an oesophageal atresia.

To diagnose a suspected tracheo-oesophageal fistula a viscid contrast medium such as propyliodone may be used. This substance does not irritate the respiratory tract; to diagnose an oesophageal atresia an opaque catheter is passed into the oesophagus.

Preparation of the child
The infant may be in an incubator, in which case this is transported to the X-ray department. Otherwise, he is wrapped up warmly and taken to the X-ray department by a nurse. The infant should be dressed in warm clothes without buttons, and his hands and feet should be kept warm with mittens and bootees to prevent loss of heat. Suction or aspiration equipment should be available to prevent aspiration of saliva. He should be placed in the position which will minimise the possibility of aspirating saliva. For example, his head is kept lower than his chest, lying on his side, or he is kept upright to allow drainage of saliva into the pouch or the oesophagus. The saliva is aspirated from the pouch through a fine catheter which is left in position.

Requirements

1. Spoon.
2. 2 ml syringe and withdrawing needle.
3. Oesophageal catheter or radiopaque catheter.
4. Mucus extractor or suction equipment.
5. Warmed ampoule of propyliodine.
6. Paper tissues.
7. Disposal bag.

Method
Normally this examination is performed under screening when the infant is given about 1 to 2 ml of the contrast medium to swallow from a spoon. The lights are dimmed and the progress of the medium is watched on the screen. An alternative method is to lubricate the oesophageal catheter with the medium and pass it gently, watching the progress under fluoroscopic control, or to use a radiopaque catheter.

After-care of the child
If an atresia, or obstruction of the oesophagus is present, the medium should be sucked out before returning the child to the ward. The most effective method of aspiration is with direct vision when an endoscope is passed by the anaesthetist and any material is removed through an open-ended catheter attached to a suction machine.

Barium enema
A barium enema can be given to aid diagnosis. It will outline any abnormality of contour or of emptying of the lower bowel, such as occurs in Hirschsprung's disease, or idiopathic megacolon.

Preparation of the child
The preparation of the child depends on the suspected abnormality. For example, children suffering from a suspected megacolon, either congenital or acquired, may require no prior preparation of the bowel as any purgation will alter the outline and mobility of the bowel. Infants and young children who are very apprehensive should be sedated prior to the examination to prevent resistance to retrograde injection of barium and to prevent premature expulsion of the medium.

The mother or a favourite nurse should always accompany and stay with the younger child. She can do much to allay fear and permit the examination to be carried out quickly and with the least discomfort. The older child requires adequate explanation and should be accompanied by a member of the nursing staff. This is an unpleasant procedure and the child will be anxious in case he cannot retain the medium.

On the morning of the examination a normal diet is given. The child is dressed in a buttonless gown and taken to the X-ray department.

Requirements

1. Funnel, tubing, connecting rod and rectal catheter.
2. Barium sulphate mixed with normal saline to prevent water intoxication in cases of megacolon. The mixture should be at a temperature of 37.2°C.
3. Water-repellent sheet.
4. Bedpan and cover, or readily available toilet facilities.

Method
The enema is given under fluoroscopic control and the progress is observed. The barium is syphoned back after X-ray.

After-care of the child

On return to the ward, a bowel action is encouraged. If all the barium is not returned it may form solid lumps which can be extremely difficult to remove. A detergent lubricant such as Dioctylmedo is effective in removing inspissated faeces and barium.

Alternative to barium enema for constipation and faecal soiling

Constipation or faecal soiling may be investigated by barium follow-through examination after adequate purgation. At least 2 days of purgation is required, which is followed by barium sulphate orally in four divided doses, given the next day. X-rays are taken the following morning to show the size of the colon. This method has the advantage that it can be carried out while the child attends as an outpatient.

Rectal lavage

A rectal lavage is given to cleanse the rectum of faeces. It may be necessary prior to surgery on the lower bowel, or examination of the rectum.

Principles involved

1. *Use of an isotonic solution* in the maintenance of a correct water and electrolyte balance. An isotonic solution is one which has the same osmotic pressure as some other solution with which it is compared, e.g. the concentration of salts in the blood serum is 0.9 per cent and a solution of sodium chloride of the same concentration is termed an isotonic solution. Therefore, a solution of normal saline can be safely used without fear of causing fluid or electrolyte imbalance.

In an abnormally dilated colon, such as occurs in Hirschsprung's disease, there is a greater surface area than normal. If a soap and water enema, made with tap water, is given, severe shock may result from 'water intoxication'. This is due to the rapid diffusion of water into the circulation from the dilated bowel. Water intoxication is characterised by listlessness, apathy, fatigue leading to mental confusion, convulsions and coma.

2. *Speed of insertion of fluid*. It should be understood that the greater the height of the column of liquid the greater the pressure and the more rapid the flow of fluid; similarly, the lower the height of the column of liquid the slower the flow of the fluid. When the funnel is lowered to below the level of the anus syphonage will be more effective and a more rapid return of the fluid is achieved. It is essential that the flow and return should be gentle to avoid possible damage to the mucosa of the bowel and to avoid causing discomfort to the child. For an infant, the funnel should be held approximately 25 cm above the buttocks.

3. *Temperature of the fluid*. Care should be taken to ensure that the temperature of the fluid is that of body temperature and should not exceed 37.2°C. Too high a temperature would injure the mucous membrane while a low temperature could produce shock.

Preparation and care of the child

A simple explanation is necessary, giving assurance that the procedure is not painful but may be uncomfortable. Co-operation is essential and the more relaxed the child is the easier the procedure will be. It is absolutely essential that a child who is to have a repeat enema at intervals should not find the first enema traumatic so that he will be able to accept without too much objection any subsequent enema.

Two nurses should be available, one to hold the child and distract his attention with a story or some game, while the other performs the enema. If the child is distressed whether through fear or pain, the lavage should be discontinued and the fact reported.

Requirements

1. Warm normal saline, or other isotonic solution.
2. Lotion thermometer.
3. Conical funnel, length of tubing, connection and catheter of suitable size, e.g. No. 14 FG or No. 8 EG for an infant, up to No. 24 FG or No. 14 EG for a 12-year-old.
4. Swabs.
5. Lubricant, e.g. KY jelly.
6. Water-repellent sheet.
7. Container for returned fluid.
8. Tissue paper.

Method

The apparatus is assembled and the catheter is

lubricated. The child is turned on his side, lying on the water-repellent sheet. He should be covered and kept warm.

The catheter is inserted into the rectum for approximately 9 cm in an older child and about 4 cm in an infant. To note the presence of flatus, the funnel is inverted below the level of water in a basin and bubbles, which may be quite explosive, will be seen if flatus is present. The catheter is then gently inserted further and gradually withdrawn until all flatus is passed. With the catheter in the original position, and the tubing doubled to compress it and prevent any flow, the funnel is filled with fluid and lowered to expel any air. It is then raised to allow the fluid to flow in gently. Whenever the funnel is almost empty, it is lowered nearly to floor level to aid syphonage, but not inverted until all the fluid given is returned. The funnel is then inverted and the fluid emptied into a container. Half to 1 litre may be given, depending on the age and condition of the child. As the catheter is being withdrawn, the funnel is lowered to syphon back any remaining fluid. The equipment should be cleaned or disposed of according to the policy of the hospital.

After-care of the child
The child should be cleaned and left comfortable. Should he desire a bedpan or wish to go to the toilet, he should be given the satisfaction of these facilities, even though this may be considered unnecessary.

Colostomy lavage
The same equipment will be required as for rectal lavage, however, the position the child is placed in varies. The catheter should be inserted into the distal opening of the colostomy. (See Care of the stoma, p. 152).

Colonic lavage
A colonic lavage is usually performed as a preoperative preparation prior to surgery of the colon or for sigmoidoscopy. The preparation of the child and the requirements are the same as for rectal lavage, but a greater quantity of fluid is required.

Method
Commence as for rectal lavage, passing the cath-
eter approximately 20 cm to obtain flatus. A lavage is given, and when the fluid returned is clear, the child is turned on to his back, and the catheter is inserted a further 10 cm. The lavage is repeated until the fluid returned is clear. The child is then turned on to the other side and the process is repeated until the fluid returned is clear. When the catheter is being withdrawn, the funnel is kept low to allow syphonage of the return fluid. If the child is in any way distressed or in pain the procedure is discontinued and the fact reported. The amount of fluid required depends on the condition of the child and the reason for the lavage, but 1 litre is usually adequate.

When a lavage is being given to a child with Hirschsprung's disease, a greater amount of fluid may be required. This is dependent on the severity of the child's condition and the reaction to the procedure. The decision should be made by a trained nurse or by the doctor. It is unlikely that the fluid returned will be clear after the first few lavages, and this, therefore, cannot be the deciding factor. The lavage may have to be performed daily or twice daily for a period of more than a week.

Rectal examination
Rectal examination is commonly a simple digital one which is carried out in the ward or outpatient department. It is an aid to diagnosis and is a routine procedure in a child with abdominal pain. A pelvic cellulitis or a pelvic abscess which has spread from an inflamed appendix, can be felt.

Requirements
1. Disposable gloves or finger cots.
2. Swabs or paper tissues.
3. KY jelly.
4. Water-repellent sheet.
5. Clean napkin for infant.

Method
It is important to gain the child's co-operation by adequate explanations and reassurance. It is not a pleasant examination for the child who will feel embarrassed. However, it is important to ensure the he relaxes sufficiently to make the procedure easier. The older child is usually placed in the left lateral position, while the infant is placed in the dorsal position, both with knees flexed. The water-

repellent sheet or napkin is placed under the buttocks and the nurse supports and reassures the child during the examination.

Rectal biopsy

Examination of the rectal mucosa and submucosa can provide useful diagnostic information. Indications for this examination are: Hirschsprung's disease, ulcerative colitis and Crohn's disease and neural lipidoses.

Preparation of the child

Sedation should be given to all children. Occasionally general anaesthesia may be necessary in young or uncooperative children. If the child is old enough a simple explanation should be given.

Method

A proctosigmoidoscopy is performed with the child lying in the left lateral position. The warmed and lubricated instrument is gently pressed against the anus and passed into the rectum in a sacral direction. Air may be introduced to aid advancement of the instrument but it may cause some discomfort to the child. As the instrument is slowly withdrawn the rectal mucosa are examined. Biopsy can be performed by either grasp or suction.

After-care of the child

The child should be made comfortable and comforted. Observations of complications will be necessary. Although complications are rare, the following should be anticipated: perforation, bleeding and abdominal pain. The first two would be indicated by occult or overt bleeding. Measurements of temperature, pulse and respirations should be made initially hourly and, if stable, 4-hourly. Complaints of pain should be reported to the medical officer.

Colonoscopy

This is a fibreoptic examination of the whole colon performed in suspected inflammatory bowel disease and unexplained rectal bleeding. It is a useful alternative to barium enema. Endoscopic snare polypectomy and electrocoagulation for multiple haemangiomas can be performed during the examination.

Preparation of the child

1. *Bowel preparation.* A clear fluid diet is given consisting of fruit jelly and water ice. This is given from midday on the day preceding the examination. Senna syrup is given during the afternoon of the day prior to the examination. The dose is 20 ml for babies, 30 to 50 ml for 3- to 8-year-old children (this varies according to the size of the child), and approximately 60 ml for older children. Administration of senna syrup can result in several bowel actions in 1 to 6 hours. If there is no result, a phosphate enema is given on the evening preceding the colonoscopy, using hypertonic phosphate enema. Half an enema is given for children up to 2 years old and a whole one for children over 2 years of age.

2. *Sedation.* The procedure is performed while the child is under sedation. The following regimes have been suggested:

a. Chlorpromazine (1.5 mg/kg) intramuscularly 1 hour before the examination.

b. Intravenous slow administration of a combination of diazepam 2.5 to 10 mg and pethidine 10 to 50 mg for children under 8 years of age. If the examination is difficult or prolonged 'top-up' doses are given. Pethidine may cause respiratory depression; therefore naloxone should be available as an antidote.

After-care of the child

Although no complications have so far been reported, the nurse should observe the child carefully for prolonged drowsiness (when naloxone may be given). Observations of vital functions, particularly pulse and respirations, are necessary, initially hourly and, if stable, 4-hourly. The child may be restless and in pain and there may be bleeding from the rectum. Any change observed should be reported to the medical officer.

Chapter 27
Disorders of the genito-urinary system

The genito-urinary system comprises the genital organs and the urinary system, each playing a distinct part in body function.

The male genital organs include the scrotum, testes, penis and associated organs, while the female organs include the vagina, uterus, ovaries and associated structures. They are concerned with reproduction, and though the reproductive process is not developed in the child, it does function in the pubertal period. Abnormalities can occur in both sexes and these can have profound effects on future function of the reproductive organs.

The urinary system comprises the kidneys ureters, urinary bladder and urethra (male and female). The main function of the system is to maintain a balance or constancy in the composition of body fluids. This balance is achieved by the excretion of various metabolised waste products and non-metabolised substances which are in excess of the body's needs. The main regulatory organ in this system is the kidney and any disease involving the kidneys will interfere in some way with the system's ability to maintain fluid constancy. Any part of the urinary system may be affected by disease or malformation which will interfere with the function of the system as a whole.

The male genital organs

Scrotum

This pouch contains the testes with the epididymis and the origin of the vas deferens. The dartos muscle is inserted into the scrotal skin and on contraction causes wrinkling of the skin. The muscle attachment proximally originates in Colles' fascia.

Testes

These are paired structures and form the principal content of the scrotal sac, suspended by the spermatic cord.

Embryologically the testes originate at the level of the 11th and 12th thoracic vertebrae and in their migration to the scrotal sac carry their blood supply, the testicular artery, with them. Histologically, the testes vary with age and three definitive stages can be identified (infant, adult and senile). The testes are arranged into individual lobules, each containing one to three coiled seminiferous tubules which are the site of sperm production. From the site of production the sperm passes from the germinal epithelium through the tubules, ductules and rete testis into the epididymis. From the latter the sperm passes via the vas deferens to ejaculatory ducts.

Epididymis

This is a collecting system which is closely adjacent to the body of the testes. It is wider at its upper end, the globus major, but narrows distally to the globus minor which is continuous with the vas deferens.

Vas deferens

This is a tube which arises at the globus minor of the epididymis and ascends through the scrotum and inguinal canal. Histologically, the vas has a thick layer of smooth muscle.

Penis

This is the male organ of copulation and urinary excretion, comprising a root, body and extremity, or glans penis. The root is attached to the descending portions of the pubic bone by the crura, which are the extremities of the corpora cavernosa. The body consists of two parallel cylindrical bodies, the corpora cavernosa, and beneath them the corpus spongiosum, through which the urethra passes. The glans is covered with mucous membrane and ensheathed by the prepuce, or foreskin.

Disorders of male genitalia
The commonest developmental anomalies in boys include hypospadias, inguinal hernias and hydroceles, undescended testicles and disorders affecting the prepuce and glans penis.

The female genital organs

The ovaries
These are the female gonads in which the ova are formed. They are situated one on each side, in a shallow depression on the lateral wall of the pelvis. They are attached to the posterior layer of the broad ligament of the uterus by a short peritoneal fold called the mesovarium. The ova are developed from cuboidal epithelial cells covering the surface of the ovary. Columns of germinal epithelium penetrate deeply into the connective tissue of the ovary. Primary Graafian follicles are found in great numbers in the fetal ovary and in the ovaries of children. Some of these follicles will mature under the influence of the follicle-stimulating hormone during the time from puberty to the menopause.

The fallopian tubes
These are two slender ducts, one on each side, possessing a trumpet-shaped mouth with a fringed rim (fimbriated extremity). These tubes open medially into the upper part of the uterus. The fimbriated end lies in close proximity to the ovaries and the ovum enters the fallopian tube and is conveyed along the duct by the movement of the cilia in its mucosa as well as by peristaltic movement of its wall.

Uterus
This is a hollow muscular organ in which the fertilised ovum becomes embedded and in which the developing embryo and fetus are nourished. It is a pear-shaped structure, consisting of a body, fundus, isthmus and cervix. Its cavity opens into the vagina below, and into the fallopian tubes on either side above. It is supported by ligaments.

Vagina
This is a curved canal which leads downwards and forwards from the uterus to the external genital organs. The opening of the vagina is partly closed in virgins by a lamina of mucous membrane called the hymen.

The external genital organs
The parts of the external genital organs are together called the vulva and include the mons pubis, labia minora, labia majora, the vestibule and the clitoris. The latter is placed between the anterior ends of the labia minora. It corresponds to the penis in the male and consists of similar tissue.

Disorders of the female genitalia
Developmental anomalies are rare in girls; the commonest abnormality is adhesion between the labia minora. However, there are a variety of disorders occurring during adolescence; some are due to infections, while others are due to menstrual disorders.

Ambiguous sexual development
The infant may be born with indeterminate genitalia. This may be due to aberrations of the chromosomes or the gonads which results in 'intersex' problems. The abnormal appearances may be caused by abnormalities in the production of hormones, leading to adrenogenital syndrome (pseudohermaphroditism, enlargement of the clitoris; isosexual precocity in males with infantile testes; excessive growth; possible electrolyte and water disturbances, particularly in the new-born period).

Where aberration of the number and combination of the sex chromosomes is involved, there is the male and female form. In the female, one sex chromosome is absent (XO), found in Turner's syndrome; there maybe more complex mosaic patterns, e.g. XO/XXX, XO/XXY. In the male, extra chromosomes in excess of the normal number are present, e.g. in Klinefelter's syndrome, in which the chromosomal pattern is 47, XXY or 49, XXXXY.

In any case where doubt exists about the sex of the child, special investigations will be required which involve biochemical studies, chromosomal studies, and laparatomy to inspect the internal genitalia and to obtain biopsy of the gonad for microscopic and other examinations.

Kidney

Structure of the kidney

The interior of the kidney consists of an outer reddish cortex and an inner paler medulla. The inner border of the medulla shows 10 calyces into which project the medullary papillae. The medulla contains 10 to 15 pyramids which terminate in the renal papillae (Fig. 27.1).

The functional unit of the kidney is the nephron (Fig. 27.2). There are about one million of these in each kidney. These nephrons drain into the renal pelvis. Damage or destruction of the nephrons leads to renal failure, that is inability by the kidney to maintain the constancy in the composition of body fluids. The nephron consists of the following parts:

1. *Bowman's capsule* is the dilated part which contains an invaginated tuft of capillary vessels. This tuft is called the *glomerulus* and it lies in the renal cortex. The tuft is clothed in a visceral layer of epithelium which is continous with the parietal layer at the entrance of the afferent and efferent arterioles.

The basement membrane separates the visceral epithelial cells from the capillary cells. The basement membrane is the only intact structure in the filtering surface of the glomerulus. Damage to this membrane is a feature in nephrotic syndrome.

The glomerular capillaries are not simple loops, but are in the form of a freely branching anastomotic network. It is supplied with blood by an afferent arteriole and leaves the tuft by an efferent arteriole. This allows maintenance of a higher pressure than is normally found in other capillaries (70 mmHg). This high capillary pressure is necessary for the filtration function which the glomeruli help to promote.

2. The *proximal convoluted tubule* is continuous with Bowman's capsule and consists of cells with curved and brush borders. This brush border is formed by numerous microvilli which increase the area available for absorption. These proximal tubular cells are responsible for the active transport of some 80 per cent of the *sodium* filtered out of the tubular fluid into the capillary blood.

3. The *loop of Henle* is the descending and ascending limb which is continuous with the terminal part of the proximal tubule.

4. The *distal convoluted tubule*, found near the glomerulus, is continuous with the ascending limb and ends at the nearest bifurcation of the collecting duct.

5. The *collecting tubules* receive the tubular fluid from the distal convoluted tubule and converge into the papillary ducts which lead to the renal pelvis (Fig. 27.2).

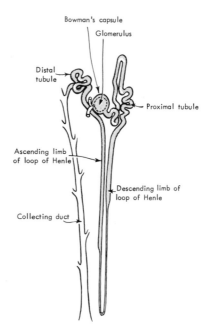

Fig. 27.2 A nephron.

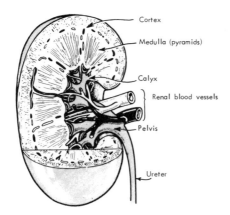

Fig. 27.1 Section through kidney.

The functions of the kidney

Urine is formed by ultrafiltration of plasma in the glomeruli. As the filtrate passes down the nephron, it is modified by the addition and/or removal of various substances. Filtered water and electrolytes are partially reabsorbed from the proximal and distal tubules and from the collecting ducts. Glucose and sodium ions are removed from the proximal tubules and substances such as ammonia, hydrogen ions and potassium ions are secreted into the distal tubules.

The glomerular filtration rate in a healthy adult is about 120 ml/min. Most of the filter is formed by the basement membrane which permits smaller molecules to pass but is impermeable to larger molecules such as those of the plasma proteins.

Reabsorption of about four-fifths of the glomerular filtrate takes place in the proximal tubules. In particular, glucose is completely reabsorbed. Impairment of sodium reabsorption causes increased fluid and electrolyte loss from the body (diuresis). The removal of bicarbonate ions from the proximal tubular fluid depends on the activity of the enzyme carbonic anhydrase.

The loop of Henle is now believed to be concerned with urinary concentration. Fluid leaving the proximal tubule is isotonic. As it passes through the loop of Henle sodium is reabsorbed, causing hypotonicity of the fluid. The concentration of the tubular fluid changes continually due to the constant movement of water and crystalloids between the tubular cells and the surrounding capillary network (Fig. 27.3).

Final adjustment takes place in the distal tubules. This is related to the metabolic needs of the body. The distal parts of the nephron are under hormonal control and adjustment will be according to circumstances. The mechanism involved is as follows. The fluid at the start of the distal tubules is hypotonic with respect to the plasma. The anti-diuretic hormone causes the distal tubular epithelium to allow passage of water and the tubular contents become isotonic with plasma. The action of aldosterone must also be considered in relation to the exchange of sodium and potassium across the tubular endothelium. Excessive aldosterone activity will lead to sodium retention and loss of potassium in the urine. Water is reabsorbed in the collecting tubules as they pass

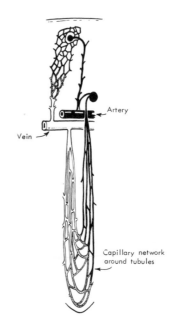

Fig. 27.3 Blood supply of nephron.

through the medulla, making the urine hypertonic.

The distal part of the nephron is also concerned in regulating the acid-base requirements of the body. During metabolism acid substances are produced, the main product being carbon dioxide. Much of this is expelled from the lungs while the remainder is dealt with in the distal part of the nephron. When the kidneys are producing an acid urine, the bicarbonate ions quickly combine with hydrogen ions in the distal tubules. Any hydrogen ions still available are buffered with ammonia and phosphate so that the acidity of the urine remains relatively fixed. The lowest urinary pH is between 4.4 and 4.5; in ordinary circumstances it is between 6 and 6.6.

Concentration and dilution of urine

The importance of the anti-diuretic hormone has been discussed above in relation to the ability of water to pass into the capillaries from the distal tubules. If it is absent, urine is excreted in a diluted, hypotonic form. If it is present, water is extracted, leaving the urine concentrated.

Endocrine function of the kidneys

The kidneys also function as an endocrine organ. They produce the hormone *erythropoietin* and the enzyme *renin*. Erythropoietin is produced by kidney tissue in response to hypoxia and thereby increases the red blood cell count. Renin forms angiotensin, which not only increases precapillary resistance and therefore renal hypertension, but also induces increased aldosterone output which leads to salt and water retention.

Composition of urine

Water (amount varies, see Table 27.1).

Urea, uric acid, total nitrogen, ammonia, chlorides, phosphate, creatinine, 17-ketosteroids.

Specific gravity 1.003 to 1.025.

Reaction — faintly acid (pH 6 to 6.6).

Renal function in the newborn infant

When the infant is born, the kidneys are fully grown with a great number of glomeruli but their function is inadequate. This is related to the glomerular 'pore' size (which is only half that of the adult) and the immaturity of the enzyme system. The newborn infant is also unable to concentrate urine and this is partly due to the shortness of the loop of Henle.

Despite the inadequacy of neonatal renal function, the healthy newborn baby is able to maintain his blood chemistry while receiving a variety of foods, some of which are physiologically unsuited. (See infant feeding, p. 212).

Drug therapy also produces problems. Some drugs may produce toxic effects. For example, phenobarbital is mainly removed from the body by the kidneys, but in the neonatal period this is not efficiently achieved and the infant becomes lethargic and even comatose. Daily dosage of antibiotics must be carefully controlled since the kidneys excrete these by glomerular filtration, and excessive dosage leads to injury to the glomeruli.

Since not all glomeruli are functioning at birth, the filtration rate will be less than the rate for the older infants, and this is achieved by the 6th week of life. Table 27.1 gives approximate amounts of urine passed in 24 hours.

Disorders of the kidney may affect any part of the nephron, for example, (a) glomerular failure due to damage to the membranes allows large quantities of plasma protein to escape with the filtrate, and (b) tubular involvement which interferes with transport of one or more substances such as glucose or amino-acids.

Although urine is formed there may be interference with its passage to the exterior. This involves other structures which are part of the urinary system.

Ureters

The ureters are two muscular tubes each leaving one kidney to enter the bladder obliquely. The upper part of the ureter is expanded. Being a muscular organ it is capable of peristaltic waves which descend the walls of the ureter at regular intervals and carry the urine into the bladder. Obstruction of the ureter will interfere with the passage of urine to the bladder. There may also be abnormalities affecting one or both ureters.

Bladder (Fig. 27.4)

The bladder is the receptacle and reservoir for the urine. It lies in the pelvis, but when full it rises into the abdominal cavity. Its muscular coat, known as the detrusor muscle, consists of three

Table 27.1

Age	Amount (ml)
1–2 days	30–60
4–5 days	70–250
6–10 days	200–300
10 days–2 months	250–450
2 months–1 year	400–500
1–2 years	500–700
3–5 years	600–1200
6–8 years	700–1300
8–14 years	800–1500

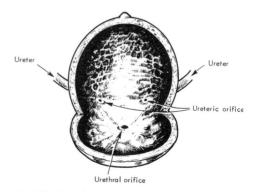

Fig. 27.4 Bladder, showing ureteric and urethral orifices.

layers. The bladder also contains a mucous and a submucous coat. Three orifices are present, two ureteric and one urethric. The muscle fibres at the neck of the bladder are thickened and constitute the internal sphincter which extends beyond the bladder to surround the commencement of the urethra.

Urethra

The urethra is a tube leading from the bladder to the exterior and its length varies with the age and sex of the child. The adult male urethra is about 18 cm long and in the adult female it is about 5 cm long. In the male, the first part of the urethra is surrounded by the prostate. The part below the prostate is the membranous urethra which is surrounded by a mass of erectile tissue. A band of circular muscle fibres surrounds the membranous urethra and constitutes the external sphincter.

Micturition

Micturition or emptying the bladder is a reflex event which involves the sacral spinal cord and the parasympathetic nerves as well as sympathetic nerves. The efferent fibres to the bladder come from both autonomic systems. Sympathetic stimulation causes the bladder to relax and the sphincter to contract. The ureteric orifice closes, the internal sphincter contracts, there is increase in the tone of the trigone and there is vasoconstriction.

The effects of parasympathetic stimulation are the relaxation of the internal sphincter, stimulation of the detrusor and emptying of the bladder.

As the bladder fills, its internal pressure slowly rises. The increased pressure leads to increased activity of the stretch receptors and causes reflex contractions of the detrusor muscle, which produces an awareness of the need to micturate. Response to this from the higher centres leads to reflex contraction of the detrusor and relaxation of the sphincters, resulting in micturition.

Interference with this mechanism leads to a variety of effects, for example retention of urine, pain and incontinence.

Disorders of the kidneys and the urinary tract

Kidney and urinary tract disorders are relatively frequent in childhood. They may be due to obstructive or non-obstructive congenital malformation of the tract and/or acquired diseases or tumours affecting any part of the system. Disorders involve renal function (kidney) and the structures associated with storage and elimination of urine (ureters, bladder and urethra).

The manifestations of renal disease vary with the age of the child. However, in all age groups major symptoms include the following:

Poor feeding (neonate, infant and young child) and anorexia in other age groups.

Vomiting — occurs in all groups.

Failure to gain weight — a feature in infants, while growth is affected in older children.

Difficulty in micturition and painful micturition with frequency will be found in all age groups.

DISTURBANCES OF MICTURITION

Disturbance may be due to the following: meatal ulceration, prepuce infection (in boys) and vaginitis (in girls). There may also be obstruction to the outflow of urine as in urethral stenosis. Observation of the act of micturition would help to establish the cause. For example, obvious discomfort (indicated by crying) during the act and a full bladder, despite passing some urine, would indicate some obstruction.

Incontinence

Bladder control during the day is usually established between the ages of 2 and 3 and at night between the third and fourth year. Occasional 'accidents' may, however, still occur, particularly when the child is preoccupied or excited. When 'wetting' persists either during the day or night after achieving bladder control, then the urine should be examined for decreased specific gravity, infection, glucose and evidence of renal disease. (See p. 562 for urine testing.) Enuresis is the term used to describe the state of uncontrolled 'wetting'.

The causes may be late maturation, a psychological disturbance such as anxiety, or local inflammation. A rare type of incontinence is found in girls, and is due to an ectopic ureter opening into the vagina or into the urethra below the external sphincter. These children show a normal voiding pattern, since one ureter empties into the bladder normally, but in addition, they have constant dribbling incontinence.

Principles of treatment and nursing management

1. Treatment, which depends on the condition is as follows:
   a. Surgical correction, e.g. for ectopic ureter.
   b. Chemotherapy for infection.
   c. Psychotherapy for the disturbed child.
2. Nursing management:
   Day care. Frequent toileting until a pattern has been established.
   Nocturnal enuresis
   a. No fluids are given before the child goes to bed. Some authorities do not believe in fluid restriction.
   b. The child is wakened during the night and toileted.
   c. Use of the incontinence pad for the older child. This incontinence pad consists of an electric device which buzzes as soon as moisture is in contact with the sensitive mechanism. The child wakens up and goes to the toilet. This method is not recommended for disturbed children.
   d. *Psychological aspect*. It is important not to make the child feel guilty or anxious about 'wetting'. He tries hard to control it and any failure only increases his anxiety. A dry bed should be recognised and rewarded; a wet bed or pants should not be punished as this only increases the feeling of indignity and anxiety. It has also been found that some cases respond favourably to hypnosis. This form of treatment is useful for children about 8 years of age. Others have been given diazepam because it is believed to be effective by reducing voluntary muscle activity at the level of the external sphincter.
3. Support and guidance for parents. The level of support will depend on the cause and the type of treatment. Where no cause can be elicited and the treatment is unsuccessful, the parents will need a great deal of help in handling their child. This is particularly important when the parents have tried hard to solve this problem. In many cases their efforts result in excessive punishment for the child, increasing the

tensions and anxiety for him and between himself and his parents.

Neurogenic incontinence

Incontinence here is due to damage of the nervous system and is found in children with spinal injury and congenital malformations such as myelomeningocele. The bladder is palpable and there is constant dribbling of urine. The type of bladder dysfunction varies depending on involvement of (1) upper motor neuron, when the sphincter is in spasm, i.e. spastic bladder, and automatic or reflex emptying develops in the child; (2) lower motor neurone, when there is constant dribbling of urine from a partially full bladder, i.e. flaccid bladder and urine can be easily expressed through the relaxed sphincter by suprapubic pressure.

Dysuria

The term means difficulty or pain on micturition. The most common cause is ammonia dermatitis leading to meatal erosion in boys and ammonia burns of the vulva in girls. Pain on micturition often leads to urinary retention as the child will tolerate a distended bladder rather than suffer the pain of passing urine.

Retention

Urine is retained in the bladder. This can be due to pain on micturition or spasm caused by local irritation of the urethra or bladder. It may also be due to mechanical obstruction caused by a small stone or crystal in the urethra.

In the chronic state, there may be dribbling overflow due to partial urethral obstruction. The cause may be a disorder of the urethral valves, congenital bladder neck obstruction or urethral stricture.

Pyuria

Pyuria is common in children with dilatation of parts of the urinary tract. It is more common in females where the short urethra allows infection to spread upwards.

Haematuria

Blood in the urine may be due to injury to the urinary tract. In little boys, bleeding from a meatal ulcer is the most common cause. Haematuria is a feature in nephritic syndrome, when it is associated with much lysis of red cells, while red cells are usually intact in nephrotic syndrome. Other causes include: neoplasm (Wilm's tumour); schistosomiasis (infection with flukes); tuberculosis; thrombocytopaenic purpura; drugs, i.e. streptomycin, suphamerazine, cyclophosphamide, and marrow depressants.

Proteinuria

In general, proteins with a molecular weight greater than 70 000 are not filtered and normal urine contains very small quantities of protein, which arise mainly from the plasma proteins. In children under 6 years of age, proteinuria generally reflects anatomic abnormalities.

Proteinuria may be classifed as pre-renal, renal and post-renal. *Pre-renal* proteinuria is caused by a general disease which affects the kidneys, and is an indication of renal damage due to a variety of conditions, e.g. heart failure, pyrexia and orthostatic albuminuria.

Proteinuria of *renal* origin is associated with disease of the kidneys. In different types of renal disease different degrees of proteinuria are seen. In glomerulonephritis the proteinuria is caused by leakage through the damaged glomeruli. In nephrotic syndrome there is excessive glomerular filtration and in severe cases secondary tubular damage may reduce reabsorption of protein. Excessive albumin catabolism has also been suggested as the cause of proteinuria in nephrotic syndrome.

Post-renal proteinuria is found in severe infection of the lower urinary tract, or associated with haematuria when the renal pelvis or the ureter is irritated by a stone or when there is local malignant disease.

CONGENITAL DISORDERS OF THE KIDNEY

Anomalies of the kidneys include bilateral or unilateral renal agenesis (absence of two kidneys or of one kidney). The former is incompatible with life, while the latter is usually asymptomatic. Most individuals having only one kidney have a normal life expectancy, however, there are increased hazards, such as trauma, obstruction and stone formation.

Anomalies also include that of volume and structure. The aplastic kidney shows minimal nephron formation and there may also be maldevelopment of normal renal structure. In infancy and childhood the kidneys may also be cystic when the kidneys are large and there is obstruction to urine formation and flow, leading to hydronephrosis. Some children may survive the first year of life gradually developing renal insufficiency.

Ectopic kidney

One or both kidneys may fail to ascend from the pelvis or both kidneys may lie on the same side. This condition is associated with obstruction, infection and stone formation. Treatment will be symptomatic and where necessary may include removal of the abnormal kidney (provided the other one is functioning normally).

ACQUIRED DISORDERS OF THE KIDNEY AND URINARY TRACT

Urinary tract infection

Urinary tract infection is a common condition in infancy and childhood and has a tendency to recur. It can range from asymptomatic bacteriuria to severe symptomatic pyelonephritis. Approximately 1 per cent of newborn babies develop urinary tract infection and males are as likely to develop infection as females. After the newborn period, urinary tract infection is uncommon in males until later adult life. The relatively high incidence of urinary tract infection in pre-school girls is due to excessive perineal faecal contamination, the short urethra, and infrequent and inadequate voiding. Infection in sexually active girls may be due to bacterial contamination of the bladder secondary to urethral trauma during intercourse.

Pathogenesis

The commonest urinary pathogen is *Escherichia coli*, and others include *Klebsiella* species, enterococci and micrococci — all members of the normal rectal and perineal bacterial flora.

Access of bacteria to the normally sterile bladder and kidneys appears to be retrourethral, although in the newborn infant the spread can be haematogenous. Entrance of bacteria is enhanced by poor perineal hygiene, the short female urethra, or urethral instrumentation. Once bacteria are in the bladder, the urine serves as an excellent culture medium, but infection is usually prevented by the washout effect of voiding. Natural host defences also prevent active multiplication of bacteria in the bladder, but if these break down then urinary tract infection will occur. Vesicoureteral reflux, often seen in young children with urinary tract infection, can allow bacteria to gain entry to the kidneys, with resulting pyelonephritis and renal damage.

Clinical features

Newborns may present with pyrexia, hypothermia, poor feeding, jaundice and evidence of failure to thrive.

Infants may have pyrexia, irritability, poor feeding and strong-smelling urine. Pre-school children may have abdominal pain, vomiting, pyrexia, enuresis, strong-smelling urine, dysuria or urgency.

School-age children have pyrexia, enuresis, increased frequency of micturition and pain in the flank region (below the ribs and above the ilium). Occasionally, children with bacterial urinary tract infection will present with haemorrhagic cystitis.

Investigations

1. Clean-catch mid-stream specimen of urine (p. 548).
2. Suprapubic aspiration of urine (p. 552).
3. Catheter-obtained urine — provided the first few millilitres of urine are excluded from the collection.

Principles of treatment and nursing management

1. Drug therapy will depend on drug sensitivities. A variety of antibacterial agents can be used, e.g. co-trimoxazole (a mixture of sulphamethoxazole and trimethoprim), nitrofurantoin and nalidixic acid.
2. Urine culture 2 or 3 and 10 days after the start of the treatment.
3. High fluid intake to dilute the urinary bacterial count, stimulate frequent voiding and ease dysuria.
4. If the child is seriously ill, intravenous infusion may be required and the drug given by this route.
5. Routine nursing care.

6. Observations of complications, e.g. urinary output should be monitored and signs of renal failure identified.
7. Following treatment further investigations may be required, e.g. intravenous pyelogram, micturating cystourethrogram and ultrasound.
8. Support for parents. The condition must be explained to the parents and they should be allowed to participate in the care of the child. Since enuresis is a feature of the condition, they will require reassurance and guidance in the management of the child (p. 528).

Pyelonephritis

Pyelonephritis is an infection of the renal pelvis and renal parenchyma. The infection occurs more frequently in young children (2 months to 2 years). It is caused by a variety of organisms entering via the urethra, the blood stream or lymphatics. Congenital abnormalities are important predisposing factors. The condition may be acute or chronic.

Pathophysiology

Inflammation extends throughout the cortex and medulla and several areas may be involved. The renal pelvis is congested, thickened and acutely inflamed. The tubules are primarily involved and the glomeruli are also damaged.

Clinical features

The onset may be sudden or gradual. There is either moderate or high fever (40 °C); convulsions may occur in infants and gastro-intestinal symptoms, such as anorexia, vomiting and diarrhoea, are present. There is urinary frequency and dysuria. There may be tenderness in the kidney area and in some cases there may also be oedema.

Investigations

1. Examination of urine for bacterial content:
   a. Mid-stream specimen of urine (p. 548).
   b. Bladder puncture (p. 552).
   c. Catheterisation (p. 549).
2. Examination of urine for casts, blood and protein.
3. Renal function tests (p. 556).
4. Radiographic studies, e.g. voiding, cystourethrography (p. 553).

Principles of treatment and nursing management
The aims of treatment are to clear up the primary infection and to correct surgically any congenital or acquired structural defect.

1. *Care of the young infant.* He is often acutely ill and treatment involves correction of fluid and electrolyte imbalance; modification of antibiotic dosage to prevent cumulative toxicity; correction of anomaly by surgical means.
2. *Care of the older child*:
   a. Bed-rest, particularly during the febrile period, especially if vomiting persists.
   b. Tepid sponging, if fever is high (p. 92).
   c. Encouragement of fluid intake. Small amounts should be given frequently to prevent dehydration. It is important that a fluid intake and output chart should be maintained.
   d. Antibacterial treatment. This depends on the sensitivity of the causative organisms. These include sulphonamides, e.g. sulphadimidine (extra fluid intake is essential to prevent crystal formation in the kidneys) and antibiotics, e.g. tetracycline and chloramphenicol.
   e. Urinary antiseptics. These are only used if there is infection of the urinary tract. Nitrofurantoin is useful for long-term treatment.
   f. Correction of anaemia.
3. Routine nursing care:
   a. Observations of urinary function.
   b. Urine collection and testing.
   c. Daily weighing of infants.
   d. Bathing, feeding.
4. Support for parents. If the child has some abnormality this will increase their anxiety. The level of support must be measured against the degree of involvement. The parents must be kept fully informed of the treatment and response to it and where possible, they should be encouraged to participate in the care of their child.

Glomerulonephritis
The renal glomeruli are damaged in a wide variety of diseases, but the damage may also be due to disease where the primary site are the glomeruli.

The cause is often unknown, but it is believed to be due to antigen-antibody reactions to specific bacterium which are responsible for the damage. The organism responsible is usually the beta-haemolytic streptococcus group A, but other organisms such as the pneumococcus can also play a part, often in association with other conditions. Viruses have recently also been considered a causative agent. The damage to the glomeruli occurs due to hypersensitivity reaction in the kidney which produces changes. These changes have been broadly classified as membranous and proliferative (the former shows thickened capillary walls, the latter obliterated capillaries). They may also be *diffuse*, affecting all glomeruli equally, *focal*, affecting some glomeruli, or *segmental*, affecting some parts of individual glomeruli more than other parts.

Acute glomerulonephritis
This is the most common form in childhood where the specific cause is streptococcal infection. Kidney involvement usually follows a streptococcal throat infection.

Pathophysiology
The principal change is a decrease in glomerular filtration rate without a disproportional decrease in renal blood flow, resulting in a reduced urinary output. Tubular function is generally less severely impaired.

Clinical features

1. The intensity of the disease varies, but most children are not markedly ill. The child, usually of school age, develops haematuria after recovering from tonsillitis, scarlet fever or other infection. He complains of headache and may vomit. Urinary output decreases and there is mild oedema, usually in the face. Hypertension is present and is of moderate severity. There is also moderate increase in temperature.
2. Some children show other features in addition to the above. For example, there may also be signs of cardiac involvement. The heart is enlarged and there is shortness of breath. There are electrocardiographic changes and signs of pulmonary oedema. Other children may show signs of involvement of the central nervous

system, for example there may be restlessness, stupor, convulsions, vomiting and visual disturbances and headaches may be severe. This is termed hypertensive encephalopathy and is due to constriction of the arterioles which is associated with generalised vasospasm.

Investigations

1. Urinalysis:
   a. For protein.
   b. For red blood cells.
2. Blood analysis. Increased blood urea nitrogen (BUN) and creatinine.
3. Erythrocyte sedimentation rate (ESR). This is usually raised (p. 463).
4. Antistreptolysin O titre (ASO). This is raised when a throat infection has been present. The antibody, antistreptolysin O appears in the serum about 10 days after the initial infection and persists for 4 to 6 weeks.
5. Throat swab to isolate the haemolytic streptococcus.
6. Intravenous pyelography during the early phase of the disease may demonstrate an enlarged kidney (p. 554).
7. Electrocardiogram.
8. Renal biopsy. This may be helpful if the clinical course is atypical (p. 555).

Principles of treatment and nursing management
Children suffering from acute glomerular nephritis who have a normal blood pressure and a reasonable urinary output can be treated at home. Those with signs of hypertension, oedema or oliguria should be hospitalised.

1. Bed-rest is necessary for children with hypertension and oedema and particularly for those with signs of encephalopathy and cardiac failure. Mild cases with normal blood pressure and little oedema can be allowed limited activity but should not attend school.
2. Fluids. The intake of fluids is usually restricted if the urine output is low. In some units it is limited to between 900 and 1200 ml per day. Half of the fluid intake may be milk and the other half water. Real fruit juices should be avoided since they have a high potassium content. This is important where the urinary

output is less than 200 to 300 ml daily — because of the danger of potassium retention.
3. Diet. When diuresis has occurred, and hypertension has subsided, foods such as bread, cereals, fruits, potatoes and vegetables can be given. Salt is restricted until hypertension and oedema have decreased. Protein is restricted when the blood urea nitrogen is raised and while haematuria is present. When the haematuria is microscopic, protein intake can be restarted or increased.
4. Drugs. Penicillin is the effective drug for eliminating streptococcal infection (oral or intramuscular).
5. Daily urine tests for:
   a. Blood.
   b. Protein (qualitative and quantitative) (p. 564).
6. Daily weighing as an indication of increase/decrease of oedema.
7. Recording of blood pressure (p. 460).
8. Routine nursing care.
9. Support for parents. This includes recognition of their anxiety and relieving that anxiety by giving adequate information about the condition and the progress the child is making. They will want information about the degree of renal involvement and the prospects for the future. Guidance should be given regarding convalescence, follow-up and prevention of streptococcal infection.

Nephrotic syndrome
The nephrotic syndrome is a clinical and biochemical state involving increased permeability of the glomeruli. It can occur in association with a variety of renal diseases. Characteristic signs of the disease include oedema (Fig. 27.5), proteinuria, hypoalbuminaemia and hyperlipidaemia.

The cause of the proteinuria is the increased permeability of the glomerular filter to large molecules such as protein. Most of the protein lost is albumin and this leads to hypoalbuminaemia. The effect of this protein loss in plasma is to reduce the osmotic pressure (oncotic pressure) of the plasma proteins, leading to oedema. Plasma volume may also be decreased, but a compensatory mechanism prevents this. One of the mechanisms

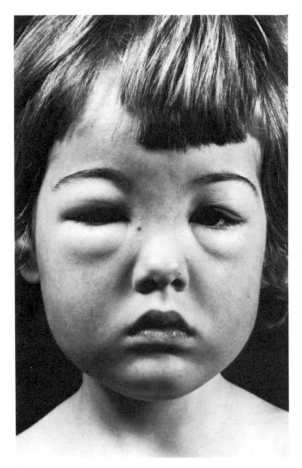

Fig. 27.5 Nephrotic oedema.

involved is the action of aldosterone and anti-diuretic hormone, which together lead to retention of salt and water by the kidney.

When hypovolaemia occurs due to loss of fluid from the intravascular compartment, there will be a rise in haemoglobin concentration and packed cell volume. If the compensatory mechanism is not effective, the hypovolaemia may progress to peripheral circulatory collapse and death. Haemo-concentration causes hyperviscosity which is a major factor in the venous thromboses which sometimes complicate the nephrotic syndrome.

Idiopathic nephrotic syndrome

The cause of this condition is not clearly under-stood, but it is believed to be the result of an immunological reaction.

Renal biopsy studies have shown glomerular changes which have been related to the various stages in this disease. These are similar to those described in glomerulonephritis (p. 532).

Clinical features

Nephrosis usually affects a young age group, the majority of cases occurring in pre-school children. Boys are more frequently affected than girls.

Oedema is one of the first symptoms, affecting the face, legs and abdomen. Swelling of the eyelids is apparent when the child wakens in the morning; this disappears during the course of the day. As the disease progresses, the swelling increases with the appearance of gross ascites.

Urinary output decreases, the child is anorexic and irritable. There is gross proteinuria and, initially, the blood pressure is normal. When glomerular failure occurs, hypertension will be present and in the terminal stages haematuria. When haematuria occurs early in the disease, the prognosis is poor. Spontaneous remission of the disease sometimes occurs.

Investigations

1. Blood analysis which indicates:
   a. Gross reduction in total serum protein to 3 to 5 g/100 ml (normal 6.5 to 8 g/100 ml).
   b. Reduction in serum albumin to about 1.2 to 2 g/100 ml.
   c. Generally normal blood urea nitrogen (BUN) and creatinine.
2. Erythrocytes sedimentation rate (ESR) which is raised during the active phase of the disease.
3. Antistreptolysin O (ASO) titre: usually normal.
4. Renal biopsy.

Principles of treatment and nursing management

1. Bed-rest is necessary during periods of severe incapacitating oedema and during intercurrent infections. It is also advisable to maintain bed-rest during diuresis when there is rapid weight loss.
2. Diet. In some units the fluid intake is reduced to 900 to 1200 ml/d and the sodium intake is limited to 2 g/d. Once diuresis has occurred and the oedema has disappeared, these restric-tions can be eased. A generous protein intake is desirable in order to minimise the persist-

ently negative nitrogen balance and tissue wastage which results from the loss of protein. The diet should contain 2 to 3 g of protein/kg of body weight/d. The anorexic child will require gentle coaxing and persuasion to ensure an adequate food intake.

3. Skin care. Massive oedema presents problems in skin care. Trauma to the skin by the frequent application of urine bags, adhesive tape or bandages must be reduced to a minimum. Urine bags and adhesive tape must be removed gently, using a solvent rather than peeling them off. The napkin area should be kept clean and dry and the scrotum should be supported with a non-constricting pad. Rubbing of the skin should be avoided, but frequent changes of position or use of a ripple bed should be considered.

4. Eye care. It is not unusual for the child's eye to be closed due to oedema of the lids and to prevent sticky eyelids, they should be swabbed with warm water (p. 114).

5. Chemotherapy:
   a. Prednisolone is widely used. It is a cortico-steroid preparation which has minimal side-effects. The doses are reduced every 10 days until the maintenance dose of 5 mg is given twice daily. Diuresis generally occurs rapidly and the drug is discontinued after 6 to 10 weeks. If the drug is continued or prolonged, side-effects can occur which include arrest of growth, osteoporosis, peptic ulcer, diabetes mellitus, convulsions and hypertension.
   b. Steroid-resistant cases can be treated with diuretics to remove the excess fluid, e.g. spironolactone and cytotoxic (immunosuppressive) drugs. The choice of these drugs is based on the presumed immunological nature of the disease. It includes drugs like 6-mercaptopurine and cyclophosphamide.

6. Management of hypovolaemic crises. The child will complain of abdominal pain and there may be vomiting and faintness. The treatment is by giving an intravenous infusion of plasma. Monitoring of pulse and blood pressure is important.

7. Prevention of infection. The nephrotic child is prone to infection by pneumococcus, though viral infections are also troublesome in children on steroids or cyclophosphamide.

8. Routine nursing care.

9. Specific nursing care:
   a. Maintenance of accurate fluid chart.
   b. Daily weighing.
   c. Recording of blood pressure (p. 460).
   d. Prevention of pressure sores (p. 94).

10. Support for parents and child. Both parents and child are often embarrassed about the appearance of the child. Understanding of these feelings is essential. The disease imposes a severe strain on the family with its periods of remissions, exacerbations and periodic admissions to hospital. The condition must be explained to the parents so that they understand the course the disease takes. It can be depressing and frustrating for them to experience the relapses necessitating hospitalisation.

11. Management of renal failure. (p. 536).

Acute renal failure

Acute renal failure exists when kidney functions become suddenly and severely impaired, leading to a reduction in urine formation. This failure of renal function may be due to pre-renal causes, e.g. hypovolaemia and diarrhoea and vomiting; renal causes, e.g. haemolytic uraemic syndrome, acute glomerulo-nephritis; or post-renal causes, when there is obstruction to the excretion of urine. Renal failure can occur when the following patho-physiological states exist:

1. There is a reduction of blood flow to the kidneys, i.e. impaired renal perfusion as in gastroenteritis, burns, haemorrhage or shock. The kidneys themselves are not damaged initially but may become so, if the primary condition persists. Dehydration from vomiting and diarrhoea is the most common cause. The blood urea level is raised.

2. There is obstruction to the outflow of urine from the kidney or collecting systems, i.e. obstruction in the lower urinary tract by stones or crystals. The extent of involvement depends on whether one or both kidneys are involved. Complete obstruction to the outflow results in cessation of glomerular filtration, partly because the pressure in Bowman's capsule rises to equal that in the glomerular capillaries and

partly because blood is shunted away from the glomeruli.

3. When the renal tissue is ischaemic due to disease or injury to the kidney itself, affecting both glomeruli and tubules. This occurs as a result of hypoxia particularly in the neonatal period.

Clinical features

The infant or child is extremely ill. Very little urine is passed (it may be as little as 50 ml in 24 hours). Nausea, vomiting and drowsiness develop. Other features presented are those of the underlying disease.

These features are due to the following events:

1. There is retention of urea and phosphate. The latter results in a fall of ionised calcium in the blood and this will lead to tetany (pedocarpal spasms). There is an increase in plasma potassium level which can lead to cardiac arrest (p. 121).
2. Water and electrolyte disturbances.
3. Metabolic acidosis due to retention of acid residues and the failure of the kidneys to manufacture bicarbonate. Severe acidosis is indicated by hyperventilation and loss of consciousness.
4. Development of anaemia. There is a decrease in haemoglobin concentration and lack of erythropoietin.

Principles of treatment and nursing management

1. Routine nursing care. Incubator care for the neonate (p. 113).
2. Intravenous infusion to replace extracellular fluid loss. Care of the child receiving an intravenous infusion (p. 448).
3. Maintenance of accurate fluid intake and output chart.
4. Daily weighing. This should be done at the same time each day.
5. Introduction of a urinary catheter and careful monitoring of all urinary output, or application of a urine bag to collect any urine passed. If the renal failure is due to burns, a bacteriostatic agent can be introduced into the bladder and kept there for half an hour and then allowed to drain.

6. Adequate calorie intake. This can be supplied intravenously as glucose solution. When a high concentration of glucose is given it is important to observe any signs of venous thrombosis.
7. Drugs. Recognition of the problems of drugs in renal failure and careful observations of side-effects.
8. Monitoring of cardiac activity. Hyperkalaemia (increased potassium level in the blood) leads to arrhythmias and cardiac arrest. Resuscitation equipment should be available (p. 118). Blood pressure should be monitored (p. 460).
9. Administration of oxygen (p. 382).
10. Care of the child on peritoneal or haemodialysis (pp. 559–561).
11. Renal transplantation in suitable cases.
12. Support for parents. Recognition of their anxiety and the need to keep them informed about the condition of their child. Provisions should be made so that they can be near their child and, if possible, participate in the care of the child.

Chronic renal failure

In acute renal failure, the nephrons are damaged, often reversibly; in the chronic form, the nephrons are progressively destroyed, leading to gradually increasing uraemia. Chronic renal failure can be due to (1) chronic pyelonephritis and glomerulonephritis of various types and (2) renal dysplasias and cystic disease of the kidney and others.

Pathophysiology

The kidney has a remarkable ability to compensate for the persistent loss of nephrons that occurs in chronic renal failure. When the glomerular filtration rate has dropped to 5 to 20 ml/min/1.73 m^2, this capacity begins to fail. This results in a variety of biochemical problems related to the major substances handled by the kidney.

Water. Defects in concentrating urine appear early in most chronic renal diseases. Polyuria is present with a urine of low specific gravity. This leads to increased water intake to meet the demands of this situation. In later stages, the ability to dilute urine may be lost, and a urine of fixed specific gravity close to that of plasma will be excreted.

Nitrogenous products. Blood urea nitrogen and serum creatinine and uric acid levels rise as the glomerular filtration rate falls.

Hydrogen ions. In chronic renal failure the ability of the kidneys to excrete hydrogen ions is considerably reduced; they therefore accumulate in the plasma, causing metabolic acidosis. *Acid-base balance* is therefore affected. There is decreased ammonia production and retention of endogenous acid.

Electrolyte imbalance. Sodium loss is increased by osmotic diuresis and by decreased capacity of the tubules to secrete hydrogen ions in exchange for sodium. Potassium retention leading to hyperkalaemia is a late problem in chronic renal failure, occurring in the oliguric phase.

Calcium. There is often defective absorption of calcium from the gut, and the rate of urinary calcium excretion may be considerably below normal. There is also resistance to the action of vitamin D, leading to renal osteodystrophy.

Clinical features

Chronic renal failure involves nearly every body system. Anaemia is usually present. It is usually normochromic and normocytic and results from decreased production secondary to diminished renal erythropoietin synthesis. Blood loss, haemolysis and nutritional deficiencies also play a part. Platelet dysfunction and other abnormalities of the coagulation system are also frequently present. Gastro-intestinal haemorrhage with haematemesis/melaena may be a problem. The central nervous system is also affected. The child may be apathetic, lethargic and confused. With advancing uraemia, the child will become comatosed.

Cardiovascular manifestations will be seen. There may be pericarditis, congestive cardiac failure and hypertension. The hypertension may relate to volume overload or to excessive renin secretion.

Nutritional deficiencies associated with anorexia can lead to impaired growth and development. The child also tends to be prone to infections and because of his debilitated state is not able to combat them.

Principles of treatment and nursing management

The aim is to improve renal function and remove the products of the patient's metabolism. This can be achieved by intermittent haemodialysis and by renal transplantation.

1. The general measures adopted will depend on the glomerular filtration rate. If this is reasonably good then dietary restrictions should not be necessary. As the rate decreases other measures such as haemodialysis will be necessary (p. 561).
2. Monitoring blood pressure (p. 460).
3. Control of infection. Antibiotics are usually given with the dose adjusted to prevent toxic effects.
4. Routine nursing management (p. 113).
5. Psychological support. As with most chronic diseases it is important that the child and his family are helped to adjust to the disease. This involves a team approach and should include not only the physician treating the child but also psychiatrists, dietician, play leader, teacher and of course nurses, all in close co-operation with the parents.

Hypertension

Hypertension in children is most commonly of renal origin, but can also be due to cardiovascular, endocrine or neurological disorders.

Pathophysiology

It is now believed that hypertension is a disorder characterised by a multifactorial derangement of regulation. It may be due to retention of salt and water. This retention may be due to excess mineralocorticoid activity or to an inability to excrete dietary sodium. It leads to increased total extracellular fluid volume and an increased cardiac output. It may also be due to overactivity of the renin-angiotensin system, which results in vasoconstriction and sodium retention. An additional factor responsible for hypertension may be the composition of the arteriolar wall. Changes occurring in these vessels include thickening of the wall and narrowing of the vessel lumen. This leads to increase of peripheral resistance resulting in increase in blood pressure.

Essential hypertension can also be found in children. The cause is not known, although it is suggested that there are genetic determinants of the tendency towards hypertension. It is important that blood pressure measurements should be taken at routine medical examinations to identify hypertension and give the appropriate treatment. Whatever the primary cause of the hypertensive state, it appears that a vicious circle sooner or later develops, in which the primary hypertension produces renal damage which in turn exacerbates the hypertension.

Diagnosis of hypertension

Accurate blood pressure measurements are important. The diagnosis is confirmed if several measurements indicate a diastolic pressure two standard deviations above the mean (Table 24.2). Blood pressure should also be monitored at home, where the child will probably be more relaxed. For the method of measuring blood pressure see page 460.

Clinical features

Milder forms of hypertension tend to be symptomless. More severe forms give rise to headache, dizziness or true vertigo. A severe form of hypertension gives rise to serious complications involving the central nervous system, when papilloedema or seizures occur. This is known as hypertensive encephalopathy. Retinal haemorrhages may also occur.

Principles of treatment and nursing management

The aim of treatment is to decrease blood pressure to near normal levels and to prevent hypotension.

1. Accurate measurement of blood pressure either by the Doppler method (using a small electronic transmitting and receiving transducer) or by using a sphygmomanometer (p. 460).
2. Medication. Vasodilating drugs such as hydralazine and diazoxide. Both drugs cause a fall in blood pressure and this may be very rapid. Diazoxide can cause occipital blindness and hyperglycaemia. In severe hypertensive crisis sodium nitroprusside may be given. It is a potent vasodilator.
3. Maintain the child in the recumbent position and monitor blood pressure every 5 to 15 minutes until it stabilises. Thereafter blood pressure should be monitored hourly.
4. Maintain an accurate fluid chart because urinary output may decrease and oedema develop secondary to sodium and water retention caused by the above drugs.
5. Observation of child and recognition of complications.
6. Provide adequate nutrition. The type of diet will depend on the underlying condition.
7. Provide routine nursing care.
8. Support for parents. The child will be acutely ill and both he and his parents will require comfort and reassurance. The condition should be explained and the parents encouraged to participate in the care of the child. If treatment has to be continued at home, explain to the parents and the child (if old enough) about any side-effects.

Tumours of the kidney

The most common malignant tumours in young children are Wilm's tumour (embryoma of the kidney) and neuroblastoma. Wilm's tumour, also known as nephroblastoma, is a tumour of embryonic origin. It spreads rapidly into renal substance, becoming adherent to adjacent structures such as the colon, the spleen or pancreas. The danger is that it may spread to the renal vein and involve other structures via the bloodstream. The tumour is most commonly seen in the first year of life.

Clinical features

An abdominal mass which is hard and heavy, is usually first noticed by the parents. Abdominal pain may be present and some cases may have haematuria. This may be due to ulceration of the tumour or to thrombosis and rupture of obstructed veins in the renal sinus. There may also be a mild fever.

Investigations

1. Intravenous pyelogram will demonstrate radiologically the presence of the tumour and confirm the presence of a second kidney (p. 554).
2. Lung fields are X-rayed to exclude secondaries.

Principles of treatment and nursing management

1. Pre-operative preparation:
   a. Routine (p. 128).
   b. Cross-matching of blood.
   c. Possible intravenous infusion.

2. Operation. This consists of removal of the kidney (nephrectomy).
3. Post-operative care:
   a. Routine care (p. 131).
   b. Position of the child. When fully conscious he is placed in the sitting position, supported by pillows.
   c. Monitoring of intravenous infusion (p. 448).
   d. Observation of urinary output.
   e. Wound and drainage care (p. 136).
   f. Feeding should not present any problem for the infant. The older child is given fluids initially and gradually introduced to a light and normal diet.
4. Radiotherapy. This is undertaken in most cases. (See p. 106 for care during radiotherapy.)
5. Drug therapy. Actinomycin D (60 to 120 μg/kg per day) may be started pre-operatively and continued in the post-operative period. The drug is given intravenously.
6. Routine nursing care.
7. Support for parents. Recognition of the parents' anxiety and the need to give adequate information to them. The medical officer will have interviewed the parents and they will be aware of the treatment and its possible consequences. Preparation for home will include advice regarding care of the child and follow-up visits.

Neuroblastoma

This is a tumour arising from the autonomic ganglia or from the adrenal medulla. It may occur at any site in which the tissue has derived from neural crest ectoderm. The majority of tumours, approximately two-thirds, arise in the adrenal medulla and in neighbouring sympathetic ganglia.

Clinical features
The tumour occurs in the first four years of life and may already exist in fetal life. Features vary according to the site and extent of involvement:

1. Adrenal tumour presents as an abdominal mass and is highly malignant.
2. Liver involvement is indicated by jaundice and vomiting.
3. Brain involvement is indicated by headaches, behaviour changes and motor involvement.
4. Bony deposits present limb pains.

In all cases, pallor (anaemia), irritability, anorexia and lethargy are presenting features. Hypertension is occasionally found and is believed to be due to secretion of pressor amines.

Principles of treatment and nursing management

1. Pre-operative care (p. 128).
2. Operation. The aim is complete excision but this is not often possible. Partial removal and subsequent radiotherapy have been successful in some cases.
3. Post-operative care:
   a. Routine care (p. 131).
   b. Monitoring of blood pressure (p. 460).
   c. Intravenous infusion (p. 448).
   d. Wound care.
4. Drugs. Cytotoxic drugs such as vincristine sulphate and cyclophosphamide are given. These drugs may cause gastro-intestinal disturbances, mouth ulceration, alopecia and bone marrow depression. Many of the side-effects are reversible once the drugs are discontinued. Vitamin B_{12} may be used as an adjunct to the conventional treatment. The reason for its use is that since vitamin B_{12} is necessary in the maturation of blood-forming tissue, it also encourages the transformation of the embryonic tumour to adult, benign tissue. The value in treatment is not universally accepted.
5. Careful assessment radiologically and repeated urine analysis.
6. Routine nursing care (p. 116).
7. Support for parents. Recognition of the distress and anxiety of the parents and the need to provide support during the long treatment. Close follow-up visits and continued care at home with full support by the community services.

Disorders of the lower urinary tract

Anomalies of the lower urinary tract occur in both male and female. Some of these anomalies are associated with imperforate anus, which include, rectourethral or rectovesical fistula in the male or a rectovaginal fistula in the female (Fig. 25.10).

Some aspects of these conditions are discussed in Chapter 26, but for more detailed information the reader is referred to more specialised books. There are, however, a number of conditions frequently encountered in paediatrics and these include: cystitis; phimosis; meatal ulcer; stenosis; hypospadias; and epispadias.

Cystitis

When the infection is confined to the bladder it is termed cystitis. It mainly occurs in girls and there may not be any demonstrable underlying abnormality. However, there may be vesicoureteric reflux or pyelonephritis. *Escherichia coli* is responsible for over 80 per cent of initial urinary tract infection. Other micro-organisms include *Pseudomonas*, *Proteus* and enterococci.

Pathogenesis

Urine secreted by normal kidneys is sterile until it reaches the distal urethra. Bacteria can reach the urinary tract by the ascending route or by haematogenous spread. The most important factor in aiding ascending infection is anatomical or functional obstruction to free urine flow. Free flow, large urine volume, complete emptying of the bladder, and acid pH are important antibacterial defences.

Investigations

1. Microscopic examination of urine. The presence of more than 10 bacteria per field in the unstained specimen suggests a bacteria count of more than 100 000/ml of urine.
2. Urine culture. The dip-slide method is usually used.
3. Chemical tests of urine. These rely on the enzymatic activity of viable bacteria.
4. Identification of micro-organisms and sensitivity tests.
5. Investigations to identify the underlying cause, e.g. X-ray and micturating cystourethrogram.

Clinical features

There is usually frequency of micturition and enuresis is present. The urine is often turbid, offensive or dark and the child experiences burning pain on voiding. There may also be lower abdominal pain. In young children there may be fever and febrile convulsions as well as vomiting and diarrhoea.

Principles of treatment and nursing management

1. It is important to obtain a specimen of urine which is representative of bladder urine. A mid-stream or clean voiding specimen can be obtained from older children, but younger children would require either a bladder puncture or bladder catheterisation. For the method of these procedures see page 547. Careful preparation and precautions will be necessary; in the male, the foreskin should be retracted to expose the meatus before urine is collected, while in the female, it is important to separate the labia manually to expose the urethral meatus during voiding and collection, so that the urine emerges as a continuous stream.
2. Medication. The choice of antibiotics should be based on the known sensitivities, e.g. cotrimoxazole, nitrofurantoin and nalidixic acid.
3. A repeat mid-stream specimen of urine should be obtained 2 to 3 days after therapy.
4. Good fluid intake and accurate fluid intake and output recording.
5. Routine nursing care.
6. Normal diet for age of the child.
7. Preparation for surgical treatment (if required). If there is vesicoureteric reflux, then reimplantation of the ureters may be performed. Vesicoureteric reflux is the commonest cause of urinary infection in children. Either in the filling phase of the bladder or during voiding, the ureterovesical valve mechanism is defective, and urine flows into the ureter; stasis follows, and infection supervenes.
8. Post-operative management aims at ensuring that there is no infection or leakage at the site of reimplant, resulting in pain and peritonitis, and that urinary output is satisfactory.
9. Guidance for parents. The condition of cystitis should be explained to them and once the child is able to go home, the need for good personal hygiene stressed. The child should be encouraged to empty the bladder before going to bed to avoid leaving residual urine in it. Follow-up examinations will be necessary for a minimum of two years.

Phimosis

Phimosis may be congenital or acquired. The foreskin in young infants cannot be retracted, because at that age it is adherent to the underlying glans. When an attempt is made to retract the foreskin forcibly, splitting of the foreskin can occur and when healing takes place, scar formation and contracture follow, for example stenosis of the preputial orifice. Ballooning of the foreskin during micturition is a feature.

Paraphimosis occurs when the phimotic prepuce is forcibly retracted and remains in that position. Oedema occurs and replacement is impossible. The swelling can become extensive, interfering with the circulation of the blood in the area.

The function of the prepuce or foreskin is a protective one, that is, it protects the glans from urine. During the first week of life, the infant's urine has a low urea concentration but this increases with the age of the child, leading to damage of the exposed glans and to meatal ulceration. It is therefore not desirable to retract the foreskin forcibly.

Principles of treatment and nursing management

1. Routine nursing care.
2. Cleanliness of the penis. The penis should be carefully washed and the infant should not be allowed to lie with a wet or soiled napkin for any length of time.
3. Phimosis may be treated by making a dorsal slit to relieve the obstruction to the outflow.
4. Paraphimosis. The aim is to reduce the oedema by:
   a. Applying a cold compress.
   b. Injecting hyaluronidase into the area. This relieves the oedema and reduction can then be carried out.
   c. Making a dorsal slit through the constricting band and then reducing the paraphimosis.
5. Circumcision. In this operation, the excess foreskin is removed. Catgut sutures are used to proximate the skin to the mucosa and to ligate the vessels.
6. Pre-operative care. Routine (p. 128).
7. Post-operative care. This operation is not without complications and observations should include evidence of bleeding. The dressing is removed when it is wet with urine and hip baths are useful to cleanse the penis and encourage healing. Frequent napkin changes are necessary.

Complications include *meatal ulceration*. This occurs as a result of ammonia burning the epithelium of the glans. The ulcer produces pain on micturition with occasional bleeding, and retention of urine may develop. Meatal ulceration can lead to *meatal stenosis*. This can be treated by meatotomy and dilatation.

8. Guidance for the parents. Clear instructions should be given to the parents when the infant or child is ready to return home. This includes hygiene of the area and recognition of any complications. They should also be given guidance in the prevention of ammoniacal dermatitis and should it occur, how to treat the condition (p. 36).

Hypospadias

In this condition the external urinary meatus lies on the posterior aspect of the penis. It is one of the commonest congenital abnormalities of the male genitalia, occurring in one in 350 male births. It may be associated with other congenital abnormalities such as the kidney, undescended testicles and genetic anomalies such as Klinefelter's syndrome.

There are varying degrees of severity, depending on the position of the urethral meatus. This may be on the glans (glandular hypospadias); at the corona (coronal hypospadias); on the shaft (penile hypospadias); at the junction of the shaft and the scrotum (penoscrotal hypospadias); and on the perineum (perineal hypospadis) (Fig. 27.6). The penis is usually also curved downwards which is more marked during erection. This chordee is due to fibrosis between the urethral meatus and the

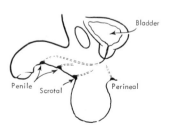

Fig. 27.6 Hypospadias (showing different positions).

glans, causing a ventral curvature. Other abnormalities are associated with hypospadias, such as deficiency in the ventral segment of the prepuce which causes a dorsal hood of redundant skin.

Embryological development of hypospadias

The development of the penis and scrotum is influenced by the testes. In the absence of the testes, the female structures of the clitoris, labia minora and labia majora dominate, but in the presence of the testes, the clitoris enlarges into the penis; the groove between the labia minora forms into the urethra and the labia majora develop into the scrotum, into which the testes subsequently descend. Hypospadias occurs when the cells of the developing testes prematurely cease androgen production, thereby interrupting the full conversion of the external genitalia into the male form.

Clinical features

The condition is easily recognised at birth. The stream of urine may be deflected downwards or splash and drip back along the shaft of the penis. The child with a penoscrotal or perineal hypospadias voids in the sitting position. In glandular or coronal hypospadias the child is able to void standing up, tilting the penis slightly upwards.

Principles of treatment and nursing management

In almost all repairs the prepuce is required as a source of extra skin. Circumcision of the neonate should therefore not be performed.

1. *Surgical correction.* This should be carried out before the child starts school to avoid social and emotional problems. The objectives of the treatment are to provide a urethra of adequate length and calibre, opening at the tip of the glans; to provide an unobstructed orifice directed forwards to prevent splashing and to provide a penis which is straight enough to permit normal sexual intercourse. The correction of the deformity is usually in two stages. The first operation is performed when the child is 3 years old to correct the chordee. The aim is to straighten the penis and prepare the way for urethroplasty. The second operation is performed some months later to bring the orifice as close as possible to the tip of the glans. This requires diversion of the urinary flow, usually through a urethrostomy temporarily created in the perineum, through which a Foley's catheter is inserted into the bladder. This allows healing of the wound. The skin of the penis is in-turned to construct a new urinary tube.

2. Pre-operative preparation (p. 128).
3. Post-operative management:
   a. The child will be on bed-rest until the catheter is removed. Care must be taken that he does not pull out the catheter. Restraint may be necessary but should be avoided if possible.
   b. Both penile and donor site wounds are kept clean and dry. Swabs should be taken if infection is suspected.
   c. Catheter care (p. 550).
   d. Examination of urine for bacterial content.
   e. Adequate fluid intake to maintain renal flow and dilute toxins.
   f. Removal of skin sutures after 5 to 7 days.
   g. The child is discharged home once the catheter has been removed and he is passing urine satisfactorily. The parents are advised about any problems regarding the wound or if the child has any difficulty passing urine.

The management of the child for the second-stage operation is much the same as that for the first stage.

1. In some units a catheter is inserted into the bladder either through a urethrostomy temporarily created in the perineum or by suprapubic catheterisation. This allows healing of the newly constructed urethra. The catheter is removed on the tenth day and the sinus closes spontaneously in 3 to 4 days.
2. Catheter care will be necessary (p. 550).
3. A foam or light cotton dressing may have been applied to the penis. This should be left undisturbed unless there is excessive bruising in the area which would indicate the presence of a haematoma. Oedema of the glans penis and especially of the prepuce is quite common but it resolves in a few days.
4. Observation of urinary flow is important when the child starts to pass urine through the newly constructed urethra. If he experiences difficulty a warm bath may help him to relax and he can

be asked to void urine into the bath. This often helps to restore confidence in his ability to pass urine and generally there is no further difficulty in voiding.

5. Observation of complications. Blockage of the catheter may occur. It can be avoided by 4-hourly catheter care and by introducing a urinary anti-septic such as co-trimoxazole. If a haematoma occurs, the child may have to return to theatre for evacuation of the haematoma. There may also be a breakdown of the repair of the urethra resulting in a fistula. In this case urine will be passed through the abnormal opening and further repair will be required four to six months later. There may also be narrowing of the new meatal opening and stricture of the urethra. This will require periodic dilatation with graduated bougies.

6. Support and guidance for the parents is very important. The condition will have been fully discussed with them but they still require reassurance and information following the correction. Since the child is young, it is advisable that a parent should be staying with him and every encouragement given to participate in the care.

Epispadias

This abnormality occurs in one in 30 000 live births. In this condition the roof of the penis is absent so that the urinary urethra is an open gutter. In its most severe form the lower abdominal wall and pubic bones are cleft from the umbilicus to the perineum, and the anterior bladder is open (exstrophy of the bladder). In this form both males and females may be affected, but it is more common in males.

In the male the abnormalities are: total epispadias, deficiencies in the corpora cavernosa, a button-like glans mounted on the junction of the crura. Often there is an inguinal hernia and undescended testicles. In the female, the two halves of the clitoris are completely separate and the vagina is frequently duplicated.

Repair of the epispadias is similar to that described for hypospadias. When the bladder is exstrophied, two surgical methods are available:

1. Diversion of urine into an ileal loop (ileal

conduit) (p. 154). The bladder mucosa are removed and the bladder muscle is sutured.

2. The bladder wall is mobilised and closed, after freeing the iliac and pubic bones to narrow the opening. The abdominal wall is then repaired. A catheter is left suprapubically to drain. Urinary continence is difficult to achieve and therefore urinary diversion is more commonly performed.

Disorders of the testis and scrotum

Descent of the testis

The testis develops on the posterior abdominal wall at the mesonephric ridge. To reach the adult position in the scrotum, it must descend. A fibrous cord form and runs from the lower pole of the testis down the posterior abdominal wall and on to the underside of the anterior abdominal wall. The latter part forms the inguinal fold. The terminal part of the fibrous cord (the gubernaculum) negotiates the layers of the anterior abdominal wall and passes into the scrotum where it ends. The function of the gubernaculum is believed to be that of anchoring the testis during the process of straightening. As it descends into the scrotum at approximately the 8th month of fetal life, it draws with it a tube of peritoneum, the processus vaginalis. The lower part of the processus vaginalis remains patent and becomes the tunica vaginalis testis. The upper part becomes a fibrous cord. If the processus remains patent throughout its length, a *congenital indirect inguinal hernia* will result. If isolated stretches of the upper part persist, a *hydrocele* results.

Both testes should be in the scrotum at birth. If the descent of the testis becomes arrested in the abdomen or inguinal canal, undescended testis (cryptorchism) results. The interstitial cells of Leydig will function normally in this position; therefore the secondary male sex characteristics will appear at puberty, but the individual will be sterile because normal spermatogenesis cannot take place in the abdominal body temperature, as it can in its normal position in the cooler scrotum.

Undescended testes (Cryptorchidism)

Undescended testes is a common disorder. It may be unilateral or bilateral and may be classified as ectopic cryptorchidism, when the testes are normal in size with a good length of spermatic cord, but have diverged from the normal path and are unable to enter into the scrotum; or true cryptorchidism, when the testes are arrested in the line of normal descent. In true cryptorchidism the testes are often small, ill-formed and relatively immobile with a short spermatic cord. A small percentage of term male newborns and many of the pre-term males have undescended testes at birth. In many cases the testes will descend by the second month with full descent by puberty. If cryptorchidism persists into adult life, failure of spermatogenesis occurs but testicular androgen production usually remains intact. Other complications possible include trauma, torsion and tumours.

Clinical features
In most infants the testes can be easily felt in the inguinal canal. The scrotum on the affected side is small. Testosterone levels are obtained and in some cases evaluation of sex chromosome abnormalities and genetic sex determination may be necessary.

Principles of treatment and nursing management
The aim of treatment is to obtain the best possible function of spermatogenesis.

1. Routine nursing care.
2. Hormone treatment. Gonadotrophic hormones are ineffective in ectopic testes and are only used when both testes are arrested in the line of normal descent.
3. Surgery. Orchidopexy is usually performed when the child is 4 to 5 years old. In boys with bilateral ectopic testes, both sides can be corrected at the one operation; in bilateral arrested testes, whichever side is more likely to be successful is operated on first.

    The spermatic cord is dissected and separated from its surroundings so that it may be lengthened sufficiently to allow the testis to reach the scrotum. A suture is placed in the lower portion of the scrotum. Sometimes this suture is attached to the upper, inner thigh with a piece of adhesive. This traction is removed in about 5 to 7 days.

If a coexistent indirect inguinal hernia is present, then herniotomy is performed at the same time as the orchidopexy.
4. Pre-operative management (p. 128).
5. Post-operative management:
    a. Routine (p. 131).
    b. Rest in bed is desirable. Discomfort usually lasts about 2 to 3 days and there may be scrotal oedema. Relief can be obtained by elevating the scrotum, raising the foot of the bed or applying a well-protected ice bag.
    c. Care of the wound and prevention of contamination of the suture line. The wound should be kept dry.
    d. Suitable occupation and prevention of excessive activity.
6. Support and encouragement for parents and child. The condition will have been discussed fully with the parents and they should be encouraged to take part in the management of the child. Anxiety about sterility and the effect on sexual behaviour should be allayed. Once the child is ready to go home, the parents should be advised about activities, such as riding a bicycle. This should be discouraged for about one to two months after operation, until the testis is fully mobile in its new position in the scrotum.

Hydroceles
A hydrocele is a painless water-filled cyst found in front of the testis. It is brightly translucent and cannot be emptied by pressure because of a 'flap valve' at its junction with the processus. The testis within it can usually be felt with ease or, when the hydrocele is tense, its shadow can be demonstrated by transillumination. A hydrocele results from excessive accumulation of normal fluid within the tunica vaginalis due to over-production caused by inflammation of the testis and its appendages, or from diminished resorption. Congenital hydrocele communicates with the abdominal cavity through a patent processus vaginalis.

Hydroceles in infants do not require surgery and all the fluid will have disappeared by the age of 1 year. In older children it may cause discomfort and affect the behaviour of the child. Surgery will then be necessary. The processus is divided at the internal inguinal ring as for an inguinal hernia.

Principles of treatment and nursing management

1. Pre-operative management (p. 128).
2. Post-operative management:
   a. Routine (p. 131).
   b. Care of the wound and prevention of contamination of the wound.
   c. Observations of complications such as bleeding into the scrotal sac and infection.
3. Support for parents. The procedure should be explained to the parents and reassurance given regarding the outcome of the operation.

Strangulated inguinal hernia

An indirect inguinal hernia can become incarcerated. A small loop of bowel becomes trapped in the hernial sac and, unless it is reduced, the blood supply can be affected. The obstruction in the sac is almost always at the level of the external inguinal ring, though in older children the obstruction is often at the internal ring. Damage to the testis can occur if the testicular vessels are compressed by a tense hernia.

Clinical features

The infant is restless and cries painfully. A swelling will be seen which is tense and tender. Local pain is replaced by generalised colicky abdominal pain, vomiting and abdominal distension; when the obstruction is complete, there will be no bowel action.

Principles of treatment and nursing management

1. Reduction of a strangulated hernia should be attempted if it has not been present for more than 12 hours. Following reduction, herniotomy is performed, usually 48 hours later to allow oedema of the sac and its investing tissue to subside.
2. Pre-operative management:
   a. Routine (p. 128).
   b. Naso-gastric tube is passed and left on free drainage.
   c. An intravenous infusion may be required to maintain fluid and elctrolyte state and in preparation for blood replacement.
3. Surgery. A small incision is made; the external ring is incised and the external oblique fascia is slit upwards and outwards. The sac is opened

and any fluid present is evacuated. The bowel is examined since in exceptional cases it can be gangrenous, when a segmental excision with anastomosis may be necessary. The hernial sac is ligated, excised and the inguinal ring repaired.

4. Post-operative care:
   a. Routine (p. 131).
   b. Continuation of intravenous infusion, if necessary.
   c. Observations for complications, i.e. bleeding, infection and drainage.
   d. Maintain gastric suction until bowel sounds return.
   e. Gradual introduction of oral feeds. For a simple herniotomy, feeds are recommenced 4 hours after surgery.
   f. Sutures are removed 7 to 10 days after the operation, depending on the condition of the wound.
5. Support for parents during the preparation of the child for theatre and subsequently during the period of the operation. Once the child has returned from theatre they should be encouraged to participate in the care of the child. If the child has had a simple herniotomy and his condition is satisfactory, then he may be allowed home later that day or the following day. The stitches can be removed at home or an appointment made for his return to hospital.

Procedures relating to the urinary system

URINARY DIVERSION

Urinary diversion may be required when there is disturbance of bladder function, failure of bladder development or tumour in the lower urinary tract. There are various types of urinary diversion, but in this book the ileal or conduit uterostomy will be described.

Principles of the operation and nursing management

The urine is diverted on to the surface of the abdominal wall, where it can be collected in a bag applied over the stoma. This method is applicable to most cases requiring a urinary diversion.

Ileal conduit

A conduit is a tube conveying fluid. An ileal conduit is a short segment of ileum, separated from the alimentary canal, which conveys urine from the ureters attached at one end to the anterior abdominal wall at the other (Fig. 7.12, p. 155). Indications for this operation are the neurogenic bladder and ectopia vesicae.

1. *Neurogenic bladder*. The common severe type is associated with myelomeningocele. Normal bladder function depends on an intact nerve supply and on the inherent properties of the bladder itself. The two functions which depend on an intact nerve supply are reflex activity and sensation. Different types can be identified, for example, (a) *facilitated neurogenic bladder* which is found when there is damage to the higher centres and the bladder empties frequently and (b) *reflex bladder* when the bladder contractions are poor and uncoordinated and emptying is inadequate.

When the bladder is totally denervated, there is no voluntary or reflex micturition. This is due to the destruction of the sacral nerve roots; sensory denervation occurs in myelomeningocele when the higher centres fail to receive adequate information regarding the state of the bladder.

When bladder dysfunction occurs with incontinence, incomplete emptying, gross vesicoureteric reflux, infection and progressive renal damage, then the urine is diverted from the bladder. Incontinence is then corrected and the renal damage is controlled.

2. *Ectopia vesicae*. The bladder opens on to the lower anterior abdominal wall as there is deficiency of tissue in this area. In addition the dorsal aspect of the urethra is open. There is constant dribbling of urine, leading to excoriation of the skin and ulceration of the mucosa.

An ileal conduit achieves urinary continence. If the anal sphincters are normal an alternative method may be used, for example anastomosis of the ureters to the sigmoid colon, that is, uretero-sigmoidostomy.

Function of the ileal conduit

The ileal segment functions as intestinal tissue and secretes, absorbs and undergoes peristaltic activity. It does not act as a storage reservoir. There may be an increase in mucous secretion, but this is not considered of significance. Absorption of fluid and electrolytes is minimised by the active emptying of the conduit by peristalsis. Metabolic acidosis from fluid and electrolyte loss is unusual.

The uretero-ileal anastomosis does not have a valvular mechanism and reflux to the kidneys can be demonstrated radiographically. The stoma may stenose; this leads to stasis in the ileal conduit which may produce metabolic changes, with bilateral hydronephrosis and consequent renal damage.

Nursing management

This involves specific nursing procedures, the aims of which are:

1. Ensuring that the stoma is functioning satisfactorily.
2. Maintenance of the appliance.
3. Care of the stoma and surrounding skin.
4. Recognition of complications.
5. Instructions and support for parents, e.g. supply of disposable bags.

The procedures are:

1. Immediate post-operative care:
   a. Routine care (p. 131).
   b. Fitting of a suitable disposable collecting apparatus. The hole in the flange must fit accurately over the stoma so that no skin is exposed to constant contact with urine. Disposable and semidisposable bags are changed at frequent intervals (p. 154).
2. Frequent routine urine tests are necessary (p. 562).
3. Bladder lavage (wash-outs) using a mild antiseptic may be required if there is persistent purulent discharge from the bladder (p. 551).
4. Recognition of complications, e.g. stricture due to granular formation. This occurs more readily if the stoma is infected. Treatment is by nursing the child in the prone position on a divided mattress, exposing the stoma and draining the urine into a container.
5. Routine nursing care.
6. Support and guidance for the parents. The emphasis here is on instruction and support regarding stoma care. The parents should be able to change the appliance and know how to care for the stoma. There should be community

involvement and the parents should feel free to contact the stoma specialist when necessary.

COLLECTION OF A URINE SPECIMEN

Examination of urine is an important aspect of diagnosis and is a means of assessing progress in conditions affecting the urinary tract and in metabolic disorders. Specimens of urine are required routinely on admission from all children and weekly thereafter, except in conditions such as nephritis and nephrosis when daily specimens are necessary.

There are various methods of collecting urine and these depend on the age of the child, the reason for the examination and the condition of the child.

Collection from infants

Requirements
A clean or sterile container.

Method
The infant may be held upside down and the spinal reflex of Perez is elicited by stroking the back along the paravertebral muscles. Spontaneous voiding usually occurs within 5 minutes (Fig. 27.7).

Method for the male infant
A urine collecting bag can be used. The napkin

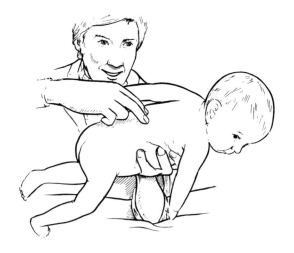

Fig. 27.7 Encouragement to void.

area is carefully cleaned with soap and water and dried thoroughly. The bag is attached ensuring that the penis is well placed in the opening of the bag. The adhesive covering should not be removed from the part which will be over the scrotum. The aperture may be enlarged to include the scrotum if leakage is occurring, but the adhesive must not become adherent to the scrotum. When urine has been passed, the adhesive part is gently eased from the skin with a solvent. It should never be pulled off as this can be painful. Any adhesive should be removed with the solvent and the infant should be left clean and comfortable.

The urine should then be emptied into a suitable container, labelled and kept in a cool place.

Method for the female infant
A disposable urine collecting bag is used.

The nurse requires a sterile dressing pack and in addition a urine collecting bag, cleansing lotion, scissors, a universal container for urine and a disposal bag.

The nurse washes and dries her hand, then she washes and dries the infant's napkin area. The hands are then washed and dried again. Using sterile swabs and cleansing lotion, the external genitalia are cleaned, working from above down either side of the labia until the area has been adequately cleansed. The direction is important and is always from above downwards to prevent the transfer of organisms from the perineum to the urethra and vagina. The area is dried gently. The protective backing is then removed from the bag and it is applied from below working upwards. The adhesive is pressed carefully to the skin starting at the bridge of skin separating the rectum from the vagina, ensuring that the adhesive is firmly attached to the skin. This type of bag has the advantage that the child need not be restrained, and indeed not be confined to bed. The bag is a double container preventing return flow thus avoiding leakage. The napkin can then be attached loosely, pinned at either side at the waist (or a disposable napkin can be used). As soon as an adequate amount of urine has been obtained, the bag is removed as described above. The urine is transferred to a suitable container, labelled, and sent to the laboratory or ward test room.

Collection from the older child

Method

For a routine examination of urine, the child is asked to pass urine into a bedpan, if a girl, or a bottle, if a boy. The urine is then transferred to a suitable container, labelled and sent to the laboratory.

It may be necessary to obtain a specimen of urine for bacterial examination when a mid-stream specimen of urine will be required.

Mid-stream specimen of urine

A mid-stream specimen of urine is the only clinically effective type of voided urine which is suitable for bacteriological examination. Usually children from the age of 4 or 5 will co-operate successfully in this procedure, if adequate explanation is given of what is required of them.

Requirements

Sterile equipment:

1. Dressing pack.
2. Foil bowl.
3. Universal container.
4. Dip slide.
5. Cleansing lotion, e.g. sterile water or sodium chloride 0.9 per cent.

Additional equipment:

6. Bedpan/urinal/collecting bag.
7. Disposal bag.

Method (for male child)

The procedure should be explained to the child as simply and clearly as possible. Whenever possible, the child should perform this procedure at the toilet.

The glans and meatus are cleansed with the cleansing lotion. The child is asked to void urine into the toilet or bed bottle and after a small amount has been passed, the flow is directed into the sterile container for the specimen. The voiding is then completed in the bed bottle. The specimen is labelled and sent to the laboratory. If the dip slide is used, it should be kept at room temperature until it is removed to the laboratory.

Method (for female child)

The procedure is explained to the child as above, but it may be easier to carry out the cleansing procedure while the child lies in bed. Two nurses may be required.

The nurse washes and dries her hands. The child is placed on the bed with her legs apart and the nurse cleanses the labia from above towards the perineum, using each swab once only. After each side has been cleaned, the centre is cleansed. If the child is old enough she can be instructed to hold her labia open during the voiding process, otherwise the nurse may do so with gloved hands. The child is instructed to void into the bedpan first and then direct the flow into a sterile container. When a small amount of urine has been obtained, the child can continue to void into the bedpan. The specimen is then labelled and sent to the laboratory (see above).

24-hour collection of urine

Method for male infant

The following are required:

1. 2-in wide Paul's tubing, length adequate to reach the container for the urine at the end of the bed, and to allow the child to be moved for bedmaking and feeding.
2. Adhesive tape.
3. Scissors.
4. Restrainers for ankles.
5. Urine collecting bag.

After a bath, or cleansing of the napkin area, the penis and scrotum are placed within the Paul's tubing, which is attached to the skin with adhesive tape.

The other end of the tubing is inserted into the collecting bag at the end of the bed. The napkin can be put on loosely, and the ankles can be restrained. By placing the bag at the end of the bed, there is no risk of it being damaged by the cot sides, and it is less likely that the bedclothes will be tucked in over the Paul's tubing. A half-hourly check should be made to ensure that drainage is satisfactory.

If Paul's tubing is not available, a Uro-bag can be used. This bag comes complete with tubing and is applied according to the method described on page 547.

Method for female infant

A simple and satisfactory method of collecting urine over a long period is by using a urine collecting bag, such as the Campbridge (Chiron) or Uro-bag. Application of the bag is as described on page 547.

Catheterisation

This is a procedure whereby the urinary bladder is emptied by means of a catheter. It is a procedure which is not without danger to the patient and is only undertaken when all other methods have failed. Catheterisation is carried out for the following reasons:

1. To aid diagnosis, e.g. diabetic coma, injury to the bladder and occasionally in urinary infection.
2. To empty the contents of the bladder, e.g. to relieve retention of urine.
3. To ascertain the amount of urine remaining in the bladder after voiding.
4. As a pre-operative measure. It is only undertaken when specifically instructed by the doctor, and is usually used as a last resort if the child has failed to empty the bladder normally.
5. As a preventive measure to avoid contamination of dressings or exposed healing areas, e.g. in burns, when the catheter is left in position.
6. To achieve an accurate measurement of urinary output when this is essential, e.g. investigation of metabolic disorders and in an unconscious child. The catheter is usually left in position.

Dangers of catheterisation

1. Infection may easily spread through faulty technique. Organisms can be introduced into the bladder leading to an upward spread of infection.
2. Poor technique may cause trauma which in turn predisposes to infection. This can be caused by the use of force in a tense child, or using too large a catheter.

   Male patients are not usually catheterised by the nursing staff, because catheterisation can easily damage the urethral valves. Therefore, the following discussion applies only to females.

Requirements

Sterile equipment:

1. Disposable sterile catheters with water-soluble lubricant. The type of catheter will depend on the reason for the catheterisation, e.g. round tip is used for non-retaining catheter, while Malecot, de Pezzer or Foley's catheters are used for self-retaining. Malecot and de Pezzer catheters are introduced with a stylet or introducer.
2. Dressing pack.
3. 3 pairs of forceps.
4. Container for catheters.
5. Container for urine.
6. Drapes.
7. Disposable gloves.

Additional equipment:

8. Measuring jug.
9. Water-soluble lubricant, e.g. KY jelly (anaesthetic lubricant for male patients).
10. Disposal bag.
11. Appropriate forms and labels.
12. Book for the child.
13. Good light, e.g. an adjustable lamp.

Preparation of the child

It is essential to have the co-operation of the child while carrying out the procedure. A child who is frightened and restless will not be easily catheterised and this increases the danger of trauma and the risk of infection. It is not difficult to pass the catheter when the child is lying quietly; it is quite another matter if she is tense or distraught. The presence of the mother can be of value here in keeping the child calm.

Method

Three nurses may be required (if available), one to hold the child's legs in the correct position, the second to hold a book propped up on the child's chest to keep the instruments out of view and read to the child, and the third is the performer. The performer washes and dries her hands and with forceps wrings out sufficient swabs placing them in a gallipot. Using the same forceps, one catheter is lubricated if desired and placed in the receiver. The child is placed in position and a good light is directed at the vulval region.

Still using forceps, the performer cleanses the labia from above towards the perineum, cleansing each side and then the centre, using each swab only once and repeating as often as necessary. These forceps are then discarded. The towels are placed in position, one covering each leg and joining over the abdomen, and the third is placed on the table between the legs up to the perineum. The container is now brought over to the table and placed on the sterile towel. The labia are now separated with the left hand (if right-handed) and only when the urethral meatus can be seen clearly (the urthral orifice is very small in small children and it lies above the vaginal orifice) is the final cleansing performed.

The catheter is then held with a gauze swab about 5 cm from the tip and is gently introduced; alternatively a glove may be worn and the tip inserted with the fingers. The end of the catheter is directed into the container and the bladder is allowed to empty slowly. The catheter is then removed gently and the labia dried. The child is then returned to bed after she has been comforted and rewarded.

Foley's self-retaining catheter
Requirements as for catheterisation, with the addition of sterile water and a 5 ml syringe.

Method
When this type of catheter has been introduced, the balloon is inflated with the appropriate amount of sterile water marked on the catheter and the bung is then firmly pushed into position. The tubing can be taped to the thigh to prevent tension and traction on the bladder.

Continuous after-care
Vulval toilet should be carried out 4-hourly and the meatus cleansed daily with a suitable antiseptic lotion, such as chlorhexidine 0.5 per cent and cetrimide 0.5 per cent.

Bladder decompression
A grossly distended bladder should not be emptied rapidly because of the danger of damage to the bladder wall. This is especially liable to occur when the distension has been over a considerable time. Distension may occur where there is some urethral obstruction, such as urethral valves or bladder neck obstruction. Where a urethral catheter is used, decompression can be carried out quite simply by clamping the catheter, releasing it every hour, and withdrawing 60 ml urine.

Decompression and drainage by methods other than the use of a urethral catheter may be necessary to ensure adequate clearance of residual urine from the bladder from a grossly hydronephrotic kidney when the distension of the pelvis and calyces causes stasis of urine resulting in infection. In such cases, suprapubic cystostomy, nephrostomy or ureterostomy has to be performed.

Suprapubic drainage
Suprapubic cystostomy is performed to drain the bladder and to divert the flow of urine from the urethra. It is useful when there is injury to the urethra, stricture of the urethra, following bladder surgery or the presence of a neurogenic bladder (p. 546).

The bladder should be distended so that it is easier to locate. If it is not already distended with urine, sterile saline can be introduced via a urethral catheter. The operation can be performed either by open operation or by puncture with a trocar and needle. When the catheter is in position, it is secured with sutures, tape or a seal system. The area is covered with a sterile dressing if necessary. To prevent tension and traction on the bladder, the catheter can be secured to the abdomen with adhesive tape. A collecting system is then attached to drain the urine from the bladder and this is continued until the child is able to void urine via the urethra, when the catheter is clamped and removed.

When a *nephrostomy* is performed, the catheter is inserted directly into the pelvis of the kidney. This is performed for the following reasons:

1. To provide drainage from the kidney.
2. To facilitate healing after operation.
3. To provide drainage when the ureter is not functioning.

The catheter can be secured to the child's side to prevent tension and traction. A collecting system is then attached to drain the urine from the kidney.

A *perineal urethrostomy* is an opening made

through the perineum into the urethra, through which a catheter is passed into the bladder. This bypass is carried out to facilitate healing of the penile urethra following plastic operation for hypospadias.

In all three types of drainage, sterile connection tubing and a collecting bag will be required and should be prepared for the child's return from theatre. Initially, restraining bands will be necessary, to ensure that the younger child, or the child recovering from anaesthesia, cannot pull out the tubing or catheter. Daily cleansing and sterilisation of tubing (or replacing with new sterile disposable tubing and collecting bag) is essential to prevent ascending infections.

Bladder irrigation

The bladder can be irrigated with a solution of antibacterial fluid to remove debris in long-standing infections, or in an endeavour to prevent infection occurring after operation or trauma. Catheterisation will be necessary if an indwelling catheter has not been already inserted. Bladder irrigation may be intermittent or continous.

When an ileal loop conduit or nephrostomy drainage are being irrigated, it must be remembered that each has a very limited capacity and not more than 15 ml fluid should be instilled at a time unless otherwise ordered. No force must be used to inject the fluid and if the child complains of pain, the procedure should be discontinued.

Continuous or intermittent bladder irrigation with a gravity apparatus

This may be ordered as a post-operative measure when there has been major surgery in the pelvic region, or in the treatment of long-standing infection. It is a more gentle form of irrigation though it is not very often used now. Figure 27.8 shows the apparatus assembled and it functions in the following way:

1. Reservoir A is filled with the measured fluid and attached to the stand. The clip on tube B is closed.
2. The clip of tube B is opened and fluid is allowed to run through the tube and any air is expelled. The clip is closed again.
3. Tube B is attached to the Y connection, which

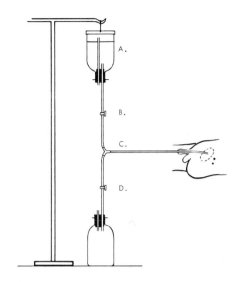

Fig. 27.8 Bladder irrigation. (See text for explanation.)

is attached to the catheter and the outlet tube D. The clip on the outlet tube is closed.
4. Open clip on tube B and allow not more than 30 ml fluid to run into the bladder. Close clip.
5. To empty the bladder, open the clip on the outlet tube D and leave it open until it is time to irrigate again.

Bladder lavage

Requirements
Sterile equipment:

1. Dressing pack.
2. Packet of drapes.
3. Bowel.
4. Hand towels.
5. Gloves.
6. Conical funnel, clip and tubing or bladder syringe.

Additional equipment:

7. Flask of chlorhexidine gluconate 1:5000 in water standing in a container of warm water.
8. Lotion thermometer in a container of chlorhexidine 0.5 per cent in alcohol 70 per cent.
9. Sterile water to rinse the thermometer.
10. Gowns and masks.
11. Measuring jug.
12. Container for returned fluid.
13. Disposal bag.

Method

Using forceps, the end of the catheter is cleansed and placed on the sterile drape. The temperature of the lotion is tested and should be 37.8 °C when given. The syringe is filled and not more than 30 ml of the lotion is injected very slowly into the bladder and retained for about a half-hour before being returned. This is repeated until the recommended amount has been given and returned. It is important to ensure that no air is injected as this causes pain and discomfort.

When a conical funnel is used, the principle is the same, but the fluid is allowed to syphon out into the funnel, which is then emptied, before introducing more fluid.

Tidal drainage using irrigating apparatus

This method is used when it is considered desirable to encourage the natural filling and emptying of the bladder. The bladder is allowed to fill to an estimated amount and emptied by syphonage.

Requirements

1. Sterile irrigating solution apparatus (Cystomat) and drainage bag.
2. Intravenous administration set and stand.
3. Flask with chlorhexidine gluconate 1:5000.
4. Bottle of chlorhexidine 0.5 per cent in cetrimide 0.5 per cent.
5. Catheter size 16 FG.

Method

1. Connect the intravenous set to the container of irrigating solution.
2. Attach the irrigating apparatus to the infusion stand below the bottle containing the irrigating solution.
3. Attach the tubing to:
   a. The catheter via a Y connection.
   b. The collecting bag.
4. Fill the apparatus with the irrigating solution.
5. Set the prescribed drip rate.
6. Remove the cap from the air vent at the top of the apparatus. The fluid level in the manometer will indicate the approximate bladder pressure.
7. Raise or lower the apparatus on the stand until the fluid in the manometer rests in the middle of the manometer scale.

8. As the irrigating solution fills the bladder, the pressure within the bladder rises inducing automatic syphonage. When the bladder has been emptied, the filling phase starts and the cycle is repeated automatically.
9. If desired, the bladder irrigation may be stopped by closing the clamp on the administration set and closing the air vent. This procedure should be performed *only* at the end of the bladder drainage phase.
10. If the system fails to function, it should be checked for blockage.

Bladder puncture (Fig. 27.9)

A bladder puncture is performed in infants and toddlers to obtain a specimen of urine for culture. It is a relatively safe procedure though some bleeding may occur from the puncture.

Requirement

Sterile equipment:

1. Dressing pack.
2. 2 ml syringe.
3. No. 21 gauge needles.
4. 20 ml syringe and No. 19 gauge needles.
5. Mediswabs.
6. Universal containers.
7. Frusemide 5 to 10 mg.

Method

If the child has passed urine, the doctor should be notified. In order to perform a successful bladder puncture, there must be enough urine in the

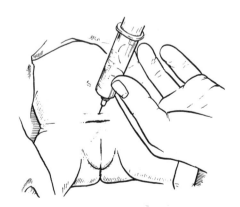

Fig. 27.9 Suprapubic aspiration.

bladder to distend it above the pubic symphysis. An injection of frusemide is given to produce diuresis.

The child lies on his back, the nurse supporting him and preventing any movement. The skin is cleansed with mediswab and the needle is introduced into the bladder. The child should be observed for any signs of distress and he should be comforted. When the urine has been obtained, the needle is removed and pressure is applied with a swab and fingers.

After-care

The child should be observed periodically to see if any bleeding or oozing has occurred. It is also important to note the time of first voiding after the procedure and to note the colour of the urine. It may be pink, but if it contains frank blood, the fact must be reported to the doctor.

Cystometrogram

This is a record obtained by measuring the pressure-volume of the bladder. It shows the rate of rise of pressure in the bladder with increasing volume, that is the tone of the bladder, the threshold value for evoking the micturition reflex, and the maximum bladder pressure achieved in the micturition contraction. For example, in neurogenic bladder, the 'tone' is high and the micturition threshold is low. It also aids diagnosis when there is obstruction at the external sphincter or at the outlet of the bladder.

Preparation of the child

The procedure should be explained to the older child and his co-operation gained. Sedation will be required for the younger child or infant. The procedure is not a painful one once the initial puncture has been performed. It is, however, tedious, taking approximately 2 hours when a series of recordings are made. It is desirable that the child's bladder is full for this investigation and it is therefore necessary to encourage him to drink fluids 1 hour prior to the test and to discourage him from voiding urine. Suitable books and toys should be provided, dependent upon the age of the child.

Method

The most accurate measurements are obtained when suprapubic percutaneous catheterisation is performed. A local anaesthetic is given unless the child has a lack of sensation below the waist, for example spina bifida or traumatic paraplegia.

Two intravenous cannulae (Intracaths) are passed directly into the bladder; one is used to fill the bladder at a physiologically accepted rate (approximately 2 ml per minute in an infant); the second catheter is used for recording purposes.

Alternatively, recordings are made after catheterisation per urethra and fluid is injected as above.

Requirements

1. Dressing pack and additional dissecting forceps for catheterisation.
2. Catheters of medium-sized intravenous cannulae (Intracaths).
3. Intravenous giving sets (two).
4. 20 ml syringe.
5. Flask with sterile water.
6. Flask with normal saline for filling bladder.
7. Recording apparatus (electronic pressure transducer).
8. Cleansing lotion.
9. Universal container.
10. Disposal bags.

After-care

1. Haematuria may be present and is usually slight, but if it persists or increases the doctor must be notified.
2. Observation of the puncture site is important to ascertain whether leakage is occurring.
3. Following the suprapubic method, catheterisation may be carried out to determine the amount of residual urine.
4. When suprapubic pressure is required to aid voiding in the paralysed child, this should be gentle to avoid leakage from the suprapubic puncture.

Cystoscopic examination

A cystoscopic examination is a visual examination of the urethra, prostatic urethra and the bladder by means of a lighted telescopic lens. It is used for the following reasons:

1. To inspect the bladder wall directly.
2. To obtain a separate specimen of urine from each kidney and evaluate renal function separately.
3. To inspect the ureteric orifices.
4. To remove calculi from the urethra, bladder and ureteric orifices.

Method and after-care

The procedure is carried out in theatre under either local of general anaesthesia. The cystoscope is passed via the urethra.

Postexamination care consists of observation of urine and voiding. The child will experience some burning sensation upon voiding and the urine will be blood-tinged. There may also be reluctance to void leading to retention of urine. Relief may be obtained by giving the child a warm Sitz-bath (38.5 to 40 °C).

Voiding cystogram

This is an X-ray examination to demonstrate the presence of urethral valves and vesicoureteric reflux.

The bladder is filled with an opaque medium and X-rays are taken when the bladder reaches its capacity. Further X-rays are taken during and on completion of voiding. Reflux of the medium into the ureters during micturition indicates incompetence of the ureto-vesical valves.

Requirements

As for catherisation (p. 549) and additional items:

1. 20 ml syringe.
2. Jug and large container.
3. Spigot or clip.
4. Warmed half-strength saline to dilute the opaque medium.
5. Adhesive tape to fix the catheter.

Preparation of the child

A suppository may be given the night before the examination to ensure that a good bowel action is achieved. There is no specific preparation on the day other than ensuring that the child understands what is being done and his part during the procedure.

Excretion pyelogram (intravenous)

Reason

This investigation is undertaken when some abnormality of the urinary tract is suspected and to demonstrate the efficiency of renal function.

Principle

The opaque medium is normally given intravenously and will be excreted by a functioning kidney a short time afterwards. X-rays are taken at 5, 10 and 20 minute intervals and outlines of the kidneys, ureters and bladder can be seen.

Requirements

1. Dressing pack.
2. Mediswabs.
3. 20 ml syringe and needles of appropriate sizes.
4. Large bore needle.
5. 1 ml syringe and needles.
6. Adrenaline or an antihistamine drug (to counteract any reaction to iodine).
7. Warmed ampoule of opaque medium and file.

Preparation of the child

Ordinary diet is given and bowel action encouraged. If necessary, a suppository may be given the evening before. On the morning of the examination, if the child is well enough, he should be allowed up to run about thus helping the bowel to be rid of gases. Fluids are withheld for 6 hours prior to the injection but dry food may be given. A straight X-ray of the abdomen is taken to exclude renal calculi. The child, if old enough, should be given an explanation of the examination and the method used.

Method

The injection is usually given into the median basilic vein by the doctor. In small infants a scalp vein may be used, or if a suitable vein is not available, the medium may be given subcutaneously and dispersal aided by hyaluronidase. Iodine sensitivity is tested by injecting a test dose of 1 ml of the substance intravenously. If no reaction occurs in half a minute, the full dose can be injected.

Subsequent to the first film after the injection, the child is given an aerated drink or the infant, a feed. This demonstrates the left kidney behind the gas bubble formed in the stomach.

When giving the medium *subcutaneously*, it is diluted with equal parts of normal saline with hyaluronidase added. The dilution depends on the strength and type of medium used. The injection is given into the lateral aspect of the thigh.

Signs of sensitivity include flushing, urticaria, nausea and vomiting and should any of these be noted, the doctor must be informed immediately.

Retrograde pyelography

Reason
If kidney function is impaired, intravenous pyelography may fail to give adequate information, and cystoscopy with retrograde pyelography can be performed.

Principle
This procedure is carried out under general anaesthesia and a cystoscope is passed into the bladder (p. 553). Ureteric catheters are passed through the cystoscope into the bladder and up each ureter to the right and left kidneys. Thus a specimen of urine from the bladder and from each kidney can be obtained. An opaque medium, amount according to age, is injected into each catheter and X-rays are taken.

Preparation and care of the child
The same preparation is necessary as for an excretion pyelogram, with the additional preparation for general anaesthesia (p. 128). It is not necessary that the child passes urine prior to the examination, as specimens of urine are to be collected. The after-care is the same as for cystoscopy (p. 554).

Renogram
This is a radioisotope study of the urinary tract. It delineates structure and function of kidneys without interfering with their normal physiological process. Radioiodine is given intravenously and the areas over the kidneys are monitored with radiation counters to reveal differences between the two kidneys with respect to blood flow, tubular function and excretion.

Although not a painful procedure, it can be frightening for the young child. Sedation may be given prior to the examination and the nurse should stay with the child throughout to comfort and reassure him.

Renoscan
In this examination a radioactive substance is given intravenously. The radionuclide injected is 5 mCi of technetium-labelled pentacetic acid and is given 20 minutes before the scan. To prevent the uptake to the thyroid gland, potassium iodide is given orally. The renoscan is useful in delineating the kidneys, and giving information of their position and size.

The care of the child is as for renogram.

Renal biopsy

Reason
This is a procedure which is an aid to diagnosis and which can give an indication as to prognosis and response to treatment in children suffering from nephritis and nephrosis. A specimen of renal tissue is obtained preferably with fluoroscopy, and examined by electron microscope.

Preparation of the child
An intravenous pyelogram is carried out beforehand to establish the position of the kidneys and treatment is given to reduce the oedema and proteinuria. Sometimes a 'marker' is placed over the proposed site of puncture and care should be taken not to remove it. The child is prepared for theatre as described on page 128.

Method
The child lies in the prone position with a sandbag under the abdomen. A renal puncture needle and a fine exploratory needle may be used to obtain renal tissue. This is collected into fixative and sent for histological examination to the pathology department.

After-care of the child
The child should remain in the prone position for about 30 minutes and pressure is applied to the

puncture site to prevent bleeding. On return to the ward the following observations are necessary:

1. Blood pressure and pulse rate are monitored hourly for the first 12 hours and 2-hourly for 24 hours thereafter.
2. The first urine voided is examined for blood. This is usually present for 24 hours following renal biopsy.
3. Any swelling or discolouration over the site should be watched for and reported. The wound is left without a dressing.
4. Any backache, shoulder pain or dysuria should be reported to the doctor.
5. If the child has previously been allowed up, he is confined to bed for 24 hours following the biopsy.

KIDNEY FUNCTION TESTS

Apart from chemical tests of the urine which the nurse can carry out in the ward, specific tests are done to determine the efficiency of the kidneys. The nurses' function is to ensure that the test is carried out according to the prescribed sequence and that all the urine passed is sent to the biochemistry department for evaluation.

The function of the kidneys has been discussed on page 526 and in gross disease of the kidneys when more than half of its substance has been destroyed, there will be evidence of inefficiency.

There is no single test of renal function and best results will be obtained by combining the results of a number of clinical tests.

Renal concentration test

This test evaluates the ability of the kidneys to concentrate urine. This ability is lost early in kidney disease affecting the tubules.

Preparation of the child
No fluids are given after 6 p.m. on the day before the test.

Method
Any urine passed during the night is saved. At 6 a.m. the child is asked to empty his bladder — this urine is added to any voided during the night. Three further specimens of urine are obtained at hourly intervals, each specimen being collected separately, and the volume and specific gravity measured. Normal range of specific gravity is 1.022 to 1.035.

Urea concentration test

The test is used to determine the efficiency of the kidneys with regard to their urea excreting function. Urea is nitrogenous waste matter, one of the end-products of protein metabolism. In this test the blood is flooded with urea.

Preparation of the child
The child has nothing to eat or drink after supper on the night prior to the test.

Method
At 6 a.m. the child empties his bladder. This constitutes specimen one. He is given a drink of 15 g of urea dissolved in 100 ml of water. He is asked to pass urine at 7 a.m., 8 a.m. and 9 a.m. Each specimen is labelled and sent to the biochemical laboratory. Three specimens of urine are necessary because the urea may act as a diuretic, giving low readings of the first two specimens. Low urinary urea concentrations are obtained in nephritis, and in these cases, the blood urea is raised. Normally, urine contains about 2 per cent of urea and if it is below 2 per cent throughout the test, the kidneys are inefficient.

Urea clearance test

The urea clearance test indicates roughly the amount of functioning tissue remaining when renal disease is present. The results are read as the percentage of available functioning renal tissue; 80 to 100 per cent is a normal reading. Percentages lower than this indicate damage to the functioning kidneys. When it decreases to 10 per cent, then the remaining tissue is insufficient and the patient is in a state of uraemia.

Preparation of the child
No special preparation is necessary. The usual diet is given during the test.

Method
Urine is collected for 24 hours. The time of commencement and completion of the collection must be accurate and recorded on the form, as an

assessment is made on the average flow per minute. A specimen of blood is obtained during the collection for blood urea estimation.

Creatinine clearance test (endogenous)

This gives an assessment of the extent of renal damage and in normal subjects is proportional to glomerular filtration. The mean normal value for endogenous creatinine clearances is 123 ($\pm$ 30 per cent) ml/min/1.73m^2 body surface area. Lower values may be normal in very young children.

Preparation of the child

The child's age, weight, height and sex must be recorded on the form. The collections of urine must be complete in volume and accurate in timing. Normal activity, diet and fluid intake are permitted on the day before the test. On the day of the test, the child should remain in bed. Breakfast should be light, avoiding meat protein. He may be given a biscuit or milk during the test if he becomes too hungry to co-operate.

Method

To ensure an adequate flow of urine, he may be given fluids to the amount of 10 ml/kg 1 hour before the test begins. During the test, which may last from about 9 a.m. to 3 p.m., he should be given drinks (about 5 ml per kg body weight) at approximately half-hourly intervals. At about 9 a.m. the child empties his bladder completely. The urine is discarded and the time recorded. All the urine passed thereafter up to about 12 noon is collected and combined as specimen A.

At about 12 noon a venepuncture is performed and 5 ml of blood is obtained and sent straight to the laboratory. All the urine passed after the end of the first collection and up to about 3 p.m. is collected and combined as specimen B. The time of voiding the last specimen is recorded accurately.

Creatinine clearance test

This is a similar test to the one described above. The method varies and is as follows:

Urine is collected for 24 hours. The first specimen of urine is discarded and any urine passed within the 24-hour period is collected. A venepuncture is performed during the collection and 5 ml of blood is obtained and sent to the biochemistry laboratory. As in the previous test, the form should contain the child's sex, age, weight and height. Normal diet is given during the test.

Addis sedimentation count

This test is carried out to determine any impairment in kidney function. A 10 ml specimen of urine is centrifuged and a drop of the sediment is examined microscopically. The following formed elements can be seen:

White cells. Occasional white cells are normally of no significance, but when present in sufficient numbers they are reported as 'pus cells'. This suggests infection and requires further investigation. Small numbers of white cells may also be seen in nephritis.

Red cells. The presence of red blood cells in the urine is known as haematuria. It may be due to injury, stones, infection or a growth. A few red blood cells may be found in normal urine, especially following catheterisation.

Casts. These are minute structures with parallel sides resembling elongated sausages in shape. They result from semi-solid material taking on the shape of the kidney tubule while passing through. An occasional hyaline (glass-like) cast may be present in the urine of normal people. The number of these casts increases in states of dehydration and in nephritis various types of casts can be seen together with a number of white and red blood cells.

Epithelial cells. These are found in the urine and are not usually indicative of disease. They are usually found after catheterisation.

Crystals. These are crystals of various salts, e.g. urates and phosphates; they are frequently seen and usually reflect the reaction of the urine and the previous diet, e.g. oxalates following ingestion of strawberries.

FIGLU (formimino-glutamic acid) excretion test

This test is carried out when folic acid deficiency or histidinaemia is suspected. Normally only small quantities of FIGLU are found. Excessive amounts are found in folic acid deficiency, while they are absent in histidinaemia, a congenital defect in which the enzyme histidase is absent.

Method
After fasting overnight, 15 g of 1-histidine mono-hydrochloride are given orally with water. Food is permitted 1 hour later. Three hours after the histidine has been given, the bladder is emptied and the urine is discarded. For the following 2 hours all urine is collected into a bottle containing 1 ml of concentrated hydrochloric acid and some thymol crystals. A pre-test specimen is also required for dilution purposes. The FIGLU is detected by electrophoresis, chromatography or using an enzyme method.

Test for steroids
The 17-ketosteroids are breakdown products of the hormones produced in the adrenal cortex and testis. The 17-ketogenic steroids are derived from the adrenal cortex only and therefore reflect its behaviour more accurately. Steroids of both types may be reduced in pituitary deficiency and are increased in tumours of the adrenal cortex, which causes virilism in females and boys. In the adreno-genital syndrome the 17-ketosteroids show the greater increase.

Method
Urine is collected for 24 hours into a bottle containing 10 ml of concentrated hydrochloric acid.

Abdominal paracentesis

Reason
This is performed to withdraw serous fluid from the peritoneal cavity. Under normal conditions this fluid is produced by the peritoneum and functions as a lubricant to the abdominal viscera. Gross increase of fluid occurs in conditions such as nephrotic syndrome, when the abdomen becomes distended (ascites) leading to respiratory difficulties. The procedure is carried out to relieve pressure symptoms, as a diagnostic measure or to inject various therapeutic agents.

Requirements

1. Dressing pack.
2. Cleansing lotions.
3. Peritoneal catheter with trocar.
4. 1 ml syringe and hypodermic needles (for local anaesthesia).
5. Scalpel and blade.
6. Dissecting forceps.
7. Skin suture needle and silk.
8. Water-repellent sheet.
9. Clip to regulate the flow.
10. Collecting bag.
11. Abdominal binder, safety pins and adhesive tape.
12. Local anaesthetic.
13. Fluid chart.
14. Disposal bag.

Preparation of the child
Sedation is usually given to help allay fear and restlessness. The child is kept in bed supported by two pillows in a position which gives the child the greatest comfort. The bladder must be emptied immediately before the paracentesis is carried out. If the child is unable to pass urine, it will be necessary to catheterise him, to ensure that the bladder is empty. When ascites is present, it is very difficult to feel the distended bladder and there is a danger of puncturing the bladder during the procedure. The child is dressed in warm, light clothing and a water-repellent sheet is placed under him. An abdominal binder is placed in position so that it can be applied as soon as the cannula is inserted.

Method
The procedure is carried out by the doctor under local anaesthesia. The catheter is introduced with the trocar but it may be necessary to make a small incision before introducing the catheter. In this case a skin suture may be inserted when the catheter is in position. The catheter is held in position with a dressing and adhesive tape.

Care during drainage
The drainage is often continued for 24 hours and the amount of fluid drained may be several litres. However, it is important not to withdraw fluid too rapidly or to remove too much at one time, because of the danger of circulatory collapse as the veins of the abdomen become refilled.

Firm pressure is maintained on the abdomen by means of the abdominal binder, which must be adjusted according to the decrease of abdominal distension. The level in the collecting bag is noted and the amount recorded, before the bag is emptied. Throughout the procedure the child must be observed carefully and any change in colour, pulse rate and rhythm and respiratory rate reported to the medical officer.

When the desired amount has been drawn off, the cannula is withdrawn. A suture may be inserted or, if the skin is less tense, a suture plaster may be used to bring the edges of the incision into apposition. The child is then made comfortable and comforted.

If the procedure is repeated, there is considerable loss of body protein and this should be replaced. However, the diet should be suitable to meet the nutritional and therapeutic needs of the child.

Peritoneal dialysis

Reasons

This is a process by which dangerous end-products of protein metabolism, or poisonous substances, can be removed from the body. Normally the kidneys remove these substances, but where renal function is severely impaired, other means, such as peritoneal dialysis, have to be used.

It is indicated in the following conditions:

1. Acute renal failure, particularly if the prognosis is good.
2. Hypertonic dehydration.
3. Drug poisoning, e.g. barbiturates.
4. Hypervolaemic (left) heart failure in culminating acute nephritis.

Principles involved

The patient's blood is separated from the dialysing fluid by a thin membrane, that is the peritoneum, which acts as a semi-permeable membrane. The peritoneum is readily permeable to small molecules, for example glucose, urea, etc. but it does not allow large molecules such as plasma protein and cells to pass through. The effective filtering area of the peritoneum is greater than the area utilised by the kidneys.

Diffusion across such a membrane occurs down the appropriate concentration gradient. For example, in renal failure, the concen-

tration of urea in the blood is high, but it is low in the dialysing fluid, therefore, urea moves from the blood into the peritoneal catheter and collecting bag. Sodium is the same concentration on both side of the membrane and therefore no movement of sodium takes place.

The solutions which are used contain sodium, calcium, magnesium, chloride, lactate and either dextrose 1.5 per cent or 7.0 per cent. The purpose of the more hyperosmolar fluid is to remove more water than is instilled (osmosis), thus removing the danger of water intoxication.

Glucose diffuses into the blood but is rapidly metabolised in the body.

Requirements

1. Dianeal administration set and peritoneal dialysis catheter.
2. 10 ml syringe and intramuscular needles.
3. 2 ml syringe and hypodermic needles.
4. Dressing pack.
5. Skin cleansing solutions.
6. Scalpel blade and handle.
7. Dissecting forceps.
8. Artery forceps.
9. Sterile water.
10. Heparin 5000 i.u. (anticoagulant).
11. Achromycin i.v. 250 mg (anti-microbial).
12. Ampoule of potassium chloride (to titrate against serum potassium).
13. Ampoule of calcium chloride.
14. Ampoule of sodium bicarbonate.
15. Files.
16. Fluid chart.
17. Adhesive tape.
18. Dialysing fluid — bottles must be accurately numbered.
19. Fluid heating coil.
20. Collecting bag.
21. Disposal bags.
22. Containers for specimen.
23. Infusion stand.

Preparation of the child

A simple explanation should be given to the child if he is old enough and conscious. It may be necessary to restrain his arms to prevent him from touching the tubing. Usually a local anaesthetic is given, but sedation may also be necessary to allay fear and restlessness. The child is asked to void urine if able, or he may have to be catheterised. An indwelling catheter may be used. This is important because of the danger of puncturing a distended bladder. The child is dressed in warm, light clothing and a water-repellent sheet is placed under him. He is made comfortable in the supine position.

Method
The skin is prepared with cleansing solution and the area, two-thirds of the way from the symphysis pubis to the umbilicus, is anaesthetised. A small cutaneous incision is made and the peritoneal catheter and introducer are pushed through the peritoneum. The trocar is removed and the catheter is directed into the pelvic gutter, until all the perforations are within the peritoneum. The catheter is then stitched into place. It is sometimes helpful to instil 50 to 150 ml of fluid as soon as the tube is introduced. This makes it easier to move the tube to the optimal position. Substances such as heparin, antibiotic and possibly potassium salts are added to the fluid.

The first bottle is set up on a drip stand and allowed to run into the peritoneal cavity, preferably warmed in a water bath en route. The volume used varies from 250 to 2000 ml according to age. The tubing and bottle are lowered to the floor and most of the fluid is generally recovered, although a small 'pool' may be left. The manoeuvre is repeated and the fluid is returned as soon as it is instilled. It is essential that an accurate chart is maintained, as for example Table 27.2.

Because of the relatively quick cycling, it is possible to improve the uraemic state rapidly and within 36 hours the blood urea should be below 100 mg/100 ml. (Normal values: new-born, 14 to 26 mg/100 ml; child, 20 to 40 mg/100 ml.)

The catheter should be removed after 36 hours and the wound stitched.

Care of the child
The temperature, pulse and respiration should be monitored hourly and any deviation from the normal must be reported. Peritoneal dialysis carries a considerable risk of peritoneal infection, fall in blood pressure and shock.

The room should be warm but overheating should be avoided. Pain and discomfort may be present due to increased volume in the peritoneal cavity and this may also cause respiratory difficulty. An abdominal binder may be applied to support the emptying peritoneal cavity.

Pressure care should also be given carefully because the child tends to remain in the same position for a considerable length of time. During the procedure, dietary treatment is continued according to the condition requiring this treatment, and with good dietary management a further dialysis may not be required for several days or a week. If no further treatment is given the stitches are removed on the 7th or 8th day.

Continuous ambulatory peritoneal dialysis
Peritoneal dialysis can be successfully performed at home. The parents and child (if old enough) will be taught how to apply the drainage equipment. Before leaving the hospital they will have been given the opportunity to set up the procedure, using aseptic technique, and shown how to change a dressing and how to apply the giving set and introduce the fluid.

They will be advised regarding changes required in their home; e.g. a room may have to be altered slightly to accommodate the equipment and should contain a sink and running water. They will also receive printed instructions detailing the procedure

Table 27.2

Time bottle started	Bottle no.	Weight of child (kg)	Volume instilled (a) (ml)	Volume removed (b) (ml)	Balance (a − b)	Overall gain or loss (ml)
10.30 a.m.	1	9.00	500	350	+150	+150
10.55 a.m.	2	9.15	500	620	−120	+30
11.20 a.m. etc.	3	9.03	500	550	−50	−20

and the observations to be made, e.g. colour of return fluid, weighing of the bag containing the return fluid and any action it may be necessary to take. For example, if the fluid is cloudy, the fact must be reported to the medical staff. The following daily observations and measurements will be required:

1. Daily weighing of the child. This should be done early in the morning with the fluid out of the abdomen.
2. The blood pressure should be measured morning and evening.
3. The child's temperature is measured daily and, if elevated, should be reported.
4. Observation of the wound and changing of the dressing every second day.
5. Specimen to be obtained for bacteriological and biochemical testing. If there is exudate from the wound or catheter, then site swabs have to be taken.
6. Observations for signs of peritonitis, e.g. if the return fluid is cloudy, or the child complains of abdominal pain or unusual discomfort and there is a rise in body temperature. The parents are advised to report any of these signs and symptoms to the hospital as quickly as possible.
7. Additional problems which may require investigation include: feeling of fullness, pain on emptying or filling, back pain, swelling of ankles, shoulder pains, breathlessness, faintness, dizziness and weakness.

Although extensive training is required before the parents feel confident to manage the procedure at home, it has been found that this method is preferred by most parents. It allows for greater freedom of movement and the child can live as normal a life as is possible under the circumstances. He can attend school and join in most of the school activities. Support is provided by the home nursing dialysis team and any problems identified can be dealt with at home or arrangements can be made for the admission of the child to hospital.

Haemodialysis

In haemodialysis, the dialysis is conducted outside the patient's body by means of an 'artificial kidney'. This is an electronic system which monitors the flow rate, temperature and contains other controls. A Scribner external shunt is made by connecting an artery to a vein with a loop of Silastic. It is then relatively easy to disconnect the loop and attach the cannulae to the arterial and venous sides of the machine (Fig. 27.10).

For long-term dialysis a subcutaneous arterio-venous fistula is created by sewing an artery in the forearm to a vein. This leads to the enlargement of neighbouring veins which do not thrombose because the blood flow is fast.

Dialysis is performed twice-weekly for periods of 6 to 8 hours.

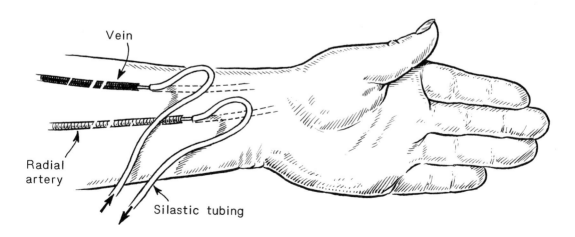

Fig. 27.10 Arterio-venous shunt for haemodialysis.

Immediate post-operative care following formation of fistula or cannulation

1. The limb is elevated to prevent oedema. Immobilisation of the arm for 2 to 3 days is advisable and movement is gradually allowed until activity can be resumed. If the cannulation is in the leg, the child is confined to bed for about 2 weeks with gradually increasing mobility.
2. The blood pressure should be checked hourly in the opposite arm. Prolonged hypotension leads to poor peripheral circulation and causes clotting in the cannula.
3. The flow of blood through the cannula is checked half-hourly by feeling the arterial pulse in the cannula and observing any colour change. If the pulse is absent or there is a colour change, to a more purple shade for example, the cannula must be declotted as soon as possible.
4. Observation of excessive staining is important and should be reported when it is noted.

Declotting of the cannula

This is performed by the medical officer.

Management of the child

1. Continuous weight monitoring is essential. The child is treated while reclining either in a bed or reclining chair which have a weight scale incorporated.
2. Position of the child. The child sits supported by pillows with the shunt arm or leg exposed and resting on sterile covers.
3. Sedation is normally not required but may be given to an anxious or restless child.
4. Psychological care. Although the majority of children accept the frequent treatments reasonably well, there are some who are depressed and require a great deal of support and encouragement. The condition and the restrictions imposed by frequent dialysis produce a great strain on the child and some find it difficult to cope with the situation. He should be allowed to express his fears and if he has difficulty in doing so, then psychiatric help may be useful.
5. Occupational therapy. The child should be occupied. Part of the time can be spent in school work, if he is able, or the play leader or nurses can help him to pass the time by reading to him or finding some game which is suitable for his age and condition.
6. Nutrition. The child receives his normal diet for his condition without extra fluids. It should be remembered that he can only use one hand and therefore food should be cut small enough so that he can manage to feed himself.
7. Prevention of infection. Superficial infections are associated with external arterio-venous shunt. This can be prevented by meticulous skin care. The danger of virus hepatitis can be minimised by limiting blood transfusions and observing the principles of aseptic technique.

Complications arising during dialysis

1. Loss of consciousness. This can occur soon after connection to the dialyser, the child first becoming pale and restless. The medical staff must be notified, the negative pressure should be reduced and the child's head lowered.
2. Convulsions may occur if the child is hypertensive.
3. Poor flow due to kinking of tubing, low blood pressure or a clot in the cannula.
4. High venous pressure, due to obstruction to venous return, e.g. clot, bends or a kink in the tubing.
5. Disconnection from the dialyser.
6. Clotting of the dialyser. This may be due to inadequate heparinisation, inadequate flow through the dialyser or low temperature of dialysate.

Examination of urine

Urine contains all the by-products of body metabolism with the exception of carbon dioxide.

Examination of the urine may reveal valuable information which can be an important source on which to base a diagnosis. Tests should be carried out accurately and if proprietary tests are used, the manufacturer's instructions should be followed.

Urine to be tested must be fresh, as changes in its composition occur when allowed to stand. For example, in glycosuria, the type of sugar alters on standing, and this will affect the result of the test.

It is also important to collect urine in clean receptacles.

General examination

The appearance of the urine is an important indication for specific tests. The colour shows the degree of concentration and depends on the amount voided. Normal urine is yellow-amber, due to the pigment urochrome. The colour varies with the specific gravity — dilute urine is straw-coloured while concentrated urine is highly coloured. Abnormally coloured urine shows the following characteristics:

1. Turbid or smoky urine, may be due to blood, fat droplets or chyle.
2. Red or red-brown urine, is due to presence of red blood cells, blood pigments.
3. Yellow-brown or green-brown, indicates presence of bile.

Volume. The volume of urine passed varies considerably in different age groups and is also dependent on the fluid intake and loss by the various routes (See fluid balance p. 223.)

Reaction (acidity or alkalinity) (pH)

The reaction of the urine reflects the ability of the kidneys to maintain normal hydrogen ion concentration in the plasma and extracellular fluid. Normal reaction is 6 (acid) but is usually within the range of 4.6 to 8.

The reaction is tested with universal test papers when the paper is dipped into the urine and the colour is compared with the colour scale provided. Litmus paper can also be used; when blue litmus paper is dipped into the the urine, it will turn red if the urine is acid.

Specific gravity

This indicates the density of particles in the urine and reflects the concentrating and diluting power of the kidneys. It is measured by floating a urinometer in the urine and reading it at eye level. The urine glass must contain sufficient amount of urine to ensure that the urinometer floats. Normal specific gravity ranges from 1.005 to 1.025.

Where there is a diminished output, as in a febrile state, the specific gravity is found to be high, while it is low when the output is high. The exception to this is in diabetes mellitus, where the output is high and the specific gravity is also high. The is due to the high sugar content.

Odour

Smell is only rarely of value. However, there are some odours which are indicative of some abnormality or disease.

1. The sweet smell of acetone found in patients suffering from diabetes mellitus.
2. Fishy odour, when there is a cystitis.
3. Ammoniacal odour — this develops when urine is allowed to stand and is due to bacterial action on urea.
4. Smell of honey — found in children suffering from phenylketonuria.

Test for chlorides

Normally chlorides are present in urine. Absence denotes chloride deficiency which may be due to loss through excessive vomiting, or to continuous gastric aspiration. Although a more accurate evaluation will be achieved in the biochemical laboratory, it is possible to perform this test at ward level. The test is called the 'Fantus' test.

Requirements

1. Test tube.
2. Pipette.
3. 20 per cent potassium chromate solution.
4. 2.9 per cent silver nitrate solution.
5. Distilled water for rinsing.

Method

1. Rinse the test tube and pipette with distilled water.
2. Place 10 drops of urine in the test tube and rinse the pipette.
3. Add 1 drop of potassium chromate and rinse the pipette.
4. Add silver nitrate drop by drop until a sharp colour change from yellow to reddish-brown occurs. Assessment of amount of chlorides is made by counting the number of drops of silver nitrate necessary for the colour change. This number is equivalent to grams of chloride per litre of urine. The normal range is between 3 and 5. In order to interpret the result, it is also

important to know the amount of urine passed in 24 hours and the specific gravity of the specimen of urine.

Test for protein

1. *Boiling test*

Some units still use this test.

Requirements

1. One test tube and holder.
2. Bunsen burner.
3. Pipette.
4. 10 per cent acetic acid.
5. Filter paper and funnel, if necessary.
6. Litmus paper or universal test papers.

Method

1. Filter urine, if cloudy.
2. Test for reaction; if alkaline, add a few drops of acetic acid.
3. Fill test tube three-quarters full of urine and boil the top 2.5 cm.
4. Compare the boiled upper part with the lower unboiled part. The presence of a white precipitate indicates the presence of albumin.

2. *Esbach's test*

This is a useful test when it is desirable to estimate the quantity of protein in the urine. It is carried out at ward level daily over a period of weeks.

Requirements

1. Urinometer.
2. Esbach's albuminometer and reagent.
3. Litmus paper.
4. 10 per cent acetic acid.
5. Collection of urine over a 24-hour period.

Method

1. The 24-hour collection of urine is well mixed and a sample taken. The specific gravity is read and if it is above 1.010 the urine is diluted with water, and the final result is multiplied by the requisite number of times. The urine must be acid. If it is alkaline a few drops of 10 per cent acetic acid are added until the reaction changes.

2. Pour the urine into the Esbach's tube until it reaches the letter 'U'.
3. Add Esbach's reagent up to the letter 'R'.
4. Lock the tube and invert gently two or three times to ensure thorough mixing of the contents.
5. Place the tube upright in the stand and leave in a constant temperature for 24 hours.
6. The reading is taken at eye level when the depth of the sediment is measured against the scale on the albuminometer. This gives the amount of protein in the urine in parts per thousand, or grams per litre.

The main constituent of the reagent is picric acid, which precipitates the protein.

Rapid screening tests

There are now commercially available a number of paper tapes or stocks impregnated with chemicals designed to test urine rapidly for albumin, glucose, acetone, blood, bilirubin, degree of acidity and the presence of phenylketonuria. Each kit contains instructions and colour charts for each substance being tested. If the Clinistix tape is used and a positive result is obtained, this must be confirmed by laboratory tests.

Clinitest (Ames Co.)

This test is used for the detection of glucose and is the method usually used by patients at home.

Requirements

Kit comprising:

1. Stand with small test tubes.
2. Pipette.
3. Water.
4. Clinitest tablets.
5. Colour chart.

Method

1. Place two drops of urine into a test tube. Rinse the dropper.
2. Add 10 drops of water.
3. Drop in one Clinitest tablet and watch the reaction. Note the 'flush' of orange, if present, as this indicates a percentage of sugar present.
4. Compare colour with the chart to estimate the amount of sugar present.

A fairly accurate quantitative test can be done using Clinitest tablets. If 3+ or less reaction is obtained, the glucose concentration can be estimated (p. 282). If 4+ or higher is obtained, dilute 10 drops of urine in a test tube with 10 drops of distilled water (or any multiple of 10 as necessary). Invert to mix well. Use five drops of this dilution to perform the above Clinitest. If a 4+ result is still obtained, make another separate dilution and repeat. Continue diluting until a 3+ result is obtained.

$$\text{Dilution factor} = \frac{\text{drops of urine} + \text{drops of water}}{\text{drops of urine}}$$

3+ result = 1 per cent sugar = 1 g/100 ml.
Sugar concentration = result × dilution factor.

For the total amount of sugar in a given specimen (e.g. 24-hour urine collection), multiply the concentration by the total volume in ml divided by 100.

Example: 24-hour urine volume of 980 ml
10 drops urine + 20 drops water gives 3+ result
Dilution factor = (10 + 20)/(10) = 3
Sugar concentration = (1 g/100 ml) × 3 = 3 g/100 ml
Total sugar = (3 g/100 ml) × (980 ml/100) = 29.4 g.

Tests for acetone and diacetic acid

1. *Ketostix, Acetest* (Ames Co.) *tablets for using the rapid screening tests*

Requirements

1. Acetest tablets.
2. Paper square.
3. Pipette.
4. Colour chart.

Method

1. Place an Acetest tablet on a clean surface, preferably a piece of white paper.
2. Put one drop of urine on the tablet.
3. Take a reading in 30 seconds and compare the colour of the tablet with the colour chart. Negative, if the tablet remains white; trace — slight purple shade; moderate — positive purple; positive — mauve.

2. *Rothera's test*
This is a very sensitive test.

Requirements

1. Ammonium sulphate crystals.
2. Two per cent sodium nitro-prusside solution, or crystals.
3. Strong ammonia.
4. Test tube.
5. Pipette.

Method

1. Place about 2 cm of ammonium sulphate crystals in the test tube and add 5 ml of urine to make a saturated solution.
2. Add 10 drops of freshly prepared solution of 2 per cent sodium nitro-prusside and mix well. Alternatively, two crystals of sodium nitro-prusside are added and the mixture is shaken well.
3. Ten drops of strong ammonia are run down the side of the test tube.
4. A purple ring will develop at the junction of the two fluids if acetone or diacetic acid is present.

Test for blood
Rapid screening test or haemastix are used.

Test for bilirubin

1. Rapid screening test.
2. *Ictotest.*

Requirements

1. Ictotest reagent tablets.
2. Pipette.
3. Special test mat.

Method

1. Place five drops of urine on a square of the special test mat.
2. Place one tablet on the centre of the moistened area.
3. Put two drops of water on the tablet with the pipette.

Results

A negative reaction shows no bluish colour change within 30 seconds. Any change of colour to pink or red should be ignored. A positive reaction is demonstrated when the mat around the tablet turns bluish-purple within 30 seconds. The amount of bilirubin present is proportional to the speed and intensity of the colour change.

Test for phenylketonuria

Requirements

Phenistix with colour scale.

Method

1. The test end is dipped into the urine and removed immediately or the test end is pressed against the wet napkin.
2. After 30 seconds the colour is compared with the colour chart. A grey to grey-green colour indicates presence and concentration of phenyl-pyruvic acid in the urine. A false positive result yielding a less stable green colour can be due to p-hydroxyphenylpyruvic acid in the urine. To avoid a false negative result the test strip should not be dropped into the urine and left there, nor pressed too firmly or too long against the wet napkin.

Ferric chloride test for phenylketonuria

Requirements

1. Ferric chloride 5 or 10 per cent aqueous solution.
2. Test tube.
3. Pipette.

Method

1. The urine must be acid.
2. Place 5 ml of urine into the test tube.
3. Add a few drops or 5 to 10 per cent ferric chloride. If phenylpyruvic acid is present a green colour will develop within 2 to 3 minutes.

Urine for bacterial counts

A specimen of urine is obtained as described on page 547. The specimen must be transferred to the laboratory immediately or else placed in the refrigerator prior to transfer to the laboratory. If a dip slide is used it must be stored at room temperature until collected or sent to the laboratory. Indication of infection depends on the number of organisms per ml, e.g. under 10 000 organisms per ml indicates absence of infection; 10 000 to 100 000/ml is doubtful; and over 100 000 per ml in three consecutive urine specimens indicates definite infection.

Chapter 28
Disorders of the skin

The skin and its appendages are complex structures which make up the toughest and firmest tissues of the body. Their functions can be affected by damage to the structure as well as by disorders. Since there are many disorders affecting the skin only the more common ones will be discussed here.

The skin consists of two layers: the epidermis, or outer layer, and the dermis, or true skin. There are also appendages to the skin which include the hair and nails.

Epidermis
The epidermis consists of keratinised epithelial cells containing fatty substances which make the skin waterproof. The superficial cells of this stratum are constantly being shed and replaced. Other cells contain an oily fluid. A third layer consists of cells containing granules which are able to refract light and help to give the white colour to the skin. A fourth layer contains cells producing melanin, a substance which acts as a protection against the effects of ultraviolet rays. The epidermis does not contain blood vessels, but lymph circulates in the intercellular spaces.

Dermis
The dermis is composed of fibrous tissue which is more dense in the superficial part than in the inner part. Two layers can be identified: the first contains sensory nerve endings, blood vessels and lymphatics; the second contains collagen fibres, elastic fibres, sebaceous and sweat glands, hair follicles and arrectores muscles.

Hypoderm
This is a transitional zone between the skin and the underlying adipose tissue. It contains fat cells as well as white and yellow connective tissue, coils of some of the sweat glands and the roots of some of the hairs.

The dermis or corium is dependent for its nourishment on the veins and lymphatics. Both myelinated and non-myelinated sensory nerves are found in the skin which contains the end-organs of many nerve fibres. These respond to sensation of heat, cold, pain, itching and light touch.

Sweat glands
Sweat glands consist of a glomerulus or secreting part and a duct. They are relatively richly supplied with blood and secrete sweat which is a slightly turbid, almost colourless fluid, containing some 99 per cent water, and small amounts of chloride, urea, ammonia, uric acid and creatinine. Different types of sweat glands are found in areas such as the genitals, anus, axillae and nipples and each of these also has a distinctive odour.

Appendages
The appendages include hair and nails. Hair is epithelial in origin and is made of modified horny cells, which arise in a complex structure, the follicle, situated in the deeper layers of the dermis. As the hair passes through the superficial layer of the dermis it is lubricated by sebum, which is the excretion of a small gland lying adjacent to the hair shaft. Its function is to lubricate the skin and to keep it supple, to act as a water repellent and to protect the skin from a dry atmosphere.

The nails consist of modified horny cells firmly united. They are formed proximally in the nail matrix. The nail bed consists of somewhat modified prickle cells to which the nail is firmly attached.

The skin owes its colour partly to the blood and partly to various pigments in the epidermis, the chief one being melanin. As an outer covering it has many functions which are not only protective in nature, but also include the following:

1. It acts as a barrier to infection provided it remains intact, but it also can destroy micro-organisms by the action of long-chain fatty acids which are present in the skin. Bacterial invasion can also be retarded by the acidity of the skin.
2. The tough resilient tissue protects the underlying tissue.
3. Skin acts as an insulator (hypoderm) and helps to regulate the body temperature. Control of body temperature is also a function of the sweat glands and the blood vessels. When it is hot, the glands secrete sweat, the evaporation of which causes cooling; the blood vessels dilate to allow loss of body heat, by increasing the flow of blood near the body's surface. When it is cold, the blood vessels constrict, reducing the blood flow and thereby reducing body heat loss.
4. Because it contains sensory nerve endings, sensations from the skin play an important part in the maintenance of health.
5. To a limited extent, the skin acts as an excretory organ removing some of the body's waste products. It therefore plays some part in maintaining fluid and electrolyte balance.
6. Under suitable conditions, the skin supplies vitamin D to the body. This vitamin is formed by the photochemical action of ultraviolet rays on a sterol which is believed to be excreted in the sebum.

Fingerprints

Fingerprints are already formed by the third month of intra-uterine life and these have important application in genetics and medicine. Each individual has his own pattern of fingerprints and this fact is used as a means of identification by the police and in some hospitals. It has also been found that in some genetic defects there are abnormal handprints or footprints. For example, in Down's syndrome (mongolism), looped fingerprints are more frequent than usual, and in Turner's syndrome there are more ridges than normal.

The skin of the newborn infant

The skin of the newborn infant is covered by a greasy substance, the vernix caseosa, which is an exaggeration of the normal protective mantle found on the skin of the adult. This substance is produced by the action of maternal sex hormones which stimulate secretion from the glands of the infant's skin. The effect of these hormones lasts for a few months after birth, but the baby's own skin glands remain relatively inactive until puberty.

The vernix should be allowed to wear off or to be removed gradually. When the skin is clear of vernix, the infant can be bathed using a good soap and drying the skin gently. Drying can be further enhanced by using a fine talcum powder. Some babies are born with a dry skin. This appears to be an inherited affection, where there is an excess of horny layer and often fewer and less active sweat glands than in normal skin.

Terminology in dermatological conditions

Many different forms of lesions are described in dermatological states which define specific disorders. These can be divided into those which do not break the skin (*primary lesion*) and those which do break the skin (*secondary lesion*).

Primary lesions

Macules
These are alterations in the colour of the skin. They vary in size and shape, and appear as stains in the skin. Macules are formed from:

1. Deposits of pigments in the skin, e.g. freckles.
2. Escape of blood into the skin, e.g. petechiae.
3. Permanent dilatation of capillary blood vessels, e.g. naevi.
4. Transitory dilatation of capillary blood vessels, e.g. erythema.

Papules
These are palpable elevations of the skin varying in diameter from about 1 to 5 mm. Their surfaces may be pointed, round or flat. They are superficial

and are formed by proliferation of the cells or exudation of fluids into the skin.

Nodules

These are similar to papules but are more deep-seated in the skin. They vary in size and are usually larger than papules. An example of subcutaneous nodules are the nodes of acute rheumatism.

Vesicles

Vesicles are small blisters formed by accumulation of fluid in the epidermis; they are usually filled with serous fluid and are present in children suffering from eczema.

Bullae or pustules

Bullae are large vesicles which may contain serum, pus or blood. They are found, for example, in pemphigus neonatorum.

Wheal

A wheal is a transient elevation of the skin caused by oedema of the dermis and surrounding capillary dilatation. It is usually associated with an allergic response to some foreign agent.

Secondary lesions

Scales

Scales are heaped up horny layers of dead epidermis, which may develop as a result of inflammatory changes. These are found in psoriasis.

Crusts

These are formed from serum, blood or pus drying on the skin. Each can be recognised by the following colours:
Red-black (blood crusts)
Yellow-green (pus crusts)
Honey-coloured (serum crusts)

Fissures

These are small cracks extending through the epidermis and exposing the dermis. They may occur in dry skin and in chronic inflammation.

Ulcers

Ulcers are lesions formed by local destruction of the whole of the epidermis and part or all of the underlying corium.

General principles in the treatment of skin disorders

The aim of treatment is to preserve or restore the physiological state of the skin. Topical treatment is often preferred because medication can be delivered in optimal concentration at the exact site where it is needed.

Water plays an important part and is found in many solutions and lotions. When the skin is hydrated, it is soft and smooth and to remain in that state, the environmental humidity must be adequate (approximately 60 per cent). If it falls, the stratum corneum shrinks and cracks; the epidermal barrier is lost and micro-organisms and irritants enter, inducing an inflammatory response. Overhydration can also occur, when the amount of water absorbed increases and the tight lipid junctions between the cells of the stratum corneum are gradually replaced by water. This can occur on napkin areas, axillae, etc.

The bases for topical preparations are:

1. Liquids:
   a. As wet dressings when they can relieve itching.
   b. With powder, when they are used as drying pastes.
   c. With oil, when they are used as vanishing cream. This penetrates quickly and allows for evaporation.
   d. Excess grease and emulsifier. Water in oil acts as emollient cream which penetrates more slowly and thereby retains moisture on the skin.
2. Oils. As ointments; these hold material on the skin for a prolonged time and prevent evaporation of water.
3. Powders. These enhance evaporation.

Many bases are used as vehicles for medication, such as lotions or ointments that serve more than one function. For example, topical adrenocorticosteroid agents have an anti-inflammatory action.

Disorders of the skin

Infantile and childhood eczema

Eczema is a term that describes any inflammatory dermatosis which is characterised by erythema, papules, vesicles, oozing, crusting and scaling in various phases of resolution. It involves the epidermis and the cutaneous vascular layer.

Inflammation is due to some irritant within the body leading to eruptions. These emanate from the capillaries. Mild cases present only with erythema and scaling but there are often vesicles and oozing (weeping wells).

There appears to be a strong hereditary factor and the condition recurs throughout life. It is also believed to be an allergic disorder. (An allergy is defined as an altered reaction of the tissues in certain individuals on exposure to agents which, in similar amounts, are innocuous to other persons.) The mechanism involved is believed to be as follows: (a) there is liberation of histamine, a powerful substance that causes smooth muscle contraction, capillary dilatation and a fall in blood pressure; (b) liberation of other substances, e.g. acetylcholine; and (c) reaction between allergens and an antibody (p. 234).

Eczema seldom appears before the second or third month of life and most cases clear spontaneously by the second or third birthday. It is more common in artificially-fed infants than in breast-fed infants.

Clinical features

Skin lesions initially appear on cheeks, forehead and scalp, but are also found on the flexor surfaces of arms and legs. Later they spread to the entire skin surface. They are very itchy and most skin changes result from scratching, rubbing and excoriation.

Principles of treatment and nursing management

1. To promote healing:
   a. Prevention of infection by isolation.
   b. Prevention of scratching by applying protective devices but not restraining the child excessively. Finger-nails should be kept short. Cotton hand mitts can be applied to the young infant.
   c. Sedation is often given to prevent scratching but should not cause drowsiness.
   d. Antihistamines are given to relieve the itchiness.
   e. Local application of hydrocortisone or corticosteroid creams are very effective. If the baby is severely affected, he can be encased in cotton bandages impregnated with the cream. The bandages may be left on for as long as a week. Older children obtain relief by applying corticosteroid (Synalar) cream to the affected lesions, but this may be absorbed through the skin.
   f. Antibiotics may be given to treat any concurrent infections.
2. Routine nursing care:
   a. Bathing — this involves the use of prescribed methods, e.g. oil may be advocated if the skin is dry and crusted.
   b. Care of the eyes. Eyes are often sticky and should be washed gently with warm saline (p. 339).
   c. Care of the napkin area and frequent napkin changes.
   d. Feeding. Normal feeds are given for the age and weight of the infant, however, if the food is believed to be the cause, then an elimination diet is prescribed, i.e. gradual introduction of food and observation of the effect.
   e. Importance of establishing a calm and loving atmosphere. Rejection can easily occur and every effort must be made not to make the child feel unwanted.
3. Support for the parents. It is often difficult for them to accept their child and be loving, but with the support from the nursing staff, they should learn how to handle him, apply ointments and also learn to accept that some form of immobilisation will be required. This support should also include community care and frequent follow-up visits either to the hospital or local clinic.

Impetigo

Impetigo is a staphylococcal infection. It starts as a small blister which dries quickly to form a scab with a moist red spreading margin. In the newborn baby it presents a pemphigus neonatorum where it is frankly bullous. As pemphigus neonatorum, it is a notifiable disease in the United Kingdom.

Principles of treatment and nursing management
1. The new-born infant should be isolated (p. 250).
2. Drugs. Antibiotics are given orally and they may also be applied locally.
3. Management of the lesions. Scabs and crusts should not be removed as healing takes place beneath them. The only exception is when the impetigo is superimposed on some other condition, such as scabies. The scabs can then be removed by applying a starch poultice every 15 minutes for 1 hour.

   The poultice is made by adding boiling water slowly to 30 g of corn starch, stirring until the whole gels. This is allowed to cool a little and is then spread on lint and is covered with a layer of gauze. The poultice is applied to the affected area and is bandaged in position. Another useful method is to dress with Lassar's paste. The paste is spread on lint and bandaged into position. It is changed once or twice a day.

   The scabs can be removed without damaging the underlying tissue.
4. Routine nursing care.
5. Support for the parents. This support aims at helping the parents to understand the cause and give guidance with regard to prevention and future care.

Psoriasis
Psoriasis is fairly common in children. It is a functional disorder which tends to be inherited.

Clinical features
The individual lesions are sharply defined. They are salmon-red in colour, surmounted by a heap of silvery scales. It chiefly affects the elbows, knees and scalp, but can occur anywhere. The condition may be precipitated by infection such as tonsillitis; emotional stress also appears to be a predisposing factor.

Investigations
Diagnosis by inspection is rarely difficult. It may, however, be confused with conditions such as seborrhoeic dermatitis or fungal infection. If any doubt exists then a skin biopsy can be performed.

Principles of treatment and nursing management
1. The aim is to achieve complete clearance, particularly of the first attack.
2. Local treatment:
   a. Dithranol paste — this is applied after a medicated bath has been given, e.g. tar. Lassar's paste with 0.5 per cent dithranol is applied to the lesions. This paste should not ooze beyond the lesions because it is activated on contact with the skin, producing an inflammatory reaction which removes the psoriasis. Treatment is repeated daily, the bath preventing a severe reaction to the dithranol. Areas which are sensitive, such as the face and scalp, can be treated with corticosteroid, but the cream should not be covered with occlusive polythene dressings because of the danger due to absorption of the drug.

      Sunlight or ultraviolet light (artificial) will produce some improvement. Bathing with tar at night, followed by ultraviolet light the next day, may be sufficient in mild cases (tar makes the skin more sensitive to light). In very severe cases, methotrexate may be given. It is believed to act by interfering with the rapid proliferation of epidermal cells. Since it is potentially toxic, haematological, renal and hepatic function must be monitored carefully.
3. Routine nursing care also includes scalp care. Special ointment is used on the scalp if lesions are present and this is removed with tar shampoo.
4. Support for the child and parents. For the older child and the adolescent, the lesions can cause embarrassment and emotional stress. The condition and treatment should be explained fully and the child as well as the parents encouraged to discuss their problems with medical and nursing staff. The parents must be shown how to apply the paste and continue the treatment at home. There should be liaison between hospital, home and the community health service so that hospitalisation can be kept to a minimum.

Scabies

Scabies is caused by the parasite *Sarcoptes scabiei*. The pregnant female burrows into the horny layer of the epidermis. Here she lays a few eggs daily which hatch out to give a multitude of immature mites which feed in the orifices of the secretory glands.

The burrows appear as whitish lines of irregular outline, at the end of which is the site of the mite. Burrows are found in flexures, between fingers, on the genitals and on the face in babies.

The condition is transmitted by intimate, warm contact and tends to affect the whole family.

Clinical features

Itchiness is a cardinal sign and on examination the above picture will be found. Scratching causes bleeding and infection superimposes the infestation.

Principles of treatment and nursing management

1. Local treatment:
   a. A warm bath is given and the skin is scrubbed using a rough flannel.
   b. After drying the skin, benzyl benzoate emulsion is applied by hand to every part of the skin, from the neck to the toes. The room should be warm and the emulsion allowed to dry before dressing the child.
   c. The child is not washed again for 48 hours; if the hands are washed, the emulsion is reapplied.
   d. A second treatment may be required.
2. The whole family has to be treated and this is usually carried out as outpatients. This involves the community health service and their task is to ensure that the parents understand the cause and how to prevent this condition from reoccurring. Guidance should be given for personal hygiene, if this is required, and it may be necessary to involve the social services, e.g if there is overcrowding in the home.

Acne

Acne is a disease of the sabaceous follicles — those follicles that have abundant sebaceous glands and lack of hair. The openings of the sebaceous glands are blocked by horny plugs (blackheads) and there is retention of sebum which is altered by organisms leading to inflammation of the surrounding tissues. This leads to pustule formation and abscesses resulting in scarring. This condition affects young adolescents causing much embarrassment and unhappiness.

Principles of treatment

1. The patient is generally treated as an outpatient. Guidance is given regarding cleanliness of the skin and the type of soap to use. Girls are advised against the use of cosmetics and face creams, since many cause low-grade acne.
2. Antibiotics are given to diminish the activity of skin bacteria. Tetracycline is concentrated in sebum and is useful in reaching the affected areas.
3. Ultraviolet light is also effective, though the mechanism is not clearly understood.

Congenital abnormalities

The infant is born with structural abnormalities. Some may be obvious from birth, others appear soon after birth. Both epidermal and dermal layers can be affected.

Abnormalities of the epidermal layer include papillomata, pigmentary macular lesions and these may be associated with moles or more extensive pigmented hairy naevi. In the dermis, there may be fibromata, neuromata and lipomata. Vascular naevi are, however, more common and these include:

1. Spider naevus. This is a dilatation of a small arteriole and its capillary tributaries. They often disappear spontaneously but can be destroyed by diathermy or phenol; the latter is applied with a pointed probe.
2. Port-wine stain. This is a dark red or purple macule. It is a diffuse dilatation of all the normal capillaries of the affected tissue in depth. It may also involve underlying organs, such as the eye and brain. There is no treatment, but cosmetic coverings can be used.
3. Strawberry haemangioma. This lesion is often present at birth. It appears as a red, rubbery nodule with a roughened surface. Both capillary and venous elements are involved. Strawberry haemangioma usually resolves, leaving only redundant skin and treatment is rarely necessary.

Chapter 29
Disorders of the skeletal-muscular system

This chapter discusses disorders affecting the bones and muscles. These disorders can be due to congenital abnormalities. The child is born with either some structural or functional abnormality, or alternatively, he can acquire it through trauma or infection. The latter involves injuries, such as fractures and dislocations or changes in bone structures.

Growth and development of bony tissues

The growth and anatomical development of the skeleton shows three important features:

1. Bony tissue develops from its embryonic beginnings from the mesenchymal cells or from a cartilagenous model via enchondral ossification. The latter is very active during prenatal life and persists until adulthood.
2. Bony tissue is subject to continuous remodelling throughout life, a balance being struck between osteogenesis (which is continuous) and osteolysis and osteoclastic resorption (bone destruction). Remodelling is also present during the period of development and it facilitates alterations of length and shape and structure. Later this remodelling adapts the bony tissue to its mechanical needs and to the effects of damage.
3. Bony tissue is strongly mineralised. Throughout the various developmental stages, mineral content plays an important part in the regulation of the equilibrium between the extra-cellular phosphate and calcium, while it is also very susceptible to the endocrine and nutritional factors impinging on these metabolic pathways. For example, vitamin A is necessary for the metabolism of cartilage and bone cells and its deficiency affects growth to varying degrees depending on age and conditions;

vitamin C is essential for new bone formation; deficiency leads to sparse vessels and few osteoblasts as well as a decrease in the amount of soluble collagen: vitamin D is necessary for the process of calcification.

Primary ossification commences at the beginning of the 8th week of embryonic life. After the rudimentary pattern is established primary bone can be recognised along the middle third in a long bone and gradual changes are seen in structure, weight and density.

Functions of bones

Bones provide the central axis and give form to the body. Many are adapted to give support to the weight of the body. They may fulfil some other functions, for examples, the thigh bones (femurs) support the weight of the body on standing, walking and running. They also act as levers which are essential for locomotion. Other bones give protection to the underlying structures, for example, the skull protects the brain; the sternum and ribs protect the heart and lungs. Other bones provide attachments for muscles and levers for speedy and efficient movements. For lever actions, bones are connected to each other by movable joints and movement is produced by muscle action.

Functions of joints

A joint or articulation is formed when two or more bones of the skeleton meet one another. In long bones the ends are the parts which form the joints, in flat bones the joints are formed at the edges and in short and irregular bones, joints may form at various parts of the surfaces (for example carpal bones).

The function of a joint is the most important

factor in determining its character and structure. In a situation where little or no movement is required between the bones, the union is of a fibrous nature, for example in the skull, or by cartilage forming a cartilaginous joint, for example in the vertebra. Where a wider range of movement is necessary, a cavity bond by a fibrous articular capsule intervenes between the bones, and a synovial joint results, for example in the knee joint.

The extent and direction of the possible movement vary in each joint and are related to the closeness and form of the opposing bones, the nature and density of the intervening tissues, the form and attachment of the ligaments surrounding it and the activity of the muscles acting on it.

Muscles

The formation of the muscle fibre syncytium with its complex system of contractile proteins involves a series of cellular interactions and biosynthetic processes which are unique in that tissue. Skeletal muscle derives from the primitive mesoderm and by the 3rd week of gestation segments begin to form. The first myotube can be recognised at about the 5th week.

The establishment of neural contacts on the fibres of developing muscles represents a critical stage in muscle development. Nerve branches ramify among the developing muscle during the 10th week and myoneural junctions begin to form during the 11th week of intra-uterine life.

The growth of skeletal muscles results both from an increase in the number of muscle fibres and from an increase in size of individual muscle fibres. The greatest increase in numbers occurs in early fetal life. The growth of muscle fibres in the late fetal, early neonatal and postnatal periods appears to be related to functional requirements.

Congenital disorders of the neuromuscular system are not uncommon and range from absence of single muscles to widespread involvement of most of the skeletal muscles of the body. Although the clinical manifestations and the muscle pathology in some of the disorders are well described, there is little knowledge of their cause. In some of these conditions hereditary factors appear to be responsible for the abnormality of muscle differentiation.

Types and functions of muscles

There are three varieties of muscle tissues: (1) striped or voluntary; (2) unstriped or involuntary; and (3) cardiac muscle. In this chapter, the skeletal, striped or voluntary muscles only will be discussed.

In order that a muscle may exercise its function of producing movement, the muscle must be attached at both of its extremities. When a muscle contracts, one of its attachments remains relatively stationary while the other is approximated to it.

Most skeletal muscles are attached to bony structures. One of the bones to which a muscle is attached is usually held more or less stationary by the other muscles. The prime mover is therefore provided with a fixed point for its contraction. The attachment of the muscle is usually called its 'origin'. The other extremity of the muscle, especially of a limb muscle, is usually attached to a bone which moves upon some type of joint when the muscle contracts; this attachment is called the 'insertion'.

In accordance with these definitions, the contraction of a muscle results in the approximation of its insertion to its origin, but the terms are arbitrary and used for convenience only. It frequently happens that the contraction of a muscle may result in the approximation of its origin to its insertion.

The voluntary muscles are attached to the bones, cartilages, ligaments, skin or to other muscles directly or through the medium of fibrous structures called tendons. Most muscles are provided with tendons at one or both extremities.

Postnatal growth of skeletal muscle

Fully differentiated muscle fibres are highly specialised cells and do not normally multiply nor are new muscle fibres differentiated after early fetal life. Skeletal muscles, however, grow in parallel with the region which they occupy. This is accomplished by enlargement of the individual fibres. During growth in length, this occurs at the end of the muscle. Active contraction and passive elongation are powerful postnatal growth stimuli. If the distance through which a muscle shortens during movement is artificially increased or decreased, then growth in length is increased or diminished. Immobilisation of a muscle in a shortened position leads to decreased growth in length, as does enervation. Increase in the work which a muscle has to perform stimulates growth in its girth.

Recognition of these features of muscle growth and activity have important implications when considering treatment and nursing management of children with skeletal abnormalities or injuries.

Aspects of orthopaedic surgery

Bone is a constantly growing tissue and is moulded by the periosteum which is firmly attached to its surface. Most long bones consist of a diaphysis (shaft of the bone) and epiphysis (end of the bone) at each end.

At birth, the ends of the bones are made of cartilage and are gradually converted into bone as growth proceeds. A special plate of cartilage between the epiphysis and diaphysis, called the epiphyseal plate, is the site of continuous growth by which the bone achieves its adult length. Between the ages of 15 and 20 years, the epiphyseal plate stops producing new bone and the epiphysis fuses to the shaft.

During the growth years the normal strains and stresses of weight-bearing may lead to unequal growth and subsequent deformity, especially if the bone suffers injury (trauma or infection). Damage, such as bone softening can occur due to lack of vitamin D (rickets.). In the use of splints and during exercise, abnormal strains may be placed deliberately on the epiphyseal lines to alter the growth of the bone artificially and thereby correct deformity. Once puberty has been reached, deformity can only be corrected by surgery, which may also be necessary when the bone deformity is congenital.

Although bone has a rich blood supply from its periosteum and marrow cavity, it has very little resistance to micro-organisms. Tendons and joints are similarly susceptible to infection, the effect of which may be permanent damage.

Skeletal defects

Skeletal defects can occur in fetal life and also after birth. For the majority there is no treatment, but for some, treatment may be surgery, splintage or manipulation, depending on the associated symptoms, for example, respiratory difficulties due to compression of the brain stem or due to funnel chest deformities.

Many skeletal defects are believed to be due to mutant genes. When the mutant is not lethal, it may be transmitted to the offspring. Other conditions may be due to defective development, while changes in chemical and physical structure of the bone can be due to factors such as trauma, nutritional inadequacy, metabolic abnormality, endocrine malfunction, neurological disorders, infections, circulatory deficiency and mechanical defects. For example, increase in circulation as seen in inflammation (rheumatoid arthritis) may cause increased growth in length; while interference with nerve supply leads to retardation of growth.

The congenital deformities which will be discussed include: talipes equino-varus, talipes calcaneo-valgus, genu varum, genu valgum and congenital dislocation of the hip. The acquired conditions include: fractures and dislocations, Perthes' disease, kyphosis and scoliosis.

CONGENITAL DEFORMITIES

Some of the deformities can be seen in relation to the position which the fetus occupies in the uterus. At first the fetus floats freely, but as it grows its movements are more restricted and it assumes a more comfortable position. It has been suggested that the resulting pressure may be partly responsible in deformities such as talipes and asymmetries.

Talipes equino-varus

The term means 'foot or ankle like that of a horse'. This is the most frequent deformity in which the foot is in plantar flexion and deviates medially,

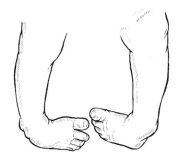

Fig. 29.1 Talipes equino-varus.

that is the deformity is concave to the midline of the body (Fig. 29.1). It may be due to hereditary factors or due to intra-uterine moulding and may be unilateral or bilateral. Three main deformities can be recognised:

1. Equinos at the ankle (the heel lies to the inner side of the midline of the ankle).
2. Inversion of the foot.
3. Adduction (drawing towards) of the forefoot.

Principles of treatment and nursing management

1. Correction of the deformity:
   a. Manipulation, which is started soon after birth and repeated at weekly or fortnightly intervals, and continued by the parents.
   b. Application of Denis Browne splints (p. 598).
   c. Wearing of special boots, i.e. once the child can stand, the outer part of the boots are raised.
   d. Wearing of night boots.
2. If there is a relapse:
   a. Manipulation under general anaesthesia.
   b. Soft tissue release operation, e.g. posterior capsulotomy and lengthening of the Achilles tendon.
   c. Plaster of Paris.
3. Routine nursing care.
4. Pre- and post-operative care:
   a. Routine (pp. 128 and 131).
   b. Specific, e.g. care of the plaster (p. 592).
5. Support for parents. Any deformity causes anxiety and initially repulsion The defect and the recommended treatment must be explained to them, particularly the role they can play in ensuring that correction is achieved. For example, they must be shown how to manipulate the foot, apply the boots and if special shoes are required they must be given clear instructions regarding reconstruction and maintenance of the shoes. Since treatment is over a prolonged period, involving perhaps financial burdens, the social services department may also be involved.

Talipes calcaneo-valgus (Fig. 29.2)
Talipes calcaneo-valgus is the term applied when there is excessive dorsiflexion of the ankle, where

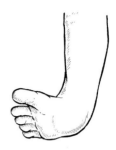

Fig. 29.2 Calcaneo-valgus.

the foot is in valgus (convex to the midline). It is believed to be caused by intra-uterine moulding, particularly during the later stages of pregnancy.

Principles of treatment and nursing management

1. Correction of the deformity:
   a. Manipulation.
   b. Fixation with plaster of Paris.
2. Routine nursing care.
3. Specific nursing care, e.g. care of the infant in a plaster (p. 592).
4. Support for parents. Parents can usually be reassured that the treatment will be effective. The majority of cases are corrected within a relatively short time, e.g. a few weeks, and there is little tendency to relapse.

Genu varum (bow-legs)
This condition occurs late in the first and second years of life. The lower leg looks bowed due to soft tissue outline, but the bones are straight. It can be seen more readily in fat children. If no other cause such as rickets is found, then the deformity will correct spontaneously.

Genu valgum (knock-knees)
This deformity occurs in the 2 to 6 years age group. It can be recognised in the standing child, when his knees touch and the medial malleoli are no more than 3 to 5 cm apart.

Principles of treatment and nursing management

1. Rickets should be excluded first; if the deformity is mild, no treatment is necessary.
2. In more severe cases it may be necessary to

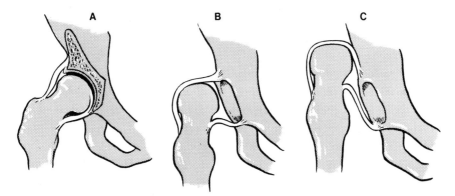

Fig. 29.3 Congenital dislocation of the hip. A, Normal. B, Soon after birth. C, Untreated at 3 years of age.

perform a tibial osteotomy, i.e. a division of the bone, allowing it to heal in a corrected position.
3. Routine nursing care.
4. Specific nursing care:
   a. Pre- and post-operative care, the latter usually includes plaster care (p. 592).

Congenital dislocation of the hip (Fig. 29.3)
Congenital dislocation of the hip occurs when the upper rim of the acetabulum fails to develop and there is malposition of the head of the femur. It is also believed that the hip is unstable at birth and the head of the femur dislocates either partially or completely. The incidence of this condition is 1.5/1000 live births with a female — male ratio of 5:1. There also appears to be a definite geographical distribution, the incidence being high in northern Italy, Brittany, the United Kingdom and Scandinavia. The condition can be unilateral or bilateral.

Anatomical appearance
The femoral head lies above and lateral to the acetabulum. As a result the capsule and ligamentus teres become elongated and also narrowed, producing an 'hour-glass' formation. The femoral head presses on the lateral acetabular brim, which becomes deformed downwards, producing a band narrowing the superior part of the acetabulum called the limbus. Because the femoral head has ridden up, there is adaptive shortening in the muscles, particularly the psoas and the adductor muscles.

Clinical features
The deformity can be detected at birth by Ortolani's test (Fig. 29.4), i.e. the flexed hip is abducted and the head of the femur slips into the acetabulum with a thud. The following features can be elicited:

1. Asymmetry of the gluteal folds (Fig. 29.5).
2. Limited ability to abduct the leg(s):
   a. Abduction is limited on the affected side to no more than 45° when the infant is lying on his back with his knees and hips flexed.

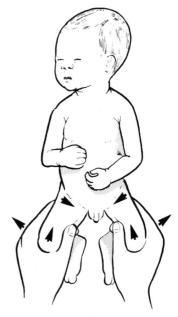

Fig. 29.4 Test for congenital dislocation of hip in the newborn.

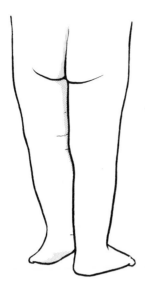

Fig. 29.5 Appearance of asymmetry of the skin, creases of the thigh.

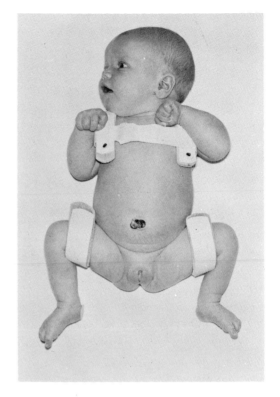

Fig. 29.6 Divaricator (Barlow's) front view.

    b. An audible click can be heard when abduction is forced.
3. If the deformity was not detected in the neonate, Trendelenburg's test can be applied to the older child when the following can be recognised. The pelvis drops on the normal side when the child stands on his affected leg and there is shortening of that leg.
4. There is delayed walking, and when it occurs it is with a limp.
5. In bilateral cases, the legs appear too short for the body, the perineum is broadened and the trochanters are prominent.

Principles of treatment and nursing management

1. Treatment is important at any age but will be more effective the earlier it is begun:
    a. *Birth to 3 months* (approx.). In the newborn infant with ligament laxity and 'dislocatable' hips, simply maintaining the thighs in abduction is sufficient to ensure a good result. The baby lies with his hips in full flexion and abduction (frog position). Abduction may be achieved by a variety of soft or rigid devices, ranging from bulky nappies and canvas slings to formal braces. Examples of splints are: Barlow's divaricator (Figs. 29.6 and 29.7), Craig and von Rosen

splints or Pavlik harness. This position can be maintained for 8 to 12 weeks. The infant can be nursed at home once the parents have been shown how to apply the device and are confident about doing so.
    b. *6 months to 1 year* (approx.). If the diagnosis is delayed, persistent dislocation causes abnormal femoral head and acetabular development. A frog plaster will be applied following manipulation and external rotation. This is reviewed in about 6 weeks. The child can be nursed at home and the parents will have been shown how to protect the plaster with a plastic adhesive so that it can be cleaned when required. The nappy is tucked under the plaster.
    c. *1 to 3 years*. Closed reduction is performed and the child is placed on an abduction frame for 3 to 4 weeks. Skin extensions are applied to both legs. Traction allows free movement and stretches the adductor tendons. The hips are abducted daily until

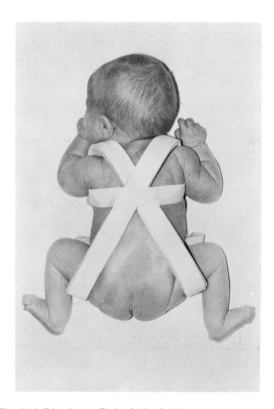

Fig. 29.7 Divaricator (Barlow's) back view.

70° of abduction is obtained. Cross-traction band is applied over the upper part of the thigh and a 2 lb weight is attached.

When the X-ray shows a satisfactory reduction, the child is placed in the frog position with the hips abducted at 60 to 90°. The situation is reassessed after 6 weeks. If the hip fails to reduce, a general anaesthetic is given and an arthrogram is performed to demonstrate an obstruction. This obstruction will have to be removed surgically.

d. *4 to 6 years.* For this age group, a high Pugh traction (p. 594) will be required and this is followed by open reduction. This involves pelvic osteotomy with femoral rotation. Further traction will be applied at low tilt to an angle of 45° and is maintained for 2 to 3 weeks.

e. *Older children.* For older children, reconstruction of the hip joint will be necessary. The child is placed on traction first and, following the reconstruction, a hip spica is applied and left on for 4 weeks.

2. Pre- and post-operative care:
   a. Routine (pp. 128 and 131).
   b. Specific, related to care of the child in a plaster cast (p. 592).
3. Routine nursing care.
4. Specific nursing care:
   a. Problems of children who are immobilised (p. 588).
   b. Play activity.
   c. Educational needs for the young child.
5. Support for parents:
   a. Recognition of their problems, with clear explanations of the initial and subsequent treatments.
   b. Co-ordination of hospital and community services to help with the physical set-up of the home and, where necessary, financial support.
   c. Need to ensure that the child and parents maintain contact with the hospital for frequent evaluation. This is important, to prevent complications in adulthood when the hips may become painful and stiff.

INFECTION AND ACQUIRED DISORDERS OF THE BONE AND JOINT

Infection of the bone and joint is transmitted via the bloodstream from a primary source elsewhere in the body, for example, throat infection, boils, etc.

Septic arthritis

The hip or knee joint are common areas to be affected. The child is ill with a high fever and a hot swollen joint which is painful on movement. This condition can be caused by organisms such as pneumococcus, staphylococcus, meningococcus or streptococcus.

Principles of treatment and nursing management
(see also treatment for osteomyelitis)

1. Appropriate antibiotic.
2. Routine nursing care.
3. Aspiration of exudate.
4. Resting of the affected part.

Osteomyelitis

Osteomyelitis is an inflammatory process involving the vascular part of a long bone. Abscess formation occurs and there is intense hyperaemia. If left untreated the infection spreads to the medulla and eventually out of the bone beneath the periosteum. The infected bone may die and form sequestra (dead bone that remains within the tissues). New bone grows and tends to form an encasement around the sequestra (involucrum). Eventually this may be punctured by numerous channels or sinuses through which pus escapes and reaches the surface.

Clinical features

The onset is often sudden following some infection. There is fever and localised pain. The child is obviously ill and reluctant to move the limb. The common sites are long bones such as the femur, tibia, humerus and radius.

Investigations

Isolation of the responsible organism by:
1. Obtaining a blood culture (in osteomyelitis).
2. Aspiration of the joint in septic arthritis. (The causative organisms may be *Straphylococcus aureus*, which is resistant to penicillin. In neonates, it may be coliforms and haemophilus.)

Principles of treatment and nursing management

1. Antibiotic therapy:
   a. Initially 'blind', i.e. before the result of the culture has been obtained, e.g. cloxacillin, erythromycin.
   b. Antibiotic on the basis of the bacteriological result.
2. Surgical intervention, e.g. release of pus, if necessary.
3. Pre-operative preparation (p. 128).
4. Post-operative management.
   a. Care of splint (p. 589).
   b. Wound care.
   c. Sedation for the relief of pain.
5. Routine nursing care:
   a. Bed-rest.
   b. Play.
   c. Schooling.
6. Support for parents. This involves recognition of their anxiety and guidance as to treatment and nursing care of the child. Treatment may be prolonged and parents can play a very active part in caring for the child.

Perthes' disease

Perthes' disease, also called Legg-Calvé-Perthes' disease or Coxa Plana, is a local disorder involving the femoral head in a process of aseptic necrosis. It occurs mainly in boys between the ages of 3 and 10 years. Unilateral hip involvement is most common, with bilateral incidence in 10 per cent of cases. The cause is unknown, though trauma is believed to be at least partly responsible.

Clinical features

There is a history of a gradual onset of pain in the hip. The pain is usually referred to the knee. A limp is always present, there is limited abduction and rotation of the hip and there is moderate muscle spasm. Four stages can be recognised and each influences the treatment to be followed:

Stage 1 (aseptic necrosis). The femoral head is damaged and there is soft tissue swelling.
Stage 2 (revascularisation). The femoral head increases in density and there are changes in the epiphysis, e.g. mottling can be seen on X-ray.
Stage 3 (reossification). New bony tissue is being formed and dead bone is removed.
Stage 4 (recovery). The head of the femur is either more flattened and some displacement persists or the head of the femur remains spherical.

Investigations

1. Joint aspirations tend to be normal.
2. Radiography. The early findings include effusion of the joint associated with widening of the joint space and periarticular swelling. Later X-rays show decreased density of the bone in and around the joint. There is also collapse or narrowing of the femoral head.

Principles of treatment and nursing management

The aim of treatment is to avoid as much femoral head distortion as possible. In the early stages, synovitis and spasm are present and can be relieved by a period in traction. The following methods can be used:

1. Pugh's traction. Skin traction is applied to each leg (p. 594).
2. Abduction frame (p. 589) (Fig. 29.8).
3. Snyder sling.
4. Use of braces such as the Toronto brace, Birmingham brace and Atlanta brace. Such braces permit limited weight-bearing, but present limitations to independent locomotion on stairs or when walking for long distances. All of them produce some form of abduction which provides a good environment for femoral head containment by positioning the lower limbs (Fig. 29.9).
5. Surgery. Derotational osteotomy whereby centering of the affected femoral head is achieved.
   a. Pre-operative management (p. 128).
   b. Post-operative care (p. 131).
6. Routine nursing care.
7. Specific care in relation to traction treatment, e.g. pressure area care and maintaining traction (p. 593).
   a. Occupation and play for the child.
   b. Educational facilities.
8. Advice to parents regarding home care of the

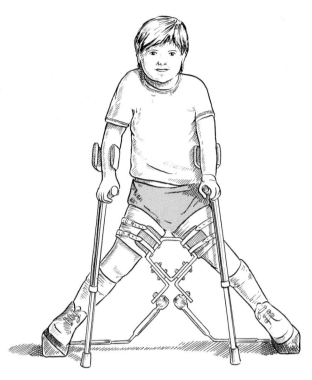

Fig. 29.9 Toronto splint.

child with braces. Before the child returns home the parents must be shown how to apply the brace and be able to do so. Frequent follow-up visits to the hospital will be necessary. If the child is of school age then he can attend school but the school authority must be notified and advice given about the brace.

If the child is to be treated by traction or on an abduction frame, then hospitalisation will be prolonged and this can produce problems for the child and his parents. If the treatment is continued at home then guidance and instructions must be given on the rational of the treatment and the importance of keeping the weight off the femoral head; maintenace of good muscle tone and good body alignment; and on how to prevent contractures.

Scoliosis

Scoliosis is a lateral curvature of the spine, which is always associated with some rotation of the involved vertebra. It may be postural or structural and is classified by its anatomic position, i.e.

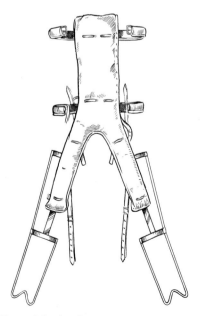

Fig. 29.8 Jones abduction frame.

thoracic, lumbar or, rarely, cervical. Postural curves are correctable while structural curves are fixed. The latter may be congenital, when there are anatomical abnormalities of one or more vertebrae; paralytic, when they are caused by muscle imbalance, e.g. following poliomyelitis, muscle dystrophies and occasionally in cerebral palsy; or idiopathic, where no cause can be found.

Scoliosis can occur at any age and is commonly classified according to the age at onset, e.g. *infantile* — up to the age of 3 years (this tends to resolve completely without treatment); *juvenile* — affecting children 3 to 9 years old and being more common than the infantile form; and *adolescent* — affecting children of 10 years and over (girls more commonly than boys).

The effects of scoliosis are cosmetic, cardio-respiratory, neurological and degenerative.

Cosmetic. The appearance of the body will be distorted: there will be loss of stature, high shoulder on convexity of curve and prominent hip on concavity of curve. It is particularly difficult for the adolescent since it threatens his self-image.

Cardio-respiratory problems can arise later in life. However, it is necessary to assess lung function pre-operatively to determine how much mechanical assistance with ventilation the patient will require in the post-operative period.

Neurological complications are usually secondary to congenital curves. Paraplegia may occur in the adolescent period and in those curves where cord pressure is possible.

Degenerative complications may include backache, which is more likely to occur in the thoracic-lumbar and lumbar region than in the thoracic region.

Principles of treatment and nursing management
The aim is to achieve a near normal curvature of the spine and the management is based on the knowledge of the likely behaviour of an individual curve. Curves of less than 20° are usually kept under observation with appropriate radiographs at regular intervals until skeletal maturity. Curves greater than 20° are treated. The methods available are:

1. Milwaukee brace (Fig. 29.10). This is a plastic corset with a well-moulded pelvic portion and vertical extensions to a circular neck assembly.

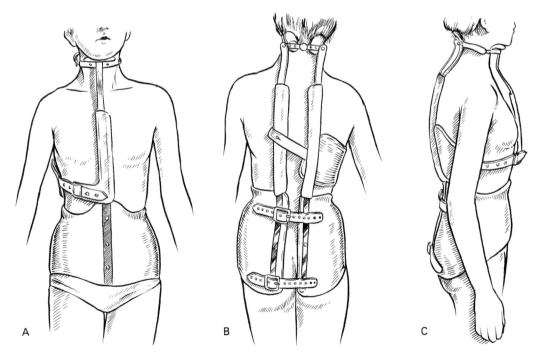

Fig. 29.10 Milwaukee jacket (brace); side, front and back views.

On the neck assembly is a throat mould and an occipital pad. The extensions or uprights are carefully adjusted so that the child, when standing erect, can just lift the chin off the throat mould. The brace is worn day and night and is removed to allow the child to have a bath. A polythene jacket (Fig. 29.11) can be worn instead of a Milwaukee brace.

2. Risser localiser cast. This is a plaster of Paris body cast applied using traction and localised pressure over the rib hump. It is a useful method for younger children.

3. Halo-pelvic traction. This is a powerful method of skeletal traction which may be used for curves which are too tight to be corrected by a plaster method.

4. Surgery. Prior to spinal fusion, Harrington rods are inserted. These consist of stainless steel rods each of which has a ratchet at one end. The hooks fit under the appropriate vertebra at the ends of the curves and the rod allows distraction, using the ratchet mechanism to lock the rod in the extended position. Another method used is insertion of a Dwyer cable which is attached to the convexity of the curve by staples to the vertebral bodies. This cable is then put under tension and this allows correction of the curvature.

Spinal fusion is the definitive treatment. It is an extensive operation involving the eradication of all the lateral vertebral joints in the affected segment of the vertebral column and re-inforcing this by bone grafts from the iliac crests. This is followed by immobilisation in plaster for a period of 6 months and a Milwaukee brace for a further 6 months.

5. Pre-operative care (p. 128).

6. Post-operative care:

   a. Routine (p. 131).

   b. Specific. The child may be nursed on a Stryker frame (Fig. 29.12). This frame allows frequent turning between supine and prone positions without disturbing spinal alignment. Training in the use of the frame is essential; it is vital to ensure that the tubings and locks are correctly manipulated and that the belts are in position around the frame to prevent slipping during the turning process. The child must be reassured throughout the procedure, because of his

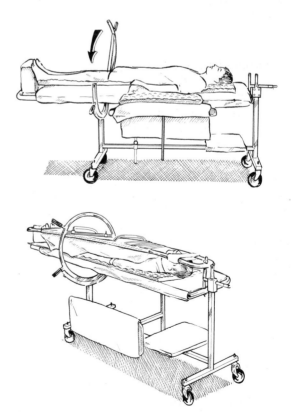

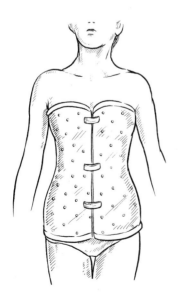

Fig. 29.11 Polythene jacket.

Fig. 29.12 Stryker frame.

fear of falling. Positional vomiting may be a problem and every effort should be made to provide diversional activity. If the child is nursed in a plaster jacket or bed then pressure area care will be necessary (p. 592).

7. Routine nursing care, which includes attention to nutrition and fluid intake, toilet needs and general cleanliness.

8. Support for parents. The condition will have been fully discussed with the parents. Throughout the child's stay in hospital, any treatment given should be explained and the parents should be encouraged to participate in the care of their child. If the child is to be nursed at home with any braces or plaster then they should feel confident about doing so. A community home nursing team would be invaluable in giving support to the parents.

Fractures

A fracture is defined as a break of a bone or cartilage. Fractures can occur in every age group, from the new-born to the elderly, but there are some people who are more liable to sustain a fracture.

Fractures form a large part of paediatric emergency admissions. Because of the resilience and springiness of children's bones, there is usually a greater degree of bending before the bone breaks. A break may therefore be incomplete and angulated (Greenstick fracture, (Fig. 29.13A). Fractures can also occur in the region of the epiphyseal plate. This area is cartilaginous and weaker than bone and is therefore liable to lead to fracture separation of an epiphysis. This type of fracture presents serious problems, for example, damage to the epiphyseal cartilage cells, or their blood supply, may interfere with growth of the bone. This damage may stop the growth of the bone or may lead to bone deformity.

Classification of fractures

A fracture may be either *simple*, where the overlying skin is intact, or it may be *compound*, where there is communication with the external skin surface. This does not necessarily mean that the bony fragments are protruding through the wound.

Fractures are further subdivided according to the character of the fracture, which in children include:

1. Fracture separation of the epiphysis.
2. Fracture through the epiphyseal plate.
3. Crushing injuries of the epiphyseal plate.
4. Incomplete fracture, where the bone is not broken completely. This is called a Greenstick fracture (Fig. 29.13A).
5. A longitudinal fracture, where the fracture line runs longitudinally along the bone.
6. A transverse fracture, where the fracture line runs at right angles to the longitudinal axis of the bone (Fig. 29.13B).
7. An impacted fracture, where one fragment is driven into the other and fixed in that position (Fig. 29.13E).

Complications of fractures

Complications of fractures may occur at the time of injury, e.g. damage to major nerves or main arteries. Other complications can arise due to infection either at the site of the fracture (if a compound fracture) or arising from infection elsewhere in the body. Late complications of fractures may be due to unsuccessful treatment or malalignment.

Infection

This follows compound fractures or open reductions. Bacteria enter the wound and travel to the soft, medullary tissue leading to osteomyelitis (p. 580).

Damage to blood vessels

Arteries carrying oxygenated blood to a limb may

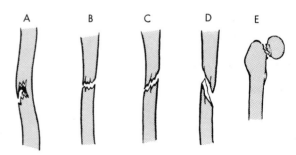

Fig. 29.13 Types of fractures. A, Greenstick (incomplete). B, Transverse (complete). C, Oblique (complete). D, Spiral (complete). E, Impacted.

be damaged by a fracture. The artery may be completely divided, in which case no blood reaches the limb. The limb will be pale, painful, pulseless, paralysed and paraesthetic. If the artery is only partly damaged, then some blood can still reach the limb and the signs of ischaemia will be limited. Circulation of blood through veins may be blocked by tight plaster or bandage. The limb becomes blue and swollen.

Damage to nerves
Nerves can be bruised, stretched or completely divided. Complete division of a nerve does not usually accompany a fracture. If it does occur it can be stitched using a very fine suture. Bruising of a nerve produces a sensation of pins and needles, and paralysis which is short-lasting. When a nerve is stretched it is ruptured, but the myelin sheath remains intact. Regeneration of nerve can take place (p. 295).

Other complications are related to the organs directly related to the injured bone/s. For example, lung damage is a complication of fracture of the ribs. The lung is punctured and, therefore, blood escapes into the thoracic cavity; this causes breathlessness and haemoptysis. A complication of skull fracture may be damage to the brain; the brain may be bruised or torn. Damage to the bladder may be associated with a fractured pelvis. The patient may not be able to pass urine or there may be haematuria; sometimes the urine escapes into the abdominal cavity causing peritonitis.

Healing of fractures
Fractured bones heal in much the same way as subcutaneous tissue. The broken area fills with blood clot which is removed by mononuclear phagocytes (macrophages). Blood vessels grow into the area, followed by migrating osteoblasts. The osteoblasts secrete collagen and mucopolysaccharides. Minerals are deposited in this material as complexes of calcium, phosphate and magnesium. This forms the provisional callus which is remodelled by osteoclasts to recover its final form, complete with Haversian canals and related structures. (Fig. 29.14).

Clinical features
Pain varies with the type of fracture and with the individual. There is localised tenderness over the fracture line and deformity is often present which is due to displacement of the fragments of bone. This takes the form of shortening of the limb, angulation or rotation of one fragment in relation to the other. Swelling and bruising accompany a fracture; this is due to the extravasation of blood and serum. There is also loss of function of the affected part.

Principles of treatment and nursing management
The treatment and nursing management will have as their main objectives:

1. Prevention of deformity.
2. Allowing growth to proceed as normally as possible.

To achieve these objectives, the following methods of treatment may be employed:

1. Reduction of the fracture. This aims at correction of displacement. For example, excessive overriding is reduced while a gentle traction is exerted on the limb. Some overriding is considered acceptable to allow for growth. However, reduction is not always necessary, e.g. in fracture of the upper end of the humerus. Reduction is performed under a general anaesthetic.
2. Immobilisation of the fracture. Plaster of Paris is the usual method as it gives good fixation, but splints are also used in combination with traction. Displaced fracture of the neck of the femur is fixed by threaded pins across the fracture; this is the method for older children.
3. Use of traction to maintain the length of the femur:
   a. Skin traction, using Gallows frame for children under 3 years of age (p. 596).
   b. Skin traction with the use of Thomas' splint for children of 3 years and over (p. 593).
   c. For older children, skin traction may not be sufficient if considerable overlap of the fragments is present. Skeletal traction may be required, using a Steinman pin, which is inserted into the upper tibia, a short distance distal to the epiphyseal plate. In these cases a sliding traction is used (p. 596).

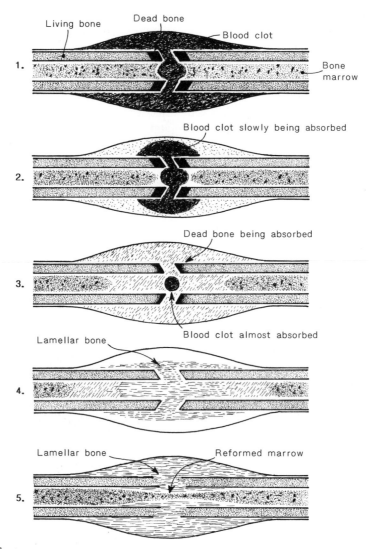

Fig. 29.14 Healing of fracture.

4. Routine pre-operative preparation (p. 128).
5. Post-operative care:
   a. Routine (p. 131).
   b. Specific, e.g. care of the child in plaster, observation of the limb (p. 591).
   c. Relief of pain.
   d. Recognition of complications. These may be *ischaemic*, due to injury of blood vessels and reduction of blood supply to the tissues; nerve palsies due to injury to nerves associated with the fracture and *bed sores* and *plaster sores*.
6. Routine nursing care.

7. Guidance for parents. This involves adequate information about the injury and the part they can play in helping the child. If part of the treatment can be given at home, then clear instructions should be given to them (p. 590).

Rickets

Rickets is a metabolic disorder of growing bone resulting in bony deformities (Figs. 29.15 and 29.16). Rickets may be due to the following:

1. Deficiency of vitamin D due to inadequate intake.

2. Inadequate exposure to sunlight.
3. Malabsorption syndromes.
4. Fanconi's syndrome (p. 436).
5. Resistance to vitamin D as in acquired or familial hypophosphataemia.

Importance of vitamin D

Vitamin D is a fat-soluble vitamin which occurs in two forms — ergocalciferol, found chiefly in irradiated yeast as vitamin D_2, and cholecalciferol (vitamin D_3) formed in human skin by the action of ultraviolet rays of sunlight and also found in fish liver oils and egg yolks.

Vitamin D participates in the absorption of calcium from the intestine and the mobilisation of calcium from bone. Therefore deficiency of vitamin D results in metabolic bone disease. The natural diet of infants, which consists primarily of either cow's or breast milk, is deficient in vitamin D and if there is also a lack of ultraviolet irradiation, then rickets may develop. Rickets or epiphyseal dysplasia may also develop during rapid growth. Children with dark skin (brown or black) are more susceptible to rickets due to deficiency in the synthesis of cholecalciferol in the skin.

Pathophysiology

New bone formation is initiated by the osteoblasts, which are responsible for matrix deposition and its subsequent bone formation. Mineralisation takes place in the presence of adequate calcium and phosphorus, and vitamin D is essential in the absorption of calcium in the intestine. In the absence of vitamin D there is defective calcification of growing bone and hypertrophy of the epiphyseal cartilages. New epiphyseal cartilage forms so that it increases in width (hypertrophy of the epiphyseal cartilages).

Clinical features

Rickets can develop in infancy but is more likely to occur in children of 1 to 2 years of age. Recently there has been an increase in the incidence of rickets in older children and adolescents from immigrant communities.

Infants with early rickets are restless and constant movement of the head of the pillow tends to denude the head of occipital hair. There is delayed closure of the anterior fontanelle, and craniotabes or reduced mineralisation of the skull at the occipital region is found in young infants. This is followed by thickening of the rib cartilages which gives the characteristic 'rickety rosary' and the rib cage also shows deformities such as 'pigeon chest'.

Bowing of the legs is marked in children who have rickets after they have begun to stand. This is due to weight-bearing which bends the bones and causes deformities such as bow-legs and knock-knees. Eruption of teeth may also be delayed and caries are prominent. Scoliosis, pelvic and other bone abnormalities may be present.

Investigations

1. Blood serum analysis (serum phosphorus is low).
2. X-ray examinations.

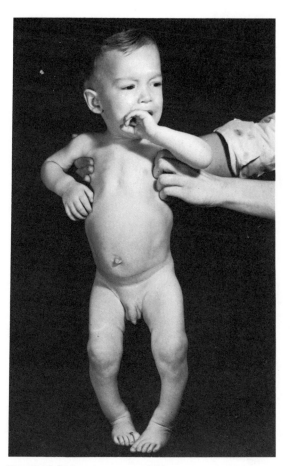

Fig. 29.15 Rickets in a young child.

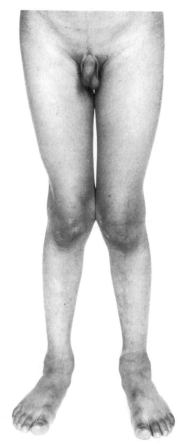

Fig. 29.16 Rickets in a young boy. Note deformities of legs.

Principles of treatment and nursing management

1. Oral dose of vitamin D (1000 to 5000 units) daily or a single dose of intramuscular cholecalciferol is given.
2. Nutrition, adequate for the age of the child, with vitamin supplements.
3. Correction of deformities.
4. Guidance for parents. If the condition is due to nutritional inadequacy, the parents should be interviewed by the dietician and the medical officer. Support and guidance should also be given by the community services, i.e. general practitioner, health visitor and child health clinic.

Orthopaedic nursing of children

There have been many changes in paediatric ortho-

paedics and although children are not confined to hospital for such long periods as in previous years, the average stay is longer than for those children suffering from some acute medical or surgical condition. The problems of hospitalisation are much the same for these children as for others and this has been discussed in Chapter 5. The major difference here is the long-term immobilisation which may be a necessary part of treatment and unless they are given adequate means to get rid of their excess energy, both mental and physical, then problems can arise. They become very easily frustrated, have temper tantrums or may become moody and withdrawn. It is in an effort to prevent such occurrences that it can be truly said that the orthopaedic ward is quite the noisiest one. It calls for ingenuity in planning to keep these children occupied and prevent boredom. The physiotherapist, play leader/occupational therapist, teachers, nurses and above all, the parents play an important part in helping the child to pass the time happily.

No child will be happy who is not allowed some measure of independence. Methods must be found to enable him whenever possible to feed himself, read his own books, and to make and create. Singing is a wonderful way of relieving feelings and should be encouraged. Equipment should be adapted to suit individual needs and requires constant reviewing. The help of the splint department is invaluable in making modifications to splints and other equipment.

General care of children

1. This includes routine nursing management of the child. The method of bathing is adjusted to the needs of the child and the areas available for normal washing.
2. Some movement is both necessary and desirable and therefore restrictions should be minimal. Standing up with a plaster will not cause any harm, provided the plaster is firmly set and functional.
3. Bed-making requires two nurses and indeed any procedure which has to be carried out on the child, should be performed by two nurses. This ensures that any movement of the child while on traction or with splints, will be achieved with the least disturbance to the child and the mechanical devices.

4. Clothing should be well fitting and suitable for the condition. It should be washable, because many children tend to crawl on the floor. For those in plaster or on traction splash pants can be used. These are tied with tapes at the side and can therefore be easily put on and taken off. Socks can be worn as the feet tend to get cold even in bed. It is also important to keep each child's shoes separate, e.g. in his locker. They should also be labelled with the child's name and only used by that child. This is an important aid in assessing the child's condition since the child will distort his own shoes and correction will be based on this distortion.

Care of the child in splints

Splints and their uses

The following splints are commonly used in children:

1. Thomas splint: used for resting limbs. It is made of iron and its ring is covered with wadding and leather. They are supplied in various sizes and lengths and the correct size should be 15 to 20 cm longer than the leg. The ring should fit close enough just to permit two fingers plus the leg inside it.
2. The caliper. This is a modification of the Thomas splint. It consists of an iron bar on each side of the leg but their ends are fixed into slots in the heel of the boot. These slots are rounded if movement of the ankle is required, but square if the foot is to be held at right angles to the leg. There is a soft leather pad behind the knee and a firmer curved pad in front is attached by straps to the side bars. The caliper is used to overcome flexion deformities of the knee, or to protect the bones of the leg in conditions such as paralysis of the quadriceps muscle. The longer the caliper is the more weight will be taken by it and the less by the leg bones. For this reason it is useful in Perthes' disease (p. 580). If greater protection is required by the thigh, a bucket-top caliper is used, where the ring is replaced by a moulded leather thigh corset.
3. Irons. This type of splint consists of either a single or double rod which runs from below the knee to the heel of the boot or shoe. The ankle is often supported with a T-strap attached to the iron. This will prevent inversion of the foot and is used in some talipes deformities or in poliomyelitis. A double iron with square heel slot will hold the foot at right angles and prevent drop foot.
4. Frames. Frames like the Thomas and Wingfield frames are made of metal and support a leather covered saddle stuffed with wool. They are used to immobilise the spine and hips or to correct kyphosis of the spine. The abduction frame is used for gradual reduction of congenital dislocation of the hip. The saddle and leg pieces are separate so that each or both legs can be abducted.
5. Plaster bed. This is more comfortable for the child than the frame. A cast is made of the child and when it is dry it is padded with gamgee and laid into a wooden frame. It is used for children suffering from tuberculosis of the spine and in paraplegia. The whole frame is then suspended from a bed frame by weights and pulleys so that the child can raise or tilt his bed.

Observation

Constant vigilance is essential so that corrective appliances are maintained in the position in which they have been placed. Pressure and friction causing redness and pain or poor alignment must be reported, treated, or corrected. This is not only important for the child confined to bed but also while he is up and about. Detection of abnormalities will be simplified if the nurse is already familiar with the normal appearance, poise, balance and alignment of the healthy child at rest, at play and in action.

It is very important, particularly in the initial phase, when the active child is confined to bed, to observe the amount of urine passed and the regularity of bowel movements. Fluid intake should be adequate and the diet should contain fruit and other high-fibre foods to ensure regular bowel actions. Vomiting too can be troublesome and should it occur it must be reported.

Feeding

The nutritional needs of the child must be satisfied. If vomiting occurs, meals may be given in small quantities but more frequently. Hot plates must not be placed on paralysed limbs, where absence of sensation could result in severe burns. The head may be raised slightly with a small pillow, and the position of the child modified to permit independent manipulation of a cup or plate. Special cups or feeders may be necessary to make drinking easier. Adequate fluid intake is essential, in order to prevent the formation of stones in the renal pelvis. This can occur where children have to be kept lying in bed for long periods, and kidneys are prevented from excreting liberated calcium salts.

Sanitary rounds

Two nurses are required to insert and remove bedpans from a child who is being treated by traction. One nurse raises the child's pelvis and supports his limbs, while the other nurse inserts the bedpan. As soon as the child has completed his toilet, two nurses will be required to remove the bedpan and give the necessary assistance. The external genitalia must be cleaned after voiding and defaecation.

Where the foot of the bed is elevated, urine may trickle upwards. To prevent this happening, the child should be assisted to assume the best possible position to urinate. This can be achieved by supporting the pelvis and holding the urinal. (See nursing care for patient with a Thomas bed splint, p. 596).

Care of appliances

Appliances, walking machines, and wheel chairs are inspected daily for wear and tear and if necessary should be sent for repair immediately. Crutches are examined to make sure that they are safe for use and of the correct size, as children quickly outgrow these. Padded splints require regular examination so that sores are not caused by exposed edges. Any appliance worn by a child with a paralysed limb requires the utmost care and attention because the child is unlikely to complain. Leather which becomes continuously contaminated with urine or faeces will harden and crack readily causing excoriation of the skin. The leather should be treated frequently with leather soap and thoroughly dried. If necessary it may be covered with some waterproofing material. If the Thomas splint is covered with synthetic material, it can be cleaned with Savlon.

Children who are allowed up

Here the nurse's responsibility includes supervision and observation of the following: (1) to ensure that the child walks and sits correctly with the appliance; (2) to ensure that the appliance is in the correct position; and (3) to give constant encouragement and allay any fears the child may have when he is using the appliance.

Preparation for home

The majority of children can be nursed adequately at home where the rehabilitating process continues. While in hospital, the parents take some part in some of the nursing functions and may well be competent in managing the appliance. The parents should be interviewed by the consultant and the full implications of the condition and treatment should be explained to them. It may be necessary to modify the home, bed, table, bath and chairs to accommodate the child. The medical social worker will be able to assist and give advice about the financial help to which they may be entitled or the special educational provisions available for their child. Physiotherapy will be started in hospital to teach balance, increase muscle power, to prevent contractures and to teach the child to walk. This will be continued on an outpatient basis and therefore appointments must be made before the child is discharged. Any behaviour problems related to the deformity should be recognised and help should be offered so that the child may find it easier to accept his disability. The parents too may require help and they should be encouraged to express their fears and anxiety, their hopes and desires so that help can be given and they can learn to accept their child's limitation.

The following advice should be given to the parents:

1. To avoid tripping and to make manipulation of the appliance safe, there should not be any obstacles such as rugs on the floor.
2. Space should be provided to encourage walking and crawling activities.
3. Advice should also be given regarding the type of toys which will be of benefit to the child and also amuse him, e.g. tricycle.

When the child is allowed home with a plaster of Paris splint, the following points should be made clear:

1. The plaster must be kept dry. Guidance should be given as to how this can be achieved.
2. The plaster must be kept free from cracks. If cracks are present, the hospital should be notified. Meanwhile the child should be kept in bed until the plaster has been repaired. This applies particularly to hip and leg plasters.

If the child has been treated as an emergency, as in cases of fractures, and allowed home, the parents must be told what to do and watch for and when to notify the hospital:

1. Any interference with circulation; the limb should be pink and warm to touch.
2. Persistence and increase in swelling; swelling may persist for 24 hours but should not increase.
3. Presence and intensity of pain; some pain may be present initially but it should gradually become less.
4. Loss of movement; the child should be able to move fingers and toes.
5. Irritation.

Children must be prevented from placing foreign bodies, e.g. buttons and coins, into the plaster, which could easily cause pressure sores. If the plaster has been applied to a leg, the child must not be allowed to bear weight on it for 72 hours.

Lifting a child in hip spica
After the first 48 hours, once the hip spica is dry, it is important that the child should spend at least 4 hours of the day in the prone position. Turning the child requires great care. Support is necessary under the hip and the upper part of the leg. Lifting one leg only or lifting the lower part of the plaster may cause cracking of the plaster below the knee.

The parents should also be shown what exercises to give to the child, for example, wriggling the toes of the affected limb and vigorous exercises of the unaffected limb. They should also be shown how to keep the plaster clean, how to place the child on a bedpan and how to remove the bedpan.

Application of plaster of Paris
Plaster of Paris is a fine powder derived from calcium sulphate. When the dry powder is mixed with water, a chemical reaction takes place and the powder sets into a solid cake. Final hardening occurs by the drying off of excessive quantities of water. During setting it becomes warm. Prepared bandages must be kept absolutely dry and stored in damp-proof containers.

Plaster of Paris may be applied after the reduction of a fracture, after surgical treatment of a soft tissue wound, or to retain the position of the limb or spine following operation on a bone or joint.

Requirements
1. Large rubber or plastic sheet.
2. Two deep bowls or buckets containing water at 36.8 °C.
3. Plaster bandages, assorted sizes.
4. Plaster wool (Orthoband).
5. Strong scissors and plaster knife.
6. Large plaster shears and small plaster cutters.
7. Tape measure.
8. Gauze bandages, 10 and 15 cm.
9. Body wipe and towel.
10. Plastic apron.
11. Rubber boots.
12. Collar and cuff ('Seton' or made to measure using calico bandage and felt; broad arm sling and safety pin) (for upper limbs).

Method
The limb or area to be treated is covered with Orthoband plaster wool and should include joints and any bony points which will be covered with plaster of Paris. The plaster bandage should then be immersed in the warm water until the bubbles cease to rise from it. The bandage is then lifted out and squeezed gently. With the loose end separated, the bandage is applied over the plaster wool, bandaging slowly up the limb so that each turn of bandage is covered by half the width on the next turn. The bandage should be rolled on without being pulled. The plaster thickness should be even throughout and wet plaster should not touch the skin. When sufficient plaster bandage has been applied, the doctor will mould the plaster with his hands and smooth it. A smooth plaster does not get dirty as quickly as a rough one.

To allow the plaster to dry, the child should be turned every 2 hours for small plaster casts, and every 4 hours for a hip spica (though initially 2-hourly turning may be required for hip spica). Artificial heat is not necessary and is not recommended because of the danger of the plaster cracking, but a free circulation of air is important. A plastered limb should be elevated on pillows and left uncovered. When a hip spica or a full leg plaster has been applied, the whole limb must be supported to prevent the plaster cracking at the groin. Weight-bearing should not be permitted until the plaster is fully set. This may take approximately 72 hours.

After-care

Circulation. The most important immediate complication to watch for is restriction of venous return. The fingers and toes must be left uncovered and inspected repeatedly during the first few hours.

The following must be watched for and reported immediately:

1. Loss of feeling and movement. This may be due to a blocked artery and damage to nerves. The pulse cannot be felt in that area and there will be local pallor.
2. The fingers or toes though pink may be swollen. Failure to flush after applying digital pressure indicates interference with circulation.
3. If the distal parts are bluish it also indicates interference with the circulation.

Prevention of pressure sores. Pieces of cotton wool or other substances should not be stuffed in at the ends of the plaster as this can be a source of pressure on the skin. When a hip spica has been applied the napkin should not be placed between the plaster and the skin. The napkin area must be cleaned and dried properly and this should include the area beneath the plaster.

Localised pain can be due to a plaster sore which has developed as a result of constant pressure of hard plaster against a badly padded bony area.

Irritation. This may be due to skin reaction and can be very distressing.

Cracks in the plaster. This will render the plaster useless and it is always advisable to renew the plaster rather than repair it.

Removal of plaster cast

This requires considerable physical effort and care must be taken not to injure the skin with the plaster shears. Plaster should not be removed while the child is anaesthetised because he then cannot indicate when the shears are nicking his skin. An explanation should be given to the child so that he can co-operate effectively. Small bites must be taken and the blades kept clean.

Some hospitals use an electric cutter for bi-valving or removing plaster instead of plaster shears. The cutters are not without danger and their use requires skill, good tactile appreciation and utmost care, so that the operator will know when the cutter has penetrated the plaster. As a precaution against cutting the child's skin, it is advisable to insert a cutter blade between the plaster and the patient's skin. Two people will be required, one to operate the cutter, and the other to hold the child to prevent any sudden movement. The noise of the motor can be frightening for the child and he will require constant reassurance.

After removal of the plaster, the skin should be cleaned gently and powdered with dusting powder.

Requirements

1. Plaster shears of appropriate size.
2. Electric cutter.
3. Metal spatula.
4. Scissors.
5. Adhesive tape.
6. Crepe bandages of appropriate sizes.
7. Plaster benders.
8. Face masks (these are worn by patient and staff to prevent inhalation of plaster dust).
9. Body wipe and towel.

The dorsal slab

These are plaster of Paris slabs which encircle three-quarters of the forearm. They are secured with bandages wound around, completely encircling the forearm while the plaster is still wet. The advantage of this appliance is that the plaster can be loosened easily if swelling is extensive and likely to interfere with the circulation. It is useful in a displacement of the distal radial epiphysis.

Batchelor plaster of Paris
A Batchelor plaster of Paris splint can be applied and is used in the continuation of the treatment of congenital dislocation of the hip. It follows a frog plaster which is used first for external rotation. Plaster of Paris is applied with the hips in full abduction and if the head of the femur is pointing too far forwards and not medially into the acetabulum, the child's legs have to be put into internal rotation to point the femoral neck at the acetabulum. In these cases rotational osteotomy is performed to allow the neck to point correctly, but rotating the shaft and knee forwards again. The plaster of Paris splint extends from the groin to the ankle and the legs are connected by a wooden bar, applied above the ankles (Fig. 29.17).

Requirements are the same as for application of plaster of Paris with the addition of a wooden bar.

After-care
Nursing presents few problems. Once the plaster has dried (p. 592) the child will soon show eagerness to move herself about the floor and reach for her own toys.

The divaricator (Barlow's type)
This splint is used instead of plaster of Paris in the treatment of congenital dislocation of hips in infants up to about 3 months of age. The splint is made of malleable metal and is covered with chamois leather. It is moulded to the figure of the child, fitting over the shoulders and under the thighs. The legs are held in abduction by winding the covered metal straps around the legs (Figs. 29.6 and 29.7 pp. 578–9).

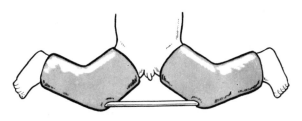

Fig. 29.17 The Batchelor plaster.

Nursing care
This is a useful splint to use at home or in the hospital. The napkin can be changed easily and, because of its lightness, the infant can be lifted and nursed without difficulty. It is important to ensure that the hip is at 90° or above at all times. While the splint is in position care should be taken to prevent the straps from chafing the skin. This can occur particularly at the top of the calf behind the knee and at the side of the neck. The skin can be moved a little each day to prevent damage due to pressure and friction. If the splint becomes soiled or alters its shape, a new splint should be applied.

Some splints are covered with vinyl and this may irritate some infants. This can be treated effectively with zinc and castor oil cream and placing a fine layer of gauze between the skin and the splint.

The divaricator (Craig's type)
This is an adjustable splint made of plastic material with padded edges. It is used as a continuation to the Barlow splint for infants over 3 months of age, suffering from congenital dislocation of the hip. The napkin is placed lengthwise on the infant and held in position by the splint. Napkin changes and cleaning of the area can be carried out without any difficulty.

Application of skin extension
The application of skin extension may be required for fixed traction or for use with weights and pulley, in the treatment of the following:

1. Perthes' disease of the hip — traction frees the head of the femur from the acetabulum.
2. Frame fixation for aiding reduction of the congenital dislocation of the hip (not used so often now).
3. To reduce a fracture of the femur in conjunction with the Thomas splint.
4. To gently reduce contracture of the knee by applying the traction below the knee.
5. To rest a diseased hip or limb.
6. It is applied to a baby's legs when the gallows extension is used to reduce a fracture of the femur.

Action of long axis traction (Fig. 29.18)
When the adhesive extension is applied to the skin

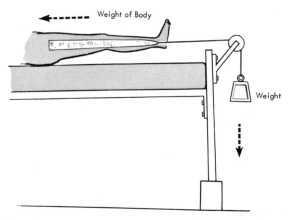

Fig. 29.18 Skin traction (pull on the leg is from the skin).

and fixed or anchored by the tapes to the end of the bed splint, or when the tapes with weights added pass over a pulley, the pull is transferred from the skin to the muscles and then to the bone. To this pull there must be an opposing force. If applied to the legs in preparation for reducing the congenital dislocation of the hip, the head of the femur is gently pulled downwards nearer the acetabulum. If applied to the legs in the treatment of Perthes' disease of the hip, it frees the head of the femur from the acetabulum, or in a fractured femur, the pull aims to keep the limb at full length thereby preventing shortening.

Preparation of the bed

The cot or bed should have a solid base or a fracture board is placed beneath the mattress. The foot of the cot or bed should be elevated (this provides the counter force) and the child should have no more than 2 pillows. Pulleys are attached to the end of the bed for sliding (free) traction. A hook may be used in place of the pulley if fixed traction is ordered.

Requirements

1. Shaving tray (if necessary).
2. Disposable razor.
3. Swabs.
4. Soap.
5. Warm water.
6. Water-repellent sheet.

Method of shaving limb

Gentle handling of the limb is essential and a second nurse should be available. The water-repellent sheet is placed beneath the limb. In wet shaving, soap is applied liberally all over the limb (dry shaving is often carried out). The skin is held taut and the hair removed by drawing the razor downwards in the direction of the hair growth. There must be no cuts or scratches. The limb is then washed and dried thoroughly.

Trolley to contain the following requirements
(sliding traction)

1. Drape.
2. Tincture benzoin compound spray.
3. 2 strips of white lint.
4. 4 adhesive extension strips with strapped ends and 2 wooden spreaders with 2 wooden pegs (for adhesive skin traction).
5. 2 lengths of Ventfoam of appropriate width with 2 metal spreaders (for non-adhesive skin traction).
6. 2 crepe bandages of required size.
7. Adhesive tape and scissors.
8. 2 weight cans containing the appropriate weight.
9. Orthopaedic cord.
10. 2 pulley attachments (bed or cot).

Requirements for fixed traction

1. Drape.
2. Tincture benzoin compound spray.
3. 2 strips of white lint.
4. 2 adhesive extensions with webbing taped ends, or 1 length of Ventfoam of appropriate width with 1 metal spreader and orthopaedic cord.
5. 4 crepe bandages of appropriate sizes.
6. Calico slings 10 and 15 cm wide (made from bandages).
7. Large curved safety pins (to hold the calico slings).
8. 2 × 15 cm Orthoband bandages or roll of gamgee tissue.
9. Adhesive tape.
10. Scissors.
11. Thomas splint of required size (see below for measurements) Fig. 29.19.

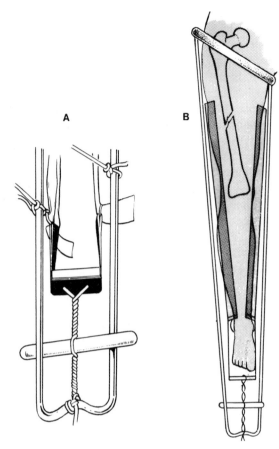

Fig. 29.19 The Thomas splint. A, The Spanish windlass which is tightened by outward rotation. B, The splint as used for fixed traction.

12. Hook attachment for the cot or bed.
13. Wooden board 15 × 10 cm (if required to support the ring).

Measurements for the Thomas splint
To ensure that the correct size of splint is applied the following measurements should be taken:

1. Measure around the thigh at the head of the femur and add 2.5 cm.
2. Measure from the head of the femur to the heel and add 15 to 30 cm according to the size of the child.

Method for making extension strips

Measurements
1. *Above knee traction.* Measure from the tip of

the great trochanter to the lateral malleolus and subtract 2.5 cm or less according to the size of the child. This will be the outer extension strip. Measure the inside of the leg from the adductor tendon in the groin to the medial malleolus and subtract 2.5 cm. This will be the inner extension strip and the measurements should ensure that the adhesive does not adhere to the external genital area.

2. *Below knee traction.* Measure from the head of the fibula to the lateral malleolus. Both extension strips are of equal lengths.

3. *Measurements for fractures of the upper third, mid-shaft and lower third of the femur.* The measurements are taken from the approximate level of the lower fragment to the malleoli and 2.5 cm are subtracted.

To make extensions for fixed traction
The required lengths are measured, allowing 3.75 cm or more, adhesive plaster or Ventfoam to enclose the orthopaedic cord. The adhesive plaster is cut into, to a depth of 2.5 cm on both sides, 3.75 cm from the end. This leaves 2.5 cm on the centre. The orthopaedic cord is placed in the centre and the cut sides are folded over it. This is then stitched securely. The ends of the approximated plaster are then fixed neatly back. The prepared extension should be held up by the orthopaedic cord and neatly notched on both side to ensure better fixation. The lengths of the outer and inner strips should be clearly marked.

To make extensions for sliding traction
The required lengths are measured, allowing 20 cm additional lengths, which act as a strap to secure the extensions to the spreader. The extension plaster is then cut into, to a depth of 2.5 cm on both sides, 20 cm from the end. This leaves 2.5 cm in the centre. The cut ends are folded over, leaving a strong double tape. The ends of the tape are folded neatly back. If they are used for a baby, the extensions should be cut to shape along the contours above the ankle.

To apply long axis traction
If the child is old enough, an explanation of the appliance should be given. The anklet is applied with an additional 0.5 cm in width, and it should

not be too tight. A drape is placed under the child's legs to protect the bed clothes. The medial and lateral aspects of the legs are sprayed with tincture benzoin compound and left for a few minutes to become 'tacky'. The measured and prepared lengths of extension plaster are applied to the lateral and medial parts of the leg, beginning just above the malleoli and smoothing them upwards. A few nicks in an oblique line at the knee may provide a smoother extension strip. An assistant should hold the limb, supporting the heel with the left hand and holding the forefoot with the right hand. In some units, a neutral position is maintained on the limb, while others advocate a pull on the limb. Care should be taken to avoid any overlapping of the extension strip over the tibial crest at the front as this could interfere with the function of the traction and may lead to the formation of pressure sores. Crepe bandages are applied using a figure of eight method below the knee and spiral turns above the knee, covering the thigh.

If a Thomas splint is used for fixed traction, a pad is placed above the popliteal space behind the knee, to maintain 5 to 10° flexion of the knee joint. The foot of the bed is elevated to provide counter-action by the rest of the body.

Weight and pulley traction

The buckles of the wooden spreader are fixed between the ends of the adhesive extensions. Sufficient room is left to allow the foot to move and exercise. There must be no pressure from the spreader and toggles near the sole of the foot. The extension cord is folded in the centre and pushed as a loop through the hole in the spreader. The cord is then secured with a spatula and adhesive and placed over the pulley at the foot of the bed. The correct weight is added and care is taken that the weights are securely fixed.

Care of the child

The child is nursed on his back. Since the purpose of the traction is to ensure approximation and healing of a fracture, or to correct and aid healing at a joint, the angle of the bed should be such that the weight of the child's body functions as a counter-traction. One pillow is usually adequate but more can be given provided an adequate angle is maintained. Opportunities for play should be provided and the child, if old enough, should be encouraged to feed himself. A tray cloth and rimmed plates should be given; the latter prevents spillage of food.

Care of the pressure areas is essential and should be carried out at frequent intervals. The healthy limb should be massaged, washed and dried to prevent wastage of muscles and formation of pressure sores. If a sliding traction is used, the nurse must observe that the appliance is functioning correctly and that the weight is not obstructed in any way either by knots in the cord, by being caught in the pulley or lying on the floor.

When giving a bedpan, two nurses are required, one to grasp the pelvis and raise the child up, the other to insert the bedpan. The same manoeuvre is necessary when removing the bedpan. After use of the bedpan, the external genitalia and perineum must be washed and dried carefully taking care that the splint ring does not become soiled. The older child can pull himself on to a bedpan with the aid of a monkey pole suspended from above.

Care of the ring area. The skin should be moved every 2 hours to vary the area bearing pressure and the area should be washed, dried and lightly powdered.

Care of the extension. The crepe bandages should be removed daily to ensure that the extension strapping is smooth and adhering to the skin. The skin should be examined for any signs of sensitivity, for example, redness and itching, and signs of scratching. The bandages are then reapplied, care being taken that they are not applied too tightly and that the foot is of good colour and moves normally.

Gallows traction

This form of traction is employed in the treatment of fracture of the femur in infants and children under 2 years of age. The appliance consists of a frame like a doorway, which is attached to the bed or cot. The legs are held vertically and are suspended by extension strapping to the horizontal bar of the frame. The buttocks are slightly raised off the bed and the hips are flexed to a right angle. This position provides the two forces necessary for traction (Fig. 29.20).

The same materials are required as for skin trac-

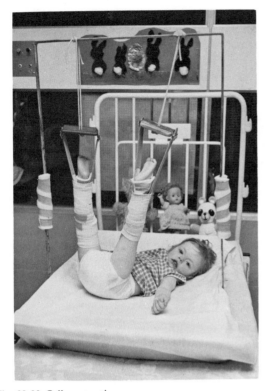

Fig. 29.20 Gallows traction.

tion (fixed) with the addition of a metal frame. Weights are usually not required but should be available in case they are required for weight and pulley (sliding) traction.

Nursing care presents few problems and the small child is usually very comfortable while lying in this position. Pressure care is easily provided. Napkin changes should be carried out as follows: the nurse should place her hands under the child's axillae, supporting his head, and pull him gently upwards and backwards. This will maintain the position of traction. The napkin area is cleaned and dried and preventive pressure care is given to all the dependent areas. A clean napkin is then applied and the child is repositioned. Areas such as the scapulae and the back of the head require attention to prevent chafing due to friction. The hair should be brushed and combed regularly to prevent matting.

When bottle feeding the small infant, the head and shoulders should be raised during feeding and the infant helped to expel any air he may have swallowed. The toddler can have a pillow under his head during meal times and a spouted feeder or beaker for drinking.

The toddler must be given toys to play with; these should be placed within easy reach of the child and every opportunity used to talk and play with him.

The child may be allowed home on a gallows stretcher frame. The parents must be given clear instructions regarding the care of the child, maintenance of traction and the correct position. Both parents should be shown how to handle the child and be able to do so under supervision while still in hospital.

Cervical halter traction (head traction)
This form of traction is applied when there is interlocking of the interarticular facets of the vertebrae as in dislocation of the cervical spine, acute torticollis and infections of the cervical spine. A soft leather harness, fitting under the chin and occiput, is used (Glisson's sling). A spreader separates the two sides and a cord is attached to this. Sliding traction is used.

Requirements

1. Bed with a solid base or fracture board.
2. Elevator to raise the head of the bed.
3. Pulley and weights (up to 4 kg).
4. Leather harness.
5. Orthopaedic cord and spreader.
6. Metal bar with hooks for attachment of a head band.

Care of the child
The chin requires great care; it should be washed and dried carefully. Talcum powder can be applied to absorb moisture but care should be taken to flake off any excess to prevent caking. Care of the chin is carried out at least three times a day. At other times it is sufficient to loosen the strap for a few minutes. During chin care the head must be held steady by another nurse so that the effect of the traction is not lost.

During meal times, a napkin should be tucked temporarily under the chin covering the leather to protect it. A leather strap which has been allowed to get damp or soiled will cause friction and can damage the skin. Initially, fluids or soft foods are given to keep chewing to a minimum. Fluids can be given with a flexible straw.

Toys and books should be readily available to keep the child occupied and amused, while a mirror placed in a suitable position over the child's head enables him to see what is happening in the ward. Movement of the legs is encouraged and regular pressure area care is necessary.

The position of the weights should be checked frequently to ensure that they have not become entangled at the head of the bed or that the feet are resting against the foot of the bed. In either case traction would be lost.

Erb's paralysis

Erb's paralysis is due to traction on the upper trunk of the brachial plexus during a difficult delivery of the baby. This leads to paralysis of the deltoid, biceps, supraspinatus, intraspinatus and the supinators of the forearm. The arm hangs by the side of his body and is flaccid, showing the characteristic 'porter's hand'.

Treatment

Most cases recover within one month and are treated by placing the arm in a position where its paralysed muscles are not stretched. For example, the baby's arm is held upwards by fixing the baby's sleeve to the pillow. If recovery does not occur within a month, a splint is made to hold the arm in full external rotation and abduction at the shoulder with right-angled flexion of the elbow and full supination of the forearm.

An acrylic splint can be made which is padded and applied by the doctor.

Nursing care

The axilla is examined for chafing. The arm is washed with soap and water, dried gently and thoroughly dusted with talcum powder. The splint is then reapplied. Physiotherapy is given daily. This is commenced as soon as possible to prevent contractures. Each joint is put through a full range of its own movements.

Home care

The parents are instructed how to change and reapply the splint and to encourage abduction and external rotation as the child grows. A coloured

ball or rattle which the baby can see will act as inducement to move the affected arm. The healthy arm may be slipped out and lightly bandaged to the body for short periods, this will encourage movement and exercise of the paralysed arm.

Denis Browne foot splints for talipes (Fig. 29.21)

Denis Browne foot splints are used for correction of talipes equino-varus (p. 575). Treatment is commenced soon after birth, preferably within 8 days. The feet are manipulated daily and as soon as a partial correction has been obtained the splints are applied.

The splints consist of simple angled strips of aluminium. They are lined with adhesive felt and the feet are strapped to them with Elastoplast (2.5 cm wide), starting at the base of the toe-nail and continuing without any gaps to the top of the splint.

Requirements

1. Prepared Denis Browne splints.
2. Transverse bar.
3. Screws and bolts.
4. Spanner, correct size to fit the screws and bar to the foot piece.
5. Elastoplast 2.5 cm wide and 75 cm long.
6. Adhesive felt 1 cm thick.

Application

A clinical photograph is taken before manipulation and application of the splint. The baby is placed at the foot of the table with a small pillow placed

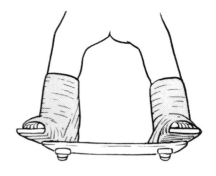

Fig. 29.21 Denis Browne splints.

below his head. The nurse separates the baby's legs and grasps the calf of the leg in both hands, thereby protecting the knee from strain. The inversion and abduction of the foot is corrected first and the plantar-flexion last.

The surgeon places a small piece of adhesive felt over the talus. The sole piece is then applied to the foot and is bandaged with Elastoplast into the correcting position. The leg pieces project outwards from the leg. These, when bandaged to the leg, pull the foot into eversion. The sole pieces are then fitted to the cross-bar pointing outwards in as much external rotation as possible.

The toes should be pink and, after removal of digital pressure, the skin should flush quickly with blood. If the toes are not pink the feet should be elevated and, should this fail, the bar between the splints can be removed or it may be necessary to remove the splints. It often takes 12 to 14 daily manipulations to achieve a corrected position. For each manipulation, the old splint is removed with blunt pointed scissors. The feet, which are red and swollen, are washed with Phisohex, dried, manipulated and splinted again. The splints are kept in the corrected position day and night.

Once overcorrection has been obtained, usually after 10 to 14 days, the child is allowed home.

Advice to the parents

The parents are asked to observe the toes and contact the hospital at once should anything abnormal occur. It should be explained to them that there may be some swelling of the toes, but they should be pink and flush readily after removal of digital pressure. Gross swelling and discolouration should be reported at once.

The baby is brought back for manipulation once a week until he is walking. He is then given boots with reduced heels and a raise on the outer part of the sole and wears night splints.

The parents are taught to manipulate the foot/feet into the corrected position daily. If this is not carried out regularly, the foot will return to its abnormal position and it may be necessary to perform a soft tissue correction or medial release by operative means. In severe cases a wedge of bone may have to be removed from the outer side of the tarsus in addition to the soft tissue operation. Correction and healing is provided by applying a plaster which is left on for 3 months.

Glossary

Abduction Muscular action drawing one part away from another.

Absorption The process of movement across the cell membrane of substances which become incorporated into the cell.

Accommodation Focusing the eye. At rest a normal eye is focused at infinity, i.e. for distant vision. For near vision, the ciliary muscle round the lens contracts, and the lens becomes rounder and optically more powerful.

Acetabulum Hemispherical socket in the bone at either side of the pelvis to fit the head of the femur.

Acetyl-choline One of the neuro-transmitters released at the ends of nerve fibres to set off an impulse in an adjacent nerve cell.

Achalasia Failure of the mechanism producing relaxation of a sphincter, leading to dilatation and muscular hypertrophy of the part immediately above the sphincter.

Acholuric jaundice Jaundice without bile in the urine.

Acid A substance which liberates hydrogen ions in solution; substance which contains hydrogen which may be replaced by a metal to form a salt.

Acidosis Alteration of the acid/alkaline balance of the blood and tissue fluid towards acidity.

Active transport The movement of materials across cell membranes against a concentration gradient.

ACTH Adrenocorticotrophic hormone formed in the anterior lobe of the pituitary body. It acts on the cortex of the adrenal glands to promote the secretion of corticosteroids.

Adduction Muscular action drawing one part inwards towards another.

Adenine A purine base, occurring in nucleic acid which plays a part in the formation of the genetic code.

Adsorption The concentration of a substance at the surface of a solid or liquid.

Aerobic Requiring air or available oxygen to live or grow.

Afferent Leading towards the centre, conveying from the periphery to a central point, e.g. blood vessel or nerve fibre.

Agar-agar A gelatinous substance obtained from seaweed used to solidify nutrient media for bacterial cultures.

Agenesis Without development.

Agranulocytosis A condition in which the bone marrow stops producing neutrophils, leaving the body unprotected against bacteria and other foreign organisms.

Albumin The most abundant of the proteins dissolved in blood, the principal factor in maintaining the osmotic pressure of the blood.

Alkali In general, a compound in solution which can take up or accept hydrogen ions; often a substance that dissociates to release hydroxyl ions.

Alkalosis A shift in the ratio of acid to alkali in the blood towards an excess of alkali. It can be due to loss of acid from the stomach through vomiting or excessive elimination of carbon dioxide.

Allele Alternative form of a gene for a particular trait, e.g. defective form of haemoglobin.

Allergen Any substance capable of producing allergy.

Allergy The body's response to a substance or substances of protein or non-protein character, usually when these substances do not cause harm.

Alopecia Loss of hair, baldness.

Alpha The first letter of the Greek alphabet. In physics, alpha particles are positively charged particles, a close combination of two neutrons and two protons (Helium nucleus) which are emitted from radioactive substances.

Amino-acids Chemically simple substances of which proteins are composed. A carboxyl acid which contains the amino-group — NH_2. These acids are fundamental to life. There are approximately 23 amino acids.

Anaesthesia Absence of sensation, either in the whole body (general) or in part (local anaesthesia).

Androgen Any substance acting as a male sex hormone.

Angioma A tumour composed of blood vessels, e.g. a naevus.

Angiotensin A polypeptide circulating in the blood. If the blood flow in the kidney decreases, the kidneys secrete *renin* which reacts with angiotensin to produce angiotensin II. This produces vasoconstriction and leads to a marked increase in total peripheral resistance. Angiotensin also brings about the release of aldosterone from the adrenal cortex.

Anion Negatively charged ion which during electrolysis is attracted towards the anode.

Anoxaemia Deficiency of oxygen in the blood.

Anoxia Lack of oxygen.

Antibiotic Chemical substance produced by micro-organisms such as moulds and bacteria, which are capable of destroying bacteria or preventing their growth.

Ataxia Failure to co-ordinate the actions of various muscles involved in performing a movement, usually without loss of muscular power.

Atelectasis Incomplete expansion of a lung usually applied to the infantile type.

Autolysis Digestion of cells or products by enzymes which have originated from within the cells themselves.

Axon A fibre projecting from the cell body of a neuron and conducting impulses towards the dendrites of the next neuron.

Basal ganglia The core of grey matter (nerve cells) at the centre of the cerebral hemispheres.

BCG (Bacille Calmette-Guerin) A vaccine against tuberculosis. Calmette and Guerin were two French bacteriologists.

Behaviourism An American school of psychology which viewed psychology as the study of only observable, objectively measurable behaviour.

Beta rays A stream of beta particles which possess greater penetration power than alpha rays.

Bilirubin Chief pigment of bile, derived from haemoglobin and formed in the reticulo-endothelial tissue.

Biliverdin The oxidation product of bilirubin.

Blastula A hollow ball of cells which forms in the very early embryonic development of animals.

Brachycephalic Having a short head.

Buffer Buffers are substances which, by their presence in solution, increase the amount of acid or base that must be added to cause a change of pH.

Calciferol Vitamin D$_2$ formed by the action of ultraviolet radiation on Ergosterol. It controls the deposition of calcium compounds in the body.

Canthus The angle formed by the junction of the eyelids.

Carbonic acid (H$_2$CO$_3$) A very weak acid probably formed in small amounts when carbon dioxide dissolves in water.

Centrifuge Apparatus for separating particles from a suspension by rotating the tubes rapidly about a central point. The suspended particles are forced outwards by centrifugal force, and collect at the bottom of the tubes.

Chelation Formation of a closed ring of atoms by the attachment of compounds. Chelating agents are used for 'locking up' unwanted metal ions.

Chromatography A method of chemical analysis; gas or paper chromatography can be used.

Chromosomes Thread-like bodies found in the nuclei of living cells, the molecules of which carry the genetic code. They consist of nucleoproteins, the nucleic acid being DNA.

Clonus Spasm with violent successive muscular contractions.

Cytotoxic agents Drugs that suppress cell reproduction or mitosis. Rapidly growing cells or cancer cells are more susceptible to these drugs.

Dead space Air passages (nose, pharynx, trachea, bronchi) through which inspired air passes on its way to the alveoli. The air in this space takes no part in respiration.

Defibrillation Restoration of rhythmical heart beat by electrical stimulation.

Dextran Carbohydrate, chemically like starch and cellulose, given to restore the volume of the blood in severe shock. Dextran molecules are too large to escape from the blood vessels so they retain the necessary water.

Dextrose Grape-sugar; glucose.

Dialysis Selective diffusion through a membrane serving as a molecular filter; small molecules, e.g. salts, pass through, while large ones, e.g. proteins, do not.

Diplegia Paralysis of both arms or both legs.

Diplopia Double vision; failure to superimpose the images recorded from the two eyes. It is nearly always due to imbalance of the eye muscles.

Dominant Character that needs to be inherited only from one parent.

Ductus arteriosus A blood vessel joining the pulmonary artery to the aorta, enabling blood to bypass the lungs. Found in the fetus until birth.

Dura mater The outer fibrous covering of the brain and the spinal cord.

Dysphagia Difficulty in swallowing.

Dyspnoea Difficulty in breathing due to factors such as airway resistance, decreased compliance.

ECHO A group of viruses (Enteric Cytopathic Human Orphan).

Ego According to Freud, that part of the self or personality that keeps in touch with the material world; the conscious mind.

Embryo In human biology, an unborn offspring from the time of fertilisation until the time when it can be recognised as unmistakably human at about 2 months' gestation.

Endoderm A layer of cells at a very early stage in the development of an embryo.

Extravasation Leakage of fluid from a vessel into the surrounding tissues.

Fibrillation Rapid uncoordinated twitching of muscle fibres; atrial fibrillation occurs in the muscle of the atria and ventricular fibrillation occurs in the muscle of the ventricle.

Focal seizure An epileptic manifestation of a restricted nature due to irritation of a localised area of the brain and is often associated with scarring, tumour or inflammation of that area.

Foramen ovale Opening between the right and left atria; closes soon after birth, but may remain open in some congenital heart abnormalities.

Friedreich's ataxia A hereditary spinocerebellar degenerative disease beginning in childhood with signs of ataxia, diminished or absent deep tendon reflexes, positive Babinski's sign, speech disturbance, etc.

Frustration The condition that results when an impulse to act or the completion of an act is blocked or thwarted, preventing the satisfaction of achievement.

Fundus (oculi) The posterior portion of the interior of the eye.

Funnel chest A deformity of the sternum, costal cartilages, and anterior portion of the ribs, producing a depression of the lower part of the chest.

Gammaglobulin A broad classification for immunoglobulins of differing molecular weights and related proteins which are of similar chemical structure, many of which have known antibody activity.

Ganglion A group of nerve cell bodies, usually located outside the brain and spinal cord.

Gene A hereditary factor; the unit of transmission of hereditary characteristics, capable of self-production which usually occupies a definite locus on a chromosome, though some genes are non-chromosomal.

Genetic code Consisting of nucleotides which permit the translation of specific gene DNA and messenger RNA molecules into proteins of specific amino-acid sequence. The code is triplet and degenerate; each amino-acid found in protein is coded for by more than one triplet, e.g. Alanine CCG, UCG.

Gestational age The age of a conceptus calculated from the first day of the last menstrual period to any point in time thereafter, but usually not calculated beyond the first few months of life after birth.

Gluten A mixture of gliadin and glutelin types of proteins found in seeds of cereal; produces cohesiveness to dough.

Head circumference Occipito-frontal circumference. An important measurement in the diagnosis of hydrocephalus and as a means of assessing its arrest or progress.

Hirschsprung's disease A disease caused by the absence of mesenteric ganglion cells in a segment of the rectum or distal colon resulting in spasm of the affected part and dilatation of the bowel proximal to the affected part. This leads to constipation.

Hunter's syndrome Mucopolysaccharidosis, transmitted as X-linked recessive; similar in appearance to Hurler's syndrome, but milder.

Hyaline A clear, structureless, homogeneous material occurring normally in the matrix of cartilage, vitreous body, mucin, glycogen. Found pathologically in degeneration of connective tissue and epithelial cells.

Icterus neonatorum Jaundice of the new-born usually due to increased rate of breakdown of erythrocytes, but may also be due to decreased ability to conjugate and excrete bilirubin.

Immunosupressive An agent, such as chemicals, drugs or X-rays, for suppressing immunological reactions, as in auto-immune diseases or for enhancing successful tissue grafts.

Incubation period The period of time required for development, as in symptoms of disease after infection, or of altered reactivity after exposure to an allergen.

Incubator A small chamber with controlled oxygen, temperature and humidity for small and pre-term new-born babies or small ill babies, requiring special care.

Intention tremor A tremor of the limbs, which may be coarse or jerky, fairly regular, usually brought on and intensified by voluntary movement and ceasing at rest. Associated with cerebellar lesions.

Intraventricular heart block Prolongation of the QRS complex of the electrocardiogram, not classical for bundle branch block.

Intubation The introduction of a tube into a hollow organ, to keep it open, especially into the larynx to ensure passage of air.

Intussusception The receiving of one part within another; especially, the invagination, slipping or passage of one part of the intestine into another, occurring usually in young children.

Isotonic solution A solution that causes no change in the tone of a tissue, such as erythrocytes, immersed in the solution.

Isotope An element that has the same atomic number as another but a different atomic weight, e.g. $I^{126\ 904}$, I^{131}. (I = Iodine.)

Keloid, Cheloid A fibrous hyperplasia (excessive tissue formation) usually at the site of a scar, elevated, rounded, firm, and with ill-defined borders.

Kernicterus Bilirubin pigmentation of grey matter of the central nervous system, especially basal ganglions, accompanied by degeneration of nerve cells; occurring as complication of erythroblastosis fetalis.

Kernig's sign (V. M. Kernig, Russian physician 1840–1917) Pain and spasm of the hamstring muscles. When the patient is in the supine position, the thigh is flexed at the hip and an attempt is made to extend the leg at the knee, which causes pain and spasm of the hamstring muscles; a positive sign in meningeal irritation.

Ketogenic diet A diet in which an excessive proportion of the allotted calories is derived from fats, which are reduced to ketones. The resulting acidosis causes H^+ to move into cells and K^+ out decreasing the electrical activity of nerve cells.

Klinefelter's syndrome The clinical syndrome of hypogonadism including enlarged mammary tissue in the male and small testicles. The Y chromosome is associated with more than one X chromosome.

Kyphosis Angular curvature of the spine, the convexity of the curve being posterior usually situated in the thoracic region.

Lanugo The soft hair that covers the fetus from about the fifth month of gestation.

Locus In genetics, the position a particular gene occupies on the chromosome.

Lower motor neurone disease An injury to the cell bodies or axons of lower motor neurons, characterised by flaccid paralysis of the muscles, diminished or absent reflexes; progressive muscle atrophy.

Lowe's syndrome Oculocerebrorenal syndrome; blindness, mental retardation.

Malabsorption Defective absorption of nutritive substances from the alimentary canal.

Maladjustment A state of faulty or inadequate conformity to one's environment, due to the inability to adjust one's desires, attitudes, or feelings to social requirements.

Manometer An instrument for measuring the pressure of liquids and gases.

Marfan's syndrome (A. B. J. Marfan, French paediatrician) An inherited disorder of connective tissue; manifested by skeletal changes such as abnormally long, thin extremities, high arched palate, defects of spine and chest; ocular changes. (Homocystinuria.)

Mean corpuscular volume An expression, in absolute terms, of the average volume of the individual erythrocyte, calculated from the equation

$$MCV = \frac{haematocrit\ (per\ cent) \times 10}{erythrocyte\ count\ (10^6/mm^3)}$$

and stated in cubic microns per cell.

Microcytic anaemia Any anaemia in which the erythrocytes are smaller than normal.

Micrognathia Abnormal smallness of the jaws, especially of the lower jaw (Pierre-Robin Syndrome).

Nephrogenic diabetes insipidus Diabetes insipidus which is unresponsive to vasopressin, because of inability of the renal tubules to reabsorb water; it is usually congenital, inherited as an autosomal dominant trait, affecting males more frequently, but may occur in chronic renal insufficiency.

Neurogenic bladder A urinary bladder in a state of dysfunction due to lesions of the central or peripheral nervous system.

Neurosis One of the two major categories of emotional maladjustments, due to unresolved conflicts, anxiety being its chief characteristic. There is usually no gross disorganisation of personality in relation to external reality; there may be some impairment of thinking and judgement.

Nocturnal enuresis Involuntary urination at night during sleep, by a person in whom bladder control may normally be expected to be achieved.

Nystagmus An involuntary rapid movement of the eyeball which may be horizontal, vertical, rotatory or mixed; may be due to neurogenic myopathic, labyrinthine or ocular causes.

Oculocerebrorenal syndrome A familial hereditary affection of males, characterised by retardation of growth, mental retardation, hypotonia, mild and severe acidosis, characteristic eye changes — cataracts and glaucoma. Believed to be transmitted as an X-linked characteristic. (Lowe's syndrome.)

Opisthotonus A position adopted when the head and lower limbs are bent backwards and the back is arched forward by a tetanic spasm of the muscles of the back; seen in severe meningeal irritation.

Opsonin A substance occurring in blood serum which prepares bacteria for phagocytosis.

Panic An extreme state of anxiety which may lead to total inaction or more often to precipitate unreasonable acts.

Paradoxical respiration A condition in which the lung fills on expiration and empties on inspiration, seen with open pneumothorax and diaphragmatic paralysis.

Primary tuberculosis The reaction to the first implantation of tubercle bacilli in the body. It consists of a caseous focal reaction in the parenchyma of the organ and in the regional lymph node or nodes. The most frequent site is the lung.

Pulmonary oedema An effusion of fluid into the air sacs and interstitial tissue of the lungs, producing severe dyspnoea; most commonly due to left heart failure.

Quarantine The limitation of freedom of movement of such susceptible persons or animals as have been exposed to communicable disease, for a period of time equal to the longest usual incubation period of the disease to which they have been exposed.

Refraction The deviation of a ray of light from a straight line in passing obliquely from one transparent medium to another of different density.

Refractive error A defect of the eye which prevents parallel light rays from being brought to a single focus precisely on the retina.

Resorption The disappearance of all or part of a process, tissue, or exudate by biochemical reactions that may involve dissolution, lysis, absorption and/or other actions.

Rorschach test A psychological test in which the subject describes what he sees on a series of 10 standard inkblots of varying designs and colours. The subject's responses indicate personality patterns, originality of thought, emotional conflict, etc.

Schizophrenia A group of psychotic disorders, characterised by fundamental alterations in concept formations with misinterpretation of reality and associated disturbances in behaviour and intelligence. There is withdrawal from reality, responses are inappropriate and there is often hallucination and delusion.

Separation anxiety The apprehension, fear or psychosomatic complaints observed in children on being separated from significant persons or familiar surroundings.

Steatorrhoea Fatty stools, found in conditions such as coeliac disease, fibrocystic disease of the pancreas.

Thoracic stomach Congenital herniation of the stomach above the diaphragm due to imperfect development of the diaphragm.

Tracheostomy The formation of an opening into the trachea performed for the insertion of a tracheostomy tube.

Umbilical hernia A hernia occurring through the umbilical ring due to weakness of the rectus abdominis muscles.

Upper motor neuron Any descending efferent neuron having its cell body in the motor cortex and essential to fine voluntary muscular activity.

Upper motor neuron lesion An injury to the cell body or axon of an upper motor neuron, resulting in spastic paralysis of the muscle involved, hyperactive deep reflexes, but diminished or absent superficial reflexes. There is little or no muscle atrophy, absence of reaction of degeneration and the presence of pathological reflexes.

Uraemia A complex biochemical abnormality occurring in kidney failure; characterised by chronic acidosis, and a variety of systemic and neurological symptoms and signs.

Vaccine A preparation administered to induce immunity in the recipient; may be a suspension of living or dead organisms or a solution of either pollens or viral or bacterial antigens.

Valgus Usually, denoting an abnormal turning away from the midline of the body, as in talipes valgus.

Varus Usually, denoting an abnormal turning inward toward the midline of the body, as in talipes varus and coxa vara.

Vitamin Any of a group of organic compounds present in variable, minute quantities in natural foodstuffs, required for normal growth and maintenance of life of animals and man, who, as a rule, are unable to synthesise these compounds. They are essential for transformation of energy and for the regulation of the metabolic processes.

Word-blindness Alexia; an individual who is unable to recognise or comprehend written or printed words.

World Health Organization (WHO) A specialised agency of the United Nations' Organization whose broad purposes in the international health field are to assist governments upon requests in the field of health; to promote standards, provide information and foster research in the field of health; to foster and promote child health, maternal and mental health and it has authority to make sanitary and quarantine regulations to set standards for purity and potency of biological and pharmaceutical products.

Bibliography

Baldwin, A. L. (1980) *Theories of Child Development*, 2nd edition. New York: John Wiley and Sons.

Baron, D. N. (1978) *A Short Textbook of Chemical Pathology*, 3rd edition. London: Unibooks, Hodder and Stoughton.

Bates, S. (1971) *Practical Paediatric Nursing*. London: Blackwell Scientific Publications.

Bell, G. H., Emslie-Smith, D. & Paterson, C. R. (1976) *Textbook of Physiology and Biochemistry*, 9th edition. Edinburgh: Churchill Livingstone.

Belman, B. A. .& Kaplan, G. W. (1981) *Genitourinary problems in Paediatrics*. Philadelphia: W. B. Saunders.

Birrell, J. F. (1960) *The Ear, Nose and Throat Diseases of Children*. London: Cassell.

Bocock, E. J. & Parker, M. J. (1972) *Microbiology for Nurses*. London: Baillière Tindall.

Bourne, L. & Ekstrand, B. (1973) *Psychology and its Meaning*. Illinois: Dryden Press.

Bower, T. G. R. (1979) *Human Development*. Oxford: W. H. Freeman and Co.

Bowlby. J. & Fry, Margery (1965) *Child Care and the Growth of Love*. Harmondsworth, Middx: Penguin.

Bowley, A. H. (1961) *The Psychological Care of the Child in Hospital*. Edinburgh: Livingstone.

Broadribb, V. (1973) *Foundation of Paediatric Nursing*, 2nd edition. Toronto: J. B. Lippincott.

Brunner, J. S., Jolly, A. & Sylva, K. (Eds.) (1978) *Play, its Role in Development and Evolution*, Ch. 6, 18, 35, 53, 62, 71. Harmondsworth, Middx: Penguin.

Brunner, L. S. & Suddarth, D. S. (1974) *The Lippincott Manual of Nursing Practice*, Ch. 23–39. Toronto: J. B. Lippincott.

Burke, S. R. (1976) *The Composition and Function of Body Fluids*, 2nd edition. St Louis: Mosby.

Burns, J. K. (1975) *Birth Defects and their Causes*.

Butler, N. R. & Alberman, E. D. (1969) *Perinatal Problems*. Edinburgh: Livingstone.

Cameron, J. M. & Rae, L. J. (1975) *Atlas of the Battered Child Syndrome*. Edinburgh: Churchill Livingstone.

Chinoy, E. (1967) *Society: An Introduction to Sociology*. Toronto: Random House.

Clegg, A. & Megson, B. (1976) *Children in Distress*. Harmondsworth, Middx: Penguin.

Craig, O. (1977) *Childhood Diabetes and its Management*. London: Butterworth.

Craigmyle, M. B. L. & Presley, R. (1975) *Embryology*, 2nd edition. London: Baillière Tindall.

Cranston, W. I. (1966) Temperature regulation. *British Medical Journal*, 2, 69.

Crelin, E. S. (1973) *Functional Anatomy of the Newborn*. New Haven: Yale University Press.

Davie, R., Butler, N. Goldstein, H. *et al.* (1972) *From Birth to Seven*. (A report of the National Child Development Study.) Harlow: Longman.

Davis, J. A. & Dobbing, J. (1974) *Scientific Foundations of Paediatrics*, Ch. 18, 20, 21, 22. London: Heinemann (Medical Books Ltd).

De Louvois, J. (1976) *Selected Topics in Clinical Bacteriology*. London: Baillière Tindall.

Dennison, W. M. (1974) *Surgery in Infancy and Childhood*, 3rd edition. Edinburgh: Churchill Livingstone.

Donaldson, M. (1978) *Children's Minds*. London: Fontana.

Eccles, J. C. (1964) *The Physiology of Synapses*. New York: Academic Press.

Edgerton, R. (1979) *Mental Retardation*. London: Fontana.

Ellis, H. (1976) *Clinical Anatomy*, 6th edition. London: Blackwell Scientific Publications.

Emery, A. E. H. (1975) *Elements of Medical Genetics*, 4th edition. Edinburgh: Churchill Livingstone.

Emery, A. E. H. (1983) *Medical Genetics*, 8th edition. Edinburgh: Churchill Livingstone.

Erikson, E. H. (1968) *Identity, Youth and Crisis*. London: Faber.

Erikson, E. H. (1974) *Childhood and Society*. Harmondsworth, Middx: Penguin.

Feldman, S. & Ellis, H. (1975) *Principles of Resuscitation*, 2nd edition. London: Blackwell Scientific Publications.

Fochtmann, D. & Foley, G. V. (Eds.) (1982) *Nursing Care of the Child with Cancer*. (Association of paediatric oncology nursing.) Boston: Little, Brown and Co.

Forfar, J. O. & Arneil, G. C. (1984) *Textbook of Paediatrics*, 2nd edition. London: Churchill Livingstone.

Foss, B. (Ed.) (1975) *New Perspectives in Child Development*. Harmondsworth, Middx: Penguin.

Gardner, E. K. & Shelton, B. (1967) *The Intensive Therapy Unit and the Nurse*. London: Faber.

Gesell, A., Amatruda, C. S., Castner, B. M. & Thompson, H. (1939) *Biographics of Child Development*. London: Hamish Hamilton.

Gesell, A. & Amatruda, C. S. (1947) *Developmental Diagnosis*. London: Hoeber.

Gibbens, J. (1954) *The Care of Children from 1 to 5*, 5th edition. London: Churchill.

Gillies, R. R. (1975) *Lecture Notes on Medical Microbiology*, 2nd edition. London: Blackwell Scientific Publications.

Gold, E. R. & Butler, N. R. (1972) *ABO Haemolytic Disease of the Newborn*. Bristol: John Wright and Sons Ltd.

Gregory, G. A. (Ed.) (1981) *Respiratory Failure in the Child*. Edinburgh: Churchill Livingstone.

Haller, J. A. (1967) *The Hospitalised Child and His Family*. London: Oxford University Press.

Hallman, G. L. & Cooley, D. A. (1975) *Surgical Treatment of Congenital Heart Disease*, 2nd edition. Philadelphia: Lea, Febiger.

Hamilton, W. (1972) *Clinical Paediatric Endocrinology*. London: Butterworth.

Hampton, J. R. (1973) *The E.C.G. Made Easy*. Edinburgh: Churchill Livingstone.

Harries, J. T. (1977) *Essentials of Paediatric Gastro-enterology*. Edinburgh: Churchill Livingstone.

Harris, A. I. *et al*. (1972) *Handicapped and Impaired in Great Britain*. London: H.M.S.O.

Harvey, S. & Hales-Tooke, A. (1972) *Play in Hospital*. London: Faber.

Hilgard, E. & Atkinson, R. (1972) *Introduction to Psychology*. New York: Harcourt, Brace and World.

Holt, J. (1970) *How Children Fail*. Harmondsworth, Middx: Pelican

Holt, J. (1973) *How Children Learn*. Harmondsworth, Middx: Pelican.

Horstmann, D. M. (1969) Viral infections in pregnancy. *Yale Journal of Biology and Medicine*, 2, 99–112.

Hubner, P. (1977) *Nurses' Guide to Cardiac Monitoring*. London: Baillière Tindall.

Illingworth, R. S. (1980) *The Development of the Infant and Young Child*, 7th edition. Edinburgh: Churchill Livingstone.

Illingworth, R. S. & Illingworth, C. (1977) *Babies and Young Children*, 6th edition. Edinburgh: Churchill Livingstone.

James, J. A. (1972) *Renal Disease in Childhood*. St Louis: Mosby.

Jones, P. (1976) *Clinical Paediatric Surgery, Diagnosis and Management*. London: Blackwell Scientific Publications.

Jones, P. G. & Campbell, P. E. (1976) *Tumours of Infancy and Childhood*. London: Blackwell Scientific Publications.

Jones, R. B. (Ed.) (1976) *Child Care, Health and Development*, Vol. 2, No. 4.

Jordan, S. C. & Scott, O. (1981) *Heart Disease in Paediatrics*. 2nd edition. London: Butterworth.

Kemble, J. V. Harvey & Lamb, B. E. (1984) *Plastic Surgical and Burns Nursing*. London: Baillière Tindall.

Kelman, G.tR. (1980) *Physiology, A Clinical Approach* 3rd edition. Edinburgh: Churchill Livingstone.

Kempe, H. C., Silver, H. K. & O'Brian, D. (1984) *Current Paediatric Diagnosis and Treatment*. Los Altos, California: Lange.

Kuzenko, J. (1976) *Asthma in Children*. London: Pitman.

Lenneberg, E. (Ed.) (1964) *A Biological Perspective of Language*. Cambridge, Massachusetts: MIT Press, 65–88.

Lissauer, T. (1982) *Paediatric Emergencies*. Lancaster: MTP Press.

Lloyd de Mause (Ed.) (1976) *The History of Childhood*.

Lorber, J. (1975) Isosorbide in treatment of infantile hydrocephalus. *Archives of Disease in Childhood*, 50, 431.

Lowbury, *et al*. (Ed.) (1981) *Control of Hospital Infection, A Practical Handbook*. London: Chapman and Hall.

Ludman, H. (1969) *Ear, Nose and Throat Diseases, Principles of Patient Care*. London: Pitman Medical and Scientific Publications.

Marlow, D. R. & Sellew, G. (1977) *Textbook of Paediatric Nursing*. Philadelphia: W. B. Saunders.

Marshall, S. (1967) *Ear, Nose and Throat Nursing*. Nurses' Aid Series. London: Baillière Tindall.

McLaren, D. & Burnam, D. (Eds.) (1976) *Textbook of Paediatric Nutrition*, Ch. 11 — Water and electrolytes. Edinburgh: Churchill Livingstone.

McLennan, D. S. & Burman, D. (1982) *Textbook of Paediatric Nutrition*. Edinburgh: Churchill Livingstone.

McNaught, A. B. & Callander, R. (1975) *Illustrated Physiology*, 3rd edition. Edinburgh: Churchill Livingstone.

Medical Research Council (1955) *Lancet*, 2, 5.

Millar, S. (1968) *The Psychology of Play*. Harmondsworth, Middx: Pelican.

Nash, E. D. F. (1981) *The Principles and Practice of Surgery for Nurses and Allied Professions*, 7th edition. London: Edward Arnold.

Noble, E. (1967) *Play and the Sick Child*. London: Hutchison.

Nurse's Reference Library Series. *Phrenic Pacing*, Ch. 9, p. 510. Intermed.

Oates, J. (Ed.) (1979) *Early Cognitive Development*, Ch. 5, 8, 18, 23. Croom Helm, London: Oxford University, Press.

Oppé, T. E. & Redstone, D. (1968) Calcium and phosphorus levels in healthy newborn infants given various types of milk. *Lancet*, 1, 1045–1048.

Piaget, J. (1924) *The Child's Conception of the World*. New York: Harcourt.

Pipes, P. L. (1981) *Nutrition in Infancy and Childhood*. St Louis: Mosby.

Pollen, A. G. (1973) *Fractures and Dislocations in Children*. Edinburgh: Churchill Livingstone.

Pringle, M. K. (1975) *The Needs of Children*. London: Hutchinson.

Purchese, G. (1977) *Neuromedical and Neurosurgical Nursing*. London: Baillière Tindall.

Reid, A. H. (1982) *The Psychiatry of Mental Handicap*. London: Blackwell Scientific Publications.

Rickham, P. P. & Johnstone, J. H. (1969) *Neonatal Surgery*. London: Butterworth.

Robertson, J. (1958) *Young Children in Hospital*. London: Tavistock.

Robertson, J. (1963) *Hospitals and Children*. N.Y. International Universities Press.

Robinson, C. H. (1972) *Normal and Therapeutic Nutrition*, 14th edition. London: Macmillan.

Roddie, I. C. & Wallace, W. F. M (1976) *The Physiology of Disease*. London: Lloyd-Luke (Medical Books).

Rose, S. (1971) *The Chemistry of Life*. Harmondsworth, Middx: Pelican.

Rutter, M. & Hersov, W. F. M. (1976) *Child Psychiatry*. London: Blackwell Scientific Publications.

Sacharin, R. M. & Hunter, M. H. S. (1969) *Paediatric Nursing Procedures*, 2nd edition. Edinburgh: Livingstone.

Sandstroem, C. I. (1969) *The Psychology of Childhood and Adolescence*. Harmondsworth Middx: Pelican.

Savage, D. R. (1968) *Psychometric Assessment of the Individual Child*. Harmondsworth, Middx: Penguin.

Scopes, J. W. & Ahmed, I. (1966) *Archives of Diseases in Childhood*, 41, 407.

Scripien, G. M., Barnard, M., Chard, M., Howe, J. & Phillips, P. J. (1975) *Comprehensive Paediatric Nursing*. Maidenhead: McGraw-Hill.

Sheridan, M. D. (1969) *Children's Development Progress N.F.E.R. Publishing Company*.

Sinclair, D. (1969) *Human Growth after Birth*, Chs. 2, 3 and 6. Oxford Medical Publications.

Smith, A. E. & Nunn, C. K. (1982) The phrenic nerve stimulator. Abstract. *Critical Care Nurse*, May/June.

Smith, J. B. (Ed.) (1983) *Paediatric Critical Care*. New York: John Wiley and Sons.

Smith, J. W. (1975) *Diseases of the Small Intestine in Childhood*. London: Pitman Medical.

Spector, W. G. (1980) *An Introduction to General Pathology*, 2nd edition. Edinburgh: Churchill Livingstone.

Stevenson, A. C., Davison, B. C. & Clare, (1976) *Genetic Counselling*, 2nd edition. London: Heinemann Medical Books Ltd.

Stone, F. H. & Koupernik, C. (1974) *Child Psychiatry for Students*, 2nd edition. Edinburgh: Churchill Livingstone.

Taylor, A. (1974) *Practical Human Cytogenetics*: Laboratory Monograph. London: Baillière Tindall.

Tierney, A. J. (Ed.) (1983) *Nurses and the Mentally Handicapped.* New York: John Wiley and Sons.

Trounce, J. R. (1977) *Pharmacology for Nurses*, 7th edition. Edinburgh: Churchill Livingstone.

Turner, P. & Richens, A. (1978) *Clinical Pharmacology*, 3rd edition. Edinburgh: Churchill Livingstone.

Valman, H. B. (Ed.) (1979) *Paediatric Therapeutics*. London: Blackwell Scientific Publications.

Vernon, P. E. (1973) *Personality Assessment*. London: Tavistock-Methuen.

Wachstein, J. (1976) *Anaesthesia and Recovery Room Technique*, 2nd edition. London: Baillière Tindall.

Wedge, P. & Prosser, H. (1973) *Born to Fail*. National Children's Bureau.

Whetnall, E. & Fry, D. F. (1964) *The Deaf Child*. London: Heinemann.

Wilkinson, A. W. (1975) *Recent Advances in Paediatric Surgery, 3*. Edinburgh: Churchill Livingstone.

Willoughby, M. L. N. (1977) *Paediatric Haematology*, Chs. 10, 18 and 20. Edinburgh: Churchill Livingstone.

Winner, H. I. (1972) *Microbiology in Patient Care*. London: Unibooks, English University Press.

Winnicott, D. W. (1964) *The Child, the Family and the Outside World*. Harmondsworth, Middx: Penguin.

Wolff, S. (1970) *Children under Stress*. Harmondsworth, Middx: Penguin.

Wright, D. (1975) *The Psychology of Moral Behaviour*. Harmondsworth: Pelican.

Zuck, D. (1969) *The Principles of Anaesthesia for Nurses*. London: Pitman Medical.

Department of Education and Science
1968 *The Education of the Visually Handicapped*
1970 *Report of the Committee on Maladjusted Children*
1975 *Educating Mentally Handicapped Children*
1980 *Prevention in Childhood of Health Problems in Adult Life* (WHO)
1980 *Towards Better Health Care for School Children in Scotland* (Scottish Home and Health Department)

Department of Health and Social Security
1959 *The Welfare of Children in Hospital*
1969 *Recommended Intakes of Nutrients for the United Kingdom*
1971 *Report of the Expert Group on Special Care for Babies*
1972 *Children with Specific Reading Difficulties*
1974 *Mentally Handicapped Children in Residential Care*
1975 *Present-Day Practice in Infant Feeding*
1976 *Fit for the Future*. The Report of the Committee on Child Health Services
1976 *Manual of Nutrition* (Ministry of Agriculture, Fisheries and Food)

Index

Abdominal paracentesis, 558
Abnormal behaviour, 319
ABO blood groups, 431
Abscess formation, 235
Absolute refractory period, 295
Accessory breath sounds, 119
Accidents, prevention of, 85
Accommodation (vision), 331
Acetazolamide, 301
Acetylcholine, 294
Achalasia of the cardia, 479
Acholuric jaundice, 436
Acid-base balance, 229
Acid-base disturbance, 229
Acne, 572
Acquired immunity, 240
Acromegaly, 272
Acute appendicitis, 495
Acutely ill child, food requirements, 216
Acute lymphoblastic leukaemia, 444
Acute mastoiditis, 346
Acute monocytic/myeloblastic leukaemia, 445
Acute myocarditis, 422
Acute nephritis, diet in, 219
Acute pancreatitis, 506
Acute pericarditis, 423
Acute renal failure
  care of the child, 113
  diet in, 220
Acute rheumatic heart disease, 421
Acute stomatitis, 474
Addis sedimentation count, 557
Addison's disease, 279
Adenoidectomy, 358
  complications of, 359
Adenoids, 358
  hypertrophy of, 358
Administration of medicines, 165
  guidelines, 171
  hypodermic, 174
  intramuscular, 175
  rectal, 173
  subcutaneous, 174
Admission of child, 76
  emergency, 77
  planned, 76
Adolescence, 27
Adolescent
  growth, 31

physical changes, 31
psychological development, 32
Adrenal cortex, 277
Adrenaline, 428
Adrenocortical
  insufficiency, 279
  overactivity, 279
Aeruginosa (pyocyanea), 246
Agammaglobulinaemia, 240
Age scaling, 317
Aggression, 25, 82
Aid techniques (psych.), 317
Airborne infection, 245
Air encephalography, 314
Albumin
  function of, 429
  transfusion, 449
Aldosteronism, 280
Alleles, 254
Allogeneic, 458
Allopurinol, 444
Alveolar ventilation, 367
Alveoli, 364
Amblyopia, 332
Amblyoscope, 338
Ambulation, 135
Amino-acids, essential, 191
Aminophylline, 374
Ammonia dermatitis, 529
Amniocentesis, 259
Anabolism, 8
Anaemia
  aplastic, 436
  haemolytic, 436
  hypoplastic, 435
  iron-deficiency, 435
  sickle cell, 439
Anaesthesia, 600
Anal deformities, 498
Anal fissure, 499
Anal stricture, 498
Anaphylactic shock, 428
Androgens, 278
Anencephaly, 297
Angiocardiography, 462
Angiogram, 314
Anions, 224
Anomalous pulmonary venous drainage, 412
Anorectal manometry, 493
Anorexia, 89

Anterior pituitary gland, disorders of, 271
Antidiuretic hormone (ADH), 224
Antigens, 240
Anuria, 90
Anxiety, expressions of, 321
Aortography, 463
Apgar score chart, 379
Aphasic, 91
Aphoria, 91
Apical heart beat, 104
Aplastic anaemia, 436
Aplastic kidney, 530
Apnoea, 105
  monitor, 105, 106
  treatment of, 158
Appetite, 89
Appliances, care of, 590
Arterial blood pressure, 460
  measurement by cannulation, 461
Arteriopuncture, 447
Artificial airway, 393
  prevention of complications, 395
Artificial eye
  care of, 340
  removal of, 339
  replacement of, 340
Artificial feeding, 512
Ascending reticular activating system, 296
Aseptic technique, 139, 247
Asilone, 482
A.S.O. titre, 421
Aspiration pneumonia, 378
Astigmatism, 332
Astrocytoma, 302
Asystole, 124
Ataxia, 311
Atelectasis, 378
Athetosis, 311
Atlanta brace, 581
Atrial fibrillation, 406
Atropine
  actions of, 336
  effects of, 128
Audiometry, 349
Augmented histamine test, 515
Autism, 321
Autosomes, 253
Autosomal
  dominant inheritance, 255

Autosomal (*Cont'd*)
recessive inheritance, 256
Axillary temperature, measuring of, 102

Baby bottle, sterilisation of, 42
Bacteria, 236
identification of, 237
multiplication of, 237
Bacterial
endocarditis, 423
pneumonia, 377
Balloon septostomy, 414
Barium
enema, 519
meal, 518
swallow, 518
Barlow's divaricator, 578
Barr body, 259
Barrier nursing, 250
Basal age, 317
Base (defined), 229
Batchelor plaster of Paris, 593
Bathing
infant, 34
older babies and toddlers, 36
Battered baby syndrome, 52
BCG, 245
Bedbathing, 93
Behaviour therapy, 325
Benzyl benzoate, 572
Bile, functions of, 198, 470
Bilirubin, 503
toxicity of, 437
Binet, A., 316
Biochemical disturbances, 427
Birmingham brace, 581
Bladder, 527
decompression, 550
irrigation, 551
lavage, 551
puncture, 552
Blalock-Taussig procedure, 409
Blastula, 3
Blepharitis, 335
Blood cells, development of, 430
Blood clotting, 433
groups, 431
reaction, 369
transfusion, 453
volume, 429
Bone, growth and development, 573
Bone marrow
puncture, 457
transplantation, 458
Bones, functions of, 573
Bottle feeding, 40
Bow-legs, 576
Bowlby, J, 49
Bradycardia, 104
Braces
Atlanta, 581
Birmingham, 581
Toronto, 581
Brain, 289

lobes of, 289
scan, 314
stem, 292
Breast feeding, 38
drug intake in, 38
Breath-holding attacks, 308
Breathing
measuring of, 105
rates, 105
types, 105
Bronchi, 363
Bronchial
asthma, 374
suction, 120
Bronchiolitis, 376
Bronchopneumonia, 377
Bronchoscopy, 393
Brotherston report, 58
Buffers, 229
Bullae, 569
Burn chart, 144
Burns and scalds
causes, 142
nursing management, 144
nutritional needs, 148
pathophysiology, 142
psychological care, 146
Buttocks, care of, 115

Calcium, 206
deficiency, 206
disturbance, 229
Calculation
of drug dosage, 165
of feeds, 41
Caliper, 589
Cancer
benign, 116
causes of, 116
host factors, 116
malignant, 116
Candida albicans, 474
Carbohydrates, 194
deficient intake, 197
dietary, 197
digestion and absorption, 196
excessive intake, 197
-free regimen, 218
functions of, 195
Carbon dioxide, transport of, 369
Cardiac arrest
causes, 121
signs, 121
treatment, 123
Cardiac catheterisation, 461
cycle, 404
disease, diet in, 220
failure
infant, 424
older child, 425
Cardiac massage, signs of effectiveness, 124
Cardiac operations, types of, 409
Cardiac surgery, 409

Cardiogenic shock, 427
Cardio-oesophageal chalasia, 480
Cardiospasm, 479
Cardiovascular problems, care of child, 110
Cardiovascular system, development of, 399
Care systems, 108
Carpopedal spasm, 229, 536
Case conferences, 54
CAT, 315
Catabolism, 8
Cataract, 334
Catarrhal tonsillitis, 356
Categories of disabilities, 61
Catheterisation, dangers of, 549
Cations, 224
Cattell, R.B., 318
Cells, structure of, 3, 4
Central venous pressure, 459
Cephalocaudal, 5
Cerebellum, 292
lesions of, 292
Cerebral
abscess, 411
hypoxia, 296
oedema, 301
palsy, 310
thrombosis, 411
Cerebrospinal fluid, 291
composition, 291
functions, 292
pressure of, 291
volume, 291
Cerebrum, 289
Cervical halter traction, 597
Chalazion, 335
Chemical battering, 53
Chest aspiration, 389
Chest physiotherapy (infant), 477
Cheyne Stokes breathing, 105
Child abuse, 52
consequences of, 54
Child Guidance clinic, 66
Child Health clinic, 59
Child minders, 56
Child nutrition, social factors, 189
Child rearing, 50
discipline, 51
feeding, 51
Children's apperception test, 318
Chlorhexidine gluconate, 551
Choanal atresia, 372
Christmas disease, 443
Chromatids, 256
Chromatin, 7
Chromosomes, 253
Chronic lymphocytic thyroiditis, 275
Chronic renal failure, diet in, 220
Chronological age, 317
Chylothorax, 420
Cimetidine, 485
Circumcision, 541
Cisterna magna, 313
Cisternal puncture, 313

Cleft lip and palate, 471
Cleft palate, 473
Clonic phase, 306
Clubbing of digits, 408
Coarctation of the aorta, 418
Cocci, 237
Coeliac disease, 500
  diet in, 217
Cognitive development, 24
Cold injury, 99
Collagen, 204
Collection of urine
  24 hour, 548
  older child, 548
Colonic lavage, 521
Colonoscopy, 522
Colostomy, 150, 521
  physiology of a, 151
  types of, 151
  wash out, 154, 521
Colostrum, 38
Coma, 303
Commensals, 236
Compensation (psych.), 25
Complement system, 240
Complementary feed, 40
Complex anenploidy, 257
Compliance, 367
Computerised axial tomography, 315
Concomitant squint, 333
Cones (eyes), 330
Congenital atresia of the oesophagus,
  475
Congenital hypertrophic pyloric
  stenosis, 480
Congenital cardiovascular anomalies,
  408
Congenital dislocation of the hip, 577
Congenital heart disease, social aspects,
  426
Congenital thyroid hypoplasia, 274
Conjunctival swab, 337
Conjunctivitis, 335
Constant positive airway pressure
  (CPAP), 396
Constipation, 498
  in cancer, 117
  mechanism of, 498
Contact lenses
  care of, 340
  removal of, 340
  replacement of, 340
Continuous ambulatory peritoneal
  dialysis (CAPD), 560
Control of drugs, 170
Convulsions, 305
  care of the child, 113
  physiological effects, 113
Cooley's anaemia, 438
Copper
  deficiency, 210
  toxicity, 210
Cor pulmonale, 507
Corneal ulcers, prevention of, 112
Corpus callosum, 289

Correcting lenses, 337
Corrigan's pulse, 104
Corset dressing, 140
Cortical mastoidectomy, 347
Corticotrophin deficiency, 273
Cortisol, 278
Coryza, 372
Cow's milk allergy, 215
Coxa plana, 580
Craniotabes, 587
Creatinine clearance test, 557
Cretinism, 274
Cri du chat, 326
Crista dividens, 400
Crohn's disease, 501
Cross infection, 245
Cross matching, 431
Croup, 373
Croupette, 381, 385
Crusts, 569
Cry, interpretation of, 12, 88
Cryoprecipitate, 449
Cryosurgery, 272
Cryptorchidism, 543
Curare, 294
Cushing's syndrome, 279
Cutaneous ureterostomy, 154
Cyanosis, 371
Cyanotic attacks, 411
Cyclic vomiting, 485
Cyclophosphamide, 445
Cycloplegic, 333
Cystic fibrosis, diet in, 217
Cystic fibrosis of the lungs, 376
Cystic fibrosis of the pancreas, 506
Cystometrogram, 553
Cystoscopic examination, 553
Cystitis, 540
Cytogenetics, 256
Cytosine arabinoside, 445

Day nursery, 56
Daunorubicin, 445
Deaf child, education of, 351
Deafness, 64, 347
  conductive, 349
  perceptive, 350
  screening for, 348
Death and dying, child's reaction to,
  125
Decibels, 343
Defence mechanism, 317
Defibrillation, 124
Deglutition, 355
Dehydration, 230
  hypertonic, 230
  hypotonic, 230
  isotonic, 230
  mild, 486
  moderate, 487
  severe, 487
De Lange syndrome, 328
Delayed primary repair, 479
Deletion, 257

Denial, 126, 317
Denis Browne foot splints, 598
Dental caries, 95
  causes of, 95
  prevention of, 96
Dental floss, 96
Dermis, 567
Dermatoglyphs, 328
Derotational osteotomy, 581
Desferrioxamine, 436, 439
Development
  child, 15
  emotional, 24
  fetus, 4
  hearing, 20
  intellectual, 22
  language, 20
  moral, 28
  motor, 16
  personality, 25
  sexual, 7
  social, 28
  speech, 20
  understanding, 22
  visual, 20
DNA, 253
Diabetes insipidus, 270
Diabetes mellitus, 281, 507
  diet in, 221
  psychological aspect, 283
Diaphragmatic hernia, 482
Diarrhoea
  cancer and, 117
  vomiting and, 486
Diazepam, 113, 522
Diazoxide, 538
Dietary fibre, 218
Diets in disease, 215
Diethylpropion, 215
Difficulties at school, 82
Digitalis, use of, 426
Dilutions of lotions, 164
Dioctylmedo, 520
Dioralyte, 486
Diphtheria, 357
Dipropylacetate, 307
Disaccharidase deficiency, test for, 267
Disinfectants, table of, 251
Dithranol paste, 571
Diuresis, 90
Discipline, 81
Disturbed sleep, 37
Dicrotic pulse, 104
Diminished absorption, 134
Divaricator
  Barlow's, 593
  Craig's, 593
Dominant trait, 255
Doppler method, 538
Dorsal slab, 592
Double ileostomy, 490
Down's syndrome, 327
Dressing techniques, 140
Drugs, administration of, 163
Duodenal atresia, 488

Duodenal intubation, 516
Duodenal stenosis, 489
Duodeno-duodenostomy, 488
Duodeno-jejunostomy, 488
Duplication (genetics), 257
Dwyer cable, 583
D-xylose absorption test, 517
Dying
  care of, 125
  stages of, 126
Dyslexia, 63
Dysarthria, 311
Dyspnoea, 105, 369
  alleviation of, 110
Dysphagia, 89
Dysuria, 90, 529

Ear, 341
  examination of, 352
  instillation of drops, 353
  insufflation of, 353
  mopping of, 352
  swabbing of, 352
  syringing of, 352
Echocardiography, 463
Echoencephalography, 315
Echolalia, 21, 322
Ectopia vesicae, 546
Ectopic cryptorchidism, 544
Ectopic kidney, 530
Ectopic ureter, 528
Eczema, 570
Egocentrism, 23
Electrocardiogram, 405
Electrocochleography, 354
Electroencephalography, 306
Electrolytes, 224
Electronic pacemaker, care of the child,
  463
Embryo, growth of, 3
Emotional development, 24
Encephalocele, 299
Encephalitis, 309
Encopresis, 499
Endocardial fibro-elastosis, 420
Endocrine glands, 270
  role in growth, 8
Endoscopes, 509
Endotracheal intubation, 393
Energy-controlled diet, 214
Enuresis, 90, 528
Environmental infection, 245
Eosinophil adenomas, 271
Ependymomas, 302
Epidermis, 567
Epididymis, 523
Epiglottis, 362
Epiglottitis, 362
Epilepsy, 305
Epilim, 307
Epiphyseal dysplasia, 587
Epispadias, 543
Erb's palsy, 598
Erythema marginatum, 421

Erythema nodosum, 421
Erythrocyte sedimentation rate, 463
Erythropoietin, 430, 526
Esbach's test, 564
'E' test, 334
Eustachian tube, disorders of, 344
Eversion of lids, 337
Excessive loss of tissue fluids, 134
Exchange transfusion, 454
Excretion pyelogram, 554
Exomphalos, 491
Exophthalmos, 275
Expiratory reserve volume, 367
Expiratory stridor, 119
Exposure treatment for burns, 146
Extensions
  fixed traction, 595
  sliding traction, 595
External cardiac massage, 123
External defibrillation, 124
Extrasystole, 406
Eye
  anatomy of, 330
  application of ointment, 338
  examination of, 336
  functions of, 331
  irrigation of, 339
Eyelashes, cutting of, 338
Eysenck, H.J., 318
  junior personality inventory, 318

Faecal fat excretion, 517
Faeces, 469
Failure to thrive, 32
Fallopian tubes, 524
Family disorganisation, 48
Family, functions of, 47
Family unit, 47
Fanconi's aplastic anaemia, 436
Fasting glucose and insulin test, 266
Fats
  deficient intakes, 199
  digestion and absorption, 198
  excessive intakes, 199
  food sources, 199
  functions of, 198
Feeding of children, 44, 213
  newborn baby, 212
  times of, 39
Feeds
  calculation of, 41
  preparation of, 42
Feingold diet, 221
Femoral vein puncture, 447
Ferric chloride test (phenylketonuria),
  566
Fetal circulation, 6, 399
  changes at birth, 400
Fetal haemoglobin, 431
Fetal heart beat, 399
Fetus, development of, 4
Fibrinogen, 429
FIGLU excretion test, 557
Fissures, 569

Fixation (psych.), 25, 317
Fluid content of the body, 223
Fluid intake/output recording, 114
Fluorine, 210
Fontan operation, 409
Fontanelle tap, 446
Fontanelles, 12
Food intolerance, 215
Food refusal, 213
Foley's self-retaining catheter, 550
Formimino-glutamic acid excretion test,
  557
Fractures, 584
  classification of, 584
  complications of, 584
  healing of, 585
  treatment of, 585
Frames, 589
Free diet, 214
Freeze-dried coagulation factor, 449
  fibrinogen, 449
  whole plasma, 449
Fresh whole plasma, 448
Freud, S., 317
Frustration, 25
Fungus, pathogenic, 237
Furunculosis, 345

Galactosaemia, 263
Gallows traction, 596
Gargles, 361
Gastric
  analysis, 515
  aspiration, 509
  gavage (continuous), 513
  gavage (intermittent), 513
  gavage (temporary), 512
  lavage, 511
  tubes, lubrication of, 509
  tube replacement, 479
Gastrografin, 518
Gastroenteritis, 486
Gastro-intestinal disturbance,
  care of child, 114
Gastro-oesophagostomy, 479
Gastropexy, 482
Gastroschisis, 492
Gastrostomy, 514
Gaviscon, 482
General pathology, 234
Genes, 253
Genetic
  code, 253
  counselling, 258
  engineering, 259
Genotype, 254
Gentian violet, 474
Genu valgum, 576
Genu varum, 576
Giardiasis, 508
Glandular fever, 357
Gliadin, 500
Globulin
  function, 429

Globulin (*Cont'd*)
  types, 429
Glomerulonephritis, 532
Glucagon
  function of, 471
  test, 266
Glucocorticoids, 278
Glucose
  function of, 195
  tolerance test, 266
Gluten enteropathy, 500
Gluten free diet, 501
Glycogen storage disease, 263
Glycosuria, 90, 281
Gonadotrophic hormones, 544
Gonadotrophin deficiency, 273
Gram-negative bacteria, 238
Gram-positive bacteria, 238
Grand mal, 306
Granulation tissue, 236
Granulocytes, 432
Greenstick fracture, 584
Group therapy, 325
Growth
  after birth, 8.14
  factors affecting, 5, 8
  hormone deficiency, 272
  in weight, 14
  spurt, 31
G-trisomy, 326
Guthrie's test, 266

Haematemesis, 89
Haematuria, 90, 529
Haemodialysis, 561
Haemoglobin, 431
Haemoglobin S, 431
Haemoglobinopathies, 438
Haemolytic anaemias, 436
Haemolytic disease of the newborn, 437
Haemolytic streptococci, 246
Haemophilia, 442
Haemophilia B, 443
Haemoptysis, 91, 100
Haemorrhage
  reactionary, 359
  secondary, 359
Haemostasis, 433
Hair, 567
  care of, 91
Halo-pelvic traction, 583
Handicapped child, needs of, 324
Handicapped schoolchild, care of, 61
Harrington rods, 583
Hashimoto's disease, 275
Head circumference, 12
Head injuries, 301
Head traction, 597
Heaf test, 244
Healing and repair, 235
Healing of wounds, 136
  delayed healing, 137
Hearing aids, 350
Hearing, development of, 347

Heart
  action of, 403
  block, 406
  rate, 404
  regulation of rate, 399
  structure and function, 402
Height, growth in, 14
Heimlich manoeuvre, 356
Henoch-Schoenlein, 440
Hepatic failure, 505
Hereditary spherocytosis, 436
Hermaphroditism, 7
Herniotomy, 545
Heterozygote, 255
Hiatus hernia, 482
  diet in, 217
High fibre diet, 219
Hip spica, lifting child, 591
Hirschsprung's disease, 152, 493
HLA (human leucocyte antigen), 458
Holter valve, 300
Homozygote, 255
Hordeolum externum, 336
Hospital-associated infection, 245
Hospital infection, prevention of, 246
Human leucocyte antigen system
      (HLA), 258, 458
  typing, 458
Human milk, production of, 212
Humidaire, 381, 385
Humidity, 381
Hydralazine, 538
Hydroceles, 544
Hydrocephalus, 299
  communicating, 300
  non-communicating (obstructive),
      300
Hydroencephaly, 297
Hydrolysis, 196
Hyoscine/Scopolamine, action of, 336
Hypercalcaemia, 207
Hypercapnia, 121, 369
Hypercarbia, 121
Hyperglycaemia, 281
Hyperkinetic syndromes, 323
Hypermetropia, 332
Hypernatraemia, 230
Hyperparathyroidism, 277
Hypersensitivity, 234
  tissue transplant, 235
Hypertension, 537
Hypertensive encephalopathy, 533
Hyperthermia, 99
Hyperthyroidism, 275
Hypertonic fluids, 448
Hypervitaminosis A, 200
Hypocalcaemia, 207
Hypoderm, 567
Hypoglycaemia, 272, 284
Hypokalaemia, 227
Hyponatraemia, 231
Hypoparathyroidism, 276
Hypoplastic anaemia, 435
Hypoprothrombinaemia, 202
Hypospadias, 541

Hypothalamus, 270, 290
  food centre in, 213
Hypothermia, 99
  profound, 409
Hypothyroidism, 274
Hypotonic fluids, 448
Hypovolaemic shock, 427
Hypoxia, 369

Identi-bands, 86
Identification, 129
Identity, 86
Idiopathic juvenile osteoporosis, 207
Ileal conduit, 154, 546
Ileostomy, 153
Imitative learning, 316
Immunisation, 241
Immunity, 239
Immunoglobulins, 240
Impacted wax, 345
Imperforate anus, 152, 497
Impetigo, 570
INAH, 309
Inborn errors of metabolism, 262
  steroid biosynthesis, 278
  thyroxine biosynthesis, 275
Incomitant squint, 333
Incontinence, 528
  pad (buzzer), 529
Incubator, 181
  care of, 183
  temperatures of, 158
Infant's buttocks, care of, 115, 487
Infant feeding, 37
  bottle, 40
  routine, 249
Infantile spasms, 306
Infection (defined), 236
  effects of, 239
  modes of spread, 238
Infectious diseases, 243
Infective diarrhoea and vomiting, 486
Inflammation, 235
  oedema in, 235
Infusion
  care of the child, 451
  objectives for, 448
  venepuncture, 449
  venesection, 450
Inguinal hernia, strangulated, 545
Inheritance, modes of, 254
Injection
  hypodermic, 174
  intramuscular, 175
Innate immune mechanism, 239
Inspection of wound, 132
Inspiratory reserve volume, 367
Instillation of
  ear drops, 353
  eye drops, 336
Insufflation of ear, 353
Insulin
  action of, 281
  administration of, 283

Insulin (Cont'd)
  choice of, 284
  functions of, 196, 471
  mixing of, 284
  production, 259
Integration
  functional, 63
  locational, 62
  social, 63
Intelligence, measurement of, 316
  quotient (I.Q.), 317
Intellectual development, 22
Intermittent mandatory ventilation
    (IMV), 396
Intermittent positive pressure
    ventilation (IPPV), 396
Internal D.C. defibrillation, 124
Intersex, 524
Interviewing parents, 78
Intestinal villi, 468
Intracranial pressure, increase in, 302
Intramuscular injection, 175
Intra-uterine transfusion, 455
Intravenous
  infusion, 448
  nutrition, 455
  pyelogram, 554
  saline test, 271
Intrinsic factor, 468
Introversion-extroversion, 318
Intussusception, 494
Involucrum, 580
Iron, 208
Iron-deficiency anaemia, 209, 435
Iron
  loss of, 209
  sources of, 209
Irons (splints), 589
Isolation of patients, 250
Isonicotinic acid hydrazide, 309
Isosorbide, 301
Isotonic fluids, 448

Jaundice, 503
Jejunal biopsy, 516
Jejuno-ileal atresia, 489
Jejunum, 468
Joints, functions of, 573
Jugular vein puncture, 447
Jung, Carl, 318
Juvenile diabetes mellitus, 281

Kayser-Fleischer ring, 210
Kernicterus, 437
Kernig's sign, 309
Ketamine, 394
Ketoacidosis, 281
Ketogenic diet, 221, 307
Ketosis, 199
Keystone machine, 60
Kidney, 525
  disorders of, 530
  endocrine function of, 526

functions of, 526
function tests, 556
tumours of, 538
Klinefelter's syndrome, 7, 524
Knock-knees, 576
Kwashiorkor, 193
Kyphosis, 602

Laboured breathing, 109, 110
Lactose-free regime, 218
Lactose tolerance test, 267
Language, development of, 20
Language and environment, 21
Large intestine, 469
Laryngeal stridor, 119
Laryngitis
  acute, 372
  diphtheretic, 373
  obstructive, 373
  spasmodic, 373
Laryngospasm, 373
Laryngo-tracheal-bronchitis, 373
Larynx, 362
Lassar's paste, 571
Last offices, 127
Latent squint, 333
Learning, 316
Legg-Calvé-Perthes disease, 580
Lens (es), 330
  correcting, 340
Leucine sensitivity, 285
  test, 266
Leukaemia(s), 443
  acute lymphoblastic, 444
  acute myeloblastic/monocytic, 445
  meningeal, 445
Levels of consciousness, 302
Lice, 91
Lipids, 197
Lipid storage disease, 265
Lipoid pneumonia, 509
Liver, 470
Liver biopsy, 517
Liver cell failure, 503
Liver, infections of, 504
Lobar pneumonia, 377
Locus, 254
Long axis traction, 595
  action of, 593
Long chain triglycerides, 198
Low fibre diet, 219
Lowe's syndrome, 602
L-thyroxine, 274
Lumbar puncture, 312
Lung biopsy, 390
Lung
  puncture, 390
  volumes, 366
Lungs
  functions of, 365
  structure of, 364
Lymphocytes, 433
Lymphocytic thyroiditis, 275

Macules, 568
Magnesium
  depletion, 229
  retention, 229
  sulphate (sweat test), 268
Malabsorption syndrome, 500
Maladjusted child, provision for, 65
Malnutrition, after effects, 190
Malrotation, 490
Mantoux test, 244
Marasmus, 193
Marfan's syndrome, 602
Mastoiditis, 346
Maternal deprivation, 49
Maturity, emotional, 25
MCT, 308
Meatal
  stenosis, 541
  ulceration, 541
Meatotomy, 541
Mechanical ventilator, 395
Meckel's diverticulum, 494
Meconium, 13, 89
Meconium ileus, 489
Medicines, administration of, 165
  guidelines, 171
  injections, 169
  oral, 169
  rectal, 169
Medium chain triglycerides, 198,
    308
Medulla oblongata, 292
Medulloblastoma, 302
Meibomian cyst, 335
Meiosis, 253
Melaena, 90
Melanin, 567
Mendel's first law, 258
Meningeal leukaemia, 445
Meninges, 290
Meningitis, 308
Meningocele, 297
Meningococcal meningitis, 309
Meningoencephalitis, 309
Meningomyelocele, 298
Menkes' kinky hair syndrome, 210
Mental age, 316
Mental deficiency (classification), 317
Mental handicap
  pathology of, 327
  provisions for children, 66
Mental retardation
  causes of, 326
  definition, 326
  management of child, 328
6-Mercaptopurine, 445
Mesnum, 459
Metabolic
  acidosis, 230
  alkalosis, 230
Methotrexate, 444
Metoclopramide, 518
Microbiology, 236
Microcephaly, 297
Micrognathia, 475

Micro-organisms
  classification, 236
  pathogenicity of, 241
Micturition, 528
Midbrain, 292
Mid-stream specimen of urine, 548
Milk, 38
  amount of, 39
  and drugs, 212
  production of, 38
Milwaukee brace, 582
Mineralocorticoids, 277
Minerals, 205
Mira oxygen analyser, 385
Mistaken identity, 86
Mittens, dangers of, 161
Monocytes, 433
Monosomy, 257
Moral development, 28
Morphine, 110
Mosaicism, 327
Motor development, 16
Motor neurones
  lower, 295
  upper, 295
Mouth (anatomy), 466
  care, 96
  irrigation of, 97
Mouth-to-mouth resuscitation, 122
Mouth-to-nose resuscitation, 123
Mouthwashes, 97
Munchausen syndrome, 53
Murmurs, 407
Muscles, types and function, 574
Mustard operation, 410
Mutation, 254
Myasthenia gravis, 294
Mydriatic, 333
Myelocele, 298
Myelomeningocele, 298
Myocarditis, 422
Myopia, 332
Myringotomy, 350

Nails, 567
Naloxone, 120, 522
Napkin area, care of, 36, 115
Nasal injuries, 372
Naso-duodenal/jejunal feeding, 514
Naso-gastric tube, securing of, 477
Naso-pharynx, 355
Necrotising enterocolitis, 496
Negative nitrogen balance, 192
Negativism, 29
Neonatal
  hepatitis, 503
  jaundice, 503
  pre-operative care, 161
  tetany, 276
Neonate
  maintaining pulmonary ventilation, 157
  surgical nursing principles, 156
Nephroblastoma, 538

Nephron, 525
Nephrostomy, 550
Nephrotic syndrome, 533
Nerve
  damage to, 295
  fibre, 294
  impulse, 295
  regeneration of, 295
Nervous system
  defects, 297
  tumours of, 302
Nervous tissue, structure of, 293
Neuroblastoma, 539
Neurogenic bladder, 546
  incontinence, 529
Neurological examination, 311
Neurological disorders, 296
Neurological problems, care of child, 111
Neurosis, 320
Neuroticism, 318
Newborn
  at birth, 9
  skin of, 568
Nicotinic acid (Niacin), 203
Niemann-Pick's disease, 265
Night terrors, 82
Nissen fundoplication, 482
Nitrogen balance, 192
Nodules, 569
Non-dysjunction, 257
Nose, structure and function, 362
Nostrils, clearing of, 381
Nursery schools, 55
Nutrients
  characteristics and functions, 190
  recommended intake, 134
Nutrition in acute renal failure, 113
Nutritional needs
  after surgery, 133
  of burns and scalds, 148

Obesity, 213
Objective audiometry, 354
Observations relating to:, 86–91
  coughing, 90
  defaecation, 90
  ears, 88
  eyes, 88
  facial expression, 87
  gums, 87
  mouth, 87
  nervous system, 91
  oedema, 88
  pain, 88, 118, 304
  posture, 87
  stools, 89
  tongue, 87
  urine, micturition, 90
Occlusion, 338
Ocular muscles, 331
Oculocerebrorenal syndrome, 326, 602
Oedema, 233
Oedematous child, care of, 114

Oesophageal
  atresia, 475
  gavage, 513
  tube (lubrication of), 509
Oesophagoscopy, 509
Oesophagostomy, 477, 479
Oesophagus, 467
Oliguria, 90
One-parent families, 49
Operant conditioning, 322
Ophthalmia neonatorum, 335
Opisthotonus, 309
Oral fluid supplement, 135
Oral thrush, 474
Orchidopexy, 544
Oronasal
  mask, 384
  pharyngeal suction, 386
Orthopaedic
  nursing, 588
  surgery, 575
Orthopnoea, 105
Orthostatic feeding, 475
Ortolani's test, 577
Osteogenesis, 573
Osteomyelitis, 580
Osteolysis, 573
Osteoporosis, 207
Otitis media, acute suppurative, 345
Ovaries, 524
Oxygen
  administration of, 382
  function of, 383
  tents, 384
  therapy (indications for), 383
  toxicity of, 382
  transport of, 368

Pacemakers, types of, 464
Pain, 304
  control of, 118, 305
Palate, 466
  cleft, 473
Palsy, cerebral, 310
Pancreas, 470
Pancreatitis, 506
Pancrex V forte, 508
Pandy's test, 312
Papules, 568
Para-amino-salicylic acid, 309
Parachute reflex, 11
Paradoxical respiration, 119
Paraldehyde, 307
Paralysis, 91
Paralytic ileus, 509
Paramagnetic oximeter, 386
Para-oesophageal hernia, 482
Paraphimosis, 541
Parathyroid glands, 276
Parent participation, 79
Parents, approach to, 78
Partially sighted, provisions for, 63
Paroxysmal nocturnal dyspnoea, 110
PAS, 309

Passive immunity, 241
Patent ductus arteriosus, 417
Pedocarpal spasms, 277
Pellagra, 204
Pemphigus neonatorum, 570
Penis, 523
Peptic ulcer, 485
Perception, 316
Pericardial effusion, 423
Perineal urethrostomy, 550
Periodic syndrome, 485
Peripheral circulatory failure, 427
Peritoneal dialysis, 559
Peritoneal tube, shortening of, 142
Peritonitis, 496
Peritonsillar abscess, 357
Personality, 25, 317
  assessment of, 318
  theories, 27
Perthes disease, 580
Pethidine, 167, 522
Petit mal, 306
pH (defined), 229
Pharyngeal suction, 120
Pharynx, structure and function, 355
Phenobarbitone therapy, 438
Phenotype, 254
Phenylketonuria, 262
Phenylalanine, 262
Phimosis, 541
Phlyctenular conjunctivitis, 244
Photoelectric cell analyser, 386
Phototherapy, 438
Phrenic nerve pacing, 396
  indications for, 397
Physical handicap, provisions for, 68
Piaget, J, 22
Pica, 89
Pierre-Robin syndrome, 475
Pigeon chest, 587
Pilocarpine (sweat test), 268
Pitressin, 271
  test, 271
Pituitary gland, 270
Placenta, 4, 6
Planning patient care, 107
Plasma, 429
  expanders, 449
  proteins, 429
Plaster bed, 589
Plaster cast, removal of, 592
Plaster of Paris, application of, 591
Platelets, 433
  transfusion, 448
Play
  functions of, 29
  groups, 56
  importance of, 29
  in hospital, 80
  leader, 81
  parallel, 30
  phases of, 30
  social role, 30
  solitary, 29
  therapy, 325

Pleura, 365
Pleurisy with effusion, 379
Pneumocystis carinii, 445
Pneumonia, 377
Pneumothorax, 379
Poliomyelitis, 310
Polyarthritis, 421
Polycythaemia, 411
Polysomy, 257
Polythene jacket, 583
Polyuria, 90
Pompe's disease, 263
Pons, 292
Porter's hand, 598
Port-wine stain, 572
Position of child, 380
Positive end-expiratory pressure
  (PEEP), 396
Positive nitrogen balance, 192
Post-operative nursing care, 131
  rehabilitation, 135
Potassium
  depletion, 227
  effects of, 228
  retention, 228
Pott's operation, 409
Precocious puberty, 271
Prednisolone, 444
Premedication, 128
Pre-operational period (development),
  23
Pre-operative preparation, 128
  gastric emptying, 130
Preparation
  for emergency operation, 130
  of infant feeds, 249
  for returning home, 82
Pressure areas, 94
  care of, 94
Pressure preset, 395
Pressure sores, prevention of, 592
Pre-term infant
  bathing, 184
  care of, 180
  characteristics, 178
  definition, 178
  feeding of, 184
  incidence of, 178
  oxygen administration, 183
  preservation of body temperature,
    181
  prevention of infection, 183
Prevention of
  accidents, 85
  heat loss, 131
Primary lesions (skin), 568
Primary ossification, 573
Proctosigmoidoscopy, 522
Pro-enzymes, 199
Projection, 25
Projective tests, 318
Propranolol, 110
Proprioceptors, 293
Propyliodine, 518
Protein and amino-acids, 190

Protein energy malnutrition (PEM), 193
Protein
  deficient intake, 193
  digestion and absorption, 192
  excessive intake, 193
  functions of, 191
  high biological value of, 191
  sources of, 191
  synthesis of, 192
Proteinuria, 530
Proximodistal, 5
Pseudohermaphroditism, 8
Pseudo-squint, 333
Psoriasis, 571
Psychiatric disorders, causes, 319
Psychological physiology, 296
Psychometric techniques, 318
Psychomotor seizures, 306
Psychosis, 321
Psychosomatic reactions, 320
Psychotherapy, 325
Pulmonary artery, banding of, 410
Pulmonary circulation, 364
Pulse
  measurement of, 103
  values, 103
Purpura, in newborn, 440
Pustules, 569
Pyelonephritis, 531
Pyloric stenosis, 480
Pyogenic meningitis, 309
Pyrexia, 92
  physiological effects of, 108
Pyrogenic reaction, 452
Pyrogens, 99
Pyuria, 90, 529

Quantitative protein test, 564
Queckenstedt's sign, 292
Quinsy, 357

Radioactive material, disposal of, 107
Radiotherapy, care of child, 106
Ramstedt's pyloromyotomy, 481
Rashkind procedure, 415
Rate of flow, calculation of, 452
Rationalisation, 25
Reactionary haemorrhage, 359
Reading difficulties, 63
Recessive trait, 255
Rectal
  biopsy, 493, 522
  deformities, 498
  examination, 521
  lavage, 520
  prolapse, 499
Recto-sigmoidectomy, 494
Red blood cells, 430
  control of production, 430
  count, 430
  functions of, 431
  transfusion of, 448

Reflex action, 293
  bladder, 546
Reflexes in newborn, 9
  eye, 9
  grasp, 10
  Moro, 10
  oral, 9
  placing, 10
  righting, 11
  rooting, 9
  startle, 10
  tonic neck, 10
  walking, 10
Regional enteritis, 501
Regression, 25, 82, 317
Reinforcement
  negative, 322
  positive, 322
Renal
  agenesis, 530
  biopsy, 555
  concentration test, 556
  disease, diet in, 219
  failure (acute), 535
  failure (chronic), 536
  function in newborn, 527
  osteodystrophy, 537
  water loss, 224
Renin, 527
Rennin, 468
Renogram, 555
Renoscan, 555
Replacement therapy, 143, 231
Replogle tube, 476
Repression, 25
Residual volume, 367
Respiratory
  acidosis, 230
  alkalosis, 230
  arrest, causes, 121
  arrest, signs, 121
Respiratory disorders, care of child, 109
  failure, 370
  system at birth, 369
Restraints, 86
Resuscitation, 118
Retention (urine), 529
Retinoblastoma, 334
Retrograde pyelography, 555
Retrolental fibroplasia, 383
Retropharyngeal abscess, 357
Reverse barrier nursing, 250
Reye's syndrome, 504
Rhesus blood groups, 432
Rhinitis, 372
Rickets, 586
Rickety rosary, 587
Rifampin, 309
Riley-Day syndrome, 294
Risser localiser cast, 583
Rods (eyes), 330
Rogers, Carl, 318
Rooming-in, 79
Rorschach test, 318
Rumination, 484

Ruptured stitch line, 132
Rutter, M, 50

Sage pump, 111
Salaam fits, 306
Salbutamol, 374
Salicylates, 422
Salivary glands, 466
Saturated fatty acids, 197
Scabies, 572
Scales (skin), 569
Scalp vein infusion, 449
Scarlet fever, 357
Schaffer, H. R., 50
Schizophrenia, 323
Schoolchild, health of, 59
School Health Service, 59
School nurse, 60
School refusal, 323
Schwartze operation, 347
Scissors gait, 311
Sclerema, 100
Scoliosis, 581
  adolescent, 582
  effects of, 582
  infantile, 582
  juvenile, 582
Screening test for galactosaemia, 266
Scribner external shunt, 561
Scrotal oedema, 544
Scrotum, 523
Secondary haemorrhage, 359
Seizures, types of, 306
Self-infection, 245
Sensorimotor stage, 22
Septic arthritis, 579
Sequestra, 580
Sex determination, 7
Sex-linked inheritance, 256
Sexual
  abuse, 52
  development, 7
  development (ambiguous), 524
Sham feeds, 479
Shaving limb, method of, 594
Shock, 427
  anaphylactic, 428
  cardiogenic, 427
  causes of, 427
  hypovolaemic, 427
  toxic, 428
Sickle cell anaemia, 439
Simon, T., 316
Sinus arrhythmia, 104, 406
Sinus rhythm, 406
Sinuses, 362
Skeletal defects, 575
Skeletal muscle, post-natal growth, 574
Skin
  colour of, 87
  congenital abnormalities, 572
  functions of, 568
  texture of, 87
Skin disorders, treatment of, 569

Skin extension, application of, 593
Skin grafts, 147
Sleep, 36
  disturbed, 37
Sliding hiatus hernia, 482
Sliding traction, 596
Slit lamp microscopy, 337
Small intestine, 468
Social development, 28
Sodium depletion, effects, 225
Sodium disturbance, 225
Sodium nitroprusside, 538
Sodium/potassium pump, 224
Sodium retention, 226
Solids, introduction of, 213
Spasticity, 311
Speech, development of, 20
Speech therapy, 474
Spider naevus, 572
Spina bifida, 297
Spinal cord, 292
  functions of, 293
  lesions of, 293
Spinal fusion, 583
Spirochaetes, 237
Splints
  care of child in, 589
  types of, 589
Sputum, 372
Squint, 332
  causes of, 333
  types of, 333
Starch, lactose and sucrose free diet, 218
Starch poultice, 571
Status asthmaticus, 374
Status epilepticus, 306
Steatorrhoea, 500, 502, 507
Steroid therapy, 280
Steroids, test for, 558
Stertorous breathing, 105
Stoma care, 153
Stomach, 467
  capacity of, 512
Stomahesive, 154
Stomatitis
  acute, 474
  in cancer, 117
Storage of blood, 453
Strabismus (squint), 332
Strawberry haemangioma, 572
Stress reactions, 320
Stryker frame, 583
Stye, 336
Subcutaneous infusion, 457
Subdural puncture, 313
Sucrose-free diet, 218
Sucrose tolerance test, 267
Suction
  endotracheal, 160
  nasal, 160
  oral, 160
Sudden infant death syndrome (SIDS), 105
Sugar malabsorption, 218

Suppository, introduction of, 174
Suppuration, 235
Suprapubic cystostomy, 550
Suprapubic drainage, 550
Surfactant, 368, 370
Sutures, removal of, 140
Sweat glands, 567
Sweat test
  iontophoresis, 268
  thermal, 267
Sweep test, 60
Switch operation, 416
Synapse, 293
Syngeneic transplant, 458
Syringing of ear, 352
Systematic nursing care, 107

Tachycardia, 104, 406
Talipes calcaneo-valgus, 576
Talipes equino-varus, 575
Tapeworm, 508
Tay-Sachs' disease, 265
Tear gas, effect of, 378
Teat, hole in, 43
Teeth, 467
  care of, 94
  decay of, 95
Temperature
  control of, 98
  maintenance of, 159
  measurement of, 102
  measuring, 98
Temporal lobe epilepsy, 306
Tension pneumothorax, 380
Tepid sponging, 92
Terbutaline, 374
Terminal care, 125
Test feeding, 481
Test weighing, 39
Testes, 523
  descent of, 543
  undescended, 543
Tetany, 207
Tetralogy of Fallot, 410
Thalamus, 290
Thalassaemia, 438
Therapeutic diets, 217
Thiamine (Vit. B_1), 202
  deficiency (Beriberi), 203
Thiersch operation, 500
Thomas splint, 589
  measurement for, 595
Threadworms, 508
Throat
  examination of, 360
  swab, 361
Thrombocytopenic purpura, 441
Thyroid gland, 273
Thyroidectomy, 276
Thyroid scintiphotography, 274
Tidal drainage, 552
Tidal volume, 367
Time-flow preset, 396
Toilet needs, 98

Tongue, 466
Tonic phase, 306
Tonsillectomy, 358
  complications of, 359
Tonsillitis
  acute, 356
  chronic, 357
Tonsils, 356
Toronto brace, 581
Toxic shock, 428
Trachea, 363
Tracheal suction, 120
Tracheo-oesophageal abnormalities,
  investigation of, 518
Tracheo-oesophageal fistula, 475
Tracheostomy, 386
  aspiration of, 387
  changing of tube, 388
  reasons for, 387
  removal of tube, 389
Transfusion, blood, 453
Translocation, 257
Transport of
  carbon dioxide, 369
  oxygen, 368
Transposition of the great vessels, 413
Trendelenburg's test, 578
Tricuspid atresia, 416
Trisomy, 257
Truancy, 323
Tryptic activity, examination for, 517
Tuberculous meningitis, 309
Tuberculosis, 242
Tumours of
  brain, 302
  eye, 334
  kidney, 538
Turner's syndrome, 7, 33, 524
Tympanic membrane, perforation of,
  346

Ulcerative colitis, diet in, 219
Ulcers
  peptic, 485
  skin, 569
Ultrasonic nebuliser, 382
Ultraviolet light, 571
Umbilical cord, care of, 36
Unconscious child, care of, 303
Underwater seal drainage, 390
Undescended testes, 543
Units of activity, 163
Unsaturated fatty acids, 197
Upper motor neurones, lesions of, 295
Urea clearance test, 556
Urea concentration test, 556
Uretero-sigmoidostomy, 546
Urethra, 528
Urethrostomy, 542
Ureters, 527
Urinary diversion, 154, 545
Urinary tract, infection, 530
Urine
  collection of, 547

composition of, 527
dilution factor, 565
examination of, 562, 563
odour of, 563
volume of, 527
Urine tests for
  acetone, 565
  bacterial counts, 566
  bilirubin, 565
  blood, 565
  chlorides, 563
  glucose (clinitest), 564
  diacetic acid, 565
  phenylketonuria, 566
  protein, 564
  reaction (pH), 563
  Rothera's test, 565
  specific gravity, 563
Uterus, 524

Vaccination and immunisation, 241
Vagina, 524
Vagotomy, 486
Vas deferens, 523
Vascular system, 406
Venepuncture, 446
Venesection, 450
Ventilation, methods of, 396
Ventilator, weaning from, 396
Ventricles (brain), 291
Ventricular fibrillation, 124, 406
Ventricular puncture, 313
Ventriculography, 314
Ventriculostomy, 301
Venturi mask, 384
Vernix caseosa, 568
Vesicles, 569
Vesico-ureteric reflux, 540
Vestibular apparatus, 345
Vincristine, 444
Viral meningitis, 309
Viruses, 237
Visual acuity, tests for, 337
Visual development, 20
Visual handicap, 63
Visual system of infant, 330
Vitamin A
  deficient intake, 200
  excessive intake, 200
  function of, 200
Vitamin B complex, 202
Vitamin B_{12}, 539
Vitamin C
  deficient intake, 205
  functions of, 204
Vitamin D
  deficient intake, 201
  excessive intake, 201
  function of, 201
  importance of, 587
Vitamin E
  deficient intake, 201
  excessive intake, 202
  functions of, 201

Vitamin K
    deficient intake, 202, 441
    excessive intake, 202
    functions of, 202
Vocalisation, 20
Voiding cystogram, 554
Volume preset, 395
Volvulus, 490
Vomiting, 89
    in infancy, 484
    older children, 485
    positional, 584
Von Gierke's disease, 263
Von Willebrand's disease, 443

Waldeyer's ring, 356
Ward dressings, 137
Warnock Report, 61
Water, 211
    depletion, 226
    depletion, effects of, 227

excretion test, 278
intoxication, 494, 520
loss (alimentary tract), 224
    lungs, 224
    skin, 224
requirements (table), 212
retention, 227
Water, regulation of intake, 211
Waterhammer pulse, 104
Waterhouse-Friderichsen's syndrome,
    279
Watershed dressing, 141
Waterston operation, 409
Wechsler test, 317
Weight and measures, 163
Weight and pulley traction, 596
Weight, growth in, 14
Wheal, 569
White blood cells (corpuscles), 432
    transfusion, 448
Whole blood, 448
Wilms' tumour, 538

Wilson's disease, 210
Winding, 39
Withdrawal, 321
Wound
    care, 133, 136
    dressing, 137
    healing, factors in, 236
    inspection of, 132
    types of, 136

X-chromosomes, 7, 253
X-linked dominant inheritance, 256
X-linked recessive inheritance, 256
Xanthochromic, 313
Xerophthalmia, 200

Y-chromosomes, 7, 253

Zinc, 210